THE CLINICAL PATHOLOGY
of
INFANCY

THE CLINICAL PATHOLOGY

of

INFANCY

Compiled and Edited by

F. WILLIAM SUNDERMAN, M.D., Ph.D., Sc.D.

Director, Institute for Clinical Science
Director of Education, Association of Clinical Scientists
Clinical Professor of Medicine, Jefferson Medical College
Philadelphia, Pennsylvania

and

F. WILLIAM SUNDERMAN, JR., M.D.

Director of Clinical Laboratories and
Associate Professor of Pathology
University of Florida College of Medicine
Gainesville, Florida

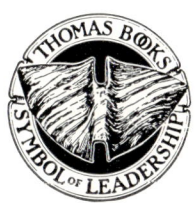

CHARLES C THOMAS • PUBLISHER
Springfield • Illinois • U.S.A.

Published and Distributed Throughout the World by

CHARLES C THOMAS • PUBLISHER

BANNERSTONE HOUSE

301-327 East Lawrence Avenue, Springfield, Illinois, U.S.A.

NATCHEZ PLANTATION HOUSE

735 North Atlantic Boulevard, Fort Lauderdale, Florida, U.S.A.

With THOMAS BOOKS *careful attention is given to all details of
manufacturing and design. It is the Publisher's desire to present books
that are satisfactory as to their physical qualities and artistic possibilities
and appropriate for their particular use.* THOMAS BOOKS *will be true
to those laws of quality that assure a good name and good will.*

Printed in the United States of America

0-5

Contributors

GONZALO E. APONTE, M.D.
Jefferson Medical College
Philadelphia, Pennsylvania

IRWIN M. ARIAS, M.D.
Albert Einstein College of Medicine
Bronx, New York City, New York

HOWARD BERK, M.D.
Beth Israel Hospital
New York City, New York

GERALD S. DEAN, M.D.
Highland Park Hospital
Highland Park, Illinois

HERBERT DERMAN, M.D.
Laboratory of City of Kingston
Kingston, New York

KURT M. DUBOWSKI, Ph.D.
University of Oklahoma
School of Medicine
Oklahoma City, Oklahoma

MARY L. EFRON, M.D.
Massachusetts General Hospital
Boston, Massachusetts

DELBERT A. FISHER, M.D.
University of Arkansas
School of Medicine
Little Rock, Arkansas

DONALD S. FREDRICKSON, M.D.
National Heart Institute, NIH
Bethesda, Maryland

ALFRED H. FREE, Ph.D.
Ames Research Laboratory
Elkhart, Indiana

HELEN M. FREE, B.S.
Ames Research Laboratory
Elkhart, Indiana

JAMES J. HARMELING, M.D.
U.S. Naval Medical School
Bethesda, Maryland

GERALD G. HOFFMAN, M.D.
Lake Forest Hospital
Lake Forest, Illinois

J. de la HUERGA, M.D., Ph.D
Grant Hospital, Northwestern
University Medical School
Chicago, Illinois

JAMES J. HUMES, M.D.
U.S. Naval Medical School
Bethesda, Maryland

JOHN P. KALTENBACH, Ph.D.
Northwestern University Medical
School, Chicago, Illinois

BERNARD J. KATCHMAN, Ph.D.
Department of Research, Miami
Valley Hospital, Dayton, Ohio

LOUIS A. KAZAL, Ph.D.
Jefferson Medical College
Philadelphia, Pennsylvania

JAMES J. LaPOLLA, M.D.
U.S. Naval Hospital
St. Albans, New York

HARRISON H. LEFFLER, M.D.
Professional Laboratories
Washington, D.C.

ANDREW E. LORINCZ, M.D.
University of Florida
College of Medicine
Gainesville, Florida

ROBERT P. MacFATE, Ph.D.
Division of Laboratories
Board of Health
Chicago, Illinois

EVELYN B. MAN, Ph.D.
Brown University, Institute
for Health Sciences
Providence, Rhode Island

ELLIOT MANCALL, M.D.
Jefferson Medical College
Philadelphia, Pennsylvania

ANDREW M. MARGILETH, M.D.
U.S. Naval Medical School
Bethesda, Maryland

MEYER W. MELICOW, M.D.
Columbia University College
of Physicians and Surgeons
New York City, New York

GORDON W. MELLA, M.D.
U.S. Naval Hospital
Bethesda, Maryland

WELLS R. MOOREHEAD, Ph.D.
University of Alabama
School of Medicine
Birmingham, Alabama

MANFORD D. MORRIS, Ph.D.
University of Arkansas
School of Medicine
Little Rock, Arkansas

MAKIO MURAYAMA, Ph.D.
National Institute of Arthritis and
Metabolic Diseases
NIH, Bethesda, Maryland

ROBERT C. NORTHCUTT, M.D.
Vanderbilt University
School of Medicine
Nashville, Tennessee

PETER C. NOWELL, M.D.
University of Pennsylvania
School of Medicine
Philadelphia, Pennsylvania

FRANK A. OSKI, M.D.
University of Pennsylvania
School of Medicine
Philadelphia, Pennsylvania

CARL M. PEARSON, M.D.
University of California
School of Medicine
Los Angeles, California

HOWARD A. PEARSON, M.D.
University of Florida
College of Medicine
Gainesville, Florida

HAROLD M. PRICE, M.D.
Armed Forces Institute of Pathology
Washington, D.C.

HOWARD QUITTNER, M.D.
University of Arkansas
School of Medicine
Little Rock, Arkansas

IRENE E. ROECKEL, M.D.
University of Kentucky
School of Medicine
Lexington, Kentucky

GRIFF T. ROSS, M.D., Ph.D.
National Cancer Institute
NIH, Bethesda, Maryland

BYRON RUSKIN, M.D.
Elmhurst, Ill.

JOSEPH C. SHERRICK, M.D.
Passavant Memorial Hospital
Northwestern University
School of Medicine
Chicago, Illinois

GEORGE W. SMETTERS, M.D.
Chicago Wesley Memorial Hospital
Chicago, Illinois

JON V. STRAUMFJORD, JR., M.D., Ph.D.
University of Alabama
School of Medicine
Birmingham, Alabama

CAROLYN R. SUNDERMAN, M.D.
University of Florida
College of Medicine
Gainesville, Florida

F. WILLIAM SUNDERMAN, JR., M.D.
University of Florida
College of Medicine
Gainesville, Florida

F. WILLIAM SUNDERMAN, M.D., Ph.D.
Institute for Clinical Science
Philadelphia, Pennsylvania

LEON N. SUSSMAN, M.D.
Beth Israel Hospital
New York City, New York

JENO E. SZAKACS, M.D.
Armed Forces Institute of Pathology
Washington, D.C.

HENRY A. TELOH, M.D.
V.A. Hospital
Coral Gables, Fla.

J. H. TJIO, Ph.D.
Laboratory of Experimental Pathology
NIH, Bethesda, Maryland

THOMAS A. WALDMANN, M.D.
National Cancer Institute
NIH, Bethesda, Maryland

RICHARD S. WEGRYN, M.D.
Stouder Memorial Hospital
Troy, Ohio

EARL B. WERT, M.D.
Mobile Infirmary
Mobile, Alabama

ROBERT E. ZIPF, M.D.
Department of Research
Miami Valley Hospital
Dayton, Ohio

ASSISTING MEMBERS OF THE ASSOCIATION OF CLINICAL SCIENTISTS

HOWARD A. BALL, M.D.*
La Mesa, California

JOSEPH S. BURKLE, M.D.
Bethesda, Maryland

ELGIN C. COWART, JR., M.D.
Washington, D.C.

MEL A. DAVIS, M.D.
Columbus, Ohio

JAMES B. HARTNEY, M.D.
Elmhurst, Illinois

E. CLIFFORD HEINMILLER, M.D.
Saginaw, Michigan

FRANK W. KONZELMANN, M.D.
Linwood, New Jersey

NORMAN C. LAW, M.S.
Bethesda, Maryland

VERNON E. MARTENS, M.D.
Washington, D.C.

ROBERT S. MELVILLE, M.D.
Bethesda, Maryland

DORA A. NEWSON, M.D.
Edmonton, Alberta, Canada

GEORGE F. STEVENSON, M.D.
Rockville, Maryland

ASHER YAGUDA, M.D.
Newark, New Jersey

*Deceased.

Preface

This book contains the edited proceedings of an Applied Seminar on the Clinical Pathology of Infancy, held in Washington, D.C. under the auspices of the Association of Clinical Scientists. In organization and format this volume is similar to the published proceedings of six previous seminars.

Lipids and the Steroid Hormones in Clinical Medicine

Measurements of Exocrine and Endocrine Functions of the Pancreas

Evaluation of Thyroid and Parathyroid Functions

Clinical Pathology of Hemoglobin, Its Precursors and Metabolites

Serum Proteins and the Dysproteinemias

Clinical Pathology of the Serum Electrolytes

The proper objectives of science are the acquisition and the communication of knowledge. The Applied Seminars of the Association of Clinical Scientists are dedicated toward these objectives. Within recent years, the acquisitions in clinical science have advanced more rapidly than the methods of communication. The Applied Seminars endeavor to minimize this inequality. It is our fervent hope that the published proceedings of the Applied Seminars will fulfill an important role in accelerating communications among clinical scientists so that the dissemination of scientific knowledge will keep pace with the acquisitions.

In editing the proceedings of the Applied Seminar on the Clinical Pathology of Infancy, judicious selection of material has been attempted. The book contains a number of newer procedures which aid in the diagnosis of various diseases of infancy and childhood and which are not currently found in textbooks of clinical pathology. These procedures include thin-layer chromatography of amino acids and sugars; measurements of pigments in amniotic fluid; measurements of erythrocyte enzymes; estimations of urinary mucopolysaccharides; and identification of chromosomal karyotypes. It is hoped that this book will assist clinical scientists in initiating these newer procedures in their own laboratories.

Our appreciation is expressed to the lecturers and assisting physicians who have generously contributed their time and energies to the success of the Applied Seminar and to the preparation of these proceedings. Our thanks are given to our publisher, and particularly to Mr. Payne E. L. Thomas and his staff for their gracious cooperation.

F. WILLIAM SUNDERMAN, M.D.

F. WILLIAM SUNDERMAN, JR., M.D.

Institute for Clinical Science
1833 Delancey Place
Philadelphia, Pennsylvania 19103

Contents

PART I – CONGENITAL BIOCHEMICAL DISORDERS IN INFANCY

PART III — CLINICAL PATHOLOGY OF SYSTEMIC DISEASES IN INFANCY

THE CLINICAL PATHOLOGY

of

INFANCY

Chapter 1

Diagnosis of Congenital Dysproteinemias

THOMAS A. WALDMANN, M.D.

Over the past decade a large number of hereditary qualitative and quantitative disorders of metabolism of the serum proteins have been described. These disorders have been of significance to the clinician in the understanding of disease, and have been of special importance to the physiologist interested in the function of the serum proteins and in their metabolic control. The pathogenesis of these protein defects is quite variable. The most common defect is a quantitative deficiency or absence of a single protein due to an isolated defect in synthesis. In other disorders there is a defect in the synthesis of a group of related proteins that share a common peptide chain or a common cell of origin. In addition, there are qualitative disorders in the synthesis of proteins with the substitution of one or more amino acid residues. In at least one disease, hypoproteinemia results from an isolated hyper-catabolism of a single protein. Finally, bulk loss of serum proteins into the gastrointestinal tract may be an hereditary disorder with onset in childhood.

The detection of the protein disorder may be made by paper electrophoresis with many of the diseases. In others, immunoelectrophoresis, quantitative immune precipitation, starch gel electrophoresis or specific assay of a biological activity of the protein may be required for diagnosis.

ANALBUMINEMIA

In 1954, Bennhold, Peters and Roth[5] described two siblings with an almost complete absence of circulating albumin. Subsequently, four other analbuminemic subjects have been reported[3, 16, 19, 27]. In view of the major functions ascribed to albumin in the transport of smaller molecules and in the maintenance of the colloid osmotic pressure of the serum, it is surprising that there were few signs or symptoms common to these patients with extreme hypoalbuminemia. Mild edema was present in five of the patients and absent in the sixth. Ease of fatigability and mild diarrhea were associated features in some of the subjects. Certain biochemical features were common to the patients, including serum albumin concentrations of 0 to 0.3 gm per 100 ml, an elevation of the total serum globulins from 4.4 to 5.7 gm per 100 ml, elevated erythrocyte sedimentation rates and elevated cholesterol concentrations of from 320 to 610 mg per 100 mil. In this disorder, there is a virtually complete defect in albumin synthesis and a marked-ly prolonged albumin survival, with half-times of survival two to three times that seen in control subjects[4, 32].

Following albumin infusions, the ery-throcyte sedimentation rate and the serum globulin and cholesterol levels returned to normal, suggesting that these abnormalities were secondary to the hypoalbuminemia. In two of the three cases studied, the survival of albu-min was still markedly prolonged fol-lowing the albumin infusions[4, 32]. This suggests that there is a defect in albu-min catabolism in association with the defect in albumin synthesis. Too few patients with analbuminemia have been reported to support any conclusions as to its pathogensis. However, this dis-order probably represents a genetically determined anomaly. The first two patients reported were siblings, the products of a consanguinous marriage. One of the subsequent cases also had consanguinity in his inheritance.

BISALBUMINEMIA

Bisalbuminemia is an example of a qualitative disorder of protein synthesis. Patients with this anomaly have a double albumin peak on electrophore-sis[7, 14, 26]. The patients have no chemical or clinical features in common other than the disorder of albumin synthesis. The electrophoresis of the serum pro-teins from patients with bisalbuminemia revealed two approximately equal peaks with a combined area equal to that of the albumin peak in normal serum. The faster moving component (Albumin A) had the same mobility as normal albu-min, while the slower moving compo-nent (Albumin B) had a mobility com-parable to an α_1-globulin. Between pH

4 and 8.3, Albumin B had a more positive charge than Albumin A equiva-lent to two protons per molecule[7, 14]. An analysis of the peptide pattern following hydrolysis with trypsin and chymotryp-sin reveals that Albumin A had the same pattern as normal albumin. Chy-motrypsin released one anomalous pep-tide from Albumin B, whereas tryspin released two anomalous peptides. These studies considered in conjunction with the electrophoretic data are consistent with the hypothesis that normal albu-min, Albumin A, and Albumin B are identical, with the exception that Albu-min B contains one anomalous lysine residue replacing an amino acid con-taining a free carboxyl group[7, 14]. Bis-albuminemia has been noted in seventy-five patients in twelve kindreds, and appears to be transmitted as a codom-inant with both the normal and abnor-mal gene being expressed.

HYPOGAMMAGLOBULINEMIA

The most complex, yet most clinically significant, group of inborn errors of protein metabolism are the hypogam-maglobulinemias. Three major classes of immuno-globulins are commonly recog-nized in man: They are the IgG- or $7S\gamma_2$-globulins, representing about 85 per cent of the γ-globulins; the IgA- or β_{2A}-globulins; and the IgM- or β_2- mac-roglobulins. Each of these fractions pos-sesses antibody activity and certain structural features in common. All are composed of four polypeptide chains including one pair of L or light chains that is common to all immuno-globulin groups, and one pair of H or heavy chains that is different with different groups providing the basis for the dis-tinctive features of the three immuno-globulin classes. The disorders of immuno-globulins may affect only one, two or all of the classes of molecules.

CONGENITAL SEX-LINKED AGAMMAGLOBULINEMIA

In 1952, Bruton described the first case of congenital sex-linked agammaglobulinemia[6]. Patients with this disorder cannot produce significant quantities of circulating antibody in response to antigenic challenge[13, 15]. There is a consequent marked reduction in the serum concentration of all three classes of immuno-globulins, with total serum γ-globulin usually below 25 mg per 100 ml. Delayed hypersensitivity is normal in most of these patients, while others have retained skin grafts for prolonged periods.

The affected patients have repeated bacterial infections, with pneumonia, septicemia, pyoderma and meningitis starting after the first six months of life after the maternal antibodies have largely been catabolized. The patients have much less difficulty with viral infection, although a few have had generalized vaccinia or fatal hepatitis. A significant percentage of the patients develop chronic sinusitis, bronchiectasis, manifestations of rheumatoid arthritis and gastrointestinal disorders. Pathologically, there is an absence of plasma cells and a generalized deficiency of lymphoid elements in the lymph nodes and spleen. The number of circulating lymphocytes is usually normal. There is an apparent absence of pharangeal lymphoid tissue. Patients with this disorder have an extreme defect in the synthesis of each of the immuno-globulins, and usually have a longer-than-normal survival of IgG and a normal survival of IgA and IgM[33].

AGAMMAGLOBULINEMIA WITH LYMPHOCYTOPENA (SWISS TYPE)

A second immuno-globulin disorder is the Swiss type agammaglobulinemia with lymphocytopenia[12, 17, 20]. This disorder affects both males and females. The patients have serious bacterial, viral and fungal infections from the first few weeks of life. They have marked growth retardation and commonly have malabsorption and colitis. All of the children with this syndrome have died in the first eighteen months of life, despite γ-globulin replacement. The patients with this syndrome have extreme hypogammaglobulinemia and significant lymphocytopenia. They do not produce antibodies to a variety of antigens and do not reject skin homografts. Pathologically, there is a complete absence of plasma cells and a marked reduction of lymphocytes in the spleen and lymph nodes. The thymus glands in most cases have been very small and show evidence of defective development[12, 20]. It has been suggested that this abnormal development of the thymus is the primary defect leading secondarily to a reduction in lymphocytes and the failure of immuno-globulin production. In some family studies, an autosomal recessive mode of inheritance has been suggested[20], while in other families the pattern is consistent with sex-linked recessive inheritance[12].

In addition to these disorders, a reduction in the concentration of all of the immuno-globulin classes is also noted in congenital non-sex-linked hypogammaglobulinemia and idiopathic acquired hypogammaglobulinemia. The clinical pattern of the congenital non-sex-linked hypogammaglobulinemia is similar to the sex-linked form. There are, however, certain distinct differences: The lymph nodes are large rather than small; and there is abundant adenoidal tissue in the non-sex-linked form[15]. The γ-globulin levels are higher in this form than in the sex-linked form.

DYSGAMMAGLOBULINEMIA

In addition to the patients with an hereditary defect in the synthesis of all the immuno-globulins, some patients have dysgammaglobulinemia, a marked defect in the synthesis of only one or two of the immuno-globulin classes. A few patients with recurrent bacterial infections have a marked deficiency of IgG and IgA and elevated levels of IgM[2, 10, 18, 23]. In some cases, this increase in γ- macroglobulin may be so severe that the electrophoretic pattern is normal and the defect may be detected most easily by immunoelectrophoresis. The majority of these patients have normal or elevated levels of γ- macroglobulin antibodies, including the isohemagglutinins. Using iodinated proteins, it has been shown that the decreased level of IgG is due to decreased synthesis with a normal survival of this protein[2].

In a second form of dysgammaglobulinemia, patients with a history of numerous bacterial infections were shown to have a normal total γ-globulin concentration and a normal level of IgG, but markedly reduced levels of IgA[1, 11] and IgM. These patients failed to develop isohemoagglutinins.

ATAXIA TELANGIECTASIA

An isolated absence of immuno-globulin A is frequently seen in the unusual disorder, ataxia telangiectasia[8, 21, 29, 30, 35]. Ataxia telangiectasia is a disease charac-

terized chiefly by cerebellar ataxia and oculo-cutaneous telangiectasia. Associated clinical findings in some patients have been recurrent sino-pulmonary infections and reticuloendothelial neoplasm. Immunogolic defects exist in many of the patients. Some patients have delayed skin homograft rejection, decreased circulating antibody response to antigenic stimulation, lymphocytopenia and thymic abnoramilities. The most striking defect is the dysgammaglobulinemia. In cases of ataxia telangiectasia studied to determine serum immuno-globulin levels twenty-two of twenty-seven showed marked reduction or absence of IgA. In one case, the IgA level was elevated. One case also had a marked reduction of IgG. Using I^{131} IgA, these patients have been shown to have an extreme defect in IgA synthesis, and, in two of five cases, an exceedingly short IgA survival, approximately one tenth of normal[29]. Thus, these patients have a combined defect of both synthesis and catabolism of IgA. The relationship of the immuno-globulin defect and the clinical features have not been elucidated. The disease is inherited as an autosomal recessive.

MYOTONIA DYSTROPHICA

Myotonia dystrophica is an hereditary progressive muscular abnormality with dominant transmittance that has an isolated hyper-catabolism of IgG[34, 36]. Patients with this disorder have weakness, wasting and myotonia, especially of the facial, neck and distal musculature. Other associated abnormalities include frontal alopecia, cataracts, gonadal atrophy, low basal metabolic rate, impaired glucose tolerance and electrocardiographic abnormalities. There is no increased incidence of infection. Patients with this disorder have a moderate depression of IgG. The reduction in IgG level has been shown to be due to hyper-catabolism of this protein with a normal rate of synthesis[34]. The patients have normal levels and rates of catabolism of IgA, IgM and albumin.

OTHER CONGENITAL VARIATIONS IN SERUM PROTEINS

There are a number of genetically determined disorders or protein metabolism in addition to the disorders of albumin and γ-globulin. Congenital afibrinogenemia is an autosomal recessive disorder with episodes of hemorrhage secondary to a defect in fibrinogen synthesis with normal fibrinogen survival[22]. Patients with Wilson's disease have an incomplete defect in ceruloplasmin synthesis in the majority of cases[25, 28]. In Tangier disease[9] and acanthocytosis[24] there is an apparent absence of serum α- and β- lipoprotein levels respectively. These syndromes have been discussed extensively elsewhere in this seminar. A number of cases of familial loss of all serum proteins into the gastrointestinal tract have been described[31]. In addition to these diseases with disorders of serum proteins, there are a number of gentically determined normal variants in serum proteins. Haptoglobins, transferrins and gammaglobulins have such genetically determined types that may be of value in the determination of paternity, in demography and in studies of the genetic orders of plasma proteins that are of

SUMMARY

There are a number of inherited disorders of plasma proteins that are of significance to the clinician. These include quantitative defects of the synthesis of a single protein, as in the syndromes of analbuminemia, Wilson's disease and acanthocytosis, defects in the synthesis of a group of related proteins, as in agammaglobulinemia, and qualitative disorders of protein synthesis, as in bisalbuminemia. Isolated disorders of protein catabolism, as in myotonia dystrophica, and disorders of protein loss, as in hereditary gastrointestinal protein loss, have also been reported.

REFERENCES

1. Barandun, S., Cottier, H., and Hassig, A.: New aspects of agammaglobulinemia and antibody deficiency syndrome. In: Immunopathology, Basel, Benno Schwabe and Co., 1958, p. 60.
2. Barth, W. F., Asofsky, R., Liddy, T. J., Tanaka, Y., Rowe, D.S., and Fahey, J. L.: An antibody deficiency syndrome: Selective immunoglobulin deficiency with reduced synthesis of γ and α immunoglobulin polypeptide chains. Amer. J. Med., 39:319, 1965.
3. Beck, G. E., and Dorta, T.: Un cas d'analbuminemia. Helv. Med. Acta, 26:764, 1959.
4. Bennhold, H., and Kallee, E.: Comparative studies on the half life of I^{131} labeled albumins and nonradioactive human serum albumin in a case of analbuminemia. J. Clin. Invest., 38:863, 1959.
5. Bennhold, H., Peters, H., and Roth, E.: Über einen Fall von kompletter Analbumineamie ohne wesentliche klinische Krankheitszeichen, Verh. Deutsch. Ges. Inn. Med., 60:630, 1954.
6. Bruton, O. C.: Agammaglobulinemia. Pediatrics, 9:722, 1952.
7. Earle, D. P., Hutt, M.P., Schmid, K., and Gitlin, D.: Observations on double albumin; a genetically transmitted serum protein anomaly. J. Clin. Invest., 38:1412, 1959.
8. Fireman, P., Boesman, M., and Gitlin, D.: Ataxia telangiectasia. A dysgammaglobulinaemia with deficient γ₁A (β₂A)-globulin. Lancet, 1:1193, 1964.
9. Fredrickson, D. S., Altrocchi, P. H., Avioli, L. V., Goodman, D. S., and Goodman, H. C.: Tangier disease. Ann. Intern. Med., 55:1016, 1961.

10. Fudenberg, H., German, J. L., III, and Kunkel, H. G.: The occurrence of rheumatoid factor and other abnormalities in families of patients with agammaglobulinemia. Arthritis Rheum., **5**:565, 1962.

11. Giedion, A., and Scheidegger, J. J.: Kongentitale Immunparese bei Fehlen spezifischer β_2-Globuline und quantitative nomalen γ-Globulinen, Helv. Paediat. Acta., **12**:241, 1957.

12. Gitlin, D., and Craig, J. M.: The thymus and other lymphoid tissues in congenital agammaglobulinemia. I. Thymic alymphoplasia and lymphocytic hypoplasia and their relation to infection. Pediatrics, **32**:517, 1963.

13. Gitlin, D., Gross, P.A.M., and Janeway, C. A.: The gammaglobulins and their clinical significance. II. Hypogammaglobulinemia. New Eng. J. Med., **260**:72, 1959.

14. Gitlin, D., Schmid, K., Earle, D. P., and Givelber, H.: Observations on double albumin. II. A peptide difference between two genetically determined human serum albumins. J. Clin. Invest., **40**:820, 1961.

15. Good, R. A., Kelly, W. D., Rotstein, J., and Varco, R. L.: Immunological deficiency diseases, Prog., Allerg., **6**:187, 1962.

16. Gordon, R. S., Jr., Bartter, F. C., and Waldmann, T.: Idiopathic hypoalbuminemias: Clinical staff conference at the National Institutes of Health. Ann. Intern. Med., **51**:553, 1959.

17. Hitzig, von W. H., Biro', Z., Bosch, H., and Huser, H. J.: Agammaglobulinämie und alymphocytose mit schwund des lymphatischen, Gewebes, Helv. Paediat. Acta, **13**:551, 1958.

18. Israël-Asselain, R., Burtin, P., and Chebat, J.: Un trouble biologique nouveau: L-agammaglobulinémie avec β_2-macroglobulinémie. Bull. Soc. Méd. Hop. Paris, **76**:519, 1960.

19. Montgomery, D. A. D., Neill, D. W., and Dowdle, E. B. D.: Idiopathic hypoalbuminaemia. Clin. Sci., **22**:141, 1962.

20. Peterson, R. D. A., Cooper, M. D., and Good, R. A.: The pathogenesis of immunologic deficiency diseases. Amer. J. Med., **38**:579, 1965.

21. Peterson, R. D. A., Kelly, W. D., and Good, R. A.: Ataxia-telangiectasia: Its association with a defective thymus, immunological-deficiency disease, and malignancy. Lancet, **1**:1189, 1964.

22. Rabe, F., and Salomon, E.: Ueber Faserstoffmangel im Blute bei einem Falle von Hämophilie. Deutsch. Arch. Klin. Med., **132**:240, 1920.

23. Rosen, F. S., Kevy, S. V., Merler, E., Janeway, C. A., and Gitlin, D.: Recurrent bacterial infections and dysgammaglobulinemia: Deficiency of 7S gamma-globulins in the presence of elevated 19S gamma-globulins. Report of two cases. Pediatrics, **28**:182, 1961.

24. Salt, H. B., Wolf, O. H., Lloyd, J. K., Fosbrooke, A. S., Cameron, A. H., and Hubble, D. V.: On having no beta-lipoprotein: A syndrome comprising a-beta lipoproteinaemia, acanthocytosis, and steatorrhoea. Lancet, **2**:325, 1960.

25. Scheinberg, I. H., and Gitlin, D.: Deficiency of ceruloplasmin in patients with hepatolenticular degeneration (Wilson's disease). Science, **116**:484, 1952.

26. Scheurlen, P. G.: Über Serumeiwessveränderungen beim Diabetes mellitus. Klin. Wschr., **33**:198, 1955.

27. Shetlar, M. R., Payne, R. W., Stidoworthy, G., and Mock, D.: Absence of serum albumin associated with rheumatoid arthritis. Ann. Intern. Med., **51**:1379, 1959.

28. Sternlieb, I., Morell, A. G., Tucker, W. D., Greene, M. W., and Scheinberg, I. H.: The incorporation of copper into ceruloplasmin in vivo: Studies with copper[64] and copper[67]. J. Clin. Invest., **40**:1834, 1961.

29. Strober, W., Wochner, R. D., Barlow, M. H., McFarlin, D. E., and Waldmann, T. A.: Immunoglobulin metabolism in ataxia telangiectasia. In preparation.

30. Thieffry, S., Arthuis, M. Aicardi, J., and Lyon, G.: L'ataxietelangiectasie. Rev. Neurol., (Paris), **105**:390, 1961.

31. Waldmann, T. A.: Protein losing enteropathy. Gastroenterology, **50**:422, 1966.

32. Waldmann, T. A., Gordon, R. S., Jr., and Rosse, W.: Studies on the metabolism of the serum proteins and lipids in a patient with analbuminemia. Amer. J. Med., **37**:960, 1964.

33. Waldmann, T. A., and Schwab, P. J.: IgG (7S gamma-globulin) metabolism in hypogammaglobulinemia: Studies in patients with defective gammaglobulin synthesis, gastrointestinal protein loss, or both. J. Clin. Invest., **44**:1523, 1965.

34. Wochner, R. D., Drews, G., Strober, W., and Waldmann, T. A.: Accelerated breakdown of immunoglobulin G (IgG) in myotonic dystrophy: An hereditary error of immunoglobulin catabolism. J. Clin. Invest., **45**:321, 1966.

35. Young, R. R., Austen, K. F., and Moser, H. W.: Abnormalities of serum gamma$_{1A}$ globulin and ataxia telangiectasia. Medicine, (Balt.), **43**:423, 1964.

36. Zinneman, H. H., and Rotstein, J.: A study of gamma-globulins in dystrophia myotonica. J. Lab. Clin. Med., **47**:907, 1956.

Hemoglobin Synthesis in the Fetus and Newborn: Diagnosis of Congenital Disturbances of Hemoglobin Metabolism

HOWARD A. PEARSON, M.D.

A century ago, Körber made the epochal observation that hemoglobin from the newborn was more resistant to denaturation by strong alkali or acid solutions than that from adults[8]. This property is still the basis of most quantitative estimations of the major fetal hemoglobin, Hgb F. However, it is now apparent that the hemoglobin of the fetus is not homogeneous. Within embryonic and fetal red cells, at various times during gestation, as many as six different varieties of hemoglobin may be detected. These are hemoglobins Gower 1, Gower 2, Barts, F, A and A_2. The polypeptide chains in these hemoglobins are listed in Table I.

The first two hemoglobins can be detected only very early in intrauterine life and may be considered as true embryonic varieties. The existence of so-called "primitive" hemoglobins has been controversial. This is largely because of technical difficulties inherent in obtaining sufficient red cells from tiny embryos. However, the careful studies of Huehns and his associates have clearly established the reality and identity of the embryonic varieties[4]. In embryos of less than two months gestation, two slow migrating hemoglobin fractions called Gower 1 and 2 are seen. In the smallest embryos examined, these two fractions accounted for nearly 40 per cent of the total hemoglobin, but after ninety days they were undetectable. Some Barts hemoglobin or γ_4 was also present.

The Gower hemoglobins were shown to contain a unique polypeptide chain, designated epsilon (ε). Epsilon chains differ considerably from other human hemoglobin chains; therefore, they are believed to result from activity of an independent genetic structural locus. Since synthesis of these chains and hemoglobins ceases very early in uterine

TABLE I THE HEMOGLOBINS OF THE HUMAN EMBRYO AND FETUS

$\alpha_2\varepsilon_2$	Hgb	Gower-2
ε_4	Hgb	Gower-1
γ_4	Hgb	Barts
$\alpha_2\gamma_2$	Hgb	F
$\alpha_2\beta_2$	Hgb	A
$\alpha_2\delta_2$	Hgb	A_2

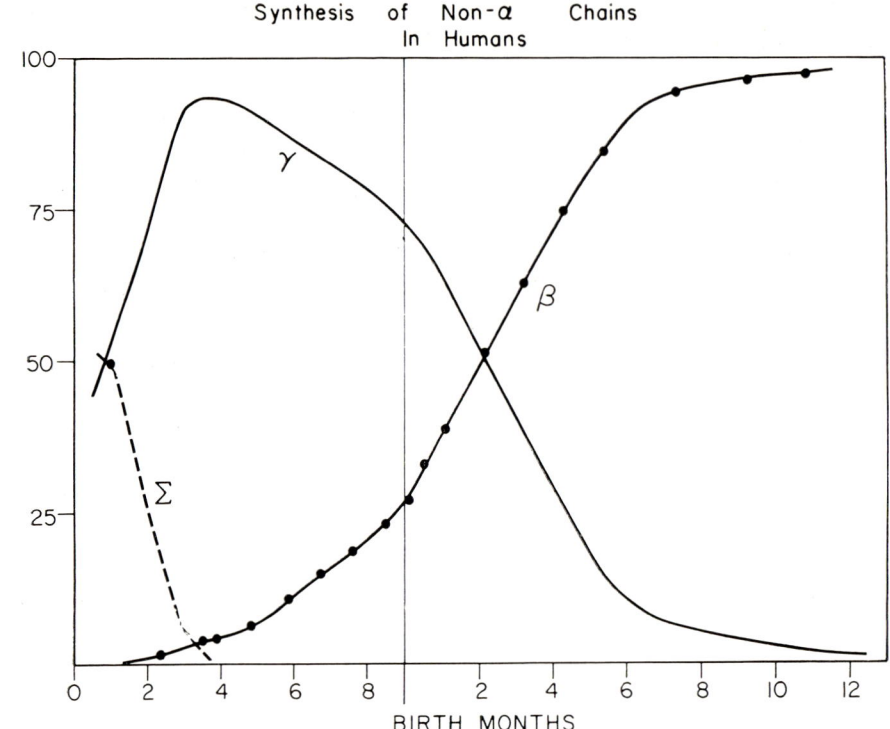

Fig. 1.   Schematic pattern of proportions of non-α-chains of hemoglobin during gestation and infancy.

life, they are mainly of theoretic interest. However, Hgb Gower 2 has also been seen in a number of newborns with the D_1 trisomy syndrome[5], indicating that genetic loci concerned with

ε-chain regulation or synthesis may be located on a D-group chromosome. This observation could also be of diagnostic value.

Figure 1 schematically depicts the

HEMOGLOBIN SYNTHESIS IN β-HEMOGLOBINOPATHY

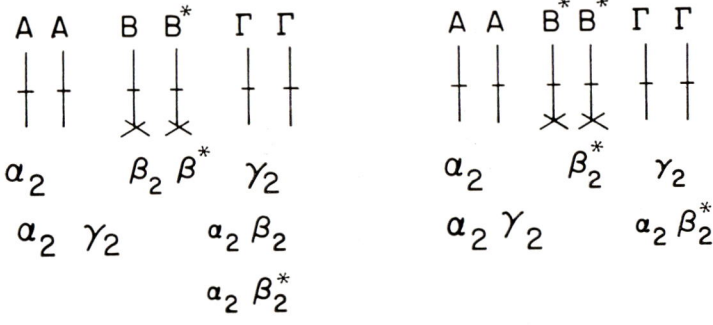

Fig. 2.   Hgb synthesis in utero of a β-hemoglobinopathy heterozygote and homozygote. The β-γ switch is indicated as a cross, blocking β-chain synthesis. The heterozygote has both Hgb A and abnormal Hgb in small amounts in addition to a preponderance of Hgb F. No Hgb A is detectable in the homozygote.

relative amounts of non-α-chains during early life. Epsilon-chain synthesis predominates initially, but rapidly declines in favor of γ-chains. Even in very early life, small amounts of Hgb A can be detected indicating activity of β-chain genes. A reciprocal relationship between β-and γ-chains is maintained. At birth, Hgb A makes up approximately 20 per cent of the total. After birth, the amount of Hgb A increases rapidly, paralleling predominant β-chain synthesis. Gamma-chain synthesis concomitantly decreases and Hgb F usually reaches the normal adult level of less than 2 per cent by six to twelve months. Exactly how this reciprocal balance between β-and γ-chain synthesis is accomplished is uncertain, although a "regulator gene" mechanism based upon models of Jacob

and Monod[7] has certain attractive features.

Symptoms of abnormal hemoglobin syndromes are not manifested at birth. This is because most of the important hemoglobin varients are due to mutant β-chain genes. This point is depicted in Figure 2. Owing to predominant γ-chain synthesis in fetal life, cord blood contains only a small proportion of the abnormal β-chain variant even in the homozygous state.

Study of hemoglobinopathies in young patients is hampered by the small amounts of abnormal hemoglobin present, and also by the intermediate electrophoretic mobility of Hgb F. As shown in Figure 3, using standard electrophoresis at pH 8.6 on starch or paper, the position of Hgb F merges with that

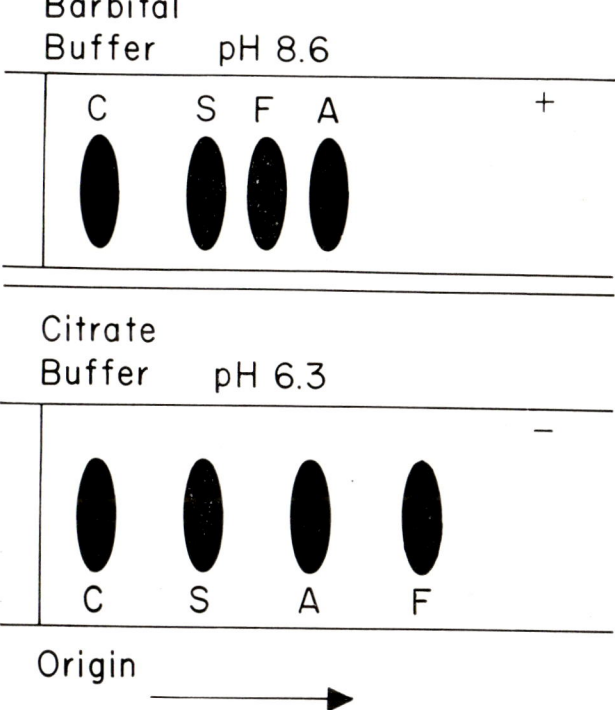

Fig. 3. Relative electrophoretic mobilities of major hemoglobins in starch electrophoresis pH 8.6 and agar electrophoresis pH 6.3. Note particularly the different mobility of Hgb F.

of Hgb A and S. A most useful technique for studying hemoglobin from young infants is agar gel electrophoresis in citrate buffer pH 6.2[10]. Methodology employed in our laboratory is appended. With this method, Hgb F has a rapid cathodal migration, moving it out of the A-S region. As shown in Figure 4, newborn twins have been studied from a family in which a previous child had sickle cell anemia. One child had three components, Hgb F, A and S. The other twin had only F and S. These children have subsequently followed typical courses of sickle cell trait and disease, respectively. A few infants with α-chain mutations have a major abnormal fetal type component $(\alpha_2^D\gamma_2)$[9].

A method which permits the detection of increased amounts of fetal hemoglobin within a single red cell is the acid elution slide technique of Betke and Kleihauer[2]. An outline of a slight modification of this simple and inexpensive test is appended. After alcohol fixation, a blood smear is immersed in a citric acid phosphate buffer at pH 3.3. Red cells containing Hgb A are eluted leaving only an empty, nonstaining

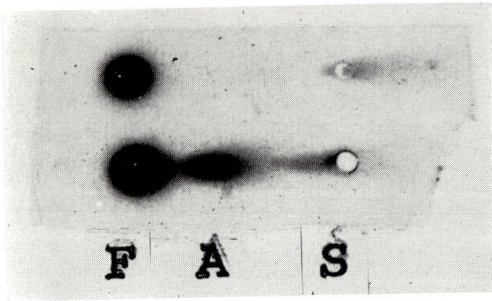

Fig. 4. Electrophoresis of cord Hgb of fraternal twins. F-S pattern on top indicates homozygous Hgb S disease. F-AS pattern beneath indicates that the child has Hgb S trait.

membrane or "ghost." Hemoglobin F resists elution by the buffer, and red cells containing significant amounts of this hemoglobin maintain normal staining properties. These differences are so apparent that as few as one in 1000 or less red cells containing Hgb F can be discerned easily in adult blood. This technique has been used on the blood of postpartum women to confirm that minute feto-maternal transfusions are usual in pregnancy.

In our laboratory, the Betke technique has been used to estimate the life span of the fetal red cell and *in vivo* Cr^{51} elution rate from fetal red cells[10]. It is also useful for determination of the efficiency of intraperitoneal transfusions given *in utero* to infants with severe erythroblastosis fetalis.

The following case summary indicates the value of the Betke method. A four-year-old child was studied because of moderate anemia. Physical examination showed that thumbs were absent. The concentration of hemoglobin was 8.0 gm per 100 ml, and the platelet count was 100,000 per cu mm. Bone marrow showed a slightly decreased cellularity. The Betke smear of the peripheral blood demonstrates a large number of red cells containing Hgb F (Fig. 5). Elevations of fetal hemoglobin have been reported to occur regularly in patients with Fanconi's hereditary aplastic anemia. This child, who has subsequently developed pancytopenia with hypoplastic marrow, confirms that disordered hemoglobin metabolism with proliferation of cells containing Hgb F may antedate the development of frank aplastic anemia[12].

Why does the fetus posses a chemically different hemoglobin? Ten years

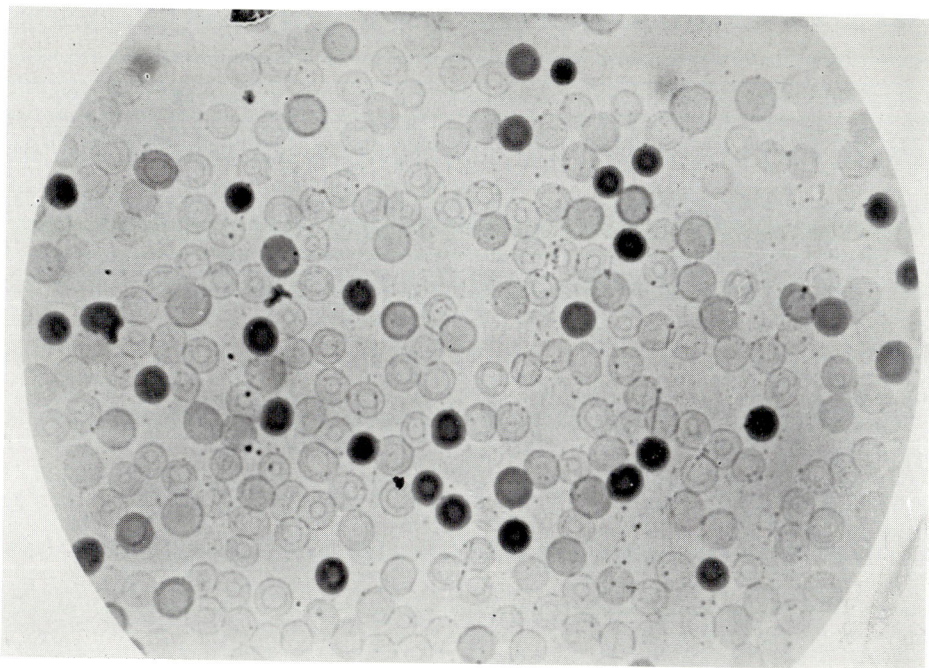

Fig. 5. Betke smear of peripheral blood on child with incipient aplastic anemia of Fanconi variety. Note the well-stained Hgb F containing RBC and the "ghost" cells from which Hgb A has been eluted.

ago the reason seemed obvious. When the oxygen dissociation curves of fetal and adult blood are compared, the fetal curve shows a higher affinity for oxygen and a more complete dissociation at low pO_2[13]. These properties would favor a transfer of oxygen from mother to fetus. It was logical to assume that these changes were due to fetal hemoglobin. However, dialyzed solutions of Hgb A and F have identical oxygen dissociation curves[1]. Therefore, the differences observed must be due to some aspect of the fetal red cell itself rather than Hgb F.

Evolutionary theories suggest that all hemoglobins evolved from a primitive myoglobin-like precursor by a process involving multiple gene duplication[6]. By this view, α-chains are evolutionarily the most primitive chain, followed by ε, γ, β and lastly the δ polypeptide chains. The same general sequence of chain appearance is seen during the development of the human embryo, fetus and infant. At the present time there is no way to confirm the thesis that developmental changes of the polypeptide chains are merely "ontogeny recapitulating phylogeny"[3]. However, there is also at the present time no definite physiologic explanation for the complex fetal-adult hemoglobin systems which occur in most vertebrate species.

METHODS

A. *Modified-Betke-Kleinhauer Method*[2].
   1. Make blood smears on glass slides.
   2. Fix in 80 per cent ethyl alcohol for five minutes.
   3. Rinse in water and dry.

4. Place slides in citric acid — phosphate buffer* at 37°C for five minutes, agitating at one minute and three minutes by lifting slide out of buffer.
5. Wash in water.
6. Giesma stain for fifteen minutes.
7. Adult red cells appear as empty "ghosts." Fetal red cells appear well hemoglobinized.

B. *Agar Gel Electrophoresis*[11].

MATERIALS

1. 0.05M citric acid-sodium citrate buffer, pH 6.2.
   Stock buffer: 147 gm sodium citrate 2H_2O in 1 liter of H_2O. Adjust to pH 6.4 with concentrated citric acid.
   Working buffer: 100 ml stock buffer, 900 ml H_2O. Adjust to pH 6.2 with concentrated citric acid.
2. Difco-Bacto agar. One gm is mixed in 100 ml of working buffer. Heat until agar disolves and solution clears, just short of boiling.
3. A mold is made from glass plate 2 in x 12 in, tightly rimmed with masking tape. The tape holds three thicknesses of Whatman #2 filter paper on each end. Twenty-five to thirty ml of agar are poured into the mold and allowed to gel.
4. Inoculation wells in middle of block are made with a #16 needle, the bevel of which is filed off. Four to six specimens may be run. Each well is filled with oxyhemoglobin solution with a glass microhematocrit tube. The concentrations of hemoglobin solutions should be 5 to 7 gm per 100 ml.

----

*Buffer
1. 0.2M $Na_2HPO_4 \cdot 7H_2O$ (26.6 parts).
2. 0.1 M citric acid (73.4 parts). Adjust pH to 3.2-3.5 with concentrated citric acid. Mix and place in 37 C incubator for thirty minutes before using.

5. Plates are sprayed with a plastic spray (Krylon-crystal clear #1302) to prevent drying of agar.
6. After inoculation and spraying, wicks are placed in two electrode tanks each filled with 450 ml of working buffer.
7. *Current*: 35 ma; 250 volts.
   Duration of run: two to four hours.
8. After electrophoresis, the agar is stained with Amido-Schwartz 10B in methanol and cleared with a solution of fifty parts methanol, fifty parts H_2O and five parts acetic acid. After staining, the agar is placed on a 3¼ x 4 cm glass slide. The agar dries as a thin film adherent to the glass.

ORDER OF SEPARATION

All hemoglobin moves to cathode. Hemoglobin F is the fastest and moves as a round spot. Hgb A, A_2, D and E move together, followed by S and C. All of these hemoglobins assume a "comet" shape.

This method is valuable as a screening test to detect the presence of Hgb S, C and F. Rates of migration are dependent on concentrations and proportions of hemoglobin, so this is not a reliable method for identification of components.

REFERENCES

1. Allen, D. N., Wyman, J., and Smith, C. I.: The oxygen equilibrium of fetal adult human hemoglobin. J. Biol. Chem., 203:81-87, 1953.
2. Betke, K., and Kleihauer, E.: Fetaler und Blubender Blutfarbstaff in Erythrozyten und Erythrroblasten von Menschlichen Feten und Neugeborenen. Blut, 4:241-249, 1959.
3. Epstein, C. J., and Motulsky, A. G.: Evolutionary origins of human proteins. In Steinberg, A. G., and Bearn, A. G. (eds.): Progress in Medical Genetics, Vol. 4. New York, Grune, 1965, pp. 85-127.
4. Huehns, E. R., Dance, N., Beaven, G. H., Keil, J. V., Hecht, F., and Motulsky, A. G.:

Human embryonic haemoglobins. Nature (London), **201**:1095-1097, 1964.

5. Heuhns, E. R., Hecht, F., Keil, J. V., and Motulsky, A. G.: Developmental hemoglobin anomalies in a chromosomal triplication D-1 trisomy syndrome. Proc. Nat. Acad. Sci. U.S.A., 89-97, 1964.

6. Ingram, V. M.: Gene evolution and the haemoglobins. Nature (London), **189**:704-708, 1961.

7. Jacob, F., and Monad, J.: Genetic regulatory mechanisms in synthesis of proteins. J. Molec. Biol., 3:318-356, 1961.

8. Körber, E.: Inaugural dissertation, Dorpat, cited by Bischoff, H. Z. Exp. Med., **48**:472-489, 1926.

9. Minnich, V., Cordonnier, J. K., Williams, W. J., and Moore, C. V.: Alpha, beta and gamma hemoglobin polypeptide chains during neonatal period with description of a fetal form of hemoglobin Dα-St. Louis. Blood, **19**:137-167, 1962.

10. Pearson, H. A.: The binding of Cr^{51} to hemoglobin. II. In vivo elution rates from Hgb CC, CS and placental red cells. Blood, **28**: 563-568, 1966.

11. Robinson, A. R., Robson, M., Harrison, A. P., and Zuelzer, W. N.: A new technique for differentiation of hemoglobins. J. Lab. Clin. Med., **50**:745-752, 1957.

12. Shahidi, N. T., Gerald, P. S., and Diamond, L. K.: Alkali resistant hemoglobin in aplastic anemia of both acquired and congenital types. New Eng. J. Med., **266**:117-120, 1962.

13. Wyman, J.: Heme proteins. Advances Protein Chem., **IV**:420-531, 1947.

Magnetic Orientation of Sickled Erythrocytes

MAKIO MURAYAMA, Ph.D.

INTRODUCTION

The effect of magnetic field on the human sickled erythrocytes was deduced and then experimentally verified[1]. A mechanism of sickled erythrocyte formation was suggested[2] which involved a linear stacking of S-hemoglobin molecules. Experimental evidence has been obtained subsequently which is consistent with this hypothesis.

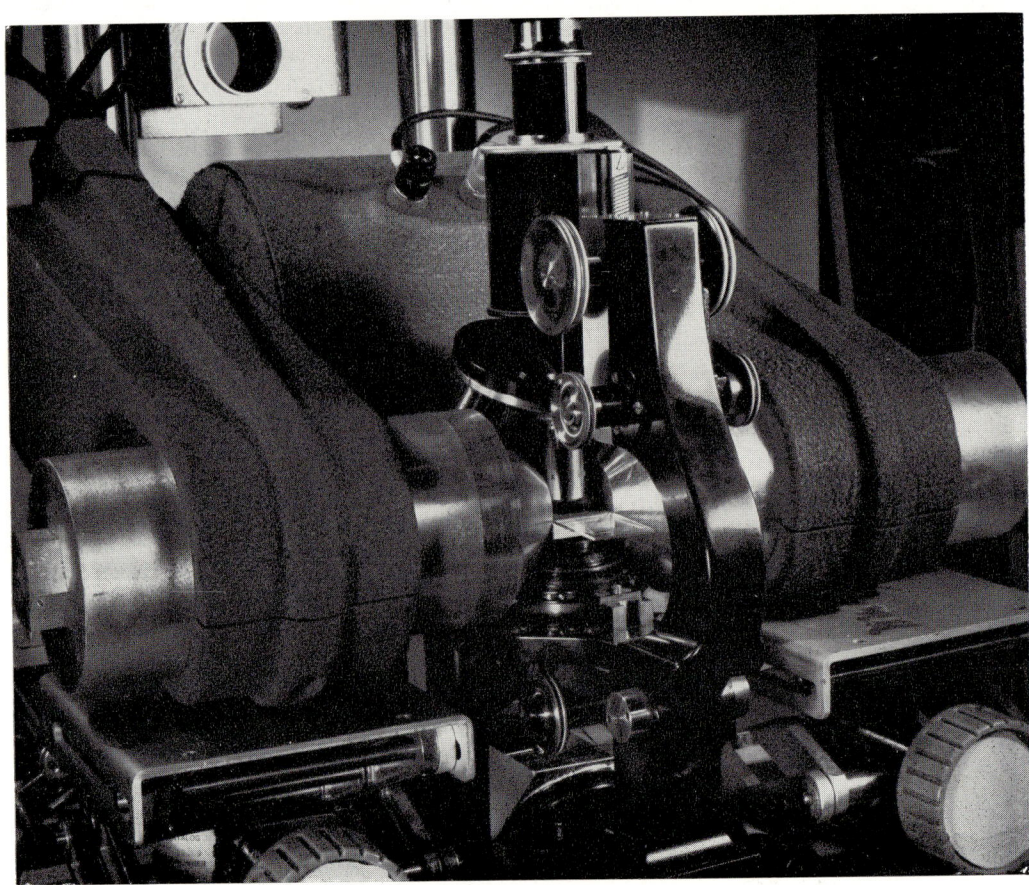

Fig. 1. Magnetic Microscope.

Michael Faraday first studied the magnetic properties of dried blood in 1845 and made a note: "Must try recent fluid blood." It is now known that dried blood contains anhydrohemoglobin which is diamagnetic. The unfinished work of Faraday was continued by Pauling and Coryell in 1936. They reported[3] that oxyhemoglobin and carbonmonoxy-hemoglobin are diamagnetic (permeability is less than 1), but, on the other hand, *deoxygenated* hemoglobin is *para-magnetic* (permeability is greater than 1 and therefore is attracted into a magnetic field). They found the value of 5.46 Bohr magneton per Fe^{++}. Therefore, they deduced that there are four unpaired electrons per heme group.

Since the sickling phenomenon takes place only upon deoxygenation, it was suggested by us that a sickled erythrocyte ought to orient itself with its long axis perpendicular to the magnetic lines of force. Earlier it had been deduced that S-hemoglobin molecules are linearly stacked along the long axis of the sickled erythrocytes. This notion was confirmed experimentally by Murayama, Olson and Jennings[4].

Apparatus (Figure 1)

1. *ALNICO magnet,* a large permanent magnet with adjustable pole pieces manufactured by General Electric Co., Schenectady, New York, Catalogue No. 7766115.

2. *Electromagnet,* similar to Catalogue No. 79641 of Central Scientific Company, Chicago, Illinois, is adequate.

3. *A compound microscope* with the fine adjustment on the objective. The stage of the microscope must be removed so that the pole pieces of the magnet can be placed in its place; a "stage" to hold a slide may be improvised from a sheet of brass or aluminum.

Reagent

Two per cent solution of *sodium dithionite.*

Procedure

1. The height of the pole pieces of a magnet is adjusted with a pair of "Lab Jacks" so that the wet preparation can be examined microscopically while it is in a magnetic field.

2. A wet preparation is made from a drop of blood of a patient known to be homozygous for S-hemoglobin.

3. The wet preparation is placed between the pole pieces, on the "stage" improvised from a sheet of brass or aluminum.

4. The microscope is focused and the orientation of the erythrocytes is observed.

Discussion

Direct evidence obtained by electron microscopy indicates that S-hemoglobin molecules stack to form molecular monofilaments and these aggregates form a "cable" of hexagonal array about its axis.[5]

To explain these observations, the following hypothesis is suggested: At the sub-molecular level the genetically introduced amino acid residue, valyl (at position 6) and the first valyl residue interact with each other by hydrophobic bonding, allowing cyclization from the 1st carbonyl to the 4th NH by hydrogen bonding. This process leads to the "key" formation in the "lock-and-key" arrangement, which allows a linear stacking of the molecules. In the normal hemoglobin molecule (Hb-A), no ring structure formation takes place. Instead,

these first six residues probably introduce a steric hindrance, thus preventing
aggregation. S-hemoglobin molecules
stack one on top of the other to form
molecular monofilaments; they aggre-
gate to form a rope or "cable" of hexagonal symmetry. The cables bundle
together to form liquid crystals of
nematic (thread-like) type. The cell
membrane simply conforms to the shape
of the liquid crystal. The water molecules leave the cell owing to change in
osmotic pressure, and the cell is said to
"sickle."

REFERENCES

1. Murayama, M.: Orientation of sickled erythrocytes in a magnetic field. Nature, (London), **206**:420-422, 1965.
2. Murayama, M.: A molecular mechanism of
   sickled erythrocyte formation. Nature, (London), **202**:258-260, 1964.
3. Pauling, L., and Coryell, C. D.: The magnetic properties and structure of hemoglobin,
   oxyhemoglobin and carbonmonoxyhemoglo-
   bin. Proc. Nat. Acad. Sci. U.S.A., **2**:210-216,
   1936.
4. Murayama, M., Olson, R. A., and Jennings,
   W. H.: Molecular orientation in horse hemoglobin crystals and sickled erythrocytes.
   Biochim. Biophys. Acta, **94**:194-199, 1965.
5. Murayama, M.: Unpublished data.

Erythrocyte Enzyme Defects in Congenital Hemolytic Anemias

FRANK A. OSKI, M.D.

It was only ten years ago that Carson and associates[11] elucidated the red cell enzymatic defect in primaquine sensitive hemolytic anemia. Since the discovery of glucose-6-phosphate dehydrogenase deficiency, many other enzyme defects have been recognized as responsible for the production of congenital non-spherocytic hemolytic anemias (Table I). In the immediate newborn period, glucose-6-phosphate dehydrogenase deficiency, pyruvate kinase deficiency and 2,3-diphosphoglycerate mutase deficiency have been recognized as being associated with significant hyperbilirubinemia and, on occasion, kernicterus. The precise role these enzymatic defects play in the causation of the congenital non-spherocytic hemolytic anemias is best appreciated after a brief review of normal red cell metabolism.

GLYCOLYSIS

The primary source of energy for the erythrocyte is derived from carbohydrate metabolism. Since glycogen is virtually absent from the cell, the red cell has no carbohydrate stores and must rely on a constant supply of carbohydrate in order to maintain a steady state of its energy potential. Glucose is the form of carbohydrate normally used by the red cell, although other monosaccharides, both hexoses and pentoses, penetrate the red cell[26]. Although glucose is the preferred carbohydrate for red cell energy production, it can also metabolize fructose and mannose almost as readily and galactose much more slowly. Carbohydrate entry and metabolism are not influenced by insulin unless the cell membrane is pretreated with chymotrypsin.

EMBDEN-MEYERHOF PATHWAY

Since the mature erythrocyte does not have a functioning Krebs cycle, the bulk

TABLE I CONGENITAL ENZYMATIC DEFECTS OF THE RED CELL RESULTING IN NON-SPHEROCYTIC HEMOLYTIC ANEMIAS

Glycolytic Enzymes
  Glucose-6-phosphate deyhdrogenase deficiency*
  Pyruvate kinase deficiency*
  2,3-diphosphoglycerate mutase deficiency*
  Triose isomerase deficiency

Non-glycolytic Enzymes
  Glutathione reductase deficiency
  Adenosine triphosphatase deficiency
  Hereditary absence of glutathione

*Recognized as a cause of neonatal jaundice.

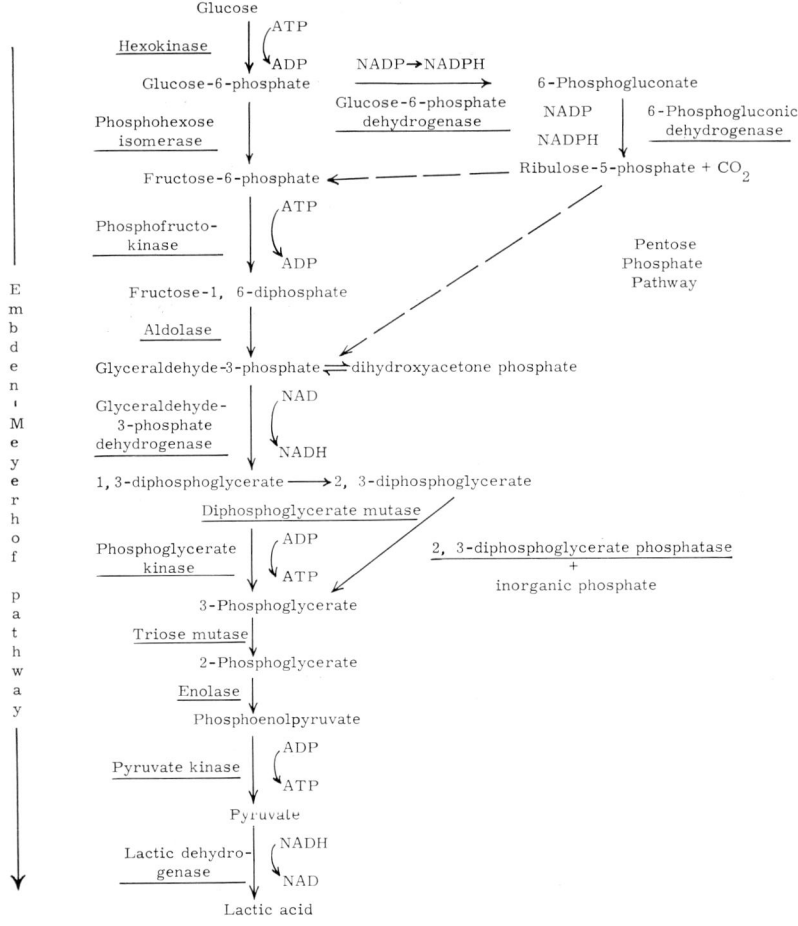

Fig. I.   Embden-Meyerhof pathway.

of glucose consumption occurs via the Embden-Meyerhof pathway, an anaerobic pathway. One mole of glucose is catabolized to two moles of lactic acid via this pathway (Fig. 1). The studies of Murphy[33] demonstrated that approximately 90 per cent of all glucose metabolized under normal conditions traverses this route. In the catabolism of one mole of glucose to two moles of lactic acid, two moles of adenosine triphosphate (ATP) are degraded to adenosine diphosphate (ADP), but four moles of adenosine diphosphate are phosphorylated to adenosine triphosphate; thus, there is a net gain of two high-energy phosphate bonds. Nicotinamide adenine dinucleotide (NAD or DPN) serves as an essential cofactor in the Embden-Meyerhof pathway. There is no net reduction or oxidation of this pyridine nucleotide during the conversion of glucose to lactic acid.

PENTOSE PHOSPHATE PATHWAY

The other 10 per cent of glucose metabolized by the red cell occurs by way of an oxidative pathway, the pentose phosphate pathway or hexose

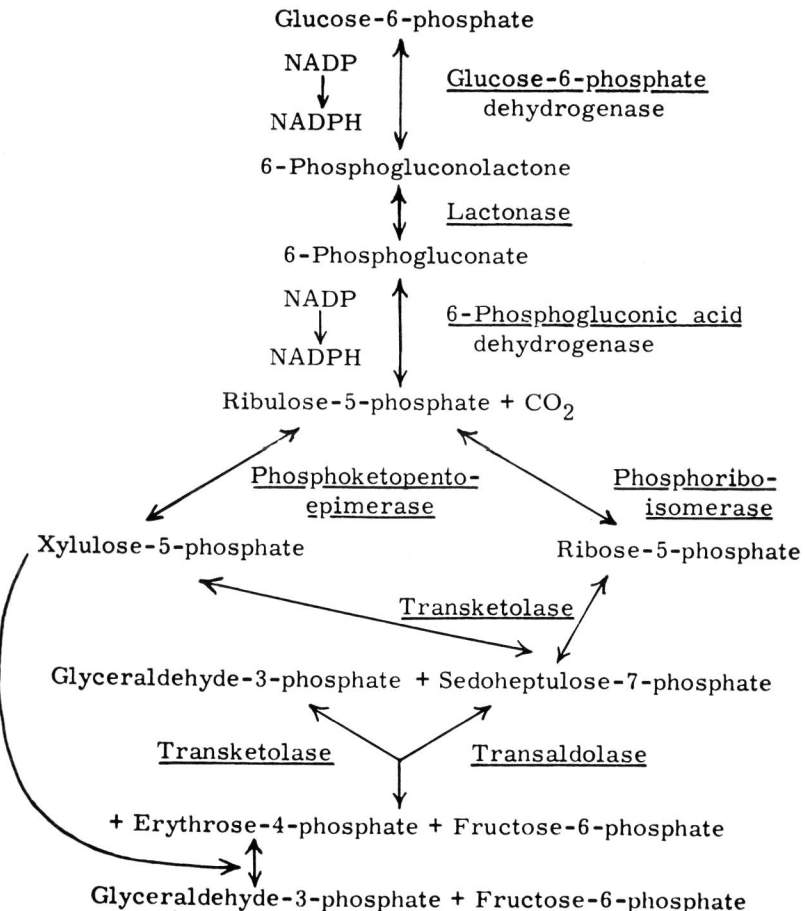

Fig. 2. Pentose phosphate pathway.

monophosphate shunt (Fig. 2). In this alternate pathway, glucose-6-phosphate undergoes oxidative decarboxylation with the consumption of oxygen and the evolution of carbon dioxide.

In the first step of this oxidative pathway, glucose-6-phosphate is oxidized to 6-phosphogluconolactone by a reaction catalyzed by the enzyme glucose-6-phopshate dehydrogenase. This enzyme in particular and this pathway in general have been the focus of extensive investigation in recent years since the demonstration by Carson[11] in 1956 that the erythrocytes of persons susceptible to acute hemolysis after ingestion of the antimalarial primaquine were deficient in glucose-6-phosphate dehydrogenase.

Unlike the Embden-Meyerhof pathway, wherein nicotinamide adenine dinucleotide serves as an essential cofactor, the pentose phosphate pathway requires nicotinamide adenine dinucleotide phosphate (NADP or TPN) as a cofactor. The reactions catalyzed by glucose-6-phosphate dehydrogenase and 6-phosphogluconic dehydrogenase (Fig. 3) require nicotinamide adenine dinucleotide phosphate and result in the generation of the reduced cofactor $NADPH_2$ (TPNH).

The pentose pathway provides the

cell with ribose-5-phosphate, which is a constituent of the vital pyridine nucleotides, nicotinamide adenine dinucleotide and nicotinamide adenine dinucleotide phosphate, and the purine nucleotides adenosine diphosphate and adenosine triphosphate. Although the mature red cell can utilize preformed purines for nucleotide synthesis, there is no pathway for *de novo* purine formation[3]. The mature red cell does, however, retain the ability for pyridine nucleotide formation[23].

Perhaps the most vital role of the pentose pathway in the mature erythrocyte is the generation of NADPH$_2$. Although there is no evidence that NADPH$_2$ oxidation serves as an energy source, it serves as a necessary cofactor in several reactions which appear vital for the preservation of red cell integrity.

NADPH$_2$ serves as a hydrogen donor in the reduction of glutathione mediated by the enzyme glutathione reductase (Fig. 3). Reduced glutathione maintains the stability of certain sulfhydryl-containing enzymes of the erythrocyte[42] as well as stabilizing hemoglobin[1]. NADPH$_2$ also plays a role in methemoglobin reduction that is mediated by the NADPH$_2$-dependent enzyme methemoglobin reductase (Fig. 3). Methemoglobin is also reduced by a NADH-dependent enzyme which appears to play a more important role in methemoglobin reduction under normal conditions[44].

It has also been demonstrated that NADPH$_2$ can directly protect hemoglobin from oxidative denaturation and that this protection need not be mediated via reduced glutathione[48].

In summary, it appears that the main function of the Embden-Meyerhof pathway is to provide adenosine triphosphate for its multiple essential functions, while the main role of the pentose pathway, by virtue of the fact that it is the only

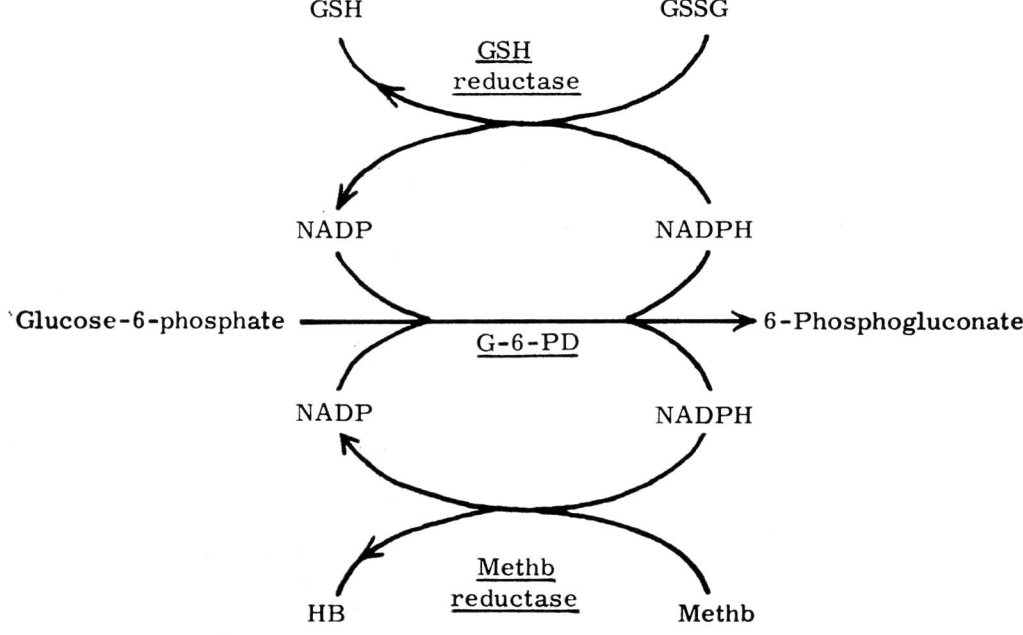

Fig. 3.   The relationship of NADPH$_2$.

source of NADPH$_2$ generation in the mature red cell, is to serve in the protection of both hemoglobin and vital enzymes from oxidative denaturation.

GLUCOSE-6-PHOSPHATE DEHYDROGENASE DEFICIENCY

While studying the mechanism of primaquine-induced hemolytic anemia, Dern and associates[15] first provided evidence that this type of drug-induced hemolysis occurred in subjects with an intrinsic abnormality of the erythrocyte. In 1956, Carson and co-workers[11] demonstrated that the major defect in the erythrocytes of these individuals was a deficiency of the enzyme glucose-6-phosphate dehydrogenase. This enzyme governs the first step in the pentose phosphate pathway.

It is now recognized that many drugs (in addition to primaquine), as well as other metabolic disturbances, may precipitate a hemolytic episode in G-6-PD-deficient individuals (Table II). The incidence of the disease, the severity of the process and the agents recognized as capable of initiating hemolysis in this condition vary among the racial and ethnic groups in which this disease occurs. Because of this genetic heterogeneity, it is necessary for any individual caring for newborns in a cosmopolitan nursery to be familiar with the variable characteristics of this deficiency state. Neonatal jaundice and kernicterus secondary to hemolytic disease has frequently been observed in G-6-PD-deficient newborns.

Mode of Inheritance and Racial Incidence

This enzyme deficiency is genetically determined and transmitted by a gene

TABLE II   A List of Some of the Agents Reported to Produce Hemolysis in Patients with G-6-PD Deficiency

Antimalarials
   Primaquine
   Pamaquine
   Pentaquine
   Plasmoquine
   Quinocide
   Quinacrine (Atabrine®)
   Quinine (C)
Sulfonamides
   Sulfanilamide
   N$_2$ Acetylsulfanilamide
   Sulfacetamide (Sulamyd®)
   Sulfamethoxypyridazine (Kynex®, Midicel®)
   Salicylazosulfapyridine (Azulfidine®)
   Sulfisoxazole (Gantrisin®)
   Sulfapyridine
Nitrofurans
   Nitrofurantoin (Furadantin®)
   Furazolidone (Furoxone®)
   Furaltadone (Altafur)
   Nitrofurazone (Furacin®)
Antipyretics and Analgesics
   Acetylsalicylic acid
   Acetanilid
   Acetophenetidin (phenacetin)
   Antipyrine [c]
   Aminopyrine [c]
   P-aminosalicylic acid
Sulfones
Others
   Dimercaprol (BAL)
   Methylene blue
   Naphthalene
   Phenylhydrazine
   Acetylphenhydrazine
   Probenecid
   Vitamin K (large doses of water-soluble analogs)
   Chloramphenicol [c]
   Quinidine [c]
   Fava beans [c]
   Chloroquine
   Orinase®
Infections
   Viral respiratory
   Infectious hepatitis
   Infectious mononucleosis
   Bacterial pneumonias
Diabetic Acidosis

[c]: Caucasians only to date.

located on the x-chromosome. Full expression of the defect therefore occurs more frequently in the hemizygous male ($\bar{x}y$) because the mutant gene ($\bar{x}$) is not balanced by a normal allele. Complete expression of the defect in the homozygous female ($\bar{x}\bar{x}$) is much less common, but great variability with respect to partial expression of the defect may be seen in the heterozygous female ($\bar{x}x$).

One explanation for the great variability in enzyme levels in the heterozygous female is that only one x-chromosome is genetically active in any cell during interphase[28]. Thus, the heterozygous female is in reality a mosaic of G-6-PD-deficient and G-6-PD-sufficient cells, and the wide range of G-6-PD values in female heterozygotes is a result of the varying proportions of somatic cells containing x-chromosomes in which either the normal or the G-6-PD-deficient x-chromosome has been "inactivated" at an early stage of cell division in the embryo. Evidence for this female G-6-PD mosaicism has been demonstrated in skin cultures by Davidson et al.[14] and in red blood cells by Beutler and Baluda[2].

Glucose-6-phosphate-dehydrogenase-deficiency is widely distributed throughout the world. Among Caucasians its incidence is highest in those groups residing in the Mediterranean area. In some areas of Sardinia, 30 per cent of males are affected. The deficiency state also occurs with great frequency among Sephardic Jews (rare among Ashkenazic Jews), Greeks and Iranians.

Mongolian groups that are known to be affected include the Chinese, Malayans, Filipinos, Indonesians and Melanesians. In the American Negro the incidence of the deficiency state is estimated to range from 9 to 13 per cent in the male and 2 to 3 per cent in the female[51]. In some parts of Africa, the incidence of the deficiency state may be close to 25 per cent. The geographic distribution of the trait closely parallels that found for falciparum malaria, and it is believed that G-6-PD deficiency may provide protection against intracellular invasion by the malarial parasite[31]. It is suggested that this enzyme deficiency may represent an example of "balanced polymorphism" where the deleterious effects of the deficiency state are balanced by the protection it affords against the severe consequences of malaria.

GENETIC HETEROGENEITY

Glucose-6-phosphate dehydrogenase deficiency is not a homogenous entity. These differences among ethnic and racial groups may be the result of several mutations occurring at the same gene locus or may reflect mutations in other genes on the x-chromosome which control the formation and structure of the enzyme.

In general, the heterogeneity of this deficiency reflects itself in variations in the degree of enzyme deficiency, differences in the types of drugs necessary to produce hemolysis, differences in the types of cells in the body also affected by the deficiency, the susceptibility to neonatal jaundice and alterations in the electrophoretic and catalytic properties of the enzyme among various racial and ethnic groups.

In the Negro, the deficiency state, in general, is milder than that observed in the Caucasian. In the Caucasian, G-6-PD deficiency has been demonstrated in the leukocytes, saliva, platelets and liver of the affected subjects, whereas, in the Negro, the deficiency has been found in the lens of the eye and the platelets. The deficiency state, however, is much more generalized, because whole body oxidation of glucose-1-C^{14} to $C^{14}O_2$ has been found to be below normal in the Negro[51].

In the newborn this genetic heterogeneity has profound clinical implications. There does not appear to be a significantly increased incidence of jaundice in Negro term infants who are G-6-PD deficient. In contrast, many instances of jaundice and kernicterus have been observed among Caucasians and Mongolians with G-6-PD deficiency.

PATHOGENESIS

The primary defect of the erythrocyte appears to be the deficiency of glucose-6-phosphate dehydrogenase (G-6-PD), the enzyme catalyzing the first step in the pentose phosphate pathway. The metabolic consequences of this deficiency, as well as other metabolic characteristics of the G-6-PD-deficient cell, are listed in Table III.

The activity of G-6-PD in the erythrocytes of the affected Negro male is approximately 10 to 15 per cent of normal, whereas in many Caucasians with the deficiency, the activity is even lower, and frequently no activity can be demonstrated.

The mechanism by which G-6-PD deficiency predisposes the cell to hemolysis is not completely understood. In these deficient cells the capacity to regenerate $NADPH_2$ (TPNH) is limited. This lack of reducing potential makes the cell vulnerable to oxidative denaturation and may result in altera-

TABLE III METABOLIC CHARACTERISTICS OF THE ERYTHROCYTES OF PRIMAQUINE-SENSITIVE AMERICAN NEGRO MALES[*]

I. *Deficient Glucose-6-Phosphate Dehydrogenase Activity; primary metabolic disorder*

II. *Other Abnormalities of the Pentose Phosphate Pathway; impaired NADPH regenerative capacity secondary to I*
  A. Diminished NADPH, increased NADP, content.
  B. Diminished responsiveness to redox dyes.
    1. Decreased oxygen consumption.
    2. Diminished rate of methemoglobin reduction.
    3. Diminished pentose formation.
    4. Diminished rate of glucose utilzation.
    5. Decreased rate of dye reduction.

III. *Abnormalities Related to the Defective Pentose Phosphate Pathway*
  A. Decreased reduced glutathione (GSH) content.
  B. Vulnerability of glutathione (GSH) to oxidation.
  C. Increased glutathione reductase activity; compensatory, or a reflection of younger RBC population.
  D. Increased methemoglobinemia during nitrite administration; insufficient NADPH for methemoglobin reduction.
  E. Susceptibility to Heinz body formation *in vivo* and *in vitro*; vulnerability of hemoglobin to oxidation.
  F. Decreased lipid content.

IV. *Abnormalities of the Embden-Meyerhof Pathway*
  A. Decreased NADH and increased NAD content.
  B. Fall in ATP content *in vitro* with acetlylphenylhydrazine; may be secondary to a deficiency of NADH and NADPH.

V. *Decreased Catalase Activity and Further Fall During Drug-Induced Hemolysis*

VI. *Normal Metabolic Characteristics*
  6-Phosphogluconic dehydrogenase, pentose content, purine nucleoside phosphorylase, transketolase, transaldolase, phosphohexose isomerase, isocritric dehydrogenase, malic dehydrogenase, acetyl cholinesterase, glyceraldehyde-phosphate dehydrogenase, adenosine triphosphate (ATP) content, lactic dehydrogenase and glutathione peroxidase.

[*]From Brewer and Tarlov, 1962.

tions in hemoglobin, vital cellular enzymes or constituients of the red cell membrane. It has been suggested that the oxidative denaturation produced by many of the hemolytic agents results from the generation of hydrogen peroxide[12]. The newborn's red cells may already be more vulnerable to damage from hydrogen peroxide because of their lowered levels of glutathione peroxidase and catalase, necessary enzymes for the detoxification of this compound.

Clinical Manifestations: Clinical Course of Hemolysis

In the adult, the clinical course of hemolysis following ingestion of a hemolytic compound has been well described[15, 25]. Following ingestion of a standard dose of 30 mg of primaquine, the hematocrit usually begins to fall between the second and fourth day and drops to its lowest level by the eighth or twelfth day. Although symptoms are uncommon in this type of experimental situation, transient jaundice may occur. Heinz bodies may be observed during the first few days of the hemolytic episode.

Clinical recovery occurs between the tenth and fortieth day, with a reticulocytosis beginning at about the fifth day and reaching a maximum ten to twenty days after drug ingestion.

More severe hemolysis may be observed if the hemolytic compound is taken in large quantities, if the patient is ill at the time of drug ingestion, or if concurrent liver or renal disease delays detoxification or excretion of the offending compound.

In contrast to the relatively mild hemolytic episode that follows primaquine ingestion is the explosive and sometimes fatal hemolytic reaction that follows ingestion of the Fava bean in G-6-PD deficient-Caucasians. Mere inhalation of the blossoms from this plant is often sufficient to initiate a severe hemolytic episode. Fava beans have not produced a hemolytic anemia in Negroes, another example of the genetic heterogeneity of this defect.

Racial Incidence

In 1960, Panizon[40] called attention to the risks of G-6-PD deficiency in the newborn period when he described eleven cases of severe jaundice in infants from Sardinia in whom there was either a family history of favism and/or glutathione instability of the erythrocytes either in the affected infant or one of the parents. Two of these infants died in the neonatal period, and five survived with severe brain damage believed to be a result of hyperbilirubinemia. In the same year, from Singapore, Smith and Vella[47] reported thirteen Chinese infants with kernicterus associated with G-6-PD deficiency, and Weatherall[53] made similar observations on four infants from the same area.

In Greece, Doxiadis and associates[16] noted that in one third of infants requiring exchange transfusions for hyperbilirubinemia, no evidence of isoimmunization could be demonstrated. When these infants were more carefully investigated, almost all were found to be G 6 PD deficient. The association of G-6-PD deficiency with neonatal jaundice has since been reported from Italy[20], Switzerland[41], Thailand[19], Israel[49], Nigeria[10], Hawaii[24], and Canada[34].

In surveys performed on Negro term infants in the United States[36, 54], no increased incidence of jaundice has been observed in the G-6-PD-deficient groups. It is our impression that G-6-PD deficiency may contribute to an increased incidence and degree of jaundice in the premature Negro infant, although statistical data is presently inadequate.

ETIOLOGY

Although the increased incidence of jaundice noted in the G-6-PD-deficient newborn is apparently the result of hemolysis, in many instances no offending drug or toxin can be incriminated as a precipitating agent. It is apparent that not all, or even the majority, of infants with G-6-PD deficiency develop significant jaundice in the newborn period. Fessas et al.[18] estimated that approximately 5 per cent of infants with G-6-PD deficiency developed clinically significant jaundice and that these cases often showed a familial pattern. This observed recurrence of severe jaundice in only certain families with G-6-PD-deficient infants led Fessas and associates[18] to speculate that an additional independent genetic factor may be operating which determines the appearance of hyperbilirubinemia. This hypothetical factor might alter the internal environment in such a manner as to produce increased red cell destruction or may impair temporarily the conjugation of bilirubin, thus making the jaundice manifest.

The chief physical findings in infants with hemolytic disease as a result of G-6-PD deficiency are jaundice, pallor or signs of kernicterus. Hepatosplenomegaly is uncommon, and when present should arouse suspicion that a second disease may also be operative, such as isoimmunization or infection.

In contrast to the jaundice caused by blood group incompatibilities, jaundice in infants with G-6-PD deficiency usually does not appear during the first twenty-four hours of life. Doxiadis and Valaes[16A], in reviewing their experience with 135 cases of neonatal G-6-PD deficiency, observed jaundice for the first time on the second day of life in fifty of these infants and on the first day of life in only twelve. The maximum bilirubin concentration was generally reached between the third and fifth day of life. Jaundice may not manifest itself until late in the first week of life, with peak levels of bilirubin occurring during the second week. It is in this relatively late-appearing jaundice that drugs or mothballs are often found responsible for the hemolytic anemia.

LABORATORY FINDINGS

Hyperbilirubinemia, variable degrees of anemia and morphologic alterations of the red cell are the chief laboratory findings in infants with hemolytic disease due to G-6-PD deficiency.

Bilirubin levels frequently exceed 20 mg per 100 ml on the third to fifth day of life, and values in excess of 50 mg per 100 ml have been observed. Levels in excess of 20 mg per 100 ml can occur in the second week of life, with resultant kernicterus.

Hemoglobin values may range from normal to as low as 7 to 8 gm per 100 ml during the first week of life. Anemia tends to be more profound in infants whose hemolysis is triggered by an exogenous agent. In some cases, both hemoglobin and reticulocyte count may be normal, again emphasizing the point that only a small proportion of a red cell population need be destroyed to produce hyperbilirubinemia in the presence of physiologic immaturity of the bilirubin conjugating and excreting mechanism in the newborn.

In general, the reticulocyte count is elevated. Morphologic abnormalities on peripheral blood smear consist of a varying number of nucleated red cells, spherocytes, poikilocytes, and crenated and fragmented cells — all findings consistent with a hemolytic anemia as a result of a metabolic derangement of the cells. With supra-vital staining techniques, red cells containing Heinz bodies can frequently be observed early in the course of the hemolytic episode. Eventually these cells are cleared by the spleen and thus may not be found. All of these morphologic abnormalities disappear when the hemolytic episode has abated.

Diagnosis

Although normal newborns have higher levels of red cell G-6-PD than do adults, this difference does not obscure the diagnosis of the deficiency state during this period of life. Glutathione levels are low, and glutathione instability is present, but these tests are not as reliable or as meaningful as studies of enzyme activity. G-6-PD-deficient newborns have markedly reduced levels of enzyme activity that can be detected by screening tests such as the decolorization test of Motulsky et al.[32] or the methemoglobin reduction test of Brewer et al.[6] These screening tests have proven reliable in the detection of the hemizygous male or the homozygous female. Direct assay of the enzyme by spectro-

photometric techniques is often necessary for precise identification of the heterozygous female.

Treatment

The basis of treatment of this condition is simple, but its application may often prove difficult. Proper care consists of recognition of the deficient patient who is potentially at risk, avoidance of hemolytic compounds in the care of these infants, careful observation for jaundice and the treatment of hyperbilirubinemia with exchange transfusions.

In nurseries in which a large percentage of the patients are from ethnic groups susceptible to spontaneous hemolysis in the neonatal period, screening procedures should be introduced to identify the infants at risk.

Potentially hemolytic agents (Table II) should not be given to G-6-PD-deficient newborns, and these compounds should also be withheld from their mothers if the child is to be breast fed. Hemolytic anemias have occurred in breast-fed infants of mothers who have ingested fava beans[17] or who have been exposed to mothballs[34, 55].

In the Negro infant there is no apparent danger from the use of naturally occurring Vitamin K_1 (Aquamephyton, Konakion®) even in doses far in excess of 1.0 mg[54]. The water-soluble Vitamin K analogs (Synkayvite®) in large doses can produce hemolysis, but in doses of 1.0 mg also appeared to have no jaundice-producing effects in the deficient Negro[54]. The safe dose for the Vitamin K analogs has not been determined for the deficient Caucasian infant. Until more information is available, it would seem advisable to adhere to the most recent recommendation of the American Academy of Pediatrics[13] and give the minimum dose (1 mg intramuscularly to the premature or full-term infant) of the least toxic preparation — Vitamin K_1.

Of considerable interest is the observation of Zinkham[54] that the administration of Vitamin K_1 or the Vitamin K analog (Synkayvite) actually reduced the maximum bilirubin level attained in the G-6-PD-deficient Negro infant. Zinkham cautions however: "Until there is conclusive proof that these large doses are necessarily beneficial, then no more than 2.0 mg of Vitamin K_1 should be given to these infants."

Following discharge of the infant from the nursery, careful instructions must be given to the parents with respect to exposure to naphthalene. These infants must not be exposed to blankets, bedclothes or diapers that have been recently removed from storage in naphthalene-containing mothballs or flakes. The parents should also be instructed to bring the child immediately to the hospital if pallor, jaundice or dark urine is noted.

When hyperbilirubinemia occurs, exchange transfusions should be performed for bilirubin levels in excess of 20 to 25 mg per 100 ml, even during the second week of life. Kernicterus occurring during the second week of life has been observed in infants with G-6-PD-deficient hemolytic anemias[34].

When a G-6-PD-deficient infant is recognized, family studies should be carried out to detect other individuals who may be at risk from the hemolytic consequences of drug therapy.

PROGNOSIS

If hyperbilirubinemia has not resulted in kernicterus, the ultimate prognosis for these infants is good. Although these G-6-PD-deficient patients will always demonstrate a slight shortening of their red cell life span[7], they will not demonstrate anemia or reticulocytosis unless stressed by drugs, infections or acidosis.

GLUCOSE-6-PHOSPHATE DEHYDROGENASE DEFICIENCY AS A CAUSE OF A CHRONIC HEMOLYTIC ANEMIA

In addition to the common variety of G-6-PD deficiency which has been somal recessive with great variation in estimated to affect 100,000,000 individuals throughout the world, there is another much rarer form of the disease which results in a chronic hemolytic anemia of the congenital, non-spherocytic type even in the absence of drug exposure.

Patients with this type of G-6-PD deficiency have a chronic anemia, reticulocytosis, a markedly shortened red cell survival and splenomegaly. These patients will also become more anemic when given drugs that initiate hemolytic episodes in the common form of G-6-PD deficiency. This disturbance is also sex-linked in its inheritance, and is much more commonly observed in patients of Northern European stock, but has recently been reported in Negroes as well[21].

Individuals with this form of congenital non-spherocytic hemolytic anemia may also present in the newborn period with evidence of hemolysis and jaundice[35, 45]. A diagnosis of this variety of the deficiency state can be arrived at only by documenting persistent anemia and reticulocytosis over a period of several months in the absence of other diseases or known causes of hemolysis.

PYRUVATE KINASE DEFICIENCY

In 1961, Valentine, Tanaka and Miwa[52] first demonstrated that a deficiency of the erythrocyte glycolytic enzyme pyruvate kinase was associated with one form of congenital non-spehrocytic hemolytic anemia.

MODE OF INHERITANCE AND RACIAL INCIDENCE

This disease is inherited as an autosomal recessive with great variation in clinical severity. The heterozygote, although generally detectable by enzyme assay, is asymptomatic. The disease has been reported chiefly in individuals of Northern European stock, particularly the Amish[5] but it has also been observed in a Mexican family[50].

PATHOGENESIS

Pyruvate kinase deficiency is an inborn error of metabolism that illustrates clearly the consequences of a block in red cell glucose metabolism. The enzyme pyruvate kinase catalyzes the conversion of phosphoenolpyruvate to pyruvate. During this step, adenosine diphosphate is converted to adenosine triphosphate, and, for every mole of glucose that enters the Embden-Meyerhof pathway, 2 moles of ATP are formed from 2 moles of ADP at this point.

As a consequence of this block, pyruvate kinase-deficient erythrocytes consume less glucose than normal erythrocytes, have low levels of ATP, and the ATP that is present in the cells falls

at an accelerated rate[38]. As a secondary consequence of this enzymatic block, these red cells have low levels of NAD. The low levels of NAD appear to be a result of the fact that decreased amounts of pyruvate are present to be converted to lactate, the step in which NADP is reduced to NAD in the presence of lactic dehydrogenase (Fig. 1).

Pyruvate kinase-deficient erythrocytes clearly illustrate the relationship between the cation pump and red cell ATP levels. Because of reduced and unstable levels of ATP, there is insufficient energy available for cation transport, and these red cells lose potassium at an accelerated rate. Their survival is shortened, and they are sequestered in both the liver and the spleen, with the liver removing the bulk of these cells.

The unstable ATP levels and the marked cation leak may be responsible for the morphologic abnormalities noted in these cells. Many irregularly contracted cells have been noted, not only in the circulation of these patients, but also upon short periods of incubation.

CLINICAL MANIFESTATIONS

A summary of some of the clinical and laboratory features of this disorder appear in Table IV. It will be noted that jaundice and anemia occur frequently in the neonatal period. Splenomegaly may be present during the first weeks of life and is almost a constant finding in later life.

LABORATORY FINDINGS

The laboratory findings include hyperbilirubinemia, anemia and reticulocytosis. Serum bilirubins in excess of 20 mg per 100 ml are not uncommon, and the hemoglobin may fall below 10 gm per

100 ml during the first week of life; values as low as 4 gm per 100 ml have been observed during the first three months of life. The reticulocyte count is above 5 per cent, and on occasion may exceed 50 per cent.

Examination of a peripheral blood smear will often reveal the presence of a small number of spherocytes, elongated oval forms, an occasional "tailed poikilocyte," and irregularly contracted cells, in addition to the macrocytosis, polychromasia and normoblastosis seen in any sever hemolytic process.

The diagnosis is made by demonstrating the enzyme deficiency by spectrophotometric assay[50]. If the infant has been transfused, the assay should be performed three to four months later, when relatively few transfused cells remain in the circulation. A presumptive diagnosis can be made by demonstrating the carrier state in the parents who are otherwise hematologically normal. The heterozygous state can be demonstrated by enzyme assay in approximately 90 per cent of carriers. A colorometric screening test has also been devised for the detection of the homozygous individuals. This test will also detect the heterozygous state in many instances[8].

A history of previously affected siblings may be present.

TREATMENT

Treatment in the newborn period is primarily directed at avoiding the neurologic complications of hyperbilirubinemia. This has been accomplished successfully by exchange transfusions. Hemoglobin values below 8 gm per 100 ml in the neonatal period may required packed cell transfusions if associated with failure to thrive or signs of circulatory failure.

Splenectomy does not "cure" these individuals as it does patients with hereditary spherocytosis. Although the anemia and reticulocytosis persists following operation, many children have benefited from this procedure by a decrease in their transfusion requirements. These infants should be transfused as often as it is clinically necessary to

TABLE IV PYRUVATE KINASE DEFICIENCY: SUMMARY OF CLINICAL AND LABORATORY FINDINGS IN TWENTY-THREE PATIENTS[4, 5, 9, 29, 38, 39, 50]*

Finding	Number of Patients
Intense jaundice in neonatal period	9/19
Hyperbilirubinemia requiring exchange transfusion	5
Jaundice noted at some time in life	21
Onset of anemia in infancy	18
Transfusions required other than at time of surgery	16
Splenomegaly	22
Splenectomy performed	14
Decreased transfusion requirements post-splenectomy	12/14
Anemia corrected post-splenectomy	0/14
Laboratory findings	
Hemoglobin (gm per 100 ml)	
4-8	9
8-11	5
11-14	1
14	1
Reticulocyte Count (per cent)	
0-5	0
5-10	5
10-20	10
20	6
Positive autohemolysis test	19/20
Partial correction with glucose	9/17

*Sex: 13 males; 29 females.

maintain relatively normal growth and activity until the age of one or two, when splenectomy may be considered. The disease is variable in its severity. Some patients may have no hematologic difficulties and will never require transfusions; therefore, it is necessary to follow these infants for some time after the neonatal period in order to determine the pattern of the disease before consideration is given to splenectomy.

DEFICIENCIES OF OTHER GLYCOLYTIC ENZYMES

2,3-Diphosphoglycerate mutase catalyzes the conversion of 1,3 diphosphoglycerate to 2,3-diphosphoglycerate (Fig. 1), and a deficiency of this enzyme has been found in association with the presence of a congenital non-spherocytic hemolytic anemia[4, 27]. The disease appears to be inherited as a Mendelian dominant and is characterized by variable degrees of anemia and reticulocytosis, intermittent jaundice and splenomegaly. The erythrocytes contain decreased quantities of 2,3-diphosphoglycerate and adenosine triphosphate associated with a slight decrease in the normal rate of glucose consumption. This deficiency state has manifested itself with jaundice in the neonatal period.

A deficiency of *triose phosphate isomerase*, another enzyme of the Embden-Meyerhof pathway, has recently been reported to be responsible for the production of a congenital non-spherocytic hemolytic anemia in two individuals[43, 46]. This deficiency, inherited as an autosomal recessive, has not as yet been reported as a cause of neonatal hyperbilirubinemia.

DEFICIENCIES OF NON-GLYCOLYTIC ENZYME AND OTHER SUBSTANCES

A *hereditary absence of glutathione* has been observed to result in a hemolytic anemia[37], although manifestations in the newborn period have not yet been described. Oort and associates[37] described a family in which four of twelve siblings suffered from a mild but well-compensated hemolytic anemia that was characterized by a virtual absence of reduced glutathione in the erythrocytes. Hemoglobins ranged from 12.5 to 14.0 gm per 100 ml, and reticulocytes from 2.9 to 5.0 per cent. Red cell reduced glutathione measured 3 to 5 mg per 100 ml of erythrocytes, as contrasted with a normal value greater than 60 mg. The cells from these patients were able to reduce oxidized glutathione normally. The basic defect in glutathione metabolism is as yet unexplained, but it appears to be either an impairment in *de novo* synthesis of this tripeptide or an inability to maintain normal amino acid exchange once the tripeptide is formed. Hereditary absence of glutathione is inherited as a recessive trait, the disease manifesting itself only in the homozygous state.

Harvald *et al.*[22] reported the finding of a deficiency of the magnesium-sodium-potassium-activated *adenosine triphosphatase* in the erythrocytes of two males with congenital non-spherocytic hemolytic anemias. In the family studies performed there was no apparent correlation between the levels of enzyme activity and the presence or absence of disease. Adenosine triphosphatase is believed to play a central role in cation transport in the erythrocytes. As yet, no studies have been reported on persons with adenosine triphosphatase deficiency to relate enzyme activity to potassium and sodium turnover in the red cell.

REFERENCES

1. Allen, D. W., and Jandl, J. H.: Oxidative hemolysis and precipitation of hemoglobin. II. Role of thiols in oxidant drug action. J. Clin. Invest., **40**:454, 1961.

2. Beutler, E., and Baluda, M. C.: The separation of glucose-6-phosphate dehydrogenase-deficient erythrocytes from the blood of heterozygotes for glucose-6-phosphate-dehydrogenase deficiency. Lancet, **1**:189, 1964.

3. Bishop, C.: Purine metabolism in human and chicken blood in vitro. J. Biol. Chem., **235**:3228, 1960.

4. Bowdler, A. J., and Prankerd, T. A. J.: Studies in congenital non-spherocytic haemolytic anaemias with specific enzyme defects. Acta Haemat. (Basel), **31**:65, 1964.

5. Bowman, H. S., and Procopir, F.: Hereditary non-spherocytic hemolytic anemia of pyruvate kinase deficient type. Ann. Intern. Med., **58**:567, 1963.

6. Brewer, G. J., Tarlov, A. R., and Alving, A. S.: Methemoglobin reduction test: A new simple, in vitro test for identifying primaquine sensitivity. Bull. W.H.O., **22**:633, 1960.

7. Brewer, G. J., Tarlov, A. R., and Kellermeyer, R. W.: The hemolytic effect of primaquine: XII. Shortened erythrocyte life span in primaquine sensitive male Negroes in the absence of drug administration. J. Lab. Clin. Med., **58**:217, 1961.

8. Brunetti, P., and Nenci, G.: A screening method for the detection of erythrocyte pyruvate kinase deficiency. Enzym. Biol. Clin. (Basel), **4**:51, 1964.

9. Brunetti, P. Puxeddu, A., Nenci, G., and Migliorini, E.: Congenital non-spherocytic haemolytic anaemia due to pyruvate-kinase deficiency. Acta Haemat. (Basel), **30**:88, 1963.

10. Capps, F. P. A., Gilles, H. M., Jolly, H., and Worlledge, S. M.: Glucose-6-phosphate dehydrogenase deficiency and neonatal jaundice in Nigeria. Lancet, **11**:379, 1963.

11. Carson, P. E., Flanagan, C. L., Ickes, C. E., and Alving, A. S.: Enzymatic deficiency in primaquine - sensitive erythrocytes. Science, **124**:484, 1956.

12. Cohen, G., and Hochstein, P.: Glucose-6-phosphate dehydrogenase and detoxification of hydrogen peroxide in human erythrocytes. Science, **134**:1756, 1961.

13. Committee on Nutrition, American Academy of Pediatrics: Vitamin K compounds and the water-soluble Analogues: Use in therapy and prophylaxis in pediatrics. Pediatrics, **28**:501, 1961.

14. Davidson, R. G., Nitowsky, H. M., and Childs, B.: Demonstration of two populations of cells in the human female heterozygous for glucose-6-phosphate variants. Proc. Nat. Acad. Sci. U.S.A., **50**:481, 1963.

15. Dern, R. J., Weinstein, I. M., LeRoy, G. V., Talmage, D. W., and Alving, A. S.: The hemolytic effect of primaquine. I. The localization of the drug induced hemolytic defect in primaquine sensitive individuals. J. Lab. Clin. Med., **43**:303, 1954.

16. Doxiadis, S. A., Fessas, P. H., Valaes, F., and Mastrokalos, N.: Glucose-6-phosphate dehydrogenase deficiency; A new aetiological factor of severe neonatal jaundice. Lancet, **1**:297, 1961.

16A Doxiadis, S. A., and Valaes, T.: The clinical picture of glucose-6-phosphate dehydrogenase deficiency in early infancy. Arch. Dis. Child., **39**:545, 1964.

17. Emanuel, B., and Schoenfeld, A.: Favism in a nursing infant. J. Pediat., **58**:263, 1961.

18. Fessas, Ph., Doxiadis, S. A., and Valaes, T.: Neonatal jaundice in glucose-6-phosphate dehydrogenase deficient infants. Brit. Med. J., **2**:1359, 1962.

19. Flatz, G., Sringam, S., and Komkris, V.: Neonatal jaundice in glucose-6-phosphate dehydrogenase deficiency. Lancet, **1**:1382, 1963.

20. Gaburro, D., Volpato, S., and Giaquinto, M.: Ictere nucleaire du nouveau-ne par defant de la G-6-PD. Sem. Hop Paris, Suppl. to Ann. Pediat., **37**:69, 1961.

21. Grossman, A., Ramanathan, K., Justice, P., Shahidi, N., and Hsia, D.: Congenital non-spherocytic hemolytic disease in Negroes associated with G-6-PD deficiency. Progr. Soc. Ped. Res., 78, 1965.

22. Harvald, B., Hanel, K. H., Squires, R., and Trap-Jensen, T.: Adenosine-triphosphatase deficiency in patients with non-spherocytic haemolytic anemia. Lancet, **2**:18, 1964.

23. Jaffe, E. R., and Gordon, E. E.: The incorporation of nicotinic acid and of nicotinamide into the pyridine nucleotides of erythrocytes and reticulocytes of rabbits in vitro. J. Clin. Invest., **42**:1017, 1963.

24. Jim, R. T. S., and Chu, F. K.: Hyperbilirubinemia due to glucose-6-phosphate dehydrogenase deficiency in a newborn Chinese infant. Pediatrics, **31**:1046, 1963.

25. Kellermeyer, R. W., Tarlov, A. R., Schrier, S. L., Carson, P. E., and Alving, A. S.: The hemolytic effect of primaquine. XIII. Gradient susceptibility to hemolysis of primaquine sensitive erythrocytes. J. Lab. Clin. Med., 58:225, 1961.

26. Le Fevre, P. G.: Sugar transport in the red blood cell: Activity relationships in substrates and antagonists. Pharmacol. Rev., 13:39, 1961.

27. Löhr, G. W., and Waller, H. D.: Zur Biochemie Einiger Angeborener Hämolytischer Anämien. Folia Haemat., 8:377, 1963.

28. Lyon, M. F.: Gene action in the x-chromosome of the mouse (Mus musculinus L.). Nature (London), 190:372, 1961.

29. Mallarme, J., and Boivin, P.: Nouvelles observations d'ectere hemolytique hereditaire non spherocytaire avec deficit in pyruvate-kinase. Proc. 9th Cong. Europ. Soc. Haemat., 787, 1963.

30. Marks, P. A., and Banks, J.: Drug induced hemolytic anemias associated with glucose-6-phosphate dehydrogenase deficiency: A genetically heterogenous trait. Ann. N.Y. Acad. Sci., 123:198, 1965.

31. Motulsky, A.: Pharmacogenetics. In Steinberg, A. G., and Bearn, A. G., (eds.): Progress in Medical Genetics, Vol. III. New York, Grune, 1964, p. 49.

32. Motulsky, A. G., and Campbell-Kraut, J. M.: Population genetics of glucose-6-phosphate dehydrogenase deficiency of the red cell. In Blumberg, B. S. (ed.): Proc. Conf. Genetic and Geographic Variations in Disease. New York, Grune, 1961, p. 159.

33. Murphy, J. R.: Erythrocyte metabolism. II. Glucose metabolism and pathways. J. Lab. Clin. Med., 55:286, 1960.

34. Naiman, J. L., and Kosoy, M. H.: Red cell glucose-6-phosphate dehydrogenase deficiency — A newly recognized cause of neonatal jaundice and kernicterus in Canada. Canad. Med. Ass. J., 91:1243, 1964.

35. Newton, W. A., Jr., and Bass, J. C.: Glutathione-sensitive chronic nonspherocytic hemolytic anemia. Arch. Dis. Child., 96:501, 1958.

36. O'Flynn, M. E. D., and Hsia, D. Y-Y.: Serum bilirubin levels and glucose-6-phosphate dehydrogenase deficiency in newborn American Negroes. J. Pediat., 63:160, 1963.

37. Oort, M., Loos, J. A., and Prins, H. K.: Hereditary absence of reduced glutathione in erythrocytes — A new clinical and biochemical entity. Vox. Sang., 6:370, 1961.

38. Oski, F. A., and Diamond, L. K.: Erythrocyte pyruvate kinase deficiency: Report of three cases. New Eng. J. Med., 269:763, 1963.

39. Oski, F. A., Nathan, D. G., Sidel, V. W., and Diamond, L. K.: Extreme hemolysis and red-cell distortion in erythrocyte pyruvate kinase deficiency. I. Morphology, erythrokinetics and family enzyme studies. New Eng. J. Med., 270:1023, 1964.

40. Panizon, F.: L'ictere grave du nouveau-ne associe a une deficience en glucose-6-phosphate dehydrogenase. Biol. Neonat., 2:167, 1960.

41. Schärer, K., Herzka, H., and Marti, H. R.: Kernicterus bei Mangee an Glukose-6-phosphat-Dehydrogenase Der Erythrocytes. Helv. Paediat. Acta, 18:148, 1962, 1963.

42. Scheuch, D., Kahrig, C., Ockel, E., Wagenknecht, C., and Rapoport, S. M.: Role of glutathione and of a self stabilizing chain of SH enzymes and substrates in the metabolic regulation of erythrocytes. Nature (London), 190:631, 1961.

43. Schneider, A. S., Valentine, W. N., Hattori, M., and Heins, H. L., Jr.: A new erythrocyte enzyme defect with hemolytic anemia—Triosephosphate isomerase (TPI) deficiency. New Eng. J. Med., 272:235, 1965.

44. Scott, E. M.: Relation of diaphorase of human erythrocytes to inheritance of methemoglobinemia. J. Clin. Invest., 39:1176, 1960.

45. Shahidi, N. T., and Diamond, L. K.: Enzyme deficiency in erythrocytes in congenital nonspherocytic hemolytic anemia. Pediatrics, 24:245, 1959.

46. Shore, M. A., Schneider, A. S., and Valentine, W. N.: Erythrocyte triosephosphate isomerase deficiency. Progr. Soc. Ped. Res., p. 23, 1965.

47. Smith, G. D., and Vella, F.: Erythrocyte enzyme deficiency in unexplained kernicterus. Lancet, 1:1133, 1960.

48. Szeinberg, A., and Marks, P. A.: Substances stimulating glucose catabolism by the oxidative reactions of the pentose phosphate pathway in human erythrocytes. J. Clin. Invest., 40:914, 1961.

49. Szeinberg, A., Oliver, M., Schmidt, R., Adam, A., and Sheba, Ch.: Glucose-6-phosphate dehydrogenase deficiency and hemolytic disease of the newborn in Israel. Arch. Dis. Child., 38:23, 1963.

50. Tanaka, K. R., Valentine, W. N., and Miwa, S.: Pyruvate kinase (PK) deficiency hereditary nonspherocytic hemolytic anemia. Blood, 19:267, 1962.

51. Tarlov, A. R., Brewer, G. J., Carson, P. G., and Alving, A. S.: Primaquine sensitivity. Arch. Intern. Med., 109:137, 1962.

52. Valentine, W. N., Tanaka, K. R., and Miwa, S.: Specific erythrocyte glycolytic enzyme defect (pyruvate kinase) in three subjects with congenital non-spherocytic hemolytic anemia. Trans. Ass. Amer. Physicians, **74**:100, 1961.

53. Weatherall, D. J.: Enzyme deficiency in haemolytic disease of the newborn. Lancet, **2**:835, 1960.

54. Zinkham, W. H.: Peripheral blood and bilirubin values in normal full-term primaquine sensitive Negro infants: Effects of vitamin K. Pediatrics, **31**:983, 1963.

55. Zinkham, W. H., and Childs, B.: A defect of glutathione metabolism in erythrocytes from patients with naphthalene-induced hemolytic anemia. Pediatrics, **22**:461, 1958.

Measurements of Erythrocyte Pyruvate Kinase and Glucose-6-Phosphate Dehydrogenase

FRANK A. OSKI, M.D.

Pyruvate Kinase

INTRODUCTION

Valentine, Tanaka and Miwa[1] were the first to demonstrate a deficiency of the glycolytic enzyme, pyruvate kinase, in the red cells of patients with a congenital non-spherocytic hemolytic anemia. Since their initial report, many other individuals with similar enzyme deficiency have been identified, and this intra-erythrocytic error of metabolism appears to be responsible for a large percentage of cases of non-spherocytic hemolytic anemia.

METHOD

The enzyme assay is dependent upon the conversion of phosphoenolpyruvate to pyruvate in the presence of adenosine diphosphate by the pyruvate kinase supplied in the hemolysate. The pyruvate formed during the reaction is converted to lactate in the presence of lactic dehydrogenase and DPNH. During this second step DPNH is converted to DPN, and this conversion is followed by measuring the change in absorbance at 340 mμ in a spectrophoto-

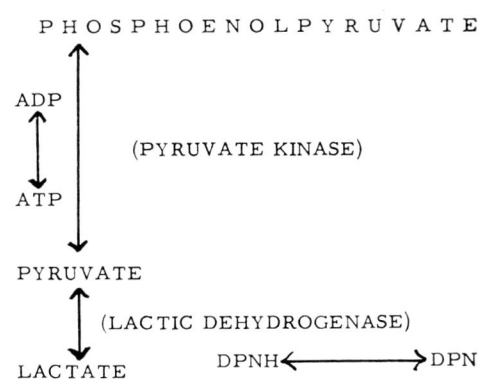

Fig. 1. Enzyme steps responsible for the conversion of phosphoenolpyruvate to lactate.

meter (Fig. 1). The procedure described below represents a slight modification of the method described by Tanaka, Valentine and Miwa[2] which was based on the method of Bücher and Pfleiderer[3].

REAGENTS

1. *Triethanolamino-HCl buffer*, 0.05 M, pH 7.5; trienthanolamine, 7.6 gm; 2N HCl, 15 ml; disodium EDTA, 2.0 gm; distilled water to 1,000 ml.

2. *Potassium chloride*, 2.25 M: KCl, 16.7 gm; distilled water to 100 ml.

3. *Magnesium sulfate*, 0.24 M; anhydrous $MgSo_4$, 2.9 gm; distilled water to 100 ml.

4. *Adenosine diphosphate*, 0.006 M: ADP (monosodium salt · 3 H_2O, Sigma) −3.02 mg per ml. Usually prepared in 10 ml quantities and dispensed in 0.5 ml aliquots for freezing.

5. *Lactic dehydrogenase* (rabbit muscle, Sigma Type II), prepared liquid. Store at 4 C. Just prior to use, 0.05 ml of LDH is diluted to 1.0 ml in distilled water so that 0.1 ml of solution will contain approximately 1,000 Bucher units.

6. *Diphosphopyridine nucleotide*, reduced (DPHN, Sigma). Just prior to use, 2 ml of TEA-HCl buffer is added to a pre-weighed vial containing 2 mg DPNH.

7. *Phosphoenolpyruvic acid*, 0.045 M: PEP, crystalline; trisodium salt (Sigma), 14.6 mg per ml of distilled water. Generally prepared in 5 ml quantities and stored frozen in 0.3 ml aliquots.

SPECIAL APPARATUS

1. *Refrigerated centrifuge.*
2. *Spectrophotometer, Beckman DU.*

PROCEDURE

1. Preparation of Hemolysate

Four to five ml of heparinized blood are centrifuged in the cold at 700 rpm for fifteen minutes to separate the red cells from the white cell and platelet rich plasma. After initial centrifugation, the red cells are washed in an equal volume of cold isotonic saline solution and then centrifuged again at 2,000 rpm. Any buffy coat is aspirated along with supernatant, and cells are washed twice more.

Following the third washing, a red cell count and white cell count are performed on this saline suspension. The white cell count should be less than 1,000 per cu mm because higher white cell counts will contribute significant pyruvate kinase activity and invalidate red cell determinations. The red cell count of the suspension should be between three and five million per cu mm.

The hemolysate is prepared by adding 0.1 ml of the red cell suspension to a solution containing 0.8 ml of TEA-HCl buffer and 1.6 ml of distilled water. The mixture is well shaken, allowed to stand for five minutes in the cold to ensure complete hemolysis and then centrifuged in the cold at 4,000 rpm for ten minutes to remove the stroma. After centrifugation the supernatant should be completely clear.

2. Assay Procedure

To each silica cuvette is added the following:

Reagent	Blank	Un-known	Final Concentration
TEA-HCl buffer	0.5	0.5	8.3×10^{-3} M
Distilled water	1.5	1.4	
2.25 M KCl	0.1	0.1	7.5×10^{-2} M
0.24 M $MgSO_4$	0.1	0.1	8.0×10^{-3} M
0.006 M ADP	0.2	0.2	4.0×10^{-4} M
Lactic dehydrogenase	0.1	0.1	1,000 Bucher units
DPNH	0.4	0.1	2.0×10^{-4} M
Hemolysate	−	0.1	
0.045 M PEP	0.1	0.1	

The reaction is initiated by adding the substrate phosphoenolpyruvate

(PEP), and the $O.D._{340}$ is recorded every two minutes for fourteen minutes. The change is linear between four and and fourteen minutes, and therefore this period is used for calculation purposes. The PEP is added at twenty- to thirty-second intervals to each of the cuvettes to allow each to be read at two-minute intervals and to allow time for any necessary blank adjustments. As DPNH is converted to DPN there will be a drop in the O.D. readings.

DISCUSSION

Values are expressed in terms of micromoles of DPNH reduced to DPN per 10^{10} RBC's per minute, under the conditions of the assay. The molar extinction coefficient of DPNH is 6.3×10^{-6}.

SOURCES OF ERROR

A false high value for pyruvate kinase activity will be obtained if significant white cell contamination is introduced into the hemolysate, because white cells contain approximately 300 times the activity of red cells and are not deficient of activity in patients with red cell deficiencies[2].

Pyruvate kinase activity may also be expressed in terms of 100 ml RBC's employing the hematocrit of the red cell suspension instead of the red count. In conditions associated with micro- cytosis, false high values will be obtained for red cell activity because more cells are introduced per volume of hemolysate than would occur in a normal individual.

False low values for activity may be obtained if the whole blood is left to stand too long before assay. Hepa- rinized blood, if refrigerated, loses negligible activity during the first twenty-four hours but begins to decline in activity between twenty-four and forty-eight hours, so should be assayed within two days of collection. If a specimen has been shipped in the mail, a control tube from a normal individual should always accompany it in order to detect possible deterioration.

False low values may also be

$$\text{Pyruvate Kinase activity (units)} = \frac{\text{O.D. per min}}{6.3} \times \frac{10^{10} \text{ RBC}}{\text{RBC per mm}^3 \times 100 \times 1/25} \times 3$$

The red count is multiplied by 100 because 0.1 ml of red cells were initially added to make the hemolysate; this is multiplied by 1/25th to account for the dilution employed before the 0.1 ml of hemolysate was used in the assay. The denominator may thus be simplified to read RBC per cu mm x 4. The entire value is multiplied by three because the final reaction volume is 3 ml and thus represents the total amount of DPNH reduced to DPN in the cuvette. The final equation may be simplified to read:

$$\frac{\text{O.D. per min}}{2.1} \times \frac{10^{10} \text{ RBC}}{\text{RBC per mm}^3 \times 4} \text{ (units)}$$

obtained if the substrates and enzymes are repeatedly thawed and refrozen or kept in storage for periods in excess of three to six months. To avoid the hazards of repeated freezing and thawing, it is recommended that these solutions be stored in aliquots that are sufficient for the performance of one or two assays.

RANGE OF VALUES

In our laboratory the normal range of values for red cell pyruvate kinase activity is 1.25 to 2.1 units per 10^{10} RBC's. Patients with the enzyme deficiency usually have values below 0.5 units of activity. The heterozygous carrier generally has red cell values between 0.6 and 1.0 units, although not in all instances is the heterozygous state detectable. Higher-than-normal adult values are seen in the newborn infant and in normal individuals with a young red cell population.

RÉSUMÉ OF CLINICAL INTERPRETATIONS

Assay of red cell pyruvate kinase activity is an essential part of the diagnostic work-up of an individual with a congenital non-spherocytic hemolytic anemia. Pyruvate kinase deficiency is inherited as an autosomal recessive disorder. Clinical manifestations are only present in the homozygous individual. These individuals generally have a history of anemia since early childhood with recurrent episodes of jaundice. Severe jaundice may be present in the newborn period and require treatment by exchange transfusion in order to avoid kernicterus. Red cell enzyme assay can only be interpreted with confidence when it is certain that a significant portion of the red cells studied are the patients and not from the donor of a recent blood transfusion.

REFERENCES

1. Valentine, W. N., Tanaka, K. R., and Miwa, S.: A specific erythrocyte enzyme defect (pyruvate kinase) in three subjects with congenital nonspherocytic hemolytic anemia. 75th Annual Meeting of the Association of American Physicians, Atlantic City, N. J., May 2, 1961, paper No. 4, Trans. Ass. Amer. Physicians, 74:100, 1961.
2. Tanaka, K. R., Valentine, W. N., and Miwa, S.: Pyruvate kinase (PK) deficiency hereditary nonspherocytic hemolytic anemia. Blood, 19:267-295, 1962.
3. Bucher, T., and Pfleider, G.: Pyruvate kinase from muscle. In Colowick, S. P., and Kaplan, N. O. (eds.): Methods in Enzymology, Vol. 1. New York, Academic Press, 1955, p. 435.

Glucose-6-Phosphate Dehydrogenase

INTRODUCTION

Glucose-6-phosphate dehydrogenase (G-6-PD) was first isolated from erythrocytes by Warburg and Christian in 1931[1]. In 1956, Carson and associates found this enzyme to be deficient in the red cells of individuals with primaquine-induced hemolytic anemias. It is now recognized that many other drugs will also precipitate a hemolytic episode in these individuals. Red cell G-6-PD deficiency is also a cause of one form of congenital non-spherocytic hemolytic anemia.

METHOD
G-6-PD catalyses the reaction:

$$\text{Glucose-6-phosphate} + \text{TPN}^+ \rightarrow \text{6-phosphogluconate TPNH} + \text{H}^+$$

The rate of formation of TPNH is a measure of the enzyme activity, and it can be followed by means of the increase in absorption at 340 mμ. One convenient method of red cell assay has been described by Zinkham[2].

Reagents

1. *Tris buffer*, 0.19 M, pH 8.0: Tris, 2.30 gm; distilled water to 90 ml. The pH is adjusted to pH 8.0 with 1 N HCl and then the final volume is brought to 100 ml.

2. *Magnesium chloride*, 0.3 M: MgCl$_2$ · 6 H$_2$O, 3.05 gm; distilled water, 50 ml.

3. *Glucose-6-phosphate solution*, 0.02 M: Dipotassium glucose-6-phosphate 3 H$_2$O (Sigma), 39 mg, is dissolved in 5 ml distilled water and divided into 0.3 ml aliquots and frozen in small tubes.

4. *Triphosphopyridine solution*, 0.002 M: TPN monosodium salt · 3 H$_2$O (Sigma), 16.4 mg, is dissolved in 10 ml distilled water and divided into 0.5 ml aliquots and frozen in small tubes.

(Note: G-6-PD and TPN are stable in the frozen state for periods up to 3 months. Each aliquot provides enough reagent to perform 2 enzyme assays.)

Special Apparatus

1. *Refrigerated centrifuge.*
2. *Spectrophotometer.*

Procedure

1. Preparation of Hemolysate

Whole blood, 4 to 5 ml is collected in heparin, and the red cells are separated and washed in the same manner as described for the pyruvate kinase assay. A hematocrit determination is performed on the well-mixed red cell suspension and then 0.1 ml of red cells are added to 1.9 ml of distilled water. The tube is well mixed, allowed to stand for five minutes in the cold, and then centrifuged at 4,000 rpm in the cold for ten minutes to remove the stroma. The supernatant should be completely clear.

2. Assay

Into two silica cuvettes pipette the following:

	Blank	Unknown
Tris buffer	1.0	1.0
MgCl$_2$	0.1	0.1
Distilled water	1.8	1.5
G-6-P	–	0.1
Hemolysate	0.1	0.1
TPN	–	0.2

The blank cuvette is set at 0 density at 340 mμ. The reaction is iniated by the addition of TPN to the unknown cuvette and the timer is started. Readings are made every two minutes for twelve minutes.

Discussion

Enzyme activity is calculated as follows:

G-6-PD activity, units per 100 ml of erythrocytes =

$$\frac{\text{O.D. change per minute}}{6.22} \times 20 \, (\text{dilution}) \times \frac{100}{\text{hematocrit}} \times 1{,}000 \times 3$$

or, simplified =

$$\frac{\text{O.D. per minute}}{2.07} \times 20 \times \frac{100}{\text{hematocrit}} \times 1{,}000$$

One unit of G-6-PD activity is defined as that amount which will produce an optical density change of 2.07 per minute in a 3.0 ml reaction mixture.

SOURCES OF ERROR

Less than normal activity will be obtained if the blood samples are not kept refrigerated prior to assay or if the TPN and G-6-PD solutions are repeatedly frozen and thawed. Heparinized whole blood if refrigerated loses no appreciable activity for periods up to twenty-four to forty-eight hours.

When using the hematocrit for purposes of calculation, higher-than-normal values will be obtained in patients with microcytosis because more red cells are introduced per unit of red cell suspension. Spuriously high values may also be obtained if signficant white cell and platelet contamination of the sample occurs.

RANGE OF VALUES

Normal range: 175 to 240 units.

The Negro deficients generally demonstrate enzyme values 10 to 15 per cent of normal while Caucasion deficients range from 0 to 10 per cent of normal. There is considerable variation in the level of enzyme activity in affected heterozygotes and a certain number of heterozygotes, documented by family studies, have red cell G-6-PD levels which fall within the range of normal.

RÉSUMÉ OF CLINICAL INTERPRETATIONS

Although under normal circumstances, the detection of the deficient individual presents no difficulties, there are occasions when the results of enzyme assay may prove misleading. This most frequently occurs just after a hemolytic episode when the oldest, most deficient red cells have been removed from the circulation and have been replaced with young erythrocytes which are high in enzyme activity. Under these conditions a deficient individual may show enzyme values in the near normal or low normal range. Because of this possibility, a reticulocyte count should be obtained. Normally with reticulocytosis, supernormal enzyme values are observed and, if in the presence of an increased number of reticulocytes, low normal values are found, a diagnosis of G-6-PD deficiency can be strongly suspected. The diagnosis can be confirmed at a later date when the mean age of the red cell population has increased.

In patients with the congenital non-spherocytic hemolytic anemia form of G-6-PD deficiency, a disease almost exclusively of Caucasians, low values for G-6-PD activity are found despite the presence of reticulocytosis.

G-6-PD values of 50 to 80 per cent of normal may be observed in hypothyroidism and values well above normal may be seen in hyperthyroidism. Values return to normal when the patient becomes euthyroid.

REFERENCES

1. Warburg, O., and Christian, W.: Uber aktivierung der robisonchen hexose-mono-phosphursaure in roten blutzellen und die gewinnung aktivierender fermentlosungen.

Biochem. Z., **242**:206-227, 1931.

2. Zinkham, W. H.: An in-vitro abnormality of glutathione metabolism in erythrocytes from normal newborns. Mechanism and clinical significance. Pediatrics, **23**:18-32, 1959.

Chapter 4

Inherited Deficiencies in Serum Enzymes

JOHN PAUL KALTENBACH, Ph.D., GERALD S. DEAN, M.D., AND
GERALD HOFFMAN, M.D.

There are two well-documented inherited deficiencies of serum enzymes: *hypophosphatasia,* which is characterized by a deficiency of serum alkaline phosphatase; and *deficiency of serum cholinesterase,* which becomes apparent when an individual receives certain anticholinesterase-types of anesthesia.

In 1952, Lehman and co-workers in London[2, 3] observed low cholinesterase activity in patients who had remained paralyzed much longer than expected after receiving the muscle relaxant, succinyldicholine. It was proposed that this condition was not due to a disease state but to an inherited factor[11]. Studies by Kalow[7, 10] in Toronto suggested that the hereditary change was an alteration of the enzyme (a qualitative change). More recently, Wetstone and co-workers[15] have presented evidence indicating that there is genetic control over the quantitative activity of this enzyme. The possibility that both a qualitative and quantitative regulation of cholinesterase may be in effect has not been ruled out.

Low levels of serum cholinesterase apparently have no deleterious effect in an otherwise normal individual. However, when such an individual is given a short duration-type muscle relaxant, such as succinyldicholine, apnea results because the succinyldicholine is not hydrolyzed.

Cholinesterase of the serum is known by a number of synonyms: e.g., serum cholinesterase; pseudocholinesterase; nonspecific cholinesterase; s-type cholinesterase; and butyrylcholinesterase. Cholinesterase will hydrolyze a number of ester-type substrates, although butyryl-choline is hydrolyzed most rapidly — much more so than acetylcholine[16]. Serum cholinesterase levels at birth are low, but gradually increase to adult levels at puberty. With advancing age, the concentrations of cholinesterase decrease again. The enzyme levels are lower in females than in males, and seem to be correlated with the body weight and amount of subcutaneous fat. Disease conditions such as nephrosis result in elevated levels of cholinesterase, whereas liver cell damage and malnutrition result in lowered levels.

Atypical cholinesterase is the general term applied to the serum cholinesterase of individuals sensitive to compounds such as succinyldicholine. Comparison of normal cholinesterase *versus* atypical cholinesterase has shown that the latter has not only a lower enzymatic rate of ester hydrolysis but a reduced affinity for substrate[8]. A common test[9] for atypical cholinesterase is to measure the hydrolysis of benzylcholine in the absence and in the presence of an inhibitor (dibucaine). The per cent inhibition is termed the dibucaine number (DN). Individuals usually fall in one of three groups according to their plasma DN. Normal values range close to DN 80; a DN below 70 is considered abnormal. A second group includes those individuals whose DN ranges around 60. A third group includes individuals with DN values under 55, ranging around 16. An explanation for these three groupings is that there are at least two cholinesterases in plasma. Thus, individuals with a DN of about 60 have a mixture of low and high activity cholinesterases and are heterozygotes for this abnormality. Persons with low DN would be homozygotes, having only the cholinesterase of low activity. The incidence of homozygotes is about 1 in 5000 persons[6].

Other methods of testing for atypical plasma cholinesterase have applied a succinylcholine number[13] or fluoride number[5]. The latter has indicated the existence of a third type of cholinesterase.

Clinically, succinyldicholine is used in anesthesiology and psychiatry. In anesthesiology, the danger of prolonged apnea may be mitigated by the use of proper artificial respiration equipment. However, this danger may not always be obvious in long operations where the patient is given additional relaxing drugs after the intubation, or where succinyldicholine is given by continuous infusion. Of greater danger is the use of succinyldicholine as a short duration muscle relaxant during electric shock treatment in the absence of adequate facilities for artificial respiration.

Individuals with atypical plasma cholinesterase may also have an altered response to such toxic compounds as the organophosphate insecticides. The atypical cholinesterase has less affinity for such esters than does normal cholinesterase, and more of the toxic material may reach the motor end plates where it will block acetylcholinesterase.

Hypophosphatasia is a rare disease which has three primary characteristics. The first, and thus its name, is a very low level of alkaline phosphatase activity. It has yet to be proved whether or not the low phosphatase activity is due to less enzyme present than normal or to an inhibitor in the serum and tissues, although mixing serum from patients with hypophosphatasia with that of normal serum has not demonstrated a nonspecific type of inhibitor. Secondly, there is an increased urinary excretion of phosphoethanolamine, presumably because the alkaline phosphatase that is present (quantitatively or qualitatively) can not hydrolyze this compound at a fast enough rate. Thirdly, there are abnormal changes in bone formation: deficient calcification; excess osteoid tissue; and irregularity of endochondral ossification[6]. The possibility that adenosine monophosphate may also be a urinary excretion product has been indicated by McCance and co-workers[12].

Fraser[4] calculates from his studies in Toronto that the incidence in that area over a ten-year period was about 1:100,-000 live births. He places hypophosphatasia patients in three groups. Group I are infants in whom bony abnormalities were present within the first six months of life. Actually, in some cases, bone lesions are present before birth[6, 12]. Group II are children in whom lesions first become apparent after six months. The severity of the disease in this group is less, although growth retardation, bone deformities and dental changes may be seen. Group III are persons in whom hypophosphatasia was first diagnosed in adult life. The symptoms found in four patients described by Fraser[4] included fragility of the long bones, mild osteoporosis, below-average height in two of the patients and low serum alkaline phosphatase.

Although low serum alkaline phosphatase is a primary characteristic of hypophosphatasia, it in itself is probably a secondary defect. The genetic lesion is probably manifest in the skeletal tissue, especially the osteoblasts[4]. Although normal in number, there is evidence that indicates that these foci, which are considered to be the main source of bone phosphatase[1], are very low in phosphatase activity in hypophosphatasia[6, 14].

From this brief discussion of the two examples of hereditary defects, it becomes apparent that the inheritance of an abnormality or disease condition is at once a mystery and a complex problem. Inherited characteristics are influenced not only by the genetic apparatus, as such, but probably also by survivors of environmental factors of many years past, e.g., great epidemics, geographic environment, nutrition, etc. It may be assumed that, for an inherited condition to occur or develop, a biochemical reaction initiated a change in the genetic mechanism. Thus, the lack of a normally occurring enzyme, or any other hereditary disorder, was probably a result of a very early change in the genetic apparatus, such as false coding in the macromolecules (DNA).

This discussion has been limited to two commonly known inherited deficiencies of serum enzymes. Enzymes affected by organ systems are discussed elsewhere in this book. There are probably other serum enzymes (lactic dehydrogenase, transaminases, etc.) whose high or low normal values may be due to hereditary factors. This would lend further evidence that the quantitative activities of enzymes are also genetically controlled. Whether or not this has an influence on our health or general function is not definitely known.

REFERENCES

1. Bourne, G. H.: The Biochemistry and Physiology of Bone. New York, Academic Press, 1956, p. 258.
2. Evans, F. T., Gray, W. S., Lehmann, H., and Silk, E.: Sensitivity to succinylcholine in relation to serum-cholinesterase. Lancet, 1: 1229-1230, 1952.
3. ———: Effect of pseudo-cholinesterase level on action of succinylcholine in man. Brit. Med. J., 1:136-138, 1953.
4. Fraser, D.: Hypophosphatasia. Amer. J. Med., 22:730-746, 1957.
5. Harris, H., and Whittaker, M.: Differential inhibition of human serum cholinesterase with fluoride: Recognition of two new phenotypes. Nature (London), 191:496-498, 1961.
6. Hsia, D. Y.: Inborn Errors of Metabolism. Chicago, Year Book Publishers, 1960, pp. 192-195.
7. Kalow, W.: Familial incidence of low pseudo-cholinesterase level. Lancet, 2:576-577, 1956.
8. Kalow, W.: Pharmacogenetics, Heredity and the Response to Drugs. Philadelphia, Saunders, 1962, pp. 69-92.
9. Kalow, W., and Genest, K.: A method for the detection of atypical forms of human serum cholinesterase. Determination of dibucaine numbers. Canad. J. Biochem. Physiol., 35:339-346, 1957.

10. Kalow, W., and Staron, N.: On distribution and inheritance of atypical forms of human serum cholinesterase as indicated by dibucaine numbers. Canad. J. Biochem. Physiol., **35:** 1305-1320, 1957.

11. Lehman, H., and Ryan, E.: The familial incidence of low pseudo-cholinesterase level. Lancet, **2:**124, 1956.

12. McCance, R. A., Fairweather, D. V. I., Barrett, A. M., and Morrison, A. B.: Genetic, clinical, biochemical and pathological features of hypophosphatasia. Quart. J. Med., **25:**523-537, 1956.

13. McComb, R. B., La Motta, R. V., and Wet- stone, H. J.: Succinylcholine number: New method for detecting atypical serum cho- linesterase. Fed. Proc., **23:**280, 1964.

14. Scaglione, P. R., and Lucey, J. F.: Further observations on hypophosphatasia. Amer. J. Dis. Child., **92:**493-495, 1956.

15. Wetstone, H. J., Honeyman, M. S., and McComb, R. B.: Genetic control of the quantitative activity of a serum enzyme in man. JAMA,**192:**165-167, 1965.

16. Whittaker, V. P.: Specificity, mode of action and distribution of cholinesterases. Physiol. Rev., **31:**312-343, 1951.

Chapter 5

Diagnosis of the Inheritable Lipidoses Seen in Infancy

DONALD S. FREDRICKSON, M.D.

Abnormal concentrations of lipids in tissues or extracellular fluid are primary manifestations of more than a dozen different mutations in man. Many of these so-called *lipidoses* are phenotypically distinguishable in infancy. Although satisfactory treatment is available for only one or two of them, their proper recognition is not merely an academic exercise. Apart from the necessity of eliminating other treatable illnesses, there remains for parents of such affected children much anxiety that can be relieved and many questions in eugenics that can be answered only when a certain diagnosis has been obtained.

This desirable objective may be missed, occasionally by a wide margin, through the influence of several rather widely held misconceptions. The first is the belief that a particular lipid can be positively identified in tissue sections by histochemical methods. In reality, the many available dyes or stains can be very helpful in indicating the presence or absence of representatives of a class of lipids, but the specificity required to distinguish one lipidosis from all others is rarely obtainable by such techniques. Likewise, except for "Gaucher cells" and certain major dif-

ferences among the leukodystrophies and between them and the other sphingolipidoses, there are few morphologic changes in either brain or viscera that positively establish the diagnosis of a given lipidosis.

Firm diagnosis of the lipidoses requires the application of certain chemical and biochemical analyses. New techniques are constantly appearing that are steadily increasing the possibility of ante-mortem diagnosis and sharpening the recognition of heterogeneity in established syndromes. The inheritable biochemical lesions themselves are becoming more accessible through development of better understanding of the relevant metabolic pathways.

The accelerated development of new methods increases the gravity of another common error. This is the failure to preserve properly tissues that are sometimes irreplaceable and often obtained with pain and peril for the patient. Generally this means preservation by freezing tissues. *Particularly it means avoiding the committal of the whole of any sample to formalin or similar solvents that destroy enzymes and other proteins and leach out certain of the lipids.* The seriousness of this cannot be overemphasized, for disregard of

TABLE I LIPIDOSES OFTEN EXPRESSED IN THE FIRST YEAR OF LIFE

Disease	Neurological Abnormalities	Hepatosplenomegaly	Marrow "Foam Cells"	Skin Lesions	Plasma Lipid Abnormalities	Special Features	Usual Requirements for Positive Diagnosis
Type I hyperlipoproteinemia (hyperchylomicronemia)[18]	0	+	+	Eruptive xanthomas	TG↑ C↑	recurrent abdominal pain; lipemia retinalis	1. demonstration of chylomicron excess on any level of dietary fat intake, and 2. decreased plasma post-heparin lipolytic activity[20]
Type II hyperlipoproteinemia (hyperbetalipoproteinemia)[18]	0	0	0	tendon and tuberous xanthomas	C↑ TG N	atherosclerosis; arcus corneae	Specific increase in plasma beta lipoproteins (S_f0-20) in patient and at least one parent
Abetalipoproteinemia[13]	0, +	0	0	0	C↓ TG↓	acanthocytosis; retinitis pigmentosa	Absence of beta lipoproteins (by immunochemical analysis)
Tangier disease (deficient alpha lipoprotein)[16]	0	+, 0	+	+, 0	C↓ TG N	enlarged, orange-yellow tonsils	1. near absence of alpha lipoproteins, and 2. cholesterol ester storage in RE tissues
Tay-Sachs disease (accumulation in neurons of monosialylotrihexoso-ganglioside)[19]	+	0	0	0	0 / 0	hyperacusis; cherry-red spot; plasma F-1, 6P aldolase deficient[2]; normal spinal fluid protein	accumulation in brain of specific "Gₒ" or "Gm2" ganglioside[28,43] (usually only possible post mortem)
Generalized gangliosidosis (accumulation of monosialo-tetrahexosoganglioside)[25,29,37,38]	+	+	+	0	0	cherry-red spot ±; vacuolations in WBC; Alder-Reilly bodies in WBC; skeletal x-ray changes (similar to Hurler's syndrome)	accumulation of gangliosides in viscera and brain
Gaucher's disease (accumulation of glucocerebrosides in viscera and brain)[15]	+ (nearly all infantile cases)	+	+	0	inconsistent	hyperacidphosphatasia	1. clear-cut identification of Gaucher cells usually adequate; 2. positive identification of glucocerebrosides in tissues for confirmation
Niemann-Pick disease (accumulation of sphingomyelin and cholesterol)[17]	+ (usually)	+	+	rare xanthomas	inconsistent	cherry-red spot ±; vacuolated WBC	increased tissue sphingomyelin

Disease	C	TG			Consider in Differential Diagnosis		
Wolman's disease (accumulation of cholesterol and glycerides)[9]	+	+	+	?	0	adrenal calcification	normal phospholipid pattern; sterol excess in tissues
Hurler's syndrome (chondroitin sulfuric acid B and heparin monosulfuric acid accumulation; two clinical forms)[12]	+	+	+	inconsistent	whitish nodules	facial, ocular and skeletal abnormalities; deafness and cardiovascular disease; Alder-Reilly bodies in WBC's	acid mucopolysaccharide excretion in urine, coupled with clinical picture
Krabbe's disease (a leukodystrophy)[18]	+	0	0	0	0	high CSF protein	morphological ascertainment
Pelizaeus-Merzbacher disease (a leukodystrophy)[18]	+	0	0	0	0	males only; early cerebellar signs; normal CSF protein	morphological ascertainment

C: cholesterol; TG: triglyceride; N: normal; ↑: increased; ↓: decreased; 0: absent.

this principle may be considered of medicolegal importance at some not-too-distant time. Precise recommendations for handling biopsies will be taken up below.

THE INFANTILE LIPIDOSES

The lipidoses that may appear between birth and age one are listed in Table I. Certain omissions from this table deserve comment. Missing are several well-known diseases accepted as lipidoses that do not — or, more accurately, have not yet been noted to — have detectable manifestations before the affected child is more than a year old. Among these diseases are metachromatic leukodystrophy (cerebroside sulfatide storage)[36], Fabry's disease or angiokeratoma corporis diffusum (ceramide trihexoside storage)[46], Refsum's syndrome or heredopathia atactica polyneuritiformis (phytanic acid storage)[27, 40], and several types (III, IV, V) of familial hyperlipoproteinemia[18]. Also not included are familial disorders that resemble lipidoses but whose metabolic derangements actually involve non-lipid substances, such as Farber's lipogranulomatosis[1], or certain xanthomatous disorders that are not familial and apparently not due to primary abnormalities in lipid metabolism, as, for example, the histiocytoses like eosinophilic granuloma.

Present in Table I, because they especially need to be considered in differential diagnosis, are three diseases or syndromes that are either clearly not lipidoses or at least not generally accepted as such. Hurler's syndrome is a disorder of mucopolysaccharide metabolism. Pelizaeus-Merzbacher disease and Krabbe's disease (or globoid-cell type leukodystrophy)[48] are two kinds of leukodystrophy that begin to show signs in infancy. In neither disease is there definite lipid accumulation, and neither has been shown to be due to an inherited defect in metabolism of a lipid; but they occur frequently enough to require consideration in diagnosis of the neuro-lipidoses.

COMMON MANIFESTATIONS

The infantile lipidoses nearly always come initially to the attention of a physician because one or more of several general manifestations are present. These are: (a) neurological abnormalities, varying from a simple "failure to thrive" to specific and severe deficits; (b) enlarged liver or spleen, usually both; (c) plasma lipid or lipoprotein abnormalities, usually lactescence (hyperglyceridemia), or sometimes high or low cholesterol concentrations; and (d) skin lesions, such as xanthomas. Sometimes all of these manifestations occur in one disease, and several are shared by many others. It will also be noted (Table I) that both vacuoles and inclusions (Alder-Reilly bodies) in the leucocytes may be observed in the peripheral blood smear in several of the diseases under consideration. They do not form a reliable basis for diagnosis.

Following the routine clinical assessment and careful exploration of the family history, one can usually separate the patients into one of two groups: that in which a plasma lipoprotein abnormality (dyslipoproteinemia) or that in which tissue lipid storage seems paramount. The discussion will now follow this major division. One should keep in mind that some of the diagnostic procedures described below, especially the qualitative analysis of plasma lipoproteins and a bone marrow aspiration, may still be useful in most patients in either group.

LIPOPROTEIN ANALYSES

Four of the diseases with which we are concerned may be called primary dyslipoproteinemias. Two are characterized by extreme elevations in concentrations of certain lipoproteins and two by the absence or near absence of different lipoproteins. Under appropriate conditions these diseases can usually be identified in a preliminary way by the modification of paper electrophoresis introduced by Lees and Hatch[22, 32] in which albumin is added to the buffer. Both paper electrophoresis and immunochemical methods are of particular value in studying infants, for diagnoses can often be firmly established using less than 0.5 ml of plasma.

The application of electrophoresis for phenotyping familial hyperlipoproteinemia has been described in detail elsewhere[18]. Five different basic lipoprotein patterns have been used to classify different syndromes. Such syndromes have not yet been shown to be specific for a single genotype, and likely they will prove to be more heterogenous. They have therefore been designated as Types I through V, nomeclature bridging the transition between older names that have lost their specificity and new terminology that will develop as the basic biochemical defects are illuminated.

SAMPLING

Both the nutritional state and manner of sample collection influence plasma lipoprotein patterns. Samples should be obtained at the maximum post-absorptive interval possible with the infant (up to 12 to 16 hours after the last feeding) and while the diet of the preceding week has been as near normal as possible. The ideal conditions also include use of 1 mg of EDTA (disodium ethylenediaminetetracetic acid) per 1 ml of blood as anticoagulant, and centrifugation and subsequent storage and shipment of the plasma at 2 to 4°. In serum obtained by allowing the clot to retract at room temperature, some lipoproteins undergo transformations that appear on immunoelectrophoresis and decrease the sharpness of the lipoprotein bands obtained by paper electrophoresis.

ELECTROPHORESIS

Electrophoresis is performed basically as described elsewhere[22] with certain modifications.

Twenty to 40 μl of plasma are loaded on pre-cut Whatman No. 1 paper in a Durrum hanging-strip cell (Beckman Instruments Corp., Palo Alto, California) and electrophoresed at room temperature for sixteen hours at 120 volts and about 7/8 ma per strip. Barbital buffer of ionic strength 0.1 pH 8.6 containing 0.001 M EDTA and 1 per cent human albumin is employed. After electrophoresis, the strips are oven dried at 100 to 110°C for one half hour, then immediately hung in a saturated solution of oil-Red-0 (National Aniline Division, Allied Chemical Co.) in 60 per cent ethanol in a vessel containing excess solid dye at the bottom to maintain saturation. They are stained for eight hours, then washed for a few minutes in running tap water and air-dried.

Plasma from a normal child should contain a sharp β-lipoprotein band and a broader α-lipoprotein band on paper electrophoresis (Fig. 1). If the sample has been obtained up to six hours after the last feeding, a small chylomicron band may be seen at the origin. A faint pre-β-lipoprotein band may also be normal. (Experience with postprandial samples from infants using the albumin-veronal buffer has not been sufficient to determine precisely what the normal pattern should be at all intervals after feeding and at each age.)

FAMILIAL HYPERLIPOPROTEINEMIA

TYPE I

There are few diseases associated with hyperlipemia (lactescent plasma due to hyperglyceridemia) in infancy. Only "idiopathic hyperlipemia"[23], or what the author and his colleagues have called Type I familial hyperlipoproteinemia[18], is a familial lipidosis in the definition employed here. The excess glycerides in plasma are overwhelmingly of exogenous (dietary) origin and are retained in large particles called chylomicrons. Thus, the presence of a lipoprotein pattern completely dominated by a chylomicron band (Figs. 1, 2) is enough for a preliminary diagnosis of this rare "fat-induced" hyperlipemia if the clinical manifestations are otherwise consistent. The swift disappearance of the chylomicron band within three to four days after fat has been withdrawn from the diet provides further support (Fig. 2) and confirmation is obtained by demonstration of low plasma post-heparin lipolytic activity (see below).

There are other means of establishing whether or not hyperlipemia is primarily due to chylomicrons. (a) A marked disproportion between the elevations in

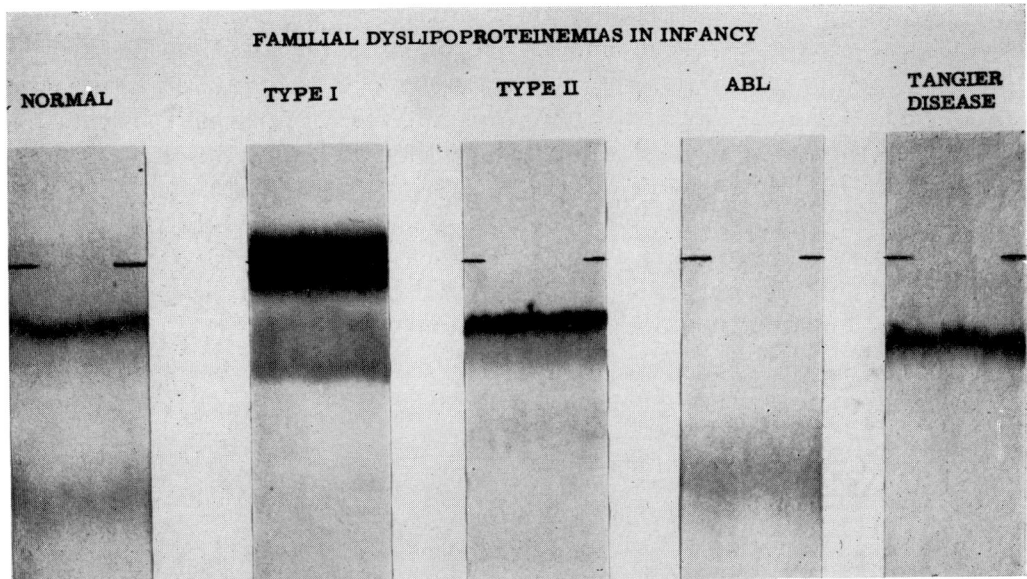

Fig. I. Electrophoretograms obtained with 20-40 μl of plasma obtained under conditions specified in the text. In contrast to the normal pattern, far left, the abnormal patterns (and the characteristic of each) is as follows, from left to right: Type I (a heavy chylomicron band at the origin); Type II (an increased β-lipoprotein band, sometimes accompanied by a modest increase in pre-β-lipoprotein); abeta-lipoproteinemia (presence of only an α_1-lipoprotein band); Tangier disease (absence of α-lipoproteins, usually a rather broad β-lipoprotein band).

plasma concentrations of cholesterol and triglycerides occurs. Chylomicrons have a very low content of cholesterol, and in infants the cholesterol concentration should be approximately 100 mg per 100 ml plus 5 per cent of the plasma glyceride concentration if hyperlipemia is due to chylomicronemia. (b) Chylomicrons readily float in plasma, due to their very low density and have a tendency to flocculate, especially when cold. If a plasma sample sits at 2 to 4° overnight, chylomicrons will form a "cream" layer at the top, leaving a fairly clear infranatant. The ultracentrifuge cannot provide a much more accurate definition than this simple test. (c) Starch block electrophoresis differentiates "particles" of alimentary glycerides into two types, *primary* and *secondary*[4]. There is some overlap between the primary particles and those of endogenous origin. (d) Polyvinylpyrrolidone density gradients achieve separations very similar to those obtained with the starch block[21]. The latter two methods are, of course, more desirable for experimental studies than for rapid screening of patients.

A patient with Type I hyperlipoproteinemia will, on a fat-poor diet, develop "endogenous" or "carbohydrate-induced" hyperlipemia (Fig. 2). Here the characteristic lipoprotein pattern includes a pre-β-lipoprotein band, often with a long trail back toward the origin[31]. Experience with hyperlipoproteinemia in young children is still very limited, but excessive pre-β-lipoprotein also seems to be characteristic of the hyperglyceridemia seen in glucose-6

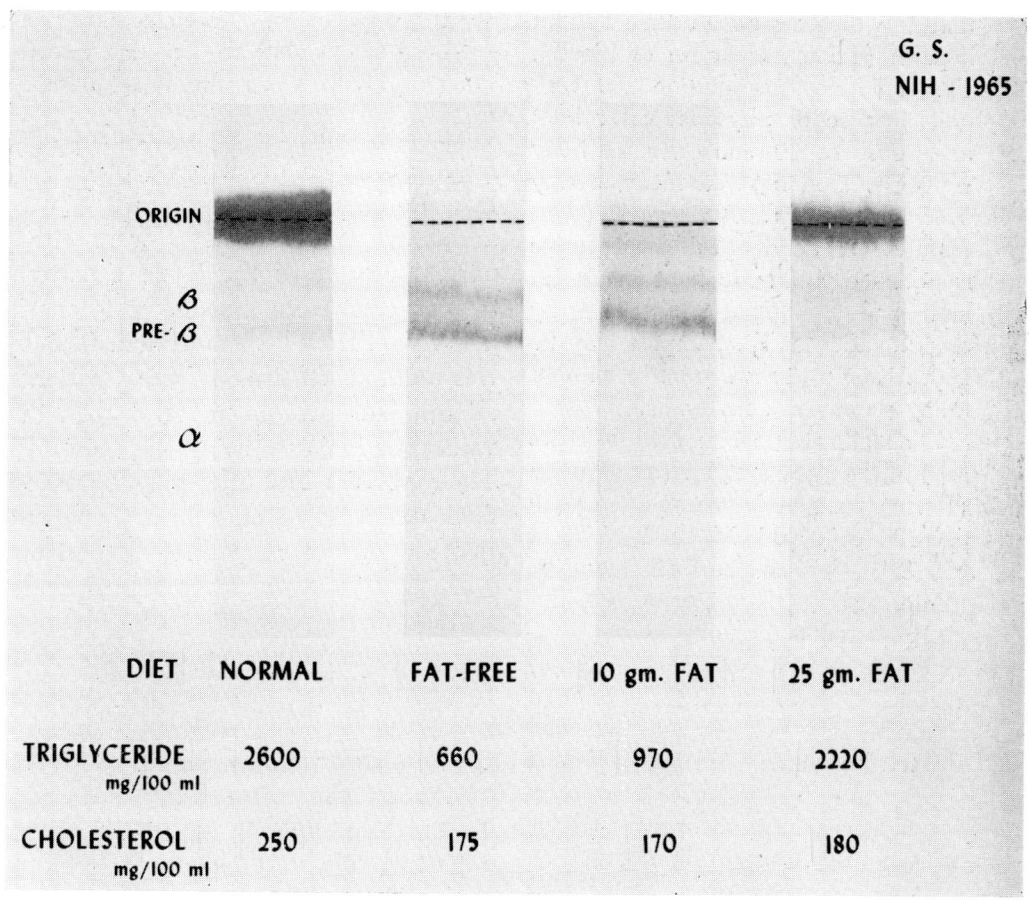

Fig. 2. An example of "carbohydrate-induced hyperlipemia" appearing in a child with Type I hyperlipoproteinemia (on "Normal" diet) after fat has been removed from her diet ("Fat-Free"). In this patient this is assumed to be due to severe defect in removing any type of glyceride rather than their excessive production from glucose. The patient's PHLA (see text) was low, 0.15μEq FFA per minute per cc plasma. Chylomicrons appear at the origin sixteen hours after 10 and 25 gm of fat have been added to diet.

phosphatase deficiency, idiopathic hypercalcemia and uncontrolled insulin-deficient diabetes mellitus[31].

LIPASE

The enzyme lipoprotein lipase seems to have an important role in catalyzing the hydrolysis of chylomicron glycerides, probably the rate-limiting step in their entry into cells. The enzyme is found in adipose tissue and vessel walls and is "displaced" into plasma by heparin. This is the basis for indirect measurement of tissue activity of the enzyme.

One assay, devised for use in presence of hyperlipemia and now tested in several hundred patients and normals, is that of Fredrickson, Ono and Davis[20]. It is performed as follows:

The patient is tested after at least one week of fat intake as near the normal as possible. Before breakfast a blood sample is collected in a chilled tube to which has been added sodium heparin (1.5 units per ml of blood). The same heparin solution 100 USP units per cc of physiological saline) at a dose of 10 units per kg body weight is then injected intravenously over a few seconds. Between 9 and 11 minutes later an identical blood sample is obtained. Both are kept in an ice bath and the plasma obtained by centrifugation at 2°. Samples may be kept frozen up to two months without losing significant activity.

The following stock solutions are used in the assay system: (a) albumin (bovine fraction V, Armour) 29 gm per 100 cc of 0.1 M $(NH_4)_2SO_4$ at pH 8.4; (b) coconut oil emulsion (Ediol, Riker Laboratories, California), diluted to contain 50 mg glyceride per ml of isotonic saline; (c) modified Dole's solution for extraction of fatty acids containing isopropyl alcohol: isooctane: 1 N H_2SO_4 (40:10:1 v/v) and 1.5 per cent w/v polyoxyethylene lauryl alcohol (Brij 35, Atlas Powder Corp., Wilmington).

Glass-stoppered tubes containing 100 mg albumin, 15 mg of the glyceride substrate and 0.2 ml of plasma in a total volume of 1.0 ml are incubated in a shaker at 37°. Duplicate tubes are removed at 5 minutes, as a "zero-time" blank, and then 15, 30 and 45 minutes thereafter. The reaction is stopped immediately by adding 5.0 ml of the modified Dole's solution. The tube is tipped once to allow mixing, allowed to stand 5 minutes and then shaken vigorously. This eliminates clumping and erratic extraction of free fatty acids (FFA) otherwise obtained with albumin in the presence of ammonium sulfate. FFA are then further extracted and titrated according to the method of Dole.[11] The FFA concentrations, less the zero-time value, are plotted against time and the slope of the line connecting them used to calculate the reaction velocity (in μEq FFA per min per ml plasma).

There should be no significant lipolytic activity in pre-heparin plasma by this method. In our experience with adults whose lipoproteins were either normal or not of the Type I pattern, 99 per cent have plasma post-heparin activity (PHLA) greater than 0.25 by this method. Of fifteen Type I patients, all but one have been lower than this value, the majority being less than 0.15. Their parents and sibs may be below 0.25 and tend to cluster in the lowest quartile of normal values. Experience with very young children is still inadequate, but the activities so far obtained appear comparable to those in older subjects. "Falsely" low activity may be present in patients with total lipoatrophy, malabsorption or severe restriction of dietary fat intake. A rare case of Type I hyperlipemia may have normal activity[20]. The test is remote from the tissue site involved and may be measuring more than one enzyme.

TYPE II

A very different syndrome from Type I is the familial hypercholesterolemia that is occasionally recognized in infants. We have termed it the Type II phenotype to distinguish it from a similar form of hypercholesterolemia (Type III), which apparently is due to a different mutation and has not yet been identified in very young children[18]. Although there is considerable likelihood that a single abnormal gene for the Type II syndrome is often expressed by hyperlipoproteinemia at birth or shortly thereafter, pediatricians are more likely to encounter the homozygous abnormal genotype. This may show up by age one to two years as tendon or tuberous xanthomas, arcus corneae and swiftly advancing atheromatous cardiovascular disease.

The Type II lipoprotein pattern features a discrete increase in β-lipoprotein (Fig. 1). Occasionally there is also a very modest rise in pre-β-lipoprotein. The plasma cholesterol and phospholipid concentrations are increased, and the glyceride concentrations are usually normal. The rise in β-lipoprotein can be quantitatively measured using the preparative or analytical ultracentrifuge although this is generally not necessary. A dense β-lipoprotein band on paper electrophoresis plus a plasma total cholesterol over 240 mg per 100 ml in a one-year-old child (over 100 to 150 in the neonatal period) is usually adequate. The plasma cholesterol can be approximated by the convenient commerical tests employing immuno-precipitation in a capillary tube. Such tests utilize an antibody that precipitates other low density lipoproteins as well as β-lipoproteins, however; and they do not specifically measure β-lipoproteins.

The best confirmatory test for the Type II syndrome is the ascertainment that one parent has the same lipoprotein abnormality. The gene is highly "penetrant" or nearly always expressed. If both parents have normal patterns and cholesterol concentrations below 250 mg per 100 ml, one must suspect that hypercholesterolemia is caused by some other disease. In infants it is often due to some type of biliary obstruction. The latter can often be recognized by a pathological increase in the α-lipoproteins seen easily by using paper electrophoresis or precipitation (next column).

HYPOLIPOPROTEINEMIA

PAPER ELECTROPHORESIS

The symptoms and signs of Tangier disease and abetalipoproteinemia (Table I) increase with age, and instances of either disease will usually be detected after the age of one year. However, the key chemical defect in plasma lipoproteins is almost certainly recognizable from the moment of birth. It can practically be diagnosed through patterns obtained by paper electrophoresis (Fig. 1).

There is no other pattern like that of abetalipoproteinemia. These patients cannot form either chylomicrons or the endogenous pre-β-lipoproteins[34], and the only lipoproteins present are those having α-mobility. So powerful a tool as the ultracentrifuge can sometimes be misleading in studying abetalipoproteinemia. In this disease, some of the α-lipoproteins float at density 1.063, the usual cutoff point between high and low density lipoproteins[34]. They may thus be interpreted as "β-lipoproteins" and the diagnosis obscured.

By contrast, the subject who is homozygous abnormal for Tangier disease has no visible α-lipoproteins by electrophoresis (Fig. 1). There is also a rather attenuated β-lipoprotein band, which represents a mixture of low density lipoproteins, for these patients cannot form pre-β-lipoproteins[35] although they do form chylomicrons. Unless one has a careful control of the color yields of the dye used, the differences between the 0 to 2 mg per 100 ml of plasma of alpha lipoprotein cholesterol in Tangier disease cannot be differentiated from the low levels of 5 to 15 mg per 100 ml secondary to a variety of conditions, including hyper-lipemia of any type.

PRECIPITATION

A number of popular methods for measuring "β-lipoproteins" by precipitating them with high molecular weight polysaccharides and similar substances are useful for screening. Not only β- but pre-β-lipoproteins and usually chylomicrons are included in the precipitate. This leaves the α-lipoproteins in solution. Precipitation can be used to reach a tentative diagnosis of Tangier disease and to screen for the heterozygous carriers, who usually have alpha lipoprotein cholesterol concentrations of less than 30 to 35 mg per 100 ml.

The following technique developed by Burstein[8] has been found[35] comparable to the ultracentrifuge in accuracy and reproducibility:

> To 3 ml of plasma add 0.15 ml 1.0 M manganese chloride and 6 mg of sodium heparin. The precipitate is allowed to form for 15 minutes and is then centrifuged in a refrigerated centrifuge for 15 minutes. The entire procedure must be carried out at 2 to 4 C. The cholesterol content remaining in the supernatant represents α-lipoprotein cholesterol. By subtracting this from the cholesterol in the starting plasma, a rough index of the low density lipoprotein concentration is obtained, in terms of its cholesterol content.

Precipitation, electrophoresis or ultracentrifugation must be used in association with immunoelectrophoresis to establish a definitive diagnosis of Tangier disease or abetalipoproteinemia.

IMMUNOELECTROPHORESIS

The immunochemical study of lipoproteins is now a major subject in itself. Commercial antisera to whole human serum, β-lipoproteins and α-lipoproteins are available for this purpose. The titers of such antibodies are quite variable, and rarely are they "pure" or specific for a single antigen. Antialbumin is perhaps the commonest contaminant. Staining of precipitation bands for lipid is therefore important to identify those due to lipoproteins. Immunoelectrophoresis, which adds the additional determinant of mobility in a charged field, is more useful than double diffusion in Ouchterlony plates. Agarose, which moves β-lipoproteins away from the well, is a better medium than agar for lipoproteins.

The immunoelectrophoretic patterns in Tangier disease and abetalipoproteinemia are shown in Figure 3. In abetalipoproteinemia, greater than tenfold concentration of plasma has revealed no precipitation line using a number of specific anti-β-lipoprotein sera[34]. Such testing has not been extended to samples from all patients with this disease, and "variants" with very low titers have not been excluded.

In Tangier disease there are very low titers of α-lipoproteins, roughly one twentieth to one fiftieth of the normal concentration[33]. Studies in progress suggest this remaining lipoprotein actually represents α-lipoprotein that differs from normal, at least in its antigenic character. This is a possible key to how the mutation producing this disease is basically expressed.

Patients with abetalipoproteinemia and Tangier disease are rare, and the plasma of each deserves intensive examination. They should never be given blood, plasma or plasma fractions

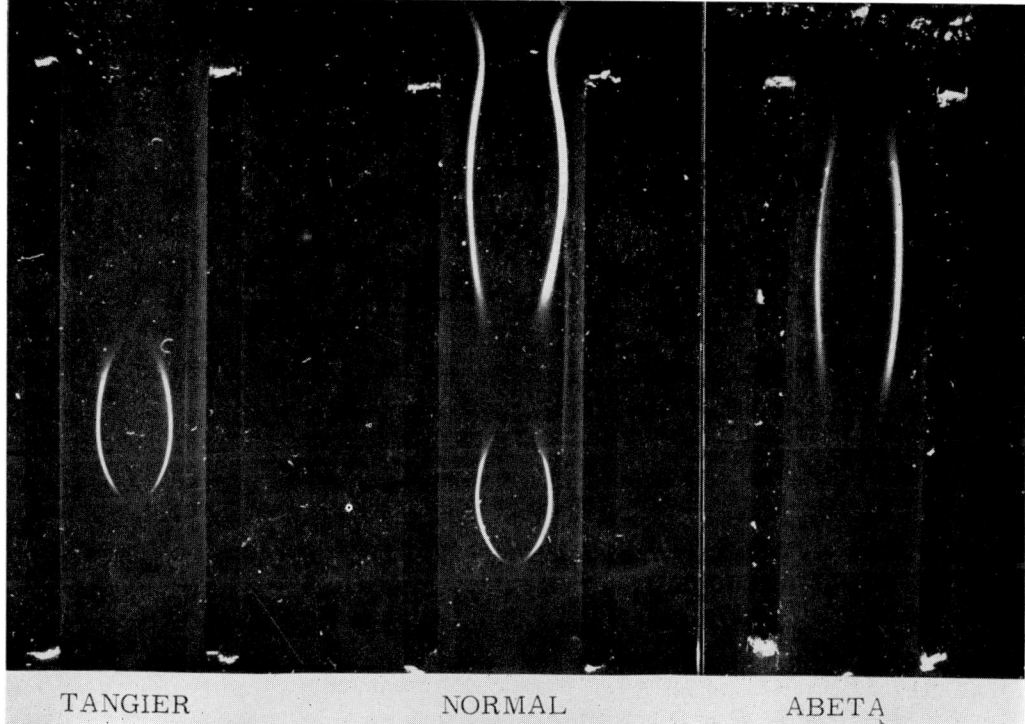

TANGIER   NORMAL   ABETA

Fig. 3. Immunoelectrophoretic patterns obtained in agarose[30] with plasma from patient with abetalipoproteinemia (right) and patients with Tangier disease (left) compared to normal subject (center). A rabbit antiserum reacting with both human α- and β-lipoproteins was used.

before a generous aliquot of their plasma has been set aside for such analyses. EDTA is the anticoagulant of choice for lipoproteins[34], and storage at 2° with added 1/1000 merthiolate is possible for a few months. Freezing alters lipoproteins, particularly their electrophoretic behavior; but frozen plasma or serum can still be used for some lipoprotein and most lipid analyses.

TISSUE LIPIDOSES

Having disposed first of the "primary dyslipoproteinemias" because they are generally easier to segregate and identify positively, we may now turn to those lipidoses in which certain tissues other than plasma must provide the lipids for chemical identification of the disease. One or two of these tissue lipidoses were thought to involve solely the nervous system; but now even Tay-Sachs disease, long a preserve of the neurologists, has been shown to include the presence of abnormal gangliosides in liver and spleen[45]. Even so, antemortem diagnosis in several of the neurolipidoses must usually be presumptive.

BONE MARROW EXAMINATION

Lipid-loaded macrophages or "foam cells" are found in the dyslipoproteinemias as well as the tissue lipidoses. The marrow should nearly always be

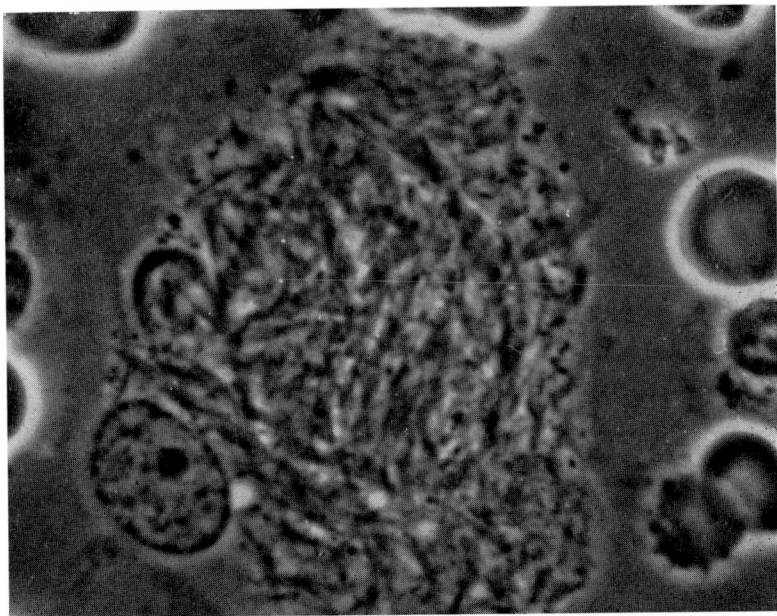

Fig. 4. The "Gaucher cell" seen in an unstained supravital preparation of bone marrow. The size can be estimated from the adjacent red cells. (Photomicrograph courtesy of Dr. George Brecher, NIH; reprinted from[12] with permission of McGraw-Hill).

examined. This includes careful search of *supra-vital* preparations which are superior to fixed and stained smears. No stain is necessary with supra-vital mounts, but phase contrast microscopy is extremely helpful. Of all the large cells with "foamy" cytoplasm that may be seen, only the "Gaucher cell" with its peculiar fibrillar cytoplasm (Fig. 4), may be considered diagnostic. The morphology of the "foam cells" seen in the other lipidoses (Fig. 5) listed in Table I is not distinctive. They all contain various granules or myelin figures, which sometimes are anisotropic; but by neither light nor electron microscopy do they provide a basis for diagnosis. There is therefore no specific entity recognized as a "Niemann-Pick" or "Tangier" cell, for example.

RECTAL BIOPSY

In the absence of hepatosplenomegaly or excisable lymph nodes, the rectal biopsy remains valuable. Involvement of neurons can often be seen early in the myenteric plexuses. The afore-mentioned limitations of histochemistry notwithstanding, some specific diagnoses can be closely approached by this technique[29].

BIOPSY OF OTHER VISCERAL TISSUES

The election to obtain tissue from sites less accessible than marrow or rectal mucosa remains an individual decision in each patient. The value of brain biopsy in these diseases is not established, but visceral biopsies can often provide a certain diagnosis. As little as 10 to 50 mg wet weight of liver or lymph node can be used to differentiate four or five of the lipidoses in Table I. A lymph node obtained under local anesthesia is preferable to open biopsy of the liver, and the latter is preferable to the spleen. Most surgeons decline to biopsy the spleen even by direct vision for fear of hemorrhage, and it is difficult indeed to justify the risks of needle biopsy of this organ to establish the nature of a lipidosis. Needle biopsy of the liver has not been used for chemical diagnosis of the lipidoses, although as techniques become more sensitive it may become useful. More than a gram of liver usually can be removed at open biopsy with only the hazard of the anesthesia. This is adequate tissue for

extensive biochemical studies. In addition to study of lipids it also provides enough for analyses of glycogen, phosphorylase, glucose-6-phosphatase or amylo-1,6 transglucosidase in the event glycogen storage has not been excluded.

Tissue obtained at biopsy must be captured in some physiological medium such as 0.15 M NaCl, kept cold, and taken directly to the pathologist. The latter is spared only an amount necessary for blocks, and this is usually placed directly in 10 per cent calcium-formalin, the fixation being quite brief for blocks to be cut as frozen sections. Both paraffin and frozen sections will be prepared for staining appropriate to determine abnormal increases in certain lipid classes[39] as well as morphological

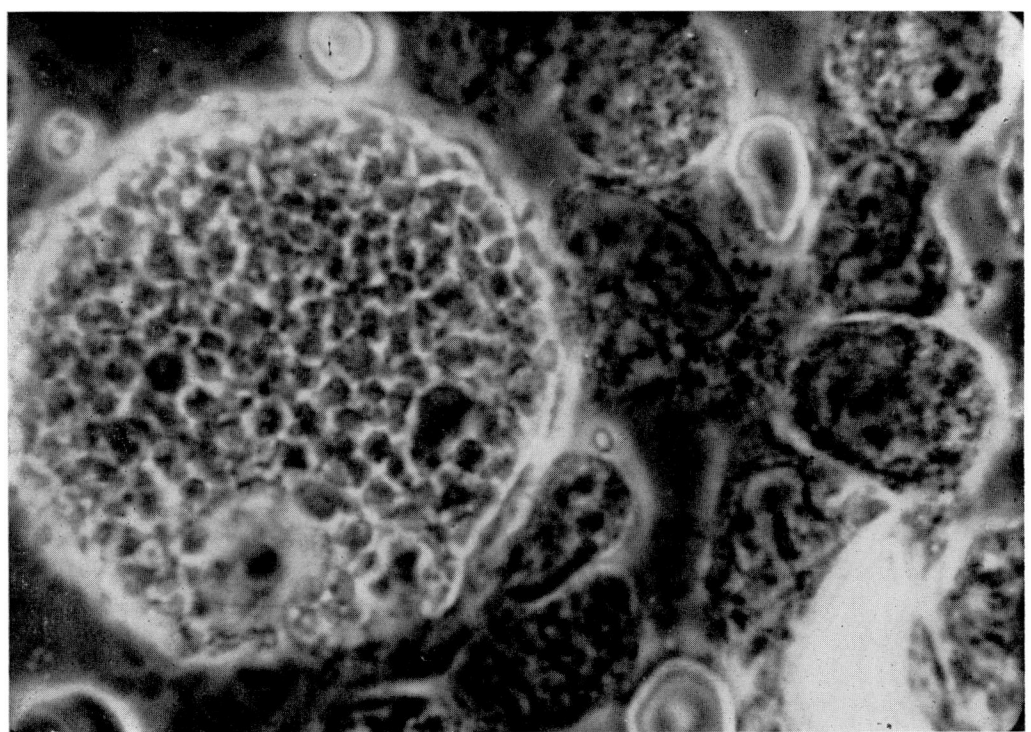

Fig. 5. Foam cell seen in bone marrow of patient with Niemann-Pick disease. The morphology is not specific for this disease. Conditions of photomicrograph as in Figure 4. (Photomicrograph courtesy of Dr. George Brecher, NIH; reprinted from[14] with permission of McGraw-Hill).

changes. The remaining tissue not to be used directly should be sealed in aliquots in plastic bags ideally placed in other containers that can be flushed with nitrogen and kept frozen at $-10°$ or lower, if possible. It should be noted that "freeze-artefacts" will render such tissues less valuable for any subsequent morphological studies.

ANALYSES

Identification of the infantile lipidoses by tissue lipid analyses requires some methods and materials not generally available or used too infrequently to be maintained by most clinical pathologists. Even among those who handle many such tissues, specialization in only one or two classes of compounds is common.

From Table I it can be seen that the minimum examination includes a qualitative assessment of the tissue content of the following: total lipids; free cholesterol; esterified cholesterol; glycerides; total phospholipids (and the relative proportion and amounts represented by sphingomyelins, lecithins, cephalins, inositides and lysolecithins); and cerebrosides. In addition, it is useful to screen for gross increases in other neutral glycolipids, sulfatides and gangliosides. The recognition of the different molecular forms these lipids may have is a special task, but one that cannot be ignored if syndromes deviating from the "classical" forms are to be identified properly. Here is a summary of a few useful screening techniques.

Extraction of Tissue. An aliquot of tissue is homogenized in 10 to 25 volumes of chloroform: methanol (2:1 v/v). This is split into a lower (chloroform) and upper (aqueous methanol) phase by adding water (10 cc per 50 cc of original chloroform-methanol). The upper phase is removed and the lower phase washed several times with .003 N CaCl$_2$[14]. The washes and original upper phase, along with any fluff at the interface, may be pooled and handled separately for analyses of gangliosides and other very polar lipids. An aliquot of the original chloroform-methanol single phase may also be saved for dialysis and screening for gangliosides by chromatography. A separate aliquot of tissue is weighed wet and then dried to constant weight solely for reference of analyses to dry tissue substance. The best control is concomitant analysis of "normal" tissue handled in the same manner.

THIN-LAYER CHROMATOGRAPHY

Certainly some of the most valuable aids in screening tissues for the characteristic chemical changes in the lipidoses are the rapid and sensitive methods for chromatography on thin layers of silicic acid[42]. Now in use is a variety of solvent systems for development and many techniques for identifying the spots. The following are several useful systems:

1. *Separation of non-polar lipids.* Either glass plates or Kodak Chromogram plastic sheets (type K301R) coated with silicic acid can be used. Development is one-dimensional in petroleum ether: diethyl ether: glacial acetic acid (90:10:1). Phospholipids remain at the origin on this system; and it is especially helpful for detecting gross changes in the content of the following commonly encountered lipids, listed in increasing R_f values: mono-glycerides; free cholesterol; diglycerides; free fatty acids; triglyc-

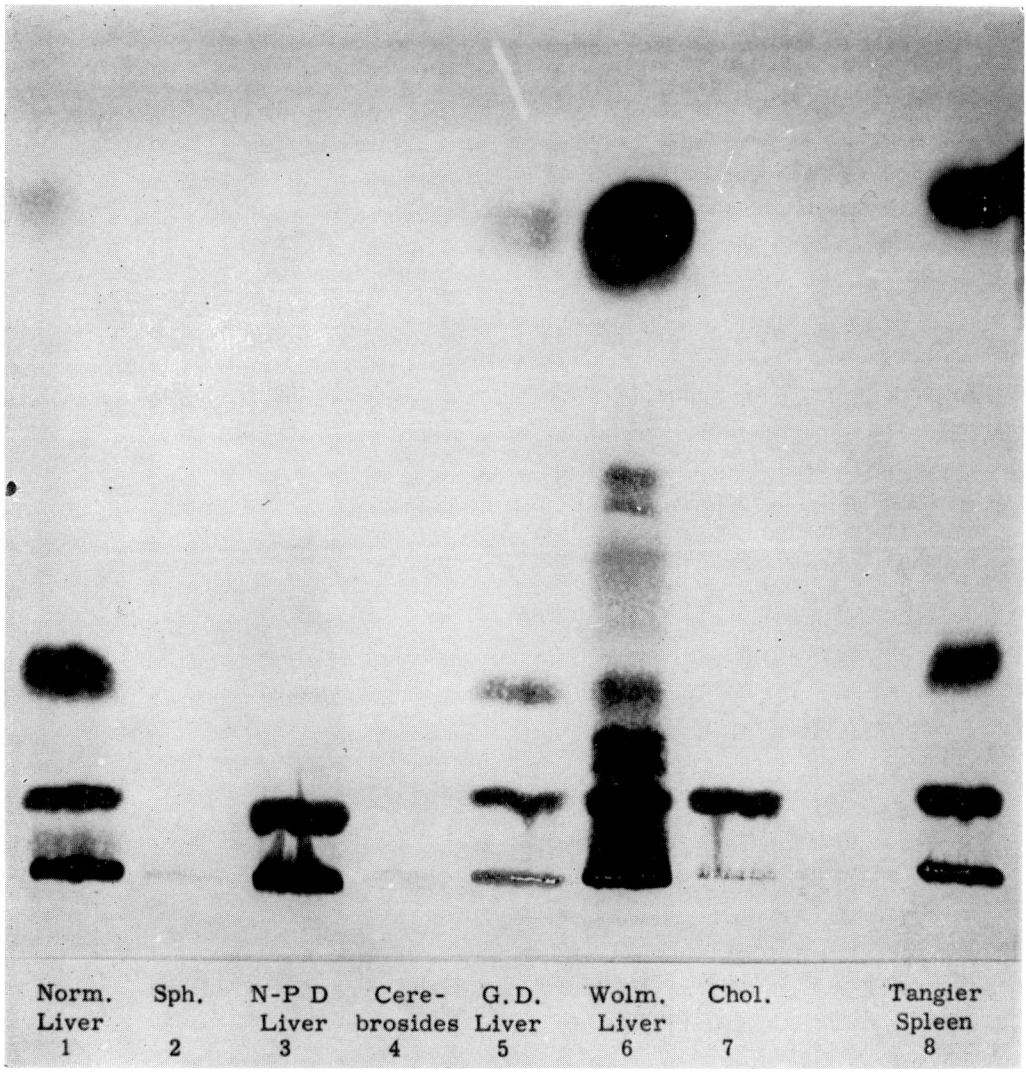

Fig. 6.   Separation of less polar lipids by thin-layer chromatography. The lipid extracts of tissues or standards run in the lanes from left to right were: (1) normal liver in which only free cholesterol and free fatty acid spots are visible above the origin; (2) sphingomyelin, which, like other phospholipids, remains at the origin; (3) liver in Niemann-Pick disease; (4) galactocerebroside, remaining at origin; (5) liver in Gaucher's disease; (6) liver in Wolman's disease; the dense spot near the front represents cholesterol esters (tissue kindly supplied by Dr. Allen Crocker, Boston); (7) free cholesterol; and (8) spleen in Tangier disease with accumulation of cholesterol esters. Development was in petroleum ether/diethyl ether/glacial acetic acid, 255/45/3 (v/v). The spots were identified by spraying with anisaldehyde and heating for twenty minutes at 120°.

erides; cholesterol esters. An example is shown in Figure 6.

2. *Quantification of different phospholipids.* Lipid extracts equivalent to 20 mg, wet weight, of normal liver (about 5 mg dry weight) are used for separations with better than 90 per cent recovery of all phospholipids. The Chromogram sheet is developed in chloroform: methanol: NH_4OH: H_2O (180:90:5:2), dried completely in a nitrogen atmosphere, and then developed in the same solvents, but now in the mixture of 120:160:5:1 (v/v)[49]. The spots are identified by iodine vapor, and each is scraped off the plastic sheet with a scalpel into a tube in which digestion and determination of phosphorus are carried out by the method of Bartlett[3]. A blank spot is similarly treated in each analysis. In Niemann-Pick disease, sphingomyelin represents greater than 10 per cent of the total phospholipids and is present in liver in concentrations exceeding 10 mg per gm of dry weight of tissue. The contrast between chromatograms of phospholipids in normal and Niemann-Pick liver is shown in Figure 7.

3. *Separation of more polar lipids.* (The author is grateful to Dr. Lars Svennerholm for instruction in the value and performance of this and the following thin-layer separations.) Separation is made on glass plates by one-dimensional development in chloroform: methanol: H_2O (65:25:4). The spots may then be identified by sprays of an anisaldehyde-sulfuric acid-acetic acid mixture[42], phosphomolybdic acid, iodine vapor or charring after spraying with sulfuric acid. This method separates sphingomyelin, lecithin, cerebrosides and other neutral

TLC SEPARATION OF LIVER PHOSPHOLIPIDS

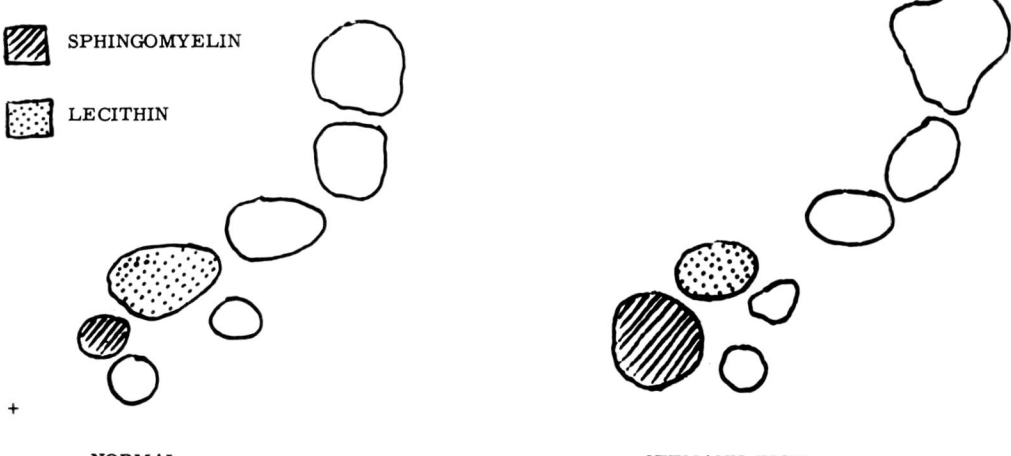

SPHINGOMYELIN

LECITHIN

+

NORMAL   NIEMANN-PICK

Fig. 7. Thin-layer chromatograms of liver-lipid extracts from a control patient and one with Niemann-Pick disease, showing separation of phospholipids. The aliquot from the Niemann-Pick patient represents less than one quarter of the liver used for the control, but the relative preponderance of sphingomyelin remains quite evident. Chromatography was carried out on Chromogram sheets according to the text under "Quantification of Different Phospholipids."

glycolipids, sulfatides, glycerides, free fatty acids, and free and esterified cholesterol. An example is shown in Figure 8. A second dimension to this system for further separations has been described by Rouser[41].

4. *Separation of gangliosides and other polar lipids.* Svennerholm[44, 45] has employed a one-dimensional development in chloroform: methanol: H_2O (55:40:8) for separation of gangliosides and related substances. These can be detected with a spray reagent made as follows: 10 ml of a stock solution of resorcinol (2 gms dissolved in 100 ml water) are added to 80 ml of concentrated hydrochloric acid containing 0.25 ml of 0.1 M copper sulfate. The volume of the reagent is made up to 100 ml with distilled water. The reagent is prepared at least four hours before use and is stable for a week when kept in the refrigerator.

OTHER ANALYSES

The usual methods employed for determining total lipids, total fatty acids, free and total cholesterol and total phospholipid phosphorus can be used on tissue extracts. Normal values need to be established by each laboratory, but some approximations to the normal lipid contents of several tissues appear in Table II.

Accurate measurement and demonstration of the structure of the glycolipids involved in some lipidoses cannot be covered here in adequate detail. They can be located through the appropriate references in Table I.

FATTY ACID PATTERNS

Tissue lipid extracts obtained from patients who do not fit well the clinical descriptions of the usual lipidoses should be examined for their content of fatty acids by gas liquid chromatography. An example of the usefulness of this technique was the recent demonstration that phytanic acid (tetramethylhexadecanoic acid) dominates the fatty acid pattern in Refsum's syndrome[29]. This disorder introduces a new chemical class of lipidoses.

TISSUE CULTURE

The use of tissue culture to study the metabolic defects in the lipidoses and to recognize the presence of the abnormal gene in the absence of clinical signs of the disease is now an exciting possibility. Among the conditions listed in Table I, tissue culture has thus far been used clinically in preliminary studies in Niemann-Pick disease[24, 47] and in Hurler's syndrome[10]. Fibroblasts cultured from Niemann-Pick tissues contain an abnormally high sphingomyelin content. This has also been observed in cells propagated from the amnions[24]. Eventually it may be possible to obtain a diagnosis at birth. Fibroblasts cultured

TABLE II SOME APPROXIMATIONS OF LIPID CONTENT IN NORMAL LIVER, SPLEEN AND LYMPH NODES

Total Lipid	Cholesterol Esters	Free Cholesterol	Total Phospholipids	Sphingo-myelin	Lecithin	Glycerides	Neutral Glycolipids
100-150*	2-5	10-15	50-90	5-10	20-50	25-50	5-15

*All measurements are in mg per gm dry weight.

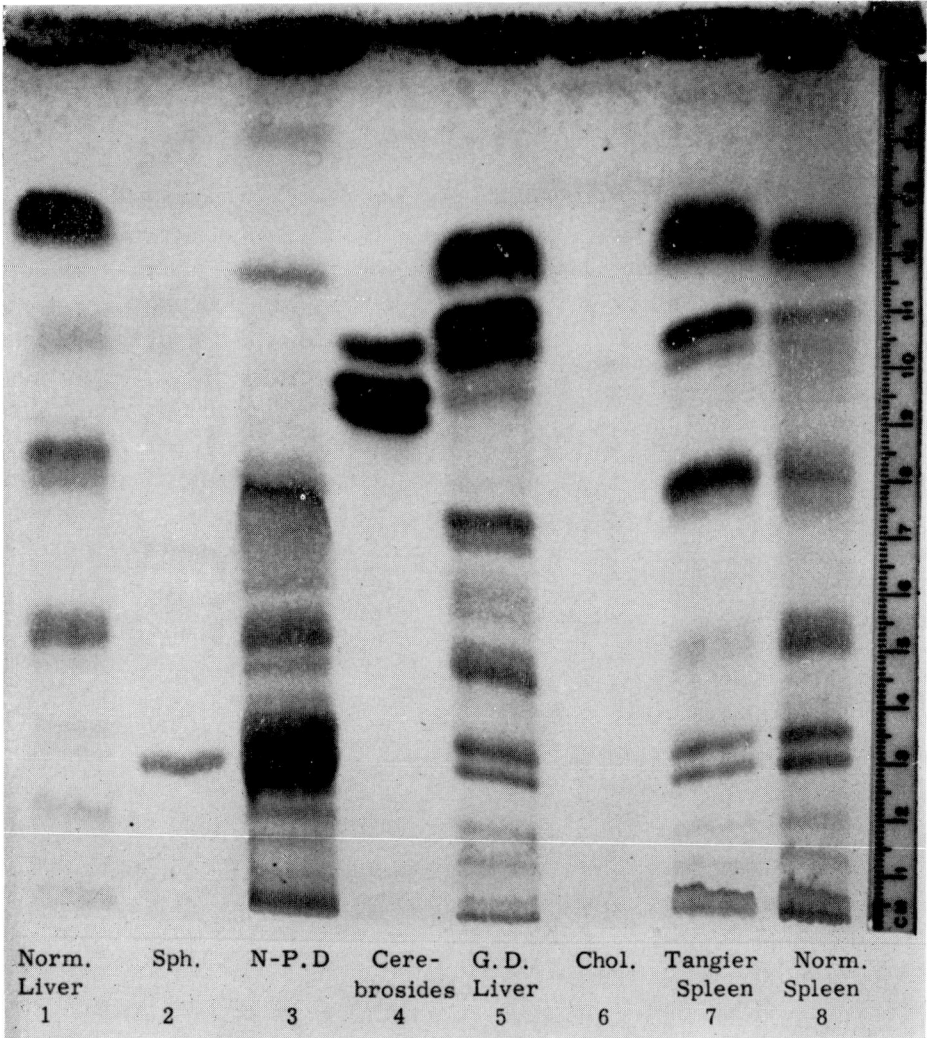

Norm. Liver	Sph.	N-P.D	Cere- brosides	G.D. Liver	Chol.	Tangier Spleen	Norm. Spleen
1	2	3	4	5	6	7	8

Fig. 8. Thin-layer chromatographic separations of some relatively polar lipids in tissues representing three of the lipidoses. The lipid extracts or standards chromatographed in each lane are as follows, from left to right: (1) normal liver; the dense spot 12.5 cm from the origin is free fatty acid; (2) pure palmitoylsphingomyelin (provided by Dr. Julian Kanfer, NIH); (3) liver from child with classical infantile form of Niemann-Pick disease, in which the excess of sphingomyelin is readily seen; (4) cerebroside standards; the three bands are interpreted to represent galacto-cerebrosides having three different types of fatty acids; (5) liver from a patient with Gaucher's disease; the characteristic abnormality, an excess of glucocerebrosides, is seen in the band 10.5 cm from the origin, an R_f comparable to the fastest moving of the cerebroside standards; (6) cholesterol standard; the sterol moves almost with the front in this system, while cholesterol esters move slightly ahead at the front; (7) spleen from an adult patient with Tangier disease and hypersplenism; the characteristic increase in cholesterol esters, which move to the front, is better demonstrated on a less polar system such as that used in Figure 6; and (8) control spleen. Development was in chloroform/methanol/H_2O (65/25/4) and the spots were identified as in Figure 6.

from both patients with Hurler's syndrome and heterozygous carriers have been shown to have abnormal metachromasia[10].

Enzyme Analyses

Positive identification of a lipidosis by demonstration of the deficiency of a specific protein is the ideal goal in diagnostics. As with other kinds of molecular diseases, this is still the exception rather than the rule in the lipid storage diseases. In Tangier disease and abetalipoproteinemia, it is likely that the elaboration of the A and B apoproteins of the lipoproteins is somehow altered by the responsible mutations. More of these diseases ultimately will be shown to be due to altered activity of a protein having enzymatic function. Recognition of deficiency of lipoprotein lipase is a helpful adjunct to diagnosis of Type I hyperlipoproteinemia; this *may* be the biochemical locus of the action of the altered gene. Enzymes catalyzing disassembly of two of the sphingolipids have very recently been characterized by Drs. R. O. Brady, J. Kanfer and D. Shapiro, and evidence obtained of their apparent deficiency in two of the lipidoses under discussion[5-7, 26]. There has not yet been time to evaluate the full significance of these findings, but it is likely that they will be of value in diagnosis and also may provide much needed discrimination between different clinical forms of the heterogeneous syndromes now identified by the eponyms, Gaucher's disease and Niemann-Pick disease.

Decreased activity of an enzyme-cleaving glucocerebroside at the glycoside bond, yielding glucose and ceramide, has been noted in spleens of three patients with the adult or non-cerebral form of Gaucher's disease[6, 7]. Measurements have not yet been made in tissues from examples of the infantile form of the disease associated with neurological abnormalities. A marked deficiency in the activity of an enzyme that splits phosphorylcholine from sphingomyelin has now been found in liver and kidney of children with the classical infantile form of Niemann-Pick disease[5, 26]. The activities in control tissues were on the average twenty times greater.

There will be more such enzymatic discoveries in the lipidoses and an increasing number of specific diseases to contend with because of them. Frozen tissues, some of them stored for several years, have made it possible to test readily the clinical significance of the identification of the enzymes cleaving glucocerebrosides and sphingomyelins. No more concrete support can be given to the plea for proper retention of tissues by those responsible for management of patients with these diseases.

REFERENCES

1. Abul-Huj, S. K., Martz, D. G., Douglas, W. F., and Geppert, L. J.: Farber's disease. Report of a case with observations on its histogenesis and notes on the nature of the stored material. J. Pediat., 61:221-232, 1962.
2. Aronson, S. M., Perle, G., Saifer, A., and Volk, B. W.: Biochemical identification of the carrier state in Tay-Sachs disease. Proc. Soc. Exp. Biol. Med., 111:664-667, 1962.
3. Bartlett, G. R.: Phosphorus assay in column chromatography. J. Biol. Chem., 234:466-468, 1959.
4. Bierman, E. L., Gordis, E., and Hamlin, J. T., III: Heterogeneity of fat particles in plasma during alimentary lipemia. J. Clin. Invest., 41:2254-2260, 1962.
5. Brady, R. O., Kanfer, J. N., Mock, M. B., and Fredrickson, D. S.: The metabolism of sphingomyelin. II. Evidence of an enzymatic deficiency in Niemann-Pick disease. Proc. Nat. Acad. Sci. U.S.A., 55:366-369, 1966.

6. Brady, R. O., Kanfer, J., and Shapiro, D.: The metabolism of glucocerebrosides. I. Purification and properties of a glucocerebroside-cleaving enzyme from spleen tissue. J. Biol. Chem., **240**:39-43, 1965.

7. Brady, R. O., Kanfer, J. N., and Shapiro: Metabolism of glucocerebrosides. II. Evidence of an enzymatic deficiency in Gaucher's disease. Biochem. Biophys. Res. Commun., **18**:221-225, 1965.

8. Burstein, M., and Samaille, J.: Sur un dosage rapide du cholesterol lié aux α- et β lipoprotéines du sérum. Clin. Chim. Acta, **5**:609, 1960.

9. Crocker, A. C., Vawter, G. F., Neuhauser, E. B. D., and Rosowsky, A.: Wolman's disease: Three new patients with a recently described lipidosis. Pediatrics, **35**:627-640, 1965.

10. Danes, B. S., and Bearn, A. G.: Hurler's syndrome: Demonstration of an inherited disorder of connective tissue in cell culture. Science, **149**:987-989, 1965.

11. Dole, V. P.: A relation between non-esterified fatty acids in plasma and the metabolism of glucose. J. Clin. Invest., **35**:150-154, 1956.

12. Dortman, A.: Heritable diseases of connective tissues: the Hurler's syndrome. In Stanbury, J. B., Wyngaarden, J. B., and Fredrickson, D. S. (eds.): The Metabolic Basis of Inherited Disease. New York, McGraw, 1965, 2nd ed., pp. 963-994.

13. Farquhar, J. W., and Ways, P.: Abetalipoproteinemia. In Stanbury et al., op. cit., pp. 509-522.

14. Folch, J., Lees, M., and Stanley, G. H. S.: A simple method for the isolation and purification of total lipides from animal tissues. J. Biol. Chem., **226**:497-509, 1957.

15. Fredrickson, D. S.: Cerebroside lipidosis: Gaucher's disease. In Stanbury et al., op. cit., pp. 565-585.

16. Fredrickson, D. S.: Familial high-density lipoprotein deficiency: Tangier disease. In Stanbury et al., op. cit., pp. 486-508.

17. Fredrickson, D. S.: Sphingomyelin lipidosis: Niemann-Pick disease. In Stanbury et al., op. cit., pp. 586-617.

18. Fredrickson, D. S., and Lees, R. S.: Familial hyperlipoproteinemia. In Stanbury et al., op. cit., pp. 429-485.

19. Fredrickson, D. S., and Trams, E. G.: Ganglioside lipidosis: Tay-Sachs disease. In Stanbury et al., op. cit., pp. 523-538.

20. Fredrickson, D. S., Ono, K., and Davis, L. L.: Lipolytic activity of post-heparin plasma in hyperglyceridemia. J. Lipid Res., **4**:24-33, 1963.

21. Gordis, E.: Demonstration of two kinds of fat particles in alimentary lipemia with polyvinylpyrrolidone gradient columns. Proc. Soc. Exp. Biol. Med., **110**:657-661, 1962.

22. Hatch, F. T.: Serum lipoproteins in coronary heart disease. In Sunderman, F. W., and Sunderman, F. W., Jr. (eds.): Serum Proteins and the Dysproteinemias. Philadelphia, Lippincott, 1964, pp. 422-429.

23. Holt, L. E., Jr., Aylward, F. X., and Timbres, H. G.: Idiopathic familial lipemia. Bull. Johns Hopkins Hosp., **64**:279-314, 1939.

24. Holtz, A. I., Uhlendorf, B. W., and Fredrickson, D. S.: Persistence of a lipid defect in tissue culture derived from patients with Niemann-Pick disease. Fed. Proc., **23**:128, 1964.

25. Jatzkewitz, H., and Sandhoff, K.: On a biochemically special form of infantile amaurotic idiocy. Biochim. Biophys. Acta, **70**:354-356, 1963.

26. Kanfer, J. N., Young, O. M., Shapiro, D., and Brady, R. O.: The metabolism of sphingomyelin. I. Purification and properties of a sphingomyelin-cleaving enzyme from rat liver tissue. J. Biol. Chem., **241**:1081-1084, 1966.

27. Klenk, E., und Kahlke, W.: Über das Vorkommen der 3.7.11.15-Tetramethyl-Hexadecansäure (Phytansäure) in den Cholesterinestern und anderen Lipoidfraktionen der Organe bei einem Krankheitsfall unbekannter genese (Verdacht auf Heredopathia atactica polyneuritiformis (Refsumsyndrom). Hoppe-Seyler Z. Physiol. Chem., **333**:133-139, 1963.

28. Kuhn, R., and Wiegandt, H.: Die Konstitution der Ganglio-N-tetraose und des Ganglioside G_I. Chem. Ber., **96**:866-880, 1963.

29. Landing, B. H., and Rubinstein, J. H.: Biopsy diagnosis of neurologic diseases in children, with emphasis on lipidoses. In Aronson, S. M., and Volk, B. W. (eds.): Cerebral Sphingolipidoses: Symposium on Tay-Sachs Disease and Allied Disorders. New York, Academic Press, 1962, pp. 1-13.

30. Landing, B. H., Silverman, F. N., Craig, J. M., Jacoby, M. D., Lahey, M. E., and Chadwick, D. L.: Familial neurovisceral lipidosis. Amer. J. Dis. Child., **108**:503-522, 1964.

31. Lees, R. S., and Fredrickson, D. S.: The differentiation of exogenous and endogenous hyperlipemia by paper electrophoresis. J. Clin. Invest., **44**:1968-1977, 1965.

32. Lees, R. S., and Hatch, F. T.: Sharper sepa-

ration of lipoprotein species by paper electrophoresis in albumin-containing buffer. J. Lab. Clin. Med., **61**:518-528, 1963.

33. Levy, R. I., and Fredrickson, D. S.: In preparation.

34. Levy, R. I., Fredrickson, D. S., and Laster, L.: The lipoproteins and lipid transport in abetalipoproteinemia. J. Clin. Invest., **45**:531-541, 1966.

35. Levy, R. I., Lees, R. S., and Fredrickson, D. S.: The nature of pre-beta (very low density) lipoproteins. J. Clin. Invest., **45**: 63-77, 1966.

36. Moser, H. W., and Lees, M.: Sulfatide lipidosis: Metachromatic leukodystrophy. In Stanbury et al., op. cit., pp. 539-564.

37. Norman, R. M., Urich, H., Tingey, A. H., and Goodbody, R. A.: Tay-Sachs disease with visceral involvement and its relationship to Niemann-Pick disease. J. Path. Bact., **78**:409-421, 1959.

38. O'Brien, J. S., Stern, M. B., Landing, B. H., O'Brien, J. K., and Donnell, G. N.: Generalized gangliosidosis. Amer. J. Dis. Child., **109**: 338-346, 1965.

39. Pearse, A. G. E.: Histochemistry—Theoretical and Applied. Boston, Little, 1960.

40. Richterich, R., van Mechelen, P., and Rossi, E.: Refsum's disease (heredopathia atactica polyneuritiformis): An inborn error of lipid metabolism with storage of 3, 7, 11, 15-tetramethyl hexadecanoic acid. Amer. J. Med., **39**:230-236, 1965.

41. Rouser, G., Galli, C., and Kritchevsky, G.: Lipid class composition of normal human brain and variations in metachromatic leucodystrophy, Tay-Sachs, Niemann-Pick, chronic Gaucher's and Alzheimer's diseases. J. Amer. Oil Chem. Soc., **42**:404-410, 1965.

42. Stahl, E.: Thin Layer Chromatography: A Laboratory Handbook. New York, Springer-Verlag-Academic Press, 1962.

43. Svennerholm, L.: The gangliosides. J. Lipid Res., **5**:145-155, 1964.

44. Svennerholm, L.: Chromatographic separation of human brain gangliosides. J. Neurochem., **10**:613-623, 1963.

45. Svennerholm, L.: Studies of gangliosides. In Aronson, S.M., and Volk, B.W. (eds.): Proceedings of the Third International Symposium on the Sphingolipidoses and Allied Diseases. New York, Pergamon, 1966.

46. Sweeley, C. C., and Klionsky, B.: Glycolipid lipidosis: Fabry's disease, In Stanbury et al., op. cit., pp. 618-632.

47. Uhlendorf, B. W., Holtz, A. I., Mock, M. B., and Fredrickson, D. S.: Persistence of a metabolic defect in tissue cultures derived from patients with Niemann-Pick disease. In Aronson and Volk (1966), op. cit.

48. Zeman, W., and Whieldon, J. A.: Clinical considerations in "Schilder's disease." Amer. J. Dis. Child., **104**:635-643, 1962.

49. Zuhowski, E., and Mock, M. B.: In preparation.

Chapter 6

Screening Measurements of Urinary Acid Mucopolysaccharides for Detection of the Hurler Syndrome

ANDREW E. LORINCZ, M.D.

INTRODUCTION

Available screening techniques for the detection of excessive urinary acid mucopolysaccharide excretion depend upon indirect measurements related to properties of these polymers or measurements of their component moieties (e.g., uronic acid, hexosamine, etc.). Because of this, the currently employed urine screening tests have their limitations. The actual isolation, fractionation and identification of acid mucopolysaccharides present in urine requires extensive facilities and procedures so that it is not practically feasible for analysis in the routine clinical laboratory[5, 8, 10]. Methodology is still being developed for the more accurate identification and characterization of excreted acid mucopolysaccharides.

Indirect screening tests for mucopolysaccharides are essentially of three types:

 I. Metachromatic staining reaction with basic dyes[1];
 II. Precipitation with acidified serum albumin[4, 11]; and
III. Precipitation of mucopolysaccharides with quaternary ammonium salts, and measurement of precipitated uronic acid[2].

The Type I spot tests which use basic dyes like Toluidine Blue or Alcian Blue are by far the simplest and cheapest to perform. However, limitations of this method are the extremely large number of false-positive tests as well as the extremely high incidence of false-negative tests which result from the interference with the metachromatic staining reaction caused by salts that may be present.

The Type III methods, which depend upon the precipitation of the polysaccharides with quaternary ammonium salts, in addition to being complex, have the further limitation that, by using the colorimetric measurement of uronic acid by the Dische Carbazole method[3], they do not give true quantitative measure of mucopolysaccharides present. The total color yield by this method for glucuronic acid, which is present in the mucopolysaccharides, chondroitin sulfuric acid-A and C, and hyaluronic acid, is much greater than for an identical amount of iduronic acid, which is the hexuronic acid present in the mucopolysaccharide chondroitin sulfuric acid-B. An even more significant limitation of any method that employs total uronic acid as an indirect quantitative measurement of mucopolysaccharide present is the fact that some polysaccharides such as keratosulfate do not contain a uronic acid moiety.

A modified method[4] of the second type, which utilizes the measurement of turbidity produced by acidified serum albumin reacting with dialyzed urine, is the recommended procedure of choice and will be described in this chapter. This method has less false-positive reactions than the metachromatic spot tests, and although less accurate as a quantitative procedure than the Type III methods, it is much simpler to perform. None of these methods permits *qualitative* identification of specific acid mucopolysaccharides present, and none of these methods are suitable for truly accurate *quantitative* measurements of mucopolysaccharides present.

METHOD

A method previously developed for the assay of hyaluronidase[6] has been modified for the detection of excessive acid mucopolysaccharide excretion in dialyzed urine. It is based on the fact that these acidic polymers react with albumin at pH 3.70 to produce turbidity. Under appropriately controlled conditions of pH, ionic strength, temperature and time, this method can be used for approximate quantitative estimations of the concentration of acid mucopolysaccharides present. It should

be noted that methods of preparation, polymer size and the qualitative character of mucopolysaccharides present will all affect the amount of turbidity produced. This is a meaningful screening test only by virtue of the fact that most individuals affected with the Hurler syndrome excrete so much more of these substances than do non-Hurler individuals[5, 7, 10, 11, 12].

REAGENTS

1. *Acid albumin reagent.* Approximately 3.3 gm NaAc · $3H_2O$, 4.6 ml glacial acetic acid and 1.0 gm Bovine serum albumin Fraction V (Pentex Corp., Kankakee, Illinois) are transferred to a one-liter volumetric flask. The solution is adjusted to pH 3.75 with concentrated HCl (approximately 1.4 ml) after dilution to volume with water. The solution is then filtered through Whatman #1 filter paper and refrigerated. The solution is allowed to come to room temperature prior to use.

2. *Acid albumin reagent blank.* Approximately 3.3 gm NaAc · $3H_2O$ and 4.6 ml glacial acetic acid are transferred to a 1 liter volumetric flask. The solution is adjusted to pH 3.75 with concentrated HCl (approximately 1.6 ml) after dilution to volume with water. The solution may be stored at room temperature.

3. *Sodium phosphate buffer.* Into a 1 liter volumetric flask are transferred 42.6 gm Na_2HPO_4, 9.0 gm NaCl and 30.0 gm citric acid ($H_3C_6H_5O_7 · H_2O$). The contents are diluted with distilled water to a volume of one liter.

STANDARD SOLUTIONS

No standard solutions are required. However, commercially available Bovine Nasal Septum Chondroitin Sulfate

(Nutrional Biochemicals Company) can be used in varying concentrations to 0.5 mg per ml to observe positive results.

Procedure

1. Six ml of urine which have been agitated to uniformly mix sediment are pipetted into a one quarter inch diameter Visking cellophane dialysis tube that has been tied in a knot at one end and pretested for leakage with distilled water.

2. After tying off filled dialysis bag at the other end and appropriate labeling of specimen, dialysis, in a volume of distilled water at least 150 times the volume of urine being dialyzed, is carried out for three to four hours or longer as desired.

3. Upon completion of dialysis, contents of dialyzed bag are transferred to a 15 ml heavy-walled centrifuge tube. Enough distilled water is added to bring the volume of the sample to double its original pre-dialysis volume, thus equalizing volume variations brought about by the dialysis procedure.

4. After mixing, centrifuge for at least ten minutes at maximum speed of clinical centrifuge to sediment any insoluble residues. Use only the clear supernatant for the turbidimetric measurement.

5. Reagents and specimens to be analyzed are set up as follows in 25 × 105 mm Coleman cuvettes:

Tube No.	Sample	Sample Volume	Phosphate Buffer	Acid Albumin Reagent*	Blank Acid Reagent
1	Distilled H$_2$O	1.5 ml	0.5 ml	10 ml	----
2	Distilled H$_2$O	1.5 ml	0.5 ml	10 ml	----
3	Unknown supernatant	1.5 ml	0.5 ml	10 ml	----
4	Unknown supernatant	1.5 ml	0.5 ml	10 ml	----
5	Unknown supernatant	1.5 ml	0.5 ml	----	10 ml
6	Unknown supernatant	1.5 ml	0.5 ml	----	10 ml

Unknown and phosphate buffer can be mixed prior to addition of the acid albumin reagent, or the acid albumin reagent blank.

*Using a stopwatch, acid albumin reagent is added to each tube at thirty-second intervals, shaking tubes to assure proper mixing as it is added.

6. Exactly ten minutes after addition of the acid albumin reagent, the optical density reading is recorded at 600 mμ, using a Coleman Jr. Spectrophotometer. The distilled water blank is used as the zero reference.

7. The average reading of Tubes 5 and 6 is subtracted from the average reading of Tubes 3 and 4. The resultant optical density reading is used as the relative quantitative measure of mucopolysaccharides present in the unknown sample.

Discussion

Tubes 5 and 6 with the acid albumin reagent blank are used to compensate for variation in urine pigment, which could contribute to the O.D. reading. In over 3000 tests on more than 1200 individuals with various types of growth and developmental retardation, the only markedly elevated O.D. readings obtained were from individuals with the Hurler syndrome. Weakly positive reactions have been found in about one third of newborn infants for the first forty-eight hours of life, and occasionally in hypothyroid children who have been started on thyroid treatment.

Sources of Error

Major sources of error are contamination of the urine specimen with semen or mucus from the genitourinary tract. Mucus contamination usually can be avoided or minimized if specimens less than 60 ml in volume are *not* accepted for analysis.

Obviously, urine dilution factors could and do affect results; however, it must be emphasized that this is only a crude quantitative screening procedure.

Range of Values

Normal range: O.D. = 0.000 to 0.020. Optical density values greater than 0.020 are usually indicative of the presence of excessive non-dialyzable glycoprotein or mucopolysaccharide polymers.

Résumé of Clinical Interpretations

Urine samples from individuals affected with the Hurler syndrome may have O.D. values as high as 0.500, and usually greater than 0.050. Only rarely have false negatives been obtained from these patients. Most of these have been limited to those with normal or near normal intelligence. Interestingly, these same specimens display a turbidity when undialyzed urine is tested.

Urine from affected children with hereditary multiple exostoses or with the nail-patella syndrome may be less than 0.030.

A more detailed description of Hurler's syndrome and diagnostic procedures helpful for establishing the diagnosis, have been reviewed by Lorincz[9].

REFERENCES

1. Berry, H. K., and Spinanger, J.: A paper spot test useful in study of Hurler's syndrome. J. Lab. Clin. Med., **55**:136-138, 1960.
2. Di Ferrante, N., and Rich, C.: The mucopolysaccharide of normal human urine. Clin. Chim. Acta., **1**:519-524, 1956.
3. Dische, Z.: A new specific color reaction of hexuronic acids. J. Biol. Chem., **167**:189, 1947.
4. Dorfman, A.: Studies on the biochemistry of connective tissue. Pediatrics, **22**:576-589, 1958.
5. Dorfman, A., and Lorincz, A. E.: Occurrence of urinary acid mucopolysaccharides in the Hurler syndrome. Proc. Nat. Acad. Sci. U.S.A., **43**:443, 1957.
6. Dorfman, A., and Ott, M. L.: A turbidimetric method for the assay of hyaluronidase. J. Biol. Chem., **172**:367-375, 1948.
7. Fried, M., and Campbell, T. N.: Excretion of urinary mucopolysaccharides in gargoylism. Proceedings of the 2nd International Congress on Mental Retardation. Vienna, 1961, Part 1. 1963, pp. 75-82.
8. Loewi, G.: Urinary excretion of acid polysaccharide in rheumatoid arthritis and other diseases. Amer. Rheum. Dis., **18**:239-243, 1959.
9. Lorincz, A. E.: Hurler's syndrome. In Carter, C. H. (ed.): Medical Aspects of Mental Retardation. Springfield, Thomas, 1965, pp. 628-650.
10. Meyer, K., Grumbach, M. M., Linker, A., and Hoffman, P.: Excretion of sulfated mucopolysaccharides in gargoylism (Hurler's syndrome). Proc. Soc. Exp. Biol. Med., **97**:275, 1958.
11. Steiness, I. B.: Acid mucopolysaccharides in urine in gargoylism. Pediatrics, **27**:112-117, 1961.
12. Teller, W. M., Burke, E. C., Rosenear, J. W., and McKenzie, B. F.: Urinary excretion of acid mucopolysaccharides in normal children and patients with gargoylism. J. Lab. Clin. Med., **59**:95-101, 1962.

Chapter 7

Genetic Errors of Glycogen Metabolism

GONZALO E. APONTE, M.D., AND
ELLIOTT L. MANCALL, M.D.

Advances in the knowledge of normal carbohydrate metabolism have made possible a more precise classification of the glycogenoses. Conversely, a better understanding of the glycogenoses is giving clearer insight of normal carbohydrate metabolism. It is true that the specific diagnosis should now be based on the determination of enzyme activity in tissue, but clinical paradoxes are being noted with increasing frequency, and the facts as seen in the patient do not always correspond to the facts in the test tube. More than one enzyme may be missing in the same patient[6, 7, 87, 142, 177, 179, 180, 186], dif-

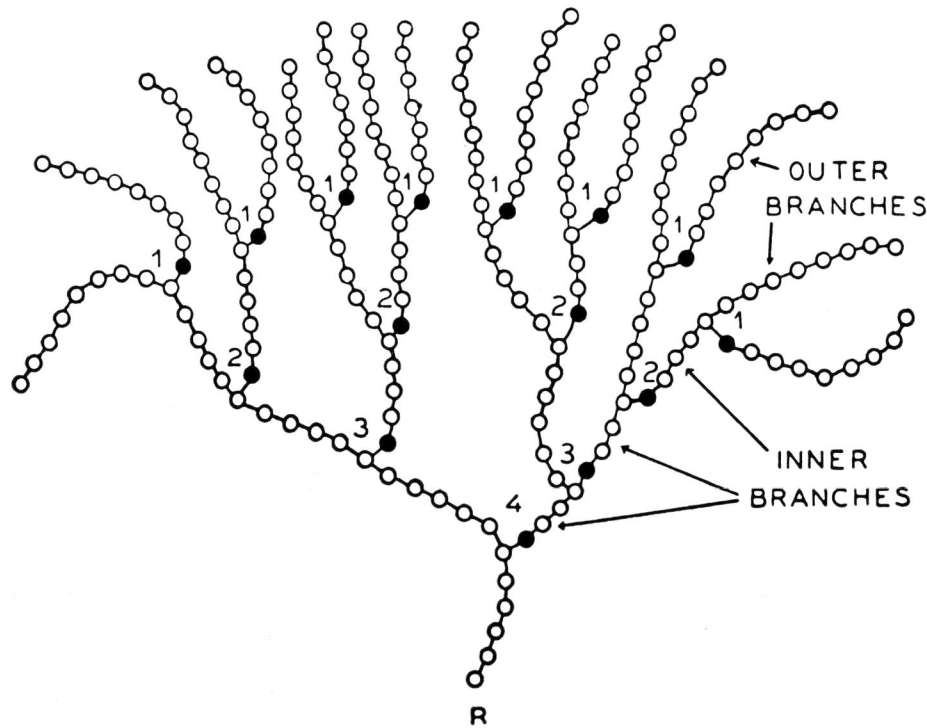

Fig. 1. Model of a segment of the glycogen molecule (Cori).

PATHWAY OF GLYCOGEN SYNTHESIS

1) $\quad$ glucose 1-phosphate $\ +$ UTP $\xrightarrow[\text{UDP-G pyrophosphorylase}]{}$ UDP-glucose

2) $\quad$ UDP-glucose $+$ polysaccharide primer $\xrightarrow[\substack{\text{a-1, 4-glucan a-4-glucosyl}\\ \text{transferase}}]{}$ glucosyl $(1,4)_{n+1}$ $+$ UDP

3) $\quad$ glucosyl $(1,4)_{n+1}$ $+$ UDP $\xrightarrow[\text{amylo-1, 4 ——— 1, 6-transglycosylase}]{}$ glucosyl 1, 4 $+$ glucosyl 1, 6

Fig. 2

ferent members of the same family may have different defects[41, 42], the clinical picture may strongly suggest a particular deficiency and yet the enzyme may be present[15, 33, 179, 203, 209], or the enzyme may seem to be inactive in the absence of the expected clinical picture.

Almost every tissue of the body can form glycogen, and the highest concentrations are found in liver and muscle. Glycogen has a branched structure (Fig. 1) of variable molecular weight. The main link between the glucose residues of the molecule is in the α-position, through carbon atoms 1 and 4. There is a smaller number of 1, 6 linkages, at the branching points. The work of Leloir[108] has delineated a pathway of glycogen synthesis independent of phosphorylase (Fig. 2). However, not all investigators agree that this view of glycogen synthesis is entirely correct, and it has not been proved beyond a doubt that phosphorylase plays no role whatever in the formation of glycogen. The 1, 4 bond is effected through the action of a transglucosylase (α-1, 4-glucan α-4-glucosyl transferase). The unit UDP glucose: transglucosylase has been termed "glycogen synthetase." The 1, 6 linkages at the branching points are formed by the action of an oligotrans-

ferase (amylo-1, 4 → 1, 6-transglycosylase), aptly called the "brancher enzyme." Such a schema focuses on glucose-1-phosphate as the basic compound controlling the reaction.

The enzymes involved in the breakdown of glycogen are listed in Table I.

TABLE I KEY ENZYMES INVOLVED IN GLYCOGEN CATABOLISM

1. Cleavage of α-1, 4 linkages:
   (a) phosphorylase (product: glucose-1-phosphate)
   (b) α-1, 4-glucosidase (product: glucose)

2. Cleavage of α-1, 6 linkages:
   a $\begin{cases} \text{amylo-1, 6-glucosidase (debranching enzyme)} \\ \text{oligo-1, 4} \to 1, \text{4-glucotransferase} \end{cases}$

3. Glucose-1-phosphate $\xrightarrow{\quad}$ glucose-6-phosphate
   phosphoglucomutase

4. Glucose-6-phosphate $\xrightarrow{\quad\quad\quad}$ glucose $\quad$ P
   glucose-6-phosphatase

The importance of phosphorylase has been recognized for a long time. It acts upon 1, 4 linkages but cannot split 1, 6 linkages. The product of phosphorylase action is glucose-1-phosphate. Phosphorylase is present in active and inactive forms, known as phosphorylase *a* and *b* respectively. The interconversion of the two forms[101] in muscle can be illustrated as follows:

$$\text{phosphorylase } a \xrightarrow[\substack{\text{dephosphorylase} \\ \text{kinase} \\ \text{(``rupturing enzyme'')}}]{} \text{2 phosphorylase } b + 4 \text{ Pi}$$

$$\text{2 phosphorylase } b + 4\text{ATP} \xrightarrow[\substack{\text{phosphorylase} \\ \text{phosphokinase}}]{} \text{phosphorylase } a + 4 \text{ ADP}$$

Muscle phosphorylase differs immunologically from hepatic phosphorylase. More recently, α-1, 4-glucosidase has been shown to play a role in the cleavage of 1, 4 bonds. Cells contain at least two different α-glucosidases, which differ in the pH of optimal activity and in intracellular localization. The enzyme absent in Type II glycogenosis is an α-glucosidase, a lysosomal enzyme with distinct acid maltase activity. The action of phosphorylase stops about four glucose units from the branching point. The partially depolymerized molecule which remains after phosphorylation is known as limit dextrin. The 1, 6 bonds are split by the action of two enzymes; or, as seems more likely, one protein with dual enzymatic activity[16]. The debranching enzyme, amylo-1, 6-glucosidase, was described first. More recently, a glucotransferase has been shown to play a role in this reaction. One or both enzymes may be inactive in Type III glycogenosis. The product of their activities is free glucose, and they are thought to account for the degradation of about 8 per cent of the glycogen molecule. The next two reactions involve the formation of glucose-6-phosphate from glucose-1-phosphate, catalyzed by phosphoglucomutase, and the liberation of glucose from glucose-6-phosphate by glucose-6-phosphatase. This is obviously a very sketchy outline

of glycogen metabolism. Much additional information can be obtained from excellent reviews of the subject[28, 48, 187].

On Table II are listed the types of genetic errors in glycogen metabolism recognized at the present. Several good reviews of the subject have appeared[28, 48, 67, 170]; the one by Hers includes descriptions of methods for assays of enzyme activity, whereas Sidbury covers the genetic aspects in detail. Assays of enzyme activity, obviously essential for a specific diagnosis, are subject to considerable error in inexperienced hands. The tissue to be analyzed should be frozen immediately and placed in a tightly sealed container. Extraneous chemicals, even sodium chloride, can interfere with the assay. In general, tissue obtained post mortem is unsatisfactory, particularly for the study of very labile enzymes such as phosphorylase. The question of how great a reduction in enzyme activity must be present in order to be significant biochemically and clinically cannot always be answered. Complete absence of enzyme activity may mean that the particular enzyme is indeed absent or that an inhibitor is present in the tissue, although the former is perhaps more likely since the disorders in question are genetic errors. There are methods to detect some of these enzymes in tissues[26, 27, 188, 189]. The presence of glycogen and its resistance or lability to

TABLE II GENETIC ERRORS OF GYCOGEN METABOLISM

| | Type | Eponym | Organs Affected | Enzyme Defect | Glycogen Content* (% wet wt) | | |
					Liver	Skel. Muscle	Heart
GLYCOGEN CATABOLISM	I	von Gierke van Creveld	liver, kidney	glucose-6-phosphatase	6-10	normal	normal
	II	Pompe	heart muscle, nervous system (generalized)	α-1, 4-glucosidase	7-11	9-13	5-9
	III	Cori Forbes	liver, muscle (generalized)	amylo-1, 6-glucosidase and/or the glucotransferase	IIIA: 12-17 IIIB: 12-17	IIIA: 4-9 IIIB: 1-2	4.5 (one case)[87]
	IV	Andersen	liver (generalized)	unknown	1.7-2.9 (one case)[5] 0.18 (one case)[174]	0.06-0.33 (one case)[5] 0.07 (one case)[174]	1.2 (one case)[174]
	V	McArdle	skeletal muscle	muscle phosphorylase	normal	2.5-5.3	normal (one case)[97]
	VI	Hers	liver	hepatic phosphorylase	usually > 12	normal	normal
	VII	————	muscle, other organs?	phosphorylase b kinase	5.8 and 16 (two cases)[7a]	3-7[7a, 67]	5.5 (one case)[7a]
GLYCOGEN SYNTHESIS	————		liver, muscle (other organs?)	"glycogen synthetase"	0.17-0.45	0.05 (one case)[138]	?

*Normal values: liver = < 5; muscle = < 1; heart = < 1.

enzymatic digestion can easily be determined histochemically[144]. Several good methods are available to measure the glycogen content of tissues[10, 23, 190, 199]. Many chemical and physical properties[137, 149] of the glycogen extracted from tissues can be studied, such as solubility[67], molecular configuration[32, 50, 90, 119], absorption spectrum in the presence of iodine[67], distribution of sedimentation coefficient[18], and rate and nature of *in vitro* degradation[50, 80].

TYPES I, III AND VI

The three types are discussed together because they have clinical and biochemical similarities, although the genetic defect is different in each. Type I (hepatorenal) glycogenosis has also been called von Gierke's disease and van Creveld's disease. Neither eponym is accurate, since there is no proof that the case reported by von Gierke[200] belonged to this group, and the patients described by van Creveld[195] later were shown to be cases of Type III glycogenosis[197]. The enzymatic defect in the latter disorder is more complex because one or two enzymatic activities may be absent in liver or muscle, or both. Although deficiency of hepatic phosphorylase has been designated as the genetic error responsible for Type VI glycogenosis, many things remain unexplained about this disorder.

TYPE I: HEPATORENAL GLYCOGENOSIS; VON GIERKE'S DISEASE; VAN CREVELD'S DISEASE

The outstanding clinical signs of Type I glycogenosis are hepatomegaly and marked obesity. Enlargement of the liver usually is first noted during infancy; and by the first year of life it is massive, extending to the iliac crest. The enlarged liver is not tender. Enlargement of the spleen is not detected in the physical examination but may be seen sometimes in the roentgenograms[14]. If abdominal distention is not too severe, the examiner often can palpate the enlarged kidneys. The nephromegaly is readily noted in the roentgenograms. As a result of marked abdominal enlargement, the child may walk with a distinctive, wide and swinging gait[48]. Although the muscles are not primarily involved, muscular weakness is a frequent finding. The severe and protracted hyperlipemia often colors the skin yellow, sometimes induces the formation of xanthomas[99, 215] and occasionally causes lipemia retinalis[47]. Retardation of somatic growth is characteristic, but the intellectual capacity is not impaired. Osteoporosis develops frequently, and in some cases the occurrence of "mushroom epiphyses"

and spontaneous fractures have been noted[48]. Other reported findings include unexplained fever, increased susceptibility to infections[170], frequent episodes of diarrhea and steatorrhea[35], hemorrhagic diathesis[1, 3, 52, 161], and hypertension[196]. For unknown reasons, the disease pursues a remarkably mild course in occasional cases[9, 14, 195].

Cori and Cori were the first to show that the abnormality in Type I glycogenosis is inactivity of glucose-6-phosphatase[33]. The enzyme, a phosphomonoesterase which acts preferentially but not exclusively on glucose-6-phosphate, is present in the human liver, kidney and small intestine. Absence of enzyme activity has been noted in the aforementioned tissues of patients with Type I glycogenosis[33, 120, 132, 210]. Fields, Epstein and Egan[47] found that enzyme activity in the jejunal mucosa of the parents was about half the value in normal adult controls. This may become a reliable test for the detection of asymptomatic heterozygous carriers of the disease. The results obtained in the assay must be corrected for activity of nonspecific phosphatases. This enzyme can also be detected histochemically[26, 27]. Many reported studies have included determinations of glycogen content in the liver, but very few have mentioned analyses of renal tissue. In the liver, the concentration of glycogen is generally in the range of 6 to 10 per cent of wet tissue (Table II). The glycogen molecule has a characteristic sedimentation coefficient[18]. Studies of glycogen degradation in homogenates have shown that, whereas in Type VI the main product is glucose, the accumulated products in Type I are phosphorylated sugars[88]. Cases have been described in

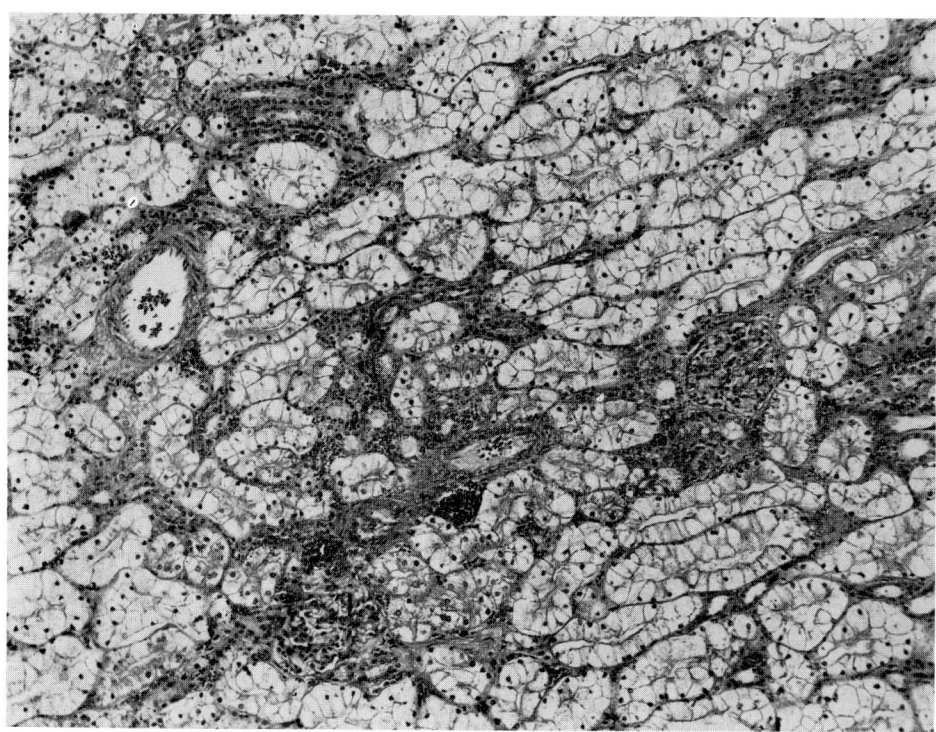

Figs. 3 and 4.   Abundant deposits of glycogen in the epithelial cells of the renal tubules and the liver, in a case of hepatorenal glycogenosis. Hematoxylin and eosin; x 85.

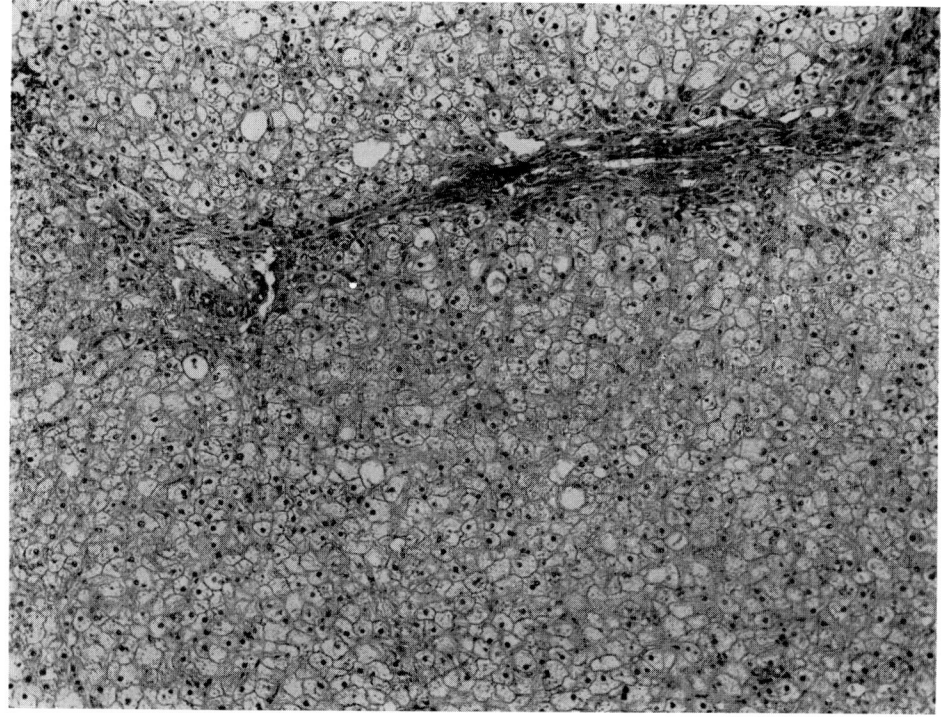

which there was coexisting deficiency of glucose-6-phosphate dehydrogenase in the liver[7, 120, 206]. However, doubt has been cast on the significance of these findings[66a], and others have actually found normal activity of the latter enzyme[20, 169].

The typical histopathologic changes are well known (Figs. 3 and 4). The deposits in liver and kidneys can be stained with Best's carmine or with the periodic-acid Schiff technique, and can be digested with diastase. Fatty liver is a common occurrence, and, in some patients, visceral or cutaneous xanthomas are found[99, 215]. An unusual but interesting post-mortem finding is the presence of nodules in the liver[74, 121]. The nodules consist of hepatic tissue and may have a higher glycogen concentration than the rest of the liver[74]. Several electron-microscope studies of the liver in Type I glycogenosis have been published[8, 155, 165]. Glycogen is found predominantly in the cytoplasm of hepatocytes and occasionally in the nucleus. The cytoplasmic deposits are diffusely dispersed and are not found within sacs, as in Type II glycogenosis. However, some Kupffer cells may contain vacuoles. Since intranuclear deposits of glycogen may occur in other diseases[147, 181], they are not a diagnostic finding.

Hypoglycemia is the basic metabolic abnormality. The concentration of blood glucose is usually near 50 mg per 100 ml, but at times is much lower. This is particularly true after an overnight fast, when the levels may be almost zero. On the other hand, the postprandial values tend to be higher than normal. Clinical signs of hypoglycemia are not too frequent, but convulsions may occur. Schulman and Saturen[161] found normal electroencephalograms in two patients, notwithstanding the fact that hypoglycemia was severe. In many patients, the severity of the hypoglycemia tends to decrease with age. Increased concentrations of glycerol may be found in the plasma[131]. The blood concentrations of phosphorylated intermediary products of glycolysis may also be increased, although normal levels are not unusual, and sometimes decreased concentrations are found[134]. Hsia[77, 78] reported that increased blood levels of glucose-6-phosphate are also found in the bloods of the parents of affected children, and suggested that this might be a way of detecting asymptomatic carriers. However, others have not been able to confirm this finding in heterozygotes[176]. It has also been claimed that the glycogen content of platelets can be used as a genetic marker[113]. It seems that the amount of glucose-6-phosphate in the liver can vary greatly. Brante and associates[14], who also have noted increased amounts of hepatic fructose-6-phosphate and fructose-1, 6-diphosphate, have discussed the possible significance of this variability.

The genetic error in carbohydrate metabolism characteristic of this disease produces other abnormalities of great clinical importance, namely, ketosis, hyperlactidemia and hyperlipemia. Many facts known about the metabolism of hexoses can provide *a priori* explanations of the latter abnormalities[76, 175], but little clinical investigation has been done to delineate the pathogenesis. Figure 5 depicts the principal pathways of hexose metabolism. The absence of glucose-6-phosphatase results in a

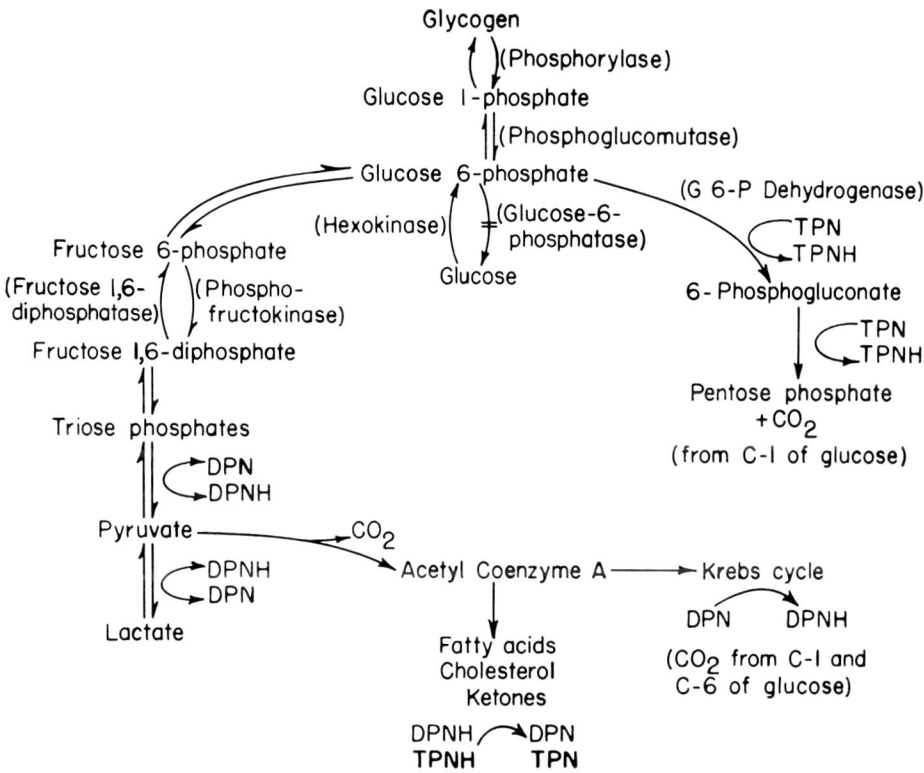

Fig. 5. Metabolic pathways of hexose metabolism.

"flooding" of the other pathways through which hexose phosphates are metabolized, and this could account for the ketosis and the high blood levels of lipids and lactic acid. Lowe and associates[115] are of the opinion that the chronic hypoglycemia causes deficiency of insulin, which in turn produces metabolic abnormalities characteristic of diabetes mellitus. Hers[67] states that the probable cause of hyperlipemia is release of fatty acids from adipose tissue as a result of chronic hypoglycemia. However, as Field[48] has pointed out, this explanation is contradicted by the fact that the majority of patients are obese.

Ketosis is said to develop in about 15 to 20 per cent of the cases[67]. Acetonuria may occur, particularly when the patient is in the fasting state and ketosis is severe. Prompt and intensive treatment may be required to avert death during such episodes. Hepatorenal glycogenosis is one of the few causes of ketonuria in the neonatal period[173]. Mason and Sly[122] were the first to report the presence of high concentrations of blood lactate and pyruvate, and others have confirmed their findings[76, 179, 180, 196]. A drop in the blood lactate and pyruvate levels after the injection of glucagon or epinephrine is the typical finding[142, 179], but exceptions have been noted[115, 134, 162]. The severity of the hyperlactidemia varies in inverse proportion to the severity of hypoglycemia. The serum concentrations of cholesterol, triglycerides and fatty acids are increased[48, 76, 180, 215]. The content of fatty solids in the serum may exceed 10 per cent by volume, and this may result in spuriously low values for sodium and certain other blood constituents. As the degree of hepatomegaly increases, hyperlipemia becomes more severe. But the diminution in the intensity of hepatomegaly sometimes noted when the patients grow older is not usually accompanied by a corresponding decrease in the serum concentration of lipids. After a meal, the serum levels of lactate, pyruvate and fatty acids decrease somewhat, but do not return to normal. The occurrence of fat embolism, perhaps a result of the hyperlipemia, has been noted[151]. Enlargement of the liver in this disease is due not only to an accumulation of glycogen within hepatocytes, but also to fatty change. No satisfactory explanation of the fatty change has been given.

The impaired glucose tolerance and the increase in serum fatty acids may be associated with high plasma levels of growth hormone[152]. High serum levels of hydrocortisone have been noted[94, 170], and in one case the half-life of serum hydrocortisone was prolonged[170]. The metabolism of glycogen and the activities of certain enzymes can be greatly affected by changes in endocrine function[2, 56, 71, 100, 104, 109, 139, 194]. Treatment of these patients with synthetic androgen preparations has been reported to have a beneficial effect[41, 42]. More studies are needed concerning the effects of hormonal activity on the clinical and biochemical expressions of glycogen-storage diseases. The disorder known as Mauriac syndrome[57, 110] is characterized by hepatomegaly, obesity, dwarfism and juvenile diabetes mellitus. It occurs only in patients inadequately treated for diabetes. Hepatic enlargement is due to the accumulation of excessive glycogen and fat. In two cases studied recently[68], the glycogen content of the liver was 12 per cent and no enzymatic abnormality was found. These patients are very susceptible to the development of ketosis, and evidence of hypercorticism has been found. Mauriac's syndrome is a disorder of glycogen storage clearly on the basis of disturbed endocrine function.

There are relatively few abnormalities of hepatic function other than those related to carbohydrate metabolism. Sometimes the thymol turbidity is elevated, occasionally markedly so. Chaptal et al.[24] found increases in serum α_2-globulins and β-globulins. Increases in the activity of serum lactic-acid dehydrogenase have been described[198]. Brante and associates[14] have noted increased plasma activity of ornithine carbamoyl transferase, an ezyme considered to be specific for hepatic tissue. The finding is evidence of increased cellular turnover in the liver. None of these abnormalities is characteristic of the disease. In spite of the fact that the renal tubules are severely affected, abnormalities of renal function occur infrequently. Nonspecific aminoaciduria[196] tends to develop, becoming severe in a few patients[48]. Glucosuria is less frequent. Although the serum calcium and plasma alkaline phosphatase are normal, the patients tend to develop hypophosphatemia. Chronic acidosis doubtless contributes to the latter change. Although the frequency and intensity of hypophosphatemia can be correlated with the degree of osteoporosis seen in roentgenograms[48], the precise relation between the two has not been sudied in detail.

Many patients with Type I glycogenosis develop hyperuricemia[76, 95, 98, 99, 178], and at least seven cases of secondary gout have been reported[75]. Two adult patients seen by Holling[74] died of gouty nephritis. Unlike the hypoglycemia, hyperuricemia tends to become more marked as the patient grows older. Several factors may contribute to the increase in serum uric acid concentration. Howell[75], as well as Jeandet and Lestradet[92], have found significant reductions in uric acid clearance in some patients. The reduction in uric acid clearance is thought to be the result of chronic hyperlactidemia. The urinary excretion of uric acid is not depressed in all patients; indeed, some develop uric acid calculi[15, 92, 93, 196]. Jeune and others[93] found the uric acid clearance to be normal or increased in five of fifteen cases. The importance of factors other than chronic hyperlactidemia has not been studied at length. In one patient, evidence was found of increased de novo synthesis of purines[75]. Chronic ketosis may be important, in view of the fact that the administration of β-hydroxybutyrate and acetoacetate to normal persons can cause retention of uric acid[55]. Chronic hypoglycemia may interfere with tubular secretion of uric acid, a process which requires glucose as a source of energy.

Harris and Cohen[60] found a greater than normal excretion of sodium and chloride in the sweat of five patients with Type I glycogenosis. They attributed this in part to the high extracellular concentrations of electrolytes induced by the hyperlipemia. However, normal electrolyte excretion was found in other cases[168, 198]; and normal values have been noted in patients with glycogenoses Types II[38], III[198] and VI[60]. The infusion of alcohol into patients with hepatorenal glycogenosis produces interesting metabolic changes[114]. The serum concentrations of lactate and free fatty acids fall to normal, hypoglycemia does not develop, no interference is noted with the removal of galactose from the blood, and the previously abnormal response to glucagon (vide infra) is corrected. These metabolic changes are just the converse of what occurs in normal persons.

Studies on the activity of glucose-6-phosphatase in the jejunal mucosas of the parents of affected children indicate that Type I glycogenosis is probably inherited as a recessive trait. There is parental consanguinity in about 10 per cent of families, and nearly 20 per cent of sibs are affected[67].

TYPE III: GENERALIZED, HEPATOMUSCULAR GLYCOGENOSIS; LIMIT DEXTRINOSIS; FORBE'S DISEASE; CORI'S DISEASE

The original case was described by Forbes[49], in 1953. The polysaccharide which accumulates in the liver and muscles has short outer chains and a high percentage of end groups. It resembles limit dextrin, the compound formed by the action of phosphorylase prior to cleavage of the α-1, 6 groups. According to Illingworth[87, 91], the outer chains tend to be shorter in muscle than in the liver, but their length varies even in samples from the same patient, and occasionally is normal. In 1956, the defect was shown to be absence of amylo-1, 6-glucosidase, the debranching enzyme[91].

The long-accepted views concerning the structure of limit dextrin were challenged by the investigations of Walker and Whelan[204], who indicated that the debranching of limit dextrin occurs as a result of the combined actions of two enzymes, amylo-1, 6-glucosidase and a transglycosylase (oligo 1, 4 → 1, 4-glucotransferase). Evidence favoring this view has been presented by others[4, 17]. The biophysical data of Brown and Illingworth[16] indicate that the two activities are associated with a single, bifunctional enzyme; i.e., there is a single protein with two different enzymatic functions. These findings have complicated considerably the original concept of the underlying abnormality in this disease[63]. At the present, four variants of Type III glycogenosis can be defined:

A: Both enzymes deficient in liver and muscle;

B: Debrancher enzyme deficient in the liver but present in muscle; glucotransferase deficient in both;

C: Debrancher enzyme deficient in muscle but present in the liver; glucotransferase present in both (one case);

D: Debrancher enzyme present in both; glucotransferase deficient in both (one case).

The clinical manifestations are milder than in Type I, and there is much more improvement with age. Hypoglycemic convulsions are not frequent. Progressive myopathy may occur, and may resemble McArdle's disease. In at least one patient, the changes in serum lactate following exercise resembled those characteristically seen in the latter disorder[135]. Increased amounts of the abnormal polysaccharide have been found in the heart[87] and are probably also present in the kidneys[67]. Although clinical manifestations of cardiac involvement are rare, abnormalities of the electrocardiograms have been seen in some cases. The child studied by Clement[30] had cardiomegaly. There is usually no clinical evidence of renal involvement. Electron microscope studies of the histopathologic changes in the liver have been reported[5, 54]. Hepatic cirrhosis with portal hypertension can develop in some patients. Starzl and associates[184] have reported on an interesting patient in whom the operation of portocaval transposition was done, not only to alleviate portal hypertension but also as an attempt at decreasing the amount of glycogen in the liver. The basis for this is experimental evidence that the procedure (in which the proximal and distal ends of the portal vein are anastomosed respectively to the distal and proximal ends of the inferior vena cava) depletes the canine liver of glycogen. The operation alleviated the portal hypertension, reduced significantly the concentration of glycogen in the liver and lead to a marked spurt of growth in the patient; but it did not change the chemical abnormalities of hepatic function.

The content of glycogen is usually 12 to 17 per cent in the liver and 4 to 9 per cent in muscle. The concentrations in muscle are distinctly higher in Type IIIA than in Type IIIB. Huijing was the first to show the presence of debrancher enzyme in normal leucocytes and its absence in the leucocytes of patients with this disease[84, 198]. Hers found that the enzyme was also deficient in the erythrocytes[197]. The studies of Steinetz et al.[185] and of Williams and associates[211] suggest that the enzyme levels in the erythrocytes and leucocytes can be used to detect heterozygotes. In the majority of cases the parents are normal, although an adult patient mentioned by Larner[105] had two children affected by the disease. The defect seems to be inherited in an autosomal recessive pattern. Familial incidence is high, and parental consanguinity has been noted[53]. Illingworth and Brown[88] have reported on twenty-four patients, twelve of whom had affected sibs. Glycogenoses of Types I and III may occur in different members of the same family[20, 87, 88, 119].

TYPE VI: HEPATIC GLYCOGENOSIS; HERS' DISEASE

In 1959, Hers[62] described three cases of glycogenosis apparently caused by subnormal activity of hepatic phosphorylase, which was reduced to about 75 per cent of normal. The glycogen content of the liver was more than 12 per cent in two patients, but it was only 2.2 per cent in the third. There was no increase in muscle glycogen. It has been difficult to pinpoint the exact nature of the defect, because the activity of hepatic phosphorylase usually has been found only partially decreased and deficiencies of other enzymes are not infrequently present. Illingworth and Brown[88] do not equate Type VI disease with deficiency of hepatic phosphorylase but include in the group patients with hepatomegaly whose livers contain more than 12 per cent glycogen in the absence of glycogen storage in other tissues, and who do not share a common enzymatic ab-

normality. About one third of their cases of glycogenosis fall in this group.

Retarded growth and hepatomegaly are often the only signs of disease during the first year of life. Some have noted an increase in the size of the liver following a bout of fever[88]. In an unusual case described by Hug et al.[83], there developed progressive brain disease. Marked obesity is not common and hemostasis is normal[170]. Hypoglycemia occurs frequently but does not produce symptoms. As in Type I glycogenosis, there is tendency to hyperglycemia following meals. Little is known about the subsequent clinical course of the disease because very few of the reported cases have been observed for a long period of time. The disorder may be inherited as a dominant trait with incomplete penetrance[86, 208].

The values for hepatic glycogen content are usually intermediate between those generally found in Types I and III. The structure of the glycogen molecule is normal, although Bueding[18] has found it has a characteristic sedimentation pattern. Upon incubation of crude liver homogenates, its rate of disappearance is slower than in Type I disease[88]. In a group of seventeen patients, only nine had decreased activity of hepatic phosphorylase[88]. Low activity of this enzyme has been detected in leucocytes[86, 208,209]; in the three original cases it was about 25 per cent of the normal. Hülsmann and associates[86] also found low levels in the mother of one patient. Wallis, Sidbury and Harris[205] found the content of glycogen in erythrocytes to be a better genetic marker than the activity of phosphorylase in the leucocytes. In other glycogenoses, the activity of this leucocytic enzyme is normal[86,

[197, 209]. Apparently, the phosphorylase in white blood cells is more closely related to hepatic phosphorylase than to the enzyme in muscle. Significant reductions in phosphoglucomutase have been noted in liver and muscle[88, 191], but the importance of this finding has not been fully assessed. Illingworth and Brown[88] also noted decreases in hepatic glucose-6-phosphatase in eleven of thirty-three cases. The histopathologic changes in the liver have been studied with the electron microscope[8, 155].

DIFFERENTIATION OF GLYCOGENOSES TYPES I, III AND VI

There is no doubt that the decisive analysis is assay of enzyme activity. There are other differences between the three disorders, some of them of definite value in their differential diagnosis but none absolutely specific. Type I tends to be more severe and is the most likely to become manifest in the neonatal period. The mean concentrations of blood glucose are lower and the hyperlipemia and hyperlactidemia are more severe. Increases in the plasma levels of non-esterified fatty acids are particularly common in Type I. Sidbury[169a] found the highest degrees of ketosis in patients with Type III disease. Hyperuricemia occurs in the three disorders, but only in hepatorenal glycogenosis is it likely to be severe or to produce secondary gout. The glycogen concentration in muscle is normal in Types I and VI, although patients with Type I disease may develop myopathy. Primary renal involvement is a feature only in Type I glycogenosis.

In typical cases of hepatorenal glycogenosis, the injection of glucagon or epinephrine fails to produce the expected increase in the concentration of blood glucose[79, 81, 161, 162]. There occurs, in turn, a characteristic increase in the level of blood lactate[76, 115]. This test is of diagnostic value, but the results are not always clear-cut (sometimes there is noted a moderate but definite increase in the blood glucose level[142] and the concentration of lactate may change little or not at all[115]). Glucagon is preferred over epinephrine because it gives fewer unequivocal results and does not produce undesirable side effects. Whereas epinephrine causes hyperglycemia by activation of the phosphorylases in liver and muscle, glucagon produces the effect by activation of the hepatic enzyme only. In normal persons, the hyperglycemia which follows the infusion of glucagon is accompanied by an increase in the activity of glucose-6-phosphatase[19]. In Type III glycogenosis, two different responses may occur. In the fasting state, there is little or no effect on the level of blood glucose, since most of the polysaccharide in liver and muscle is limit dextrin, which is not degraded by phosphorylase. However, after a meal, the molecule of glycogen is reconstituted, and, since phosphorylase activity is unimpaired, the injection of glucagon or epinephrine causes a normal or near-normal response. This dual response is the basis of the "double glucagon test"[82, 112]. A similar response has been described in patients with "glycogen synthetase" deficiency[183]. In some patients with Type III disease, glucagon may be ineffective in both the fasting and postprandial states[12]. The glycemic response to glucagon or epinephrine in Type VI is usually subnormal[62, 103], but since this glycogenosis is a heterogeneous group the test is of limited value.

The galactose tolerance test, proposed by Schwartz and associates[162], consists of the intravenous injection of 1 gm of galactose per kg body weight. Blood samples are obtained prior to injection and at intervals up to forty-five minutes or one hour later. In normal persons, there occurs a definite rise in the blood level of glucose without a change in the level of lactate. Inasmuch as this metabolic effect cannot be mediated in the absence of glucose-6-phosphatase, the administration of galactose to patients with Type I glycogenosis causes little or no rise in the concentration of blood glucose, but there occurs a definite increase in the concentration of lactate. The abnormal response to galactose is a more sensitive index of hepatorenal glycogenosis than the abnormal response in the glucagon test. In the absence of hepatic insufficiency, it is almost diagnostic. The response to fructose is also abnormal[46, 64, 70]. In Types III and VI, galactose tolerance is normal.

Small amounts of glycogen can be detected in normal erythrocytes, leucocytes and platelets. Most of the glycogen of leucocytes is found in the granulocytes[136]. Increased amounts of glycogen in cells of the peripheral blood are seen most frequently with Type III glycogenosis[172]. The glycogen content of erythrocytes can be used as a marker of heterozygosity in some families. In Type VI, the concentration is often increased, but not as markedly as in Type III. Although some investigators have also found increased amounts in cases of Type I glycogenosis[196, 201], the majority have noted normal values[15, 171, 198].

TYPE II: GENERALIZED (CARDIAC, NEUROMUSCULAR) GLYCOGENOSIS; POMPE'S DISEASE

Although the excessive tissue deposition of glycogen is generalized, by far the highest concentrations occur in striated muscles and in the nervous system. Cardiac involvement usually produces the outstanding clinical manifestations of the disease[39], which may resemble endocardial fibroelastosis, myocarditis or aberrant origin of the left coronary artery. The first reported cases of Type II glycogenosis, recorded in 1932 by Pompe[143] and (according to Hers[66]) by Bischoff[11], were examples of the "cardiac type" of disease. In other patients, the skeletal muscles and nervous system are affected more severely, giving rise to a clinical picture like amyotonia congenita. This, the "neuromuscular form" of Type II glycogenosis, was first described by Gunther, in 1939[58]. Not infrequently, the symptoms and signs indicate involvement of both the cardiovascular and neuromuscular systems[29, 51, 102].

The clinical onset is usually during the first six months of life, earlier than in the other glycogenoses. The disease has been diagnosed as early as in the neonatal period[150]. Dyspnea, cyanosis and cardiac failure are characteristic findings. Muscular weakness and hypotonicity, macroglossia, anorexia, vomiting and retardation of growth occur frequently. The retardation of growth and macroglossia may cause confusion with cretinism and Down's syndrome[29]. Ocular lesions have been described[193]. It is often stated that hepatomegaly is a rare finding. However, Ehlers and associates[43] found that enlargement of the liver had been noted in thirty-one of fifty-four reported cases. The principal cause of hepatomegaly is cardiac failure, not the excessive deposition of glycogen in the liver. The spleen is not enlarged. The metabolic abnormalities which characterize Type I glycogenosis do not occur in Type II disease. The metabolic responses to the injection of glucagon, epinephrine or galactose are normal.

In the heart, glycogen accumulates chiefly in the myocardium and produces striking hypertrophy of the ventricles. The roentgenograms typically show diffuse, globular cardiomegaly. The myocardial hypertrophy can obstruct the outflow tracts of one or both ventricles[31, 43, 73], and can cause bulging of the ventricular septum to the right[167]. The electrocardiographic abnormalities are said to be characteristic — the combination of a short P-R interval with QRS and T waves of high voltage is seen in cases of Type II glycogenosis but apparently does not occur in infants with ventricular hypertrophy due to other causes. Some cases of myocardial glycogenosis are associated with endocardial fibroelastosis (Fig. 6)[212]. Dincsoy and associates[37] found this combination in eleven of sixty-one reported cases. In the patients in whom both lesions were present, the roentgenograms often showed enlargement of the left ventricle rather than the characteristic diffuse, globular cardiomegaly. This group also had a higher mean concentration of cardiac glycogen. Endocardial accumulation of glycogen is more likely to occur when there is coexisting fibroelastosis. In occasional cases of idiopathic endomyocardial fibrosis, biopsy

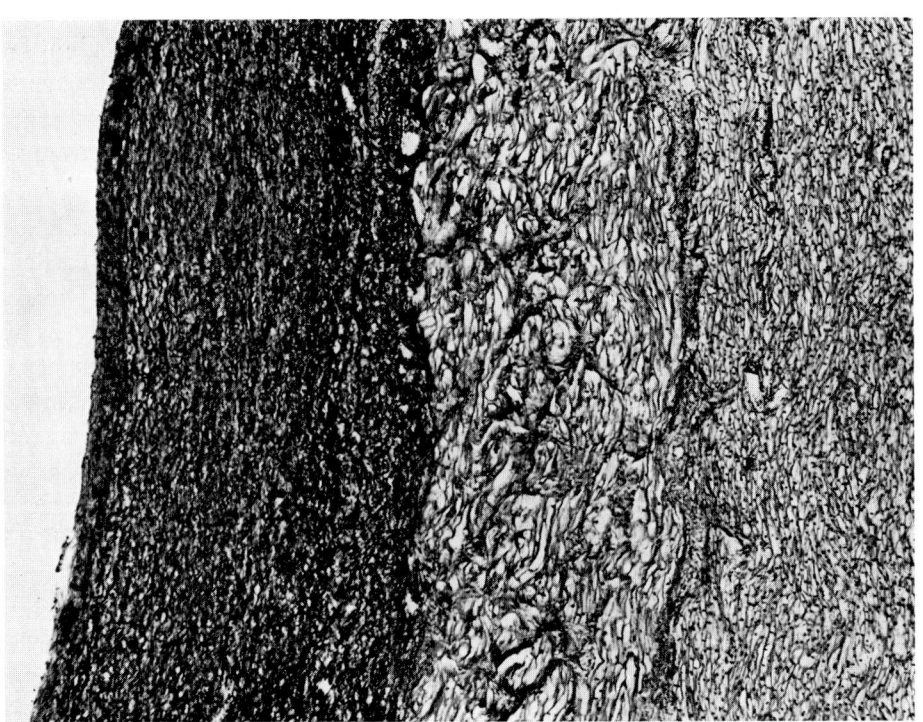

Fig. 6.   Endocardial fibroelastosis associated with myocardial glycogenosis, in a case of Pompe's disease. Weigert stain; x 50.

or postmortem studies have shown the presence of abnormally high amounts of glycogen in the myocardium[21, 125, 133]. In one case, deposits which stained with Best's carmine were seen in the heart and in other organs, but were resistant to the action of diastase. Whether or not such cases represent mild forms of cardiac glycogenosis, perhaps a *forme frustre* of the disease, can be answered unequivocally only by assays of enzyme activity in the tissue. Öckerman and Berlin[133] did assays in five such cases, from two families with idiopathic cardiomyopathy, and found normal activities of α-1, 4-glucosidase and other phosphorylytic enzymes in specimens of myocardium and skeletal muscle. In the usual case, the coarse vacuolation of myocardial fibers characteristic of cardiac glycogenosis is quite distinctive, and differs sharply from the fine vacuolation produced by other diseases. Although the myocar-

dium of the normal neonate may contain as much as 1 per cent glycogen, the amount rapidly decreases during the first few days of life[213]. This loss of myocardial glycogen is greater than normal in infants with the respiratory distress syndrome[166, 213], a loss which can be minimized or prevented by the administration of fructose[163], or by hypothermia[127]. Several histochemical studies of myocardial glycogen in neonates and infants have been published[130, 163, 166, 213, 214].

The skeletal muscles most severely affected are the tongue and the diaphragm. Although accumulation of glycogen can cause considerable distortion of the muscle fibers (Fig. 7), it does not elicit inflammation. Figures 8 and 9 illustrate characteristic lesions in the nervous system. Some have described tissue deposits of basophilic material, probably mucoprotein[164, 216], but we did not find them in a detailed study of

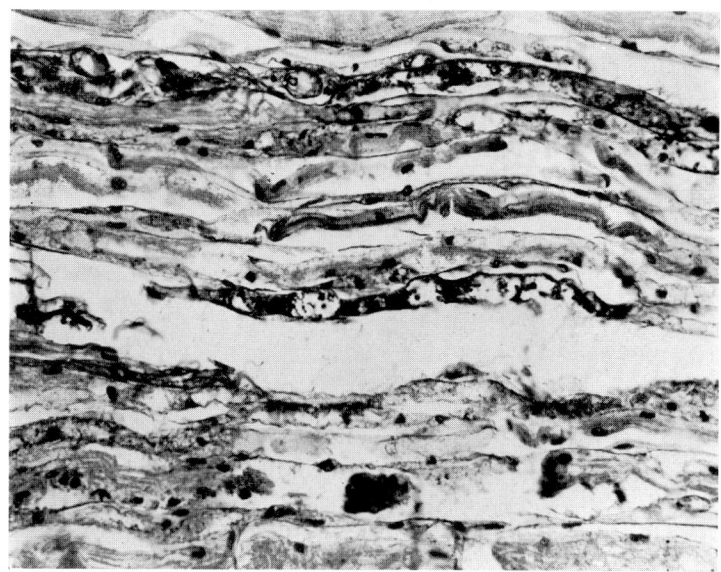

Fig. 7. Longitudinal section of gastroenemius muscle in case of Pompe's disease. There are present vacuolation and PAS-positive granules within the muscle fibers. Periodic acid-Schiff stain; x 260.

one case[118]. Additional histochemical studies of Type II glycogenosis have been reported by Crome and Zapella[36] and by us[118]. The glycogen found in this disease has a normal molecular structure and can be digested partially by incubation of tissue sections with diastase. The average concentrations of glycogen in skeletal muscle are generally higher than in the other glycogenoses which affect muscle (Table III). As a rule, the concentration of glycogen in the erythrocytes is normal.

The pathogenesis of Type II glycogenosis was clarified when Hers reported the absence of α-1, 4-glucosidase in the affected tissues[64, 65]. The enzyme cleaves the 1, 4 bonds of the glycogen molecule and has distinct maltase activity. Others have confirmed that the enzyme is inactive in the heart, muscles and liver[40, 85, 96]. The maltase activity of the erythrocytes was found to be normal[37], but it is not certain whether this activity indicates the same enzyme system. The other enzymes involved in the phosphorylytic catabolism of glycogen are normal[91]. Dincsoy and associates[37] assayed acid maltase in the umbilical cords and placentas of five newborn infants, siblings of patients with Type II glycogenosis. The four infants in whom placental and cord activity of acid maltase had been present were alive and well, whereas the only one in whom no activity was found later died of the disease. In human and rat tissues, α-1, 4-glucosidase is found within the lysosomes. Studies with the electron microscope[8, 22, 69] have shown that the excess glycogen accumulates within hepatocytes and Kupffer cells. Part of the intracellular glycogen appears scattered throughout the cytoplasm, but a large amount is also found within vacuoles enclosed by a single membrane[8, 69]. It is probable, but not proven, that these vacuoles are lyso-

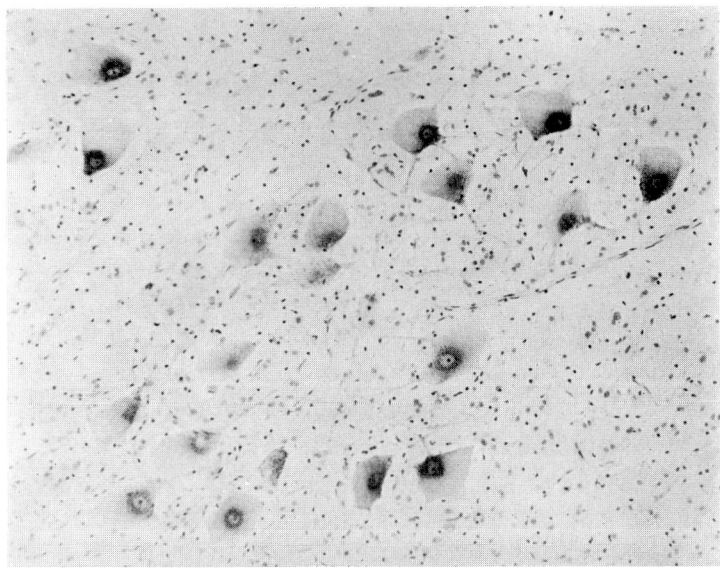

Fig. 8. Section of lumbar cord in a case of Pompe's disease. Marked ballooning of anterior horn cells is evident, with peripheral displacement of nucleus and remaining Nissl material. Cresyl violet stain; x120.

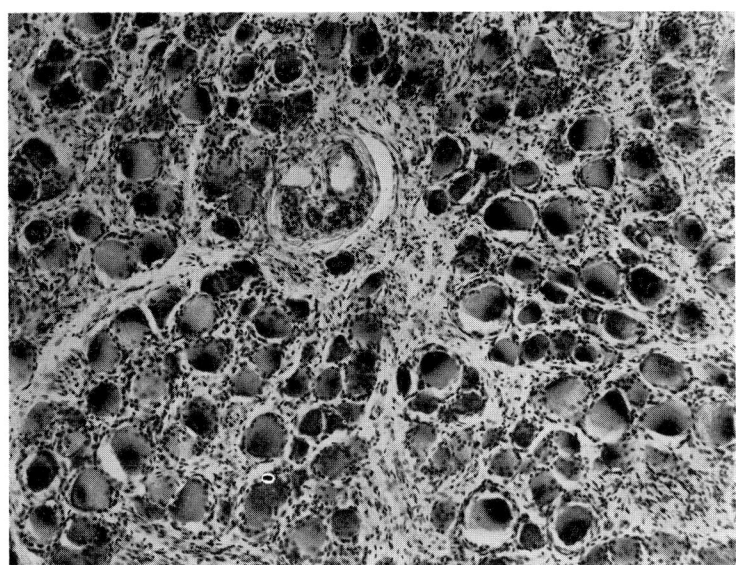

Fig. 9.   Section of distal root ganglion in a case of Pompe's disease. Many vacuolated, enlarged ganglion cells are present. Cresyl violet stain; x 90.

somes. In another study[22], it was found that although most of the intracellular glycogen in liver, kidney, smooth muscle and endothelium was located within cytoplasmic sacs, many of the deposits in the myocardium and in skeletal muscle were extra-saccular. Intra-saccular seggregation of glycogen granules has not been seen in electron-microscope studies of the other glycogenoses. The activity of acid phosphatase, another lysosomal enzyme, is reported to be increased[8, 89]. Such as singular localization isolates the glycogen granules from many cytoplasmic enzymes, including those involved in the breakdown of its molecule[66]. This explains the presence of excessive amounts of glycogen in a cell in which phosphorylase activity is normal, as well as the absence of abnormalities of carbohydrate metabolism in patients with the disease. However, it remains to be explained how the glycogen gets to the lysosomes in the first place. If Type II glycogenosis is indeed a "lysosomal disorder," it is puzzling that the excess of glycogen is not distributed in quantitative proportion to the number of lysosomes in a tissue, inasmuch as the liver has many more than cardiac or skeletal muscle. It has been suggested that the membranes are an effect, not the cause, of excessive glycogen deposition[54]. The less marked deposition of glycogen in the liver is also unusual, in view of the fact that acid maltase is about ten times more active in the liver than in muscle. As partial explanation of this discrepancy, it has been suggested that some of the hepatic glycogen may be excreted in the bile[67]. The subject of lysosomes was recently reviewed by Weissmann[207].

Sidbury[170] has reviewed the genetic pattern of Type II glycogenosis in a study of 116 patients from eighty different families. The frequency of affected infants was 47 per cent, and there was a slight but significant preponderance of affected males. In eight cases, the parents were consanguineous. The association of this disease with other hereditary or congenital abnormalities has been described in sporadic cases[25, 129, 170].

Type IV: Generalized (Hepatic) Glycogenosis; "Amylopectinosis"; Andersen's Disease

The first reported case, described by Andersen[5] in 1956, died at the age of seventeen months as a result of cirrhosis and hepatic failure. Postmortem examination of the liver disclosed not only changes characteristic of cirrhosis but also the presence of unusual pink, amorphous deposits associated with granulomatous inflammation. Further analysis of this material indicated a closer resemblance to the amylopectin of corn starch than to glycogen — it was sparingly soluble in water, the inner and outer chains of the molecule were twice as long as the chains of normal glycogen, and its spectrum showed maximal absorption at 550 mμ instead of 460 mμ. Consequently, the disorder was named amylopectinosis. Andersen examined postmortem microscopic sections of liver from two siblings of the patient who had died previously, and found similar histologic changes.

In 1962, Sidbury and associates[174] reported a second case of this disease. The clinical picture was similar, and death occurred at the age of four years. The material deposited in the liver resembled that found in Andersen's case, but was not associated with granulomatous inflammation. Similar deposits were also seen in the renal tubules, spleen, spinal cord, heart and smooth muscle. The fact that fibrosis did not

occur in association with the extra-hepatic deposits suggests, but does not prove, that the hepatic cirrhosis characteristic of Type IV glycogenosis is not merely a reactive fibrosis provoked by the formation of foreign material *in situ*. The material extracted from the liver in this case also has the same absorption spectrum as amylopectin. Whereas the biopsy material was relatively labile to the action of diastase, that obtained postmortem resisted digestion for thirty-two hours. The activity of hepatic glucose-6-phosphatase was reduced, but this has been shown to occur in patients with cirrhosis[61].

The cases of "familial metabolic disorder with storage of an unusual polysaccharide complex" reported by Craig and Uzman[34] in 1958 may be instances of this type of glycogenosis. Sidbury and associates[174] refer to an unpublished case; Recant[146] mentions another; and a third was presented at the 1965 slide seminar of the American Society of Clinical Pathologists (Fig. 10). Except for the reported presence of an abnormal glycogen in the erythrocytes[170], there is little in the clinical features of the disease that suggests a genetic defect of glycogen metabolism. The clinical picture is that of juvenile cirrhosis. The nature of the abnormality has not been found. It is assumed that there is deficiency of amylo-1, 4 → 1, 6-glucotransferase, the brancher enzyme. Hers[68] is of the opinion that such an enzymatic defect would not explain satisfactorily the molecular structure of the polysaccharide found in the tissues. He refers to an unpublished case in which large amounts of polysaccharide accumulated in the brain, although the structure and metabolism of glycogen

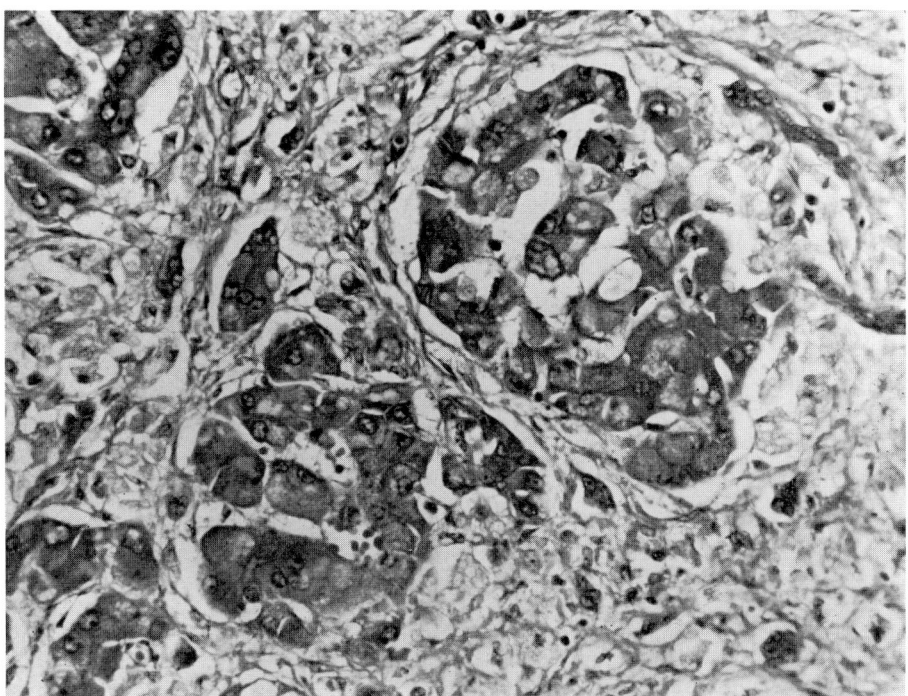

Fig. 10. Section of the liver in a case of Type IV glycogenosis (amylopectinosis). The abnormal intracellular deposits are associated with marked hepatic cirrhosis. Hematoxylin and eosin; x 250.

in the liver and muscles were normal. The findings suggest to him the existence of a defect in brain phosphorylase, which differs from the phosphorylase in liver and skeletal muscles but resembles the enzyme in smooth muscle.

TYPE V: MUSCLE GLYCOGENOSIS; McARDLE's DISEASE

The disease originally described by McArdle[123] in 1951 usually begins during childhood or adolescence and is characterized by easy muscular fatigability and cramping muscle pain following exercise. Transient myoglobinuria may occur after physical exertion. The great majority of patients are male, but cases in females have been reported, including a patient six years of age, the youngest ever reported[192]. Siblings

are frequently affected[107, 192], but the parents are asymptomatic. There is no test to detect heterozygosity. A high frequency of consanguinity has been noted[170]. Occasionally, the clinical onset is during adult life, and cramping muscular pain does not occur in all patients[44]. The occurrence of convulsions has been described[156]. In the original case, McArdle noted that the level of lactate in the blood did not rise following exercise, nor after the injection of epinephrine. The fact that the concentration of blood lactate does not rise (indeed, it may fall) after ischemic exercise has been repeatedly confirmed by others[44, 126, 128, 157, 158, 191] and is a valuable test for diagnosis. It is not absolutely specific because a similar response may occur in some patients with Type III glycogenosis[135], and, in certain undoubted cases of McArdle's disease, slight but definite rises in the blood levels of lactate and pyruvate have been noted[44, 107]. The functional capacity of the muscles is abnormally susceptible to ischemia. However, when the ischemia is removed, the blood flow in the muscle is much greater than in normal muscle after exercise of comparable intensity[123].

The concentration of blood glucose is normal and the glucose tolerance is not impaired[158]. However, the infusion of glucose markedly improves the tolerance of muscles to exercise[140]. A similar effect has been noted following the infusion of fructose[117, 140], or glucose and insulin[158]. There is a normal hyperglycemic reaction after the injection of epinephrine and, as expected, the glycemic response to glucagon is not impaired[123]. The leucocytes contain normal amounts of glycogen[158] and no defect has been found in the rate of glycolysis of incubated blood[123, 158]. As in other myopathies, the activities of serum aldolase and creatine phosphokinase may be increased[145]. The in vitro production of lactate by the erythrocytes is normal[141].

In 1959, separate reports by Schmid and Mahler[158] and by Mommaerts and associates[128] showed the nature of the defect to be inactivity or very low activity of muscle phosphorylase. Others have confirmed this, by bioassay[44, 116, 124, 126, 191] and immunoassay[45, 148, 154]. The enzyme can also be detected in muscle histochemically[44, 126, 154, 157]. The concentration of glycogen in muscle usually does not exceed 5 per cent[105, 188, 191], and occasionally it has been normal[44, 126]. The fact that much higher concentra-

tions are found in cases of Type II glycogenosis illustrates the importance of acid maltase in the degradation of muscle glycogen. The accumulated glycogen has a normal molecular structure. Apparently, it is not deposited in excess in myocardium or smooth muscle[97]. However, in a nineteen-year-old patient recently described, there were noted distinct abnormalities in the electrocardiogram[145]. Engel and associates[44] found no change in the phosphorylase of smooth muscle. Histologically, the presence of glycogen vacuoles, often as sarcolemmal blebs, is a frequent but not invariable finding. Foci of necrosis in muscle have been seen[72], but are probably an effect of excessive exercise and not a primary feature of the disease[124]. A recent electron-microscope study of two cases[160] showed that the principal change was disorganization of the myofibrils at the I band due to accumulation of glycogen in the interfibrillary spaces. A biopsy specimen studied thirty minutes after the onset of ischemic exercise disclosed changes in the mitochondria and dilatation of the sarcoplasmic reticulum.

The activities of acid maltase, amylo-1, 6-glucosidase and the kinases which activate and inactivate phosphorylase are normal[45, 105, 106, 128, 159]. The fact that UDPG pyrophosphorylase and UDPG glucotransferase are normal is good evidence that glycogen synthesis is normal[128]. However, in a case studied by Schmid and Mahler[158a], the activity of the latter enzyme was about half the normal. Although some investigators have found unaltered activity of phosphoglucomutase[105], others have found it definitely reduced[158a]. The significance of this finding has not been fully explained. Contracture of ischemic muscle in two cases did not produce a detectable decrease in ATP[153].

TYPE VII

Studies by Hers[68] on two patients with a previously unclassified form of glycogen storage disease have delineated what is very likely a new type of glycogenosis, now designated as Type VII. The defect appears to be deficiency of phosphorylase *b* kinase in muscle. The enzyme catalyzes the conversion of phosphorylase *b* to phosphorylase *a*, the active form. Activity of the enzyme in muscle was about one tenth of the normal, but in the liver it was only slightly less than in control specimens. The case recently described by Gutman and associates[59] is similar in many ways and may represent the third reported example of this disease, although assays of phosphorylase *b* kinase had not been carried out at the time of the report. The disorder was characterized by hepatic cirrhosis, splenomegaly, retarded growth, osteoporosis, renal glucosuria and changes in the electrocardiogram. The structure of glycogen was normal, and there was a normal response to the injection of epinephrine, glucagon and galactose. The activities of the enzymes known to be involved in the other glycogenoses were not affected. A recent report described the electron-microscope changes in the liver of another case[54].

DEFICIENCY OF "GLYCOGEN SYNTHETASE"
(GLYCOGEN STORAGE DEFICIENCY)

In 1963, Lewis, Spencer-Peet and Stewart[111] reported clinical and biochemical studies on identical twins who suffered from severe hypoglycemia after an overnight fast. Analyses of a liver specimen from one of the patients revealed low content of glycogen as well as absence of UDPG — glycogen transglucosylase ("glycogen synthetase"). Further studies[183] have confirmed and amplified these findings, delineating thus a new genetic error of glycogen metabolism characterized, not by excessive storage, but by glycogen depletion. The main feature of the disorder is the failure of the patient to maintain a normal concentration of blood glucose during a fast. Mental deficiency may occur in severe cases. The hypoglycemia is typically unassociated with increased secretion of epinephrine, and the administration of insulin does not cause an increase in the excretion of catecholamines and their metabolites. Intestinal absorption is normal, but the rate at which absorbed glucose is cleared from the blood is decreased. As a result, in the standard oral glucose tolerance test the levels of blood glucose are abnormally elevated two hours after feeding. There is reduction in the renal threshold for glucose and intermittent glucosuria may occur. Mild ketonuria is noted during periods of hypoglycemia, but acidosis does not usually develop. The plasma concentrations of cholesterol, phospholipids and bicarbonate are normal, and there is no evidence of hyperinsulinism. During the times of hypoglycemia, the intramuscular injection of glucagon produces little or no increase in the concentration of blood glucose. Postprandially, however, the glycemic response to glucagon is normal. It is of interest that the injection of epinephrine can raise the level of blood glucose even when glucagon has no effect. The plasma cortisol levels are moderately elevated, and ACTH can prevent hypoglycemia[182].

If the specimen of liver is obtained six hours or more after a meal, its glycogen content is found to be significantly decreased. This is associated with an increase in the content of fat, up to about 10 per cent of the wet weight. In the patients studied by Spencer-Peet and associates, the glycogen content of whole blood was decreased. The inactivity of hepatic "glycogen synthetase" is demonstrable even when glucose-6-phosphate is added to the liver homogenates, an important finding since the latter substance activates "glycogen synthetase." The enzyme was present in the erythrocytes of the patients and their parents[182]. This may mean either that the enzyme in the erythrocytes differs genetically from that in the liver, or that the inactivity of the hepatic enzyme is caused by an inhibitor.

The family studied by Spencer-Peet and associates[182] consisted of two adults and their five children. Another case was recently reported by Parr and others[138]. The patient, a female infant aged four months, had severe hypoglycemia, acidosis and hepatomegaly. The concentration of glycogen was 0.17 per cent in the liver and 0.05 per cent in muscle. Marked deficiency of "glycogen synthetase" and phosphorylase was found in specimens of liver and muscle, and the activity of muscle phosphoglucomutase was almost nil. In the postmortem examination, severe fatty change was found in the liver and the kidneys. A reported case of defective glycogen synthesis associated with leprechaunism is probably another example of this disorder[13].

REFERENCES

1. Abramson, H., and Kurtz, L. D.: Familial glycogen disease. Report of four fatal cases of the hepatic form of the disease in siblings of one family. Amer. J. Dis. Child.,72:510-520, 1946.

2. Adrouny, G. A., and Russell, J. A.: Effects of growth hormone and nutritional status on cardiac glycogen in the rat. Endocrinology, 59:241-251, 1956.

3. Alagille, D., Gabilan, J.-C., and Lelong, M.: Les anomalies plaquettaires au cours de glycogénoses hépatiques. Helv. Paediat. Acta, 18:120-137, 1963.

4. Aldullah, M., Taylor, P. M., and Whelan, W. J.: The enzymic debranching of glycogen and the role of transferase. In Whelan, W. J., and Cameron, M. P. (eds.): Control of Glycogen Metabolism. Ciba Foundation Symposium. London, Churchill, 1964, pp. 123-138.

5. Andersen, D. H.: Familial cirrhosis of the liver with storage of abnormal glycogen. Lab. Invest., 5:11-20, 1956.

6. Auerbach, V. H., and DiGeorge, A. M.: One gene, more than one enzyme? Von Gierke's disease a case in point (Abstract). Amer. J. Dis. Child., 102:578, 1961.

7. Auerbach, V. H., and DiGeorge, A. M.: Multiple enzymatic defects in glycogenoses, a challenge to the one gene one enzyme concept (Abstract). Fed. Proc., 22:650, 1963.

7a. Barker, S. A., Stacey, M., and Al-Farisi, M. A. L.: A chemical investigation of two cases of glycogen storage disease. Clin. Chim. Acta, 8:311-314, 1963.

8. Baudhuin, P., Hers, H. G., and Loeb, H.: An electron microscopic and biochemical study of type II glycogenosis. Lab. Invest., 13:1139-1152, 1964.

9. Bauer, Von B.: Über eine Sonderform der Gierkeschen Glykogenose mit Aktivitätssteigerung der α-Glukosidase in der Leber bei vollständigem Glukose-6-phosphatase-Mangel. Helv. Paediat. Acta, 19:13-28, 1964.

10. Bergström, J., Findor, J., and Hultman, E.: The contents of glycogen and potassium in human liver tissue obtained by needle biopsy. Scand. J. Clin. Lab. Invest., 13:353-354, 1961.

11. Bischoff, G.: Zum klinischen Bild der Glykogen-Speicherungskrankheit (Glykogenose). Z. Kinderheilk., 52:722, 1932.

12. Brandt, I. K., and DeLuca, V. A., Jr.: Debrancher deficiency glycogenosis: tissue specificity (Abstract). J. Pediat., 67:937, 1965.

13. Brandt, I. K., and Seidenberg, M.: Leprechaunism and defective glycogen synthesis (Abstract). J. Pediat., 63:776, 1963.

14. Brante, G. K., Kaijer, K., and Öckerman, P. A.: Glycogenosis type I (lack of glucose-6-phosphatase) in four siblings. Acta Paediat. (Suppl.), 157:3-28, 1964.

15. Briggs, J. N., and Haworth, J. C.: Liver glycogen disease. Report of a case of hyperuricemia, renal calculi and no demonstrable enzyme defect. Amer. J. Med., 36:443-449, 1964.

16. Brown, D. H., and Illingworth, B.: The role of oligo-1, 4 → 1, 4 glucotransferase and amylo-1, 6-glucosidase in the debranching of glycogen. In Whelan and Cameron, op. cit., pp. 139-150.

17. Brown, D. H., Illingworth, B., and Cori, C. F.: Combined action of oligo-1, 4 → 1, 4-glucotransferase and amylo-1, 6-glucosidase in debranching glycogen. Nature (London), 197:980-982, 1963.

18. Bueding, E., Orrell, S. A., Jr., and Sidbury, J.: Studies of storage disease glycogens. In Whelan and Cameron, op. cit., pp. 387-392.

19. Cahill, G. F., Jr., Zottu, S., and Earle, A. S.: In vivo effects of glucagon on hepatic glycogen, phosphorylase and glucose-6-phosphatase. Endocrinology, 60:265-269, 1957.

20. Calderbank, A., Kent, P. W., Larber, J., Manners, D. J., and Wright, A.: Biochemical investigation of a case of glycogen storage disease (von Gierke's disease). Biochem. J., 74:223-229, 1960.

21. Caplan, H.: A case of endocardial fibroelastosis with features of glycogen-storage disease. J. Path. Bact., 76:77-82, 1958.

22. Cardiff, R. D., and Wellings, S. R.: An electron microscopic study of Pompe's disease (Abstract). Lab. Invest., 14:599, 1965.

23. Carroll, N. V., Longley, R. W., and Roe, J. H.: The determination of glycogen in liver and muscle by use of anthrone reagent. J. Biol. Chem., 220:583-593, 1956.

24. Chaptal, J., Jean, R., and Guillaumot, R.: Glycogenic polycoria caused by deficiency of amylo-1, 6-glucosidase in the liver without muscular abnormality. Fr. Arch. Franc. Pediat., 17:1117-1125, 1960.

25. Childs, A. W., Crose, R. F., and Henderson, P. H.: Glycogen disease of the heart. Report of two cases occurring in siblings. Pediatrics, 10:208-216, 1952.

26. Chiquoine, A. D.: Distribution of glucose-6-phosphatase in the liver and kidney of the mouse. J. Histochem. Cytochem., 1:429-435, 1953.

27. Chiquoine, A. D.: Further studies on the histochemistry of glucose-6-phosphatase. J. Histochem. Cytochem., 3:471-478, 1955.

28. Ciba Foundation Symposium: Control of Glycogen Metabolism. Boston, Little, 1964.

29. Clement, D. H., and Godman, G. C.: Glycogen-disease resembling mongolism, cretinism, and amyotonia congenita. J. Pediat., 36:11-30, 1950.

30. Clément, R.: Glycogénose type III de Cori et hypoglycémie par hypersensibilité a l'insuline. Presse. Med., 72:1057-1058, 1964.

31. Cohen, J., Effat, H., Goodwin, J. F., Oakley, C. M., and Steiner, R. E.: Hypertrophic obstructive cardiomyopathy. Brit. Heart J., 26:16-32, 1964.

32. Cori, G. T.: Glycogen structure and enzyme deficiencies in glycogen storage disease. Harvey Lect., 48:145-171, 1953.

33. Cori, G. T., and Cori, C. F.: Glucose-6-phosphatase of the liver in glycogen storage disease. J. Biol. Chem., 199:661-667, 1952.

34. Craig, J. M., and Uzman, L.: A familial metabolic disorder with storage of an unusual polysaccharide complex. Pediatrics, 2:20-32, 1958.

35. Crawford, T.: Glycogen disease. Quart. J. Med., 15:285-298, 1946.

36. Crome, L., Cumings, J. N., and Duckett, S.: Neuropathological and neurochemical aspects of generalized glycogen storage disease. J. Neurol., Neurosurg., Psychiat., 26:422-430, 1963.

37. Dincsoy, M. Y., Dincsoy, H. P., Kessler, A. D., Jackson, M. A., and Sidbury, J. B., Jr.: Generalized glycogenosis and associated endocardial fibroelastosis. Report of 3 cases with biochemical studies. J. Pediat., 67:728-740, 1965.

38. diSant'Agnese, P. A.: cited by Shwachman, H.[168], p. 148.

39. diSant'Agnese, P. A., Anderson, D. H., and Mason, H. H.: Glycogen storage disease of the heart: II. Critical review of the literature. Pediatrics, 6:607-624, 1950.

40. diSant'Agnese, P. A., and Gabriel, O.: cited by Dincsoy, M. Y., et al.[37], p. 729.

41. Eberlein, W. R., Brown, B. I., and Sidbury, J. B.: Glycogen storage disease in siblings due to different enzyme defects and favorable response to treatment with fluoxymesterone (Abstract). Amer. J. Dis. Child., 102:491-492, 1961.

42. Eberlein, W. R., Illingworth, B. A., and Sidbury, J. B.: Heterogeneous glycogen storage disease in siblings and favorable response to synthetic androgen administration. Amer. J. Med., 33:20-26, 1962.

43. Ehlers, K. H., Hagstrom, J. W. C., Lukas, D. S., Redo, S. F., and Engle, M. A.: Glycogen-storage disease of the myocardium with obstruction to the left ventricular outflow. Circulation, 25:96-109, 1962.

44. Engel, W. K., Eyerman, E. L., and Williams, H. E.: Late-onset type of skeletal-muscle phosphorylase deficiency: A new familial variety with completely and partially affected subjects. New Eng. J. Med., 268: 135-137, 1963.

45. Fahn, S., Schotland, D. L., and Rowland, L. P.: McArdle's disease: Hereditary myopathy due to absence of muscle phosphorylase. Trans. Amer. Neurol. Ass., 88: 145-147, 1963.

46. Fernandes, J., and van de Kamer, J. H.: Studies on the utilization of hexoses in liver glycogen disease. Pediatrics, 35:470-481, 1965.

47. Field, J. B., Epstein, S., and Egan, T.: Studies in glycogen storage diseases. I. Intestinal glucose-6-phosphatase activity in patients with von Gierke's disease and their parents. J. Clin. Invest., 44:1240-1247, 1965.

48. Field, R. A.: Glycogen deposition diseases. In Stanbury, J. B., Wyngaarden, J. B., and Fredrickson, D. S. (eds.): The Metabolic Basis of Inherited Disease. New York, McGraw, 1960, pp. 156-207.

49. Forbes, G. B.: Glycogen-storage disease: Report of case with abnormal glycogen structure in liver and skeletal muscle. J. Pediat., 42:645-653, 1953.

50. French, D.: Structure of glycogen and its amylolytic degradation. In Whelan and Cameron, op. cit., pp. 7-24.

51. Friedman, S., and Ashe, R.: Glycogen storage disease of the heart. Clinical observations in five infants. J. Pediat., 52:635-648, 1958.

52. Gabilan, J. C.: Les glycogénoses hépatiques. Rev. Int. Hépat., 10:699-818, 1960.

53. Gabilan, J. C.: Étude génétique des glycogénoses. Sem. Hop. Paris, 40:1017-1019, 1964.

54. Garancis, J. C., Hug, G., Schubert, W. K., and Kaplan, S.: Electron Microscopy of Glycogen Storage Diseases Type II, III, VI, and VII. Presented at meeting of Amer. Soc. Clin. Path., Chicago, October, 1965.

55. Goldfinger, S., Klinenberg, J. R., and Seegmiller, J. E.: Renal retention of uric acid induced by infusion of β-hydroxybutyrate and acetoacetate. New Eng. J. Med., 272: 351-355, 1965.

56. Greengard, O., Weber, G., and Singhal, R. L.: Glycogen deposition in the liver induced by cortisone: Dependence on enzyme synthesis. Science, 141:160-161, 1963.

57. Guest, G. M.: The Mauriac syndrome. Dwarfism, hepatomegaly and obesity with juvenile diabetes mellitus (Editorial). Diabetes, 2:415-417, 1953.

58. Gunther, R.: Beitrag zur Kenntnis der Glykogenspeicherungskrankheit. Virchow. Arch. Path. Anat., 304:87, 1939.

59. Gutman, A., Rachmilewitz, E. A., Stein, O., Eliakim, M., and Stein, Y.: Glycogen storage disease. Report of a case with generalized glycogenosis without demonstable enzyme defect. Israel J. Med. Sci., 1:14-25, 1965.

60. Harris, R. C., and Cohen, H. J.: Sweat electrolytes in glycogen storage disease, type I. Pediatrics, 31:1044-1046, 1963.

61. Harris, R., and Olmo, C.: Liver and kidney glucose-6-phosphatase activity in children with normal and diseased organs. J. Clin. Invest., 33:1204-1209, 1954.

62. Hers, H. G.: Études enzymatiques sur fragments hepatiques; application à la classification des glycogenoses. Rev. Int. Hépat., 9: 35-55, 1959.

63. Hers, H. G.: Amylo-1:6-glucosidase activity in tissues of children with glycogen-storage disease. Biochem, J., 76:69P, 1960.

64. Hers, H. G.: Recent developments in the biochemistry of glycogen storage disease and fructose intolerance. Chem. Weekbl., 57:457, 1961.

65. Hers, H. G.: Alpha-glucosidase deficiency in generalized glycogen-storage disease (Pompe's disease). Biochem. J., 86:11-16, 1963.

66. Hers, H. G.: Glycogen storage disease, type II. In Whelan and Cameron, op. cit., pp. 354-363.

66a. Hers, H. G.: in a discussion of paper by Manners, D. J., op. cit., p. 333.

67. Hers, H. G.: Glycogen storage disease. In Levine, R., and Luft, R. (eds.): Advanced Metabolic Disorders, Vol. I. New York, Academic Press, 1964, pp. 1-44.

68. Hers, H. G.: Future trends in the investigation of glycogen storage disease. Israel J. Med. Sci., 1:6-8, 1965.

69. Hers, H. G., Bandhium, P., and Loeb, H.: An electron microscopic and biochemical study of type II glycogenosis. Lab. Invest., 13:1140-1152, 1964.

70. Hers, H. G., and Malbrain, H.: cited by Field, R. A.[48], p. 181.

71. Hess, W. C., Shaffran, I. P., and Everitt, E. L.: Effect of cortisone on liver phosphorylase activity. Proc. Soc. Exp. Biol. Med., **103**:695-697, 1960.

72. Hockaday, T. D. R., and Downey, J. A.: McArdle's syndrome. Lancet, **1**:1185, 1962.

73. Hohn, A. R., Lowe, C. U., Sokal, J. E., and Lambert, E. C.: Cardiac problems in the glycogenoses with specific reference to Pompe's disease. Pediatrics, **35**:313-319, 1965.

74. Holling, H. E.: Gout and glycogen storage disease. Ann. Intern. Med., **58**:654-663, 1963.

75. Howell, R. R.: The interrelationship of glycogen storage disease and gout. Arthritis Reum., **8**:780-785, 1965.

76. Howell, R. R., Ashton, D. M., and Wyngaarden, J. B.: Glucose-6-phosphatase deficiency glycogen storage disease. Studies on the interrelationships of carbohydrate, lipid, and purine abnormalities. Pediatrics, **29**:553-565, 1962.

77. Hsia, D. Y. Y.: Blood glucose-6-phosphate in heterozygous carriers and patients with liver glycogen disease (von Gierke's disease). Nature (London), **192**:266-267, 1961.

78. Hsia, D. Y. Y., and Kot, E. G.: Detection of heterozygous carriers in glycogen storage disease of the liver (von Gierke's disease). Nature (London), **183**:1331-1332, 1959.

79. Hubble, D.: Glucagon and glycogen storage disease of the liver. Lancet, **1**:235-237, 1954.

80. Hug, G.: Degradation of glycogen in tissues from generalized glycogen storage disease. Biochim. Biophys. Acta, **47**:271-274, 1961.

81. Hug, G.: Glucagon tolerance test in glycogen storage disease. J. Pediat., **60**:545-549, 1962.

82. Hug, G., Krill, C. E., Jr., Perrin, E. V., and Guest, G. M.: Cori's disease (amylo-1, 6-glucosidase deficiency) — report of a case in a Negro child. New Eng. J. Med., **268**:113-120, 1963.

83. Hug, G., Schubert, W. K., and Shwachman, H.: Imbalance of liver phosphorylase and accumulation of hepatic glycogen in a girl with progressive disease of the brain. J. Pediat., **67**:741-750, 1965.

84. Huijing, F.: Amylo-1, 6-glucosidase activity in normal leucocytes and in leucocytes of patients with glycogen storage disease. Clin. Chim. Acta, **9**:269-272, 1964.

85. Huijing, F., van Creveld, S., and Losekoot, G.: Diagnosis of generalized glycogen-storage disease (Pompe's disease). J. Pediat., **63**:984-987, 1963.

86. Hülsmann, W. C., Oei, T. L., and van Creveld, S.: Phosphorylase activity in leucocytes from patients with glycogen-storage disease. Lancet, **2**:581-583, 1961.

87. Illingworth, B.: Glycogen storage disease. Amer. J. Clin. Nutr., **9**:683-690, 1961.

88. Illingworth, B., and Brown, D. H.: Glycogen storage diseases, types III, IV and VI. In Whelan and Cameron, op. cit., pp. 336-349.

89. Illingworth, B., and Cori, C. F.: Glucose-6-phosphatase and pyrophosphatase activities of homogenates of livers from patients with glycogen storage disease. Biochem. Biophys. Res. Commun., **19**:10-14, 1965.

90. Illingworth, B., and Cori, G. T.: Stucture of glycogens and amylopectins. III. Normal and abnormal human glycogen. J. Biol. Chem., **199**:653-660, 1952.

91. Illingworth, B., Cori, G. T., and Cori, C. F.: Amylo-1, 6-glucosidase in muscle tissue in generalized glycogen storage disease. J. Biol. Chem., **218**:123-129, 1956.

92. Jeandet, J., and Lestradet, H.: L'hyperlactacidémie, cause probable de l'hyperuricémie dans la glycogénose hépatique. Rev. Franç. D'Etud. Clin. Biol., **6**:71-72, 1961.

93. Jeune, M. A., Charrat, A., and Bertrand, J.: Polycorie hépatique hypéruricemie et goutte. Arch. Franc. Pediat., **14**:897-909, 1957.

94. Jeune, M. A., François, R., Bertrand, J., and Jarlot, B.: Sur certaines modifications biologiques et sur l'evolution lointaine de las polycorie glycogenique hépatique à propos de 9 observations. Mod. Prob. Paediat., **4**:209-223, 1959.

95. Jeune, M., François, R., and Jarlot, B.: Contribution à l'étude des polycories glycogéniques du foie. Rev. Int. Hépat., **9**:1-33, 1959.

96. Kahana, D., Telem, Ch., Steinitz, K., and Solomon, M.: Generalized glycogenosis. Report of a case with deficiency of alpha glucosidase. J. Pediat., **65**:243-251, 1964.

97. Kirsten, W. H., and Schmid, R.: cited by Schmid, R., in a discussion of paper by J. Larner[105], p. 375.

98. Klinenberg, J. R., Alepa, F. P., Howell, R. R., and Seegmiller, J. E.: A relationship between adult glycogen storage disease and tophaceous gout. Clin. Res., **11**:221, 1963.

99. Kolb, F. O., deLalla, O. F., and Gofman, J. W.: The hyperlipemias in disorders of carbohydrate metabolism. Serial lipoprotein studies in diabetic acidosis with xanthomatosis and in glycogen storage disease. Metabolism, **4**:310-317, 1955.

100. Koulischer, N., and Pickering, D. E.: Glyco-gen-storage disease. A study on the effect of sodium 1-thyroxine and glucagon. Amer. J. Dis. Child., **91**:103-112, 1956.

101. Krebs, E. G., Gonzalez, C., Posner, J. B., Love, D. S., Bratvold, G. E., and Fischer, E. H.: Interconversion reactions of muscle phosphorylases b and a. In Whelan and Cameron, op. cit., pp. 200-210.

102. Krivit, W., Polglase, W. J., Gunn, F. D., and Tyler, F. H.: Studies in disorders of muscle. IX. Glycogen storage disease primarily affecting skeletal muscle and clinically resembling amyotonia congenita. Pediatrics, **12**:165-177, 1953.

103. Lamy, M., Dubois, R., Rossier, A., Frezal, J., Leob, H., and Blancher, G.: La glyco-génose par deficience en phosphorylase hépatique. Arch. Franc. Pediat., **17**:1-24, 1960.

104. Larner, J.: Genetic and hormonal control of glycogen metabolism. Fed. Proc., **19**:971-976, 1960.

105. Larner, J.: Glycogen storage disease, type V. In Whelan and Cameron, op. cit., p. 371.

106. Larner, J., and Villar-Palasi, C.: Enzymes in glycogen storage myopathy. Proc. Nat. Acad. Sci. U.S.A., **45**:1234-1235, 1959.

107. Lehoczky, T., Halasy, M., Simon, G., and Harmos, G.: Skeletal muscle glycogenosis in identical twins. Brit. Med. J., **2**:802, 1964.

108. Leloir, L. F., and Cardini, C. E.: Bio-synthesis of glycogen from uridine diphos-phate glucose. J. Amer. Chem. Soc., **79**:6340-6341, 1957.

109. Leonard, S. L.: The effect of hormones on phosphorylase activity in skeletal muscle. Endocrinology, **60**:619-624, 1957.

110. Lestradet, H.: Glycogénose hépatique se-condaire le syndrome de Mauriac. Sem. Hop. Paris, **40**:1030-1037, 1964.

111. Lewis, G. M., Spencer-Peet, J., and Stew-art, K. M.: Infantile hypoglycaemia due to inherited deficiency of glycogen synthetase in liver. Arch. Dis. Child., **38**:40-48, 1963.

112. Limbeck, G. A., and Kelley, V. C.: "Double-barrel" glucagon test. Correlation with en-zyme assays in limit dextrinoses. Amer. J. Dis. Child., **109**:162-164, 1965.

113. Linneveh and Löhr: cited by J. C. Gabilan[53], p. 1017.

114. Lowe, C. U., and Mosovich, L. L.: The paradoxical effect of alcohol on carbohy-drate metabolism in four patients with liver glycogen disease. Pediatrics, **35**:1005-1008, 1965.

115. Lowe, C. U., Sokal, J. E., Mosovich, L. L., Sarcione, E. J., and Doray, B. H.: Studies in liver glycogen disease. Effects of glucagon and other agents on metabolic pattern and clinical status. Amer. J. Med., **33**:4-19, 1962.

116. Mahler, R. F. and McArdle, B.: Specific enzyme defect in glycogen breakdown caus-ing a myopathy (Abstract). Quart. J. Med., **29**:638-639, 1960.

117. Mahler, R., Mellick, R. S., and Hughes, B. P.: Hereditary absence of muscle phos-phorylase (McArdle's syndrome). Lancet, **1**:1234-1235, 1962.

118. Mancall, E. L., Aponte, G. E., and Berry, R. G.: Pompe's disease (diffuse glycogeno-sis) with neuronal storage. J. Neuropath. Exp. Neurol., **24**:85-96, 1965.

119. Manners, D. J.: α-1, 4-glucosans. II. Molec-ular structure of the liver glycogen from a case of Von Gierke's disease. J. Chem. Soc., 3527-3530, 1954.

120. Manners, D. J.: Glycogen storage disease, type I. in Control of Glycogen Metabolism, Ciba Foundation Symposium; Eds.: W. J. Whelan and M. P. Cameron, London: J. & A. Churchill, Ltd., p. 371, 1964.

121. Mason, H. H., and Andersen, D. H.: Glyco-gen disease of the liver (von Gierke's dis-ease) with hepatomata. Case report with metabolic studies. Pediatrics, **16**:785-800, 1955.

122. Mason, H. H., and Sly, G. E.: Blood lactic acid in liver glycogen disease. Proc. Soc. Exp. Biol. Med., **53**:145-147, 1943.

123. McArdle, B.: Myopathy due to a defect in muscle glycogen breakdown. Clin. Sci., **10**:13-33, 1951.

124. McArdle, B.: Metabolic myopathies. The glycogenoses affecting muscle, and hypo- and hyperkalemic periodic paralysis. Amer. J. Med., **35**:661-672, 1963.

125. Mehrizi, A., and Oppenheimer, E. H.: Heart failure associated with unusual deposition of glycogen in the myocardium. Bull. Johns Hopkins Hosp., **107**:329-336, 1960.

126. Mellick, R. S., Mahler, R. F., and Hughes, B. P.: McArdle's syndrome: phosphorylase-deficient myopathy. Lancet, **1**:1045-1048, 1962.

127. Miller, J. A., Jr., Zakhary, R., and Miller, F. S.: Hypothermia, asphyxia and cardiac glycogen in guinea pigs. Science, **144**:1226-1227, 1964.

128. Mommaerts, W. F. H. M., Illingworth, B., Pearson, C. M., Guillory, R. J., and Soraydarian, K.: A functional disorder of muscle associated with absence of phosphorylase. Proc. Nat. Acad. Sci. U.S.A., **45**:791, 1959.

129. Monnet, P., Larbre, F., Ganthier, J., and Verneg, R.: Glycogénose cardiomusculaire du nourisson, essai de détermination de trouble enzymatique. Pediatrie, **15**:60-62, 1960.

130. Mowry, R. W. and Bangle, R., Jr.: Histochemically demonstrable glycogen in the human heart, with special reference to glycogen storage disease and diabetes mellitus. Amer. J. Path., **27**:611-625, 1951.

131. Öckerman, P. A.: Glycerol in plasma in glycogenosis of Cori's type I. Clin. Chim. Acta, **8**:910-913, 1963.

132. Öckerman, P. A.: Glucose-6-phosphatase in human jejunal mucosa. Lack of activity in glycogenosis of Cori's type I. Clin. Chim. Acta, **9**:151, 1964.

133. Öckerman, P. A., and Berlin, S.-O.: Biochemical studies in familial cardiomyopathy. With special reference to the differential diagnosis from known types of glycogen storage disease. Acta Med. Scand., **176**:277-285, 1964.

134. Oei, T. L.: Hexose monophosphate, pyruvate and lactate in the peripheral blood in glycogen-storage disease, type I. Clin. Chim. Acta, **7**:193-198, 1962.

135. Oliner, L., Schulman, M., and Larner, J.: Myopathy associated with glycogen deposition resulting from generalized lack of amylo-1, 6-glucosidase. Clin. Res., **9**:243, 1961.

136. Olsson, I., Dahlqvist, A., and Nordén, Å.: Glycogen content of leukocytes and platelets. Acta Med. Scand., **174**:123-127, 1963.

137. Orrell, S. A., Bueding, E. and Reissig, M.: Physical characteristics of undegraded glycogen. In Whelan and Cameron, op. cit., pp. 29-44.

138. Parr, J., Teree, T. M., and Larner, J.: Symptomatic hypoglycemia, visceral fatty metamorphosis, and aglycogenosis in an infant lacking glycogen synthetase and phosphorylase. Pediatrics, **35**:770-777, 1965.

139. Patrick, S. J. and Tulloch, J. A.: Glucose-6-phosphatase activity in human diabetes. Lancet, **1**:811-812, 1957.

140. Pearson, C. M., and Rimer, D. G.: Evidence for direct utilization of fructose in working

muscle in man. Proc. Soc. Exp. Biol. Med., **100**:671-672, 1959.

141. Pearson, C. M., Rimer, D. G., and Mommaerts, F. H. M.: A metabolic myopathy due to absence of muscle phosphorylase. Amer. J. Med., **30**:502-517, 1961.

142. Perkoff, G. T., Parker, V. J., and Hahn, R. F.: The effects of glucagon in three forms of glycogen storage disease. J. Clin. Invest., **41**:1099-1105, 1962.

143. Pompe, J. C.: Hypertrophie idiopathique du coeur. Ann. Anat. Path. (Paris), **10**:23-35, 1933.

144. Poppen, K. J., Green, D. M. and Wrenn, H. T.: The histochemical localization of potassium and glycogen. J. Histochem. Cytochem., **1**:160-173, 1953.

145. Ratinov, G., Baker, W. P., and Swaiman, K. F.: McArdle's syndrome with previously unreported electrocardiographic and serum enzyme abnormalities. Ann. Intern. Med., **62**:328-335, 1965.

146. Recant, L.: Recent developments in the field of glycogen metabolism and the diseases of glycogen storage. Amer. J. Med., **19**:610-619, 1955.

147. Rewcastle, N. B., and Humphrey, J. G.: Vacuolar myopathy. Clinical, histochemical and microscopic study. Arch Neurol. (Chicago), **12**:570-582, 1965.

148. Robbins, P. W.: Immunological study of human muscle lacking phosphorylase (Abstract). Fed. Proc., **19**:193, 1960.

149. Rosenfeld, E. L.: Animal tissue α-amylase and its role in the metabolism of glycogen. In Whelan and Cameron, op. cit., pp. 176-189.

150. Rosenstein, B. J.: Glycogen storage disease of the heart in a newborn infant. J. Pediat., **65**:126-128, 1964.

151. Rossier, A., Caldera, R., Sarrut, S., and Houllemare, L.: Les glycogénoses neonatales. Arch. Franc. Pediat., **17**:886-913, 1960.

152. Roth, J., Glick, S. M., Yalow, R. S., and Berson, S. A.: Hypoglycemia: A potent stimulus to secretion of growth hormone. Science, **140**:987-988, 1963.

153. Rowland, L. P., Araki, S., and Carmel, P.: Contracture in McArdle's disease. Stability of adenosine triphosphate during contracture in phosphorylase-deficient human muscle. Arch. Neurol. (Chicago), **13**:541-544, 1965.

154. Rowland, L. P., Fahn, S., and Schotland, D. L.: McArdle's disease. Hereditary myopathy due to lack of muscle phosphorylase. Arch. Neurol. (Chicago), **9**:325-342, 1963.

155. Salamon, J. C., Habib, R., and Bernhard, W.: Study of hepatic glycogenosis by the electron microscope. Path. Biol. (Paris), 9:1251-1264, 1961.

156. Salmon, S. E., and Turner, C. E.: McArdle's disease presenting as convulsion and rhabdomyolysis. Amer. J. Med., 39:142-146, 1965.

157. Schmid, R., and Hammaker, L.: Hereditary absence of muscle phosphorylase (McArdle's syndrome). New Eng. J. Med., 264:223-225, 1961.

158. Schmid, R., and Mahler, R. F.: Chronic progressive myopathy with myoglobinuria: demonstration of a glycogenolytic defect in the muscle. J. Clin. Invest., 38:2044-2058, 1959.

158a. Schmid, R. and Mahler, R. F.: cited by Tobin, R. B., and Coleman, W. A.[192].

159. Schmid, R., Robbins, P. W., and Traut, R. R.: Glycogen synthesis in muscle lacking phosphorylase. Proc. Nat. Acad. Sci. U.S.A., 45:1236-1264, 1959.

160. Schotland, D. L., Spiro, D., and Rowland, L. P.: Ultrastructural studies of muscle in McArdle's disease (deficiency of muscle phosphorylase). J. Neuropath. Exp. Neurol., 24:629-644, 1965.

161. Schulman, J. L. and Saturen, P.: Glycogen storage disease of the liver. I. Clinical studies during the early neonatal period. Pediatrics, 14:632-645, 1954.

162. Schwartz, R., Ashmore, J., and Renold, A. E.: Galactose tolerance in glycogen storage disease. Pediatrics, 19:585-594, 1957.

163. Scott, J. M.: Histological observations on glycogen reserves of the foetus and newborn infant. Arch. Dis. Child., 40:317-322, 1965.

164. Selberg, W.: Die Glykogenose des Säuglings unter dem Bilde einer tödlich verlaufenden cerebrospinalen Erkrankung. Z. Kinderheilk., 72:306-320, 1953.

165. Sheldon, H. M., Silverberg, M., and Kerner, I.: On the differing appearance of intranuclear and cytoplasmic glyocgen in glycogen storage disease. J. Cell Biol., 13:468-473, 1962.

166. Shelley, H. J.: Glycogen reserves and their changes at birth and in anoxia. Brit. Med. Bull., 17:137-143, 1961.

167. Sherman, F. E.: An Atlas of Congenital Heart Disease. Philadelphia, Lea & F., 1963.

168. Shwachman, H.: Sweat electrolytes in glycogen storage disease, type I (Letter to the Editor). Pediatrics, 32:148, 1963.

169. Sidbury, J. B., Jr.: Enzyme profiles in different types of glycogen storage disease (Abstract). Amer. J. Dis. Child., 102:634, 1961.

169a. Sidbury, J. B., Jr.: An evaluation of clinical studies of the assessment of different types of glycogen storage disease. (Abstract). Amer. J. Dis. Child., 102:769-770, 1961.

170. Sidbury, J. B., Jr.: The genetics of the glycogen storage diseases. In Steinberg, A. G., and Bearn, A. G. (eds.): Progress in Medical Genetics, Vol. IV. New York, Grune, 1965, pp. 32-58.

171. Sidbury, J. B., Jr., Cornlath, M., Fischer, J., and House, E.: Glycogen in erythrocytes of patients with glycogen storage disease. Pediatrics, 27:103-111, 1961.

172. Sidbury, J. B., Jr., Gitzelmann, R., and Fischer, J.: The glycogenoses. Further observations on glycogen in erythrocytes of patients with glycogenosis. Helv. Paediat. Acta, 16:506-516, 1961.

173. Sidbury, J. B., Jr., and Long, B. L.: Ketosis in infants and children. J. Pediat., 60:294-303, 1962.

174. Sidbury, J. B., Jr., Mason, J., Burns, W. B., Jr., and Ruebner, B. H.: Type IV glycogenosis. Report of a case proven by characterization of glycogen and studied at necropsy. Bull. Johns Hopkins Hosp., 111:157-181, 1962.

175. Siperstein, M. D.: Interrelationships of glucose and lipid metabolism. Amer. J. Med., 26:685-702, 1959.

176. Sokal, J. E., Fleisaner, S., Sarcione, E. J. and Lowe, C. U.: Blood glucose-6-phosphate in heterozygous carriers and patients with liver glycogen disease (von Gierke's disease). Nature (London), 192:265-266, 1961.

177. Sokal, J. E., Lowe, C. U., Saks, G. L., Leahy, M., and Stowens, D.: Liver glycogen disease in two generations of a family. Clinical studies and tissue analyses during overt disease and after apparent recovery. Amer. J. Med., 36:847-855, 1964.

178. Sokal, J. E., Lowe, C. U. and Sarcione, E. J.: Liver glycogen disease (von Gierke's disease). Arch. Intern. Med., 109:612-624, 1962.

179. Sokal, J. E., Lowe, C. U., Sarcione, E. J., Mosovich, L. L., and Doray, B. H.: Studies of glycogen metabolism in liver glycogen disease (von Gierke's disease): Six cases with similar metabolic abnormalities and responses to glucagon. J. Clin. Invest., 40:364-374, 1961.

180. Sokal, J. E., Sarcione, E. J., Mosovich, L. L., and Lowe, C. U.: Liver glycogen disease: a biochemical paradox (Abstract). Amer. J. Dis. Child., **100**:633-634, 1960.

181. Sparrow, W. T., and Ashworth, C. T.: Electron microscopy of nuclear glycogenosis. Arch. Path. (Chicago), **80**:84-90, 1965.

182. Spencer-Peet, J.: Erythrocyte glycogen synthetase in glycogen storage deficiency resulting from the absence of this enzyme from the liver. Clin. Chim. Acta, **10**:481-483, 1964.

183. Spencer-Peet, J., Lewis, G. M., and Stewart, K. M.: Glycogen synthetase deficiency. In Whelan and Cameron, op. cit., pp. 377-386.

184. Starzl, T. E., Marchioro, T. L., Sexton, A. W., Illingworth, B., Waddell, W. R., Faris, T. D., and Herrmann, T. J.: The effect of portocaval transposition on carbohydrate metabolism: experimental and clinical observations. Surgery, **57**:687-697, 1965.

185. Steinitz, K., Bodur, H., and Ârman, J.: Amylo-1, 6-glucosidase activity in leucocytes from patients with glycogen storage disease. Clin. Chim. Acta, **8**:807-809, 1963.

186. Steinitz, K., and Reisner, S. H.: Glycogen storage disease with double enzymatic deficiency. Israel Med. J., **20**:215-222, 1961.

187. Stetten, D. W., and Stetten, M. R.: Glycogen metabolism. Physiol. Rev., **40**:505-537, 1960.

188. Takeuchi, T.: Histochemical demonstration of branching enzyme (amylo-1, 4 → 1, 6-transglucosidase) in animal tissue. J. Histochem. Cytochem., **6**:208-216, 1958.

189. Takeuchi, T., and Glenner, G. C.: Histochemical demonstration of uridine diphosphate glucose-glycogen transferase in animal tissues. J. Histochem. Cytochem., **9**:304-316, 1961.

190. Templeton, M.: Microdetermination of glycogen with anthrone reagent. J. Histochem. Cytochem., **9**:670-672, 1961.

191. Thomson, W. H. S., MacLaurin, J. C., and Prineas, J. W.: Skeletal muscle glycogenosis; an investigation of two dissimilar cases. J. Neurol. Neurosurg. Psychiat., **26**:60-68, 1963.

192. Tobin, R. B., and Coleman, W. A.: A family study of phosphorylase deficiency in muscle. Ann. Intern. Med., **62**:313-327, 1965.

193. Toussaint, D., and Danis, P.: Ocular histopathology in generalized glycogenosis (Pompe's disease). Arch. Ophthal. (Paris), **73**:342-349, 1965.

194. Ulstrom, R. A., Ziegler, M. R., Doeden, D., and McQuarrie, I.: Metabolic and clinical effects of corticortropin (ACTH) on essential glycogenosis (von Gierke's disease). Metabolism, **1**:291-299, 1952.

195. van Creveld, S.: Oven een byzondere stoornis in de koolhydraatstofwisseling in den Kinderleeftijd. Nederl. Maandschr. Geneesk., **15**:349-359, 1928.

196. van Creveld, S.: The clinical course of glycogen disease. Canad. Med. Ass. J., **88**:1-15, 1963.

197. van Creveld, S., and Huijing, F.: Differential diagnosis of the type of glycogen disease in two adult patients with long history of glycogenosis. Metabolism, **13**:191-194, 1964.

198. van Creveld, S., and Huijing, F.: Glycogen storage disease. Biochemical and clinical data in sixteen cases. Amer. J. Med., **38**:554-561, 1965.

199. Verity, M. A. and Brown, W. J.: Rapid micromethod for glycogen: Application to hepatic needle biopsies. J. Lab. Clin. Med., **62**:846-852, 1963.

200. von Gierke, E.: Hepato-nephromegalia glykogenica (glykogenspeicherkrankheit der leber und nieren). Beitr. Path. Anat., **82**:497-513, 1929.

201. Wagner, R.: Studies on glycogen-storage disease-phosphorylated intermediates in the peripheral blood (Abstract). Amer. J. Dis. Child., **90**:580-581, 1955.

202. Wagner, R., Meyerriecks, N., and Sparaco, R.: Glycogen storage disease. (Phosphorylated intermediates in the peripheral blood). J. Pediat., **53**:683-691, 1958.

203. Walker, D. G., Ziai, M., and Bowman, J. E.: Three differing cases of glycogen storage disease. Arch. Dis. Child., **36**:432-438, 1961.

204. Walker, G. J., and Whelan, W. J.: The mechanism of carbohydrase action. 8. Structures of the muscle-phosphorylase limit dextrins of glycogen and amylopectin. Biochem. J., **76**:264-268, 1960.

205. Wallis, P. G., Sidbury, J. B., Jr., and Harris, R. C.: Hepatic phosphorylase defect. Studies on peripheral blood. In press, cited by J. B. Sidbury, Jr.[170].

206. Weber, G., and Harpur, E. R.: Liver enzymes in glycogen storage disease. Metabolism, **9**:880-883, 1960.

207. Weissmann, G.: Lysosomes. New. Eng. J. Med., **273**:1084-1149, 1965.

208. Williams, H. E., and Field, J. B.: Low leukocyte phosphorylase in hepatic phosphorylase-deficient glycogen storage disease. J. Clin. Invest., **40**:1841-1845, 1961.

209. Williams, H. E., and Field, J. B.: Further studies on leukocyte phosphorylase in glycogen storage disease. Metabolism, 12:464-466, 1963.

210. Williams, H. E., Johnson, P. L., Fenster, L. F., Laster, L., and Field, J. B.: Intestinal glucose-6-phosphatase in control subjects and relatives of a patient with glycogen storage disease. Metabolism, 12:235-241, 1963.

211. Williams, H. E., Kendig, E. M., and Field, J. B.: Leukocyte debranching enzyme in glycogen storage disease. J. Clin. Invest., 42:656-660, 1963.

212. Wilson, R. A., and Clark, N.: Endocardial fibroelastosis associated with generalized glycogenosis. Occurrence in siblings. Pediatrics, 26:86-96, 1960.

213. Wittels, B.: Myocardial glycogen in the fetus, infant and child. Arch. Path. (Chicago), 75:127-143, 1963.

214. Wittels, B., and Reiner, L.: Histochemical observations on glycogen in the human myocardium. Amer. J. Path., 36:55-75, 1960.

215. Zakon, S. J., Oyamada, A., and Rosenthal, I. H.: Eruptive xanthoma and hyperlipemia in glycogen storage disease (von Gierke's disease). Arch. Derm. (Chicago), 67:146-151, 1953.

216. Zellweger, H., Dark, A., and Abu Haidar, G. A.: Glycogen disease of the muscle. Report of two cases and review of the literature. Pediatrics, 15:715-732, 1955.

Chapter 8

Congenital Disorders of Hemostasis and Blood Coagulation in Infancy

LOUIS A. KAZAL, Ph.D.

Hemorrhagic diatheses are caused by the partial or complete absence or the malfunction of one or more of the components of the blood clotting or hemostatic systems. Actually, much of our knowledge of blood coagulation and hemostasis has its roots in the clinical observation of such hemorrhagic disorders, and their classification and etiology are based in turn on the development of our knowledge of the mechanisms involved.

Congenital disorders may be either acquired or hereditary. If not overt, they often are unmasked in the infant at circumcision. If this is not practiced, then dental extractions, tonsillectomies, adenoidectomies or other childhood surgeries, or traumatic episodes subsequently uncover the defect. This is especially true of hereditary disorders; obviously, the acquired congenital disorders are detected early and usually are self-limiting with proper therapy. The afflicted individual is seldom, if ever, spared the threat to his life at any age; however, it is in the early years of life that the severe form of some of the disorders is often detected and, hopefully, it is at this time that the basis for a good prognosis can be established. Early treatment and proper care have resulted in an increased longevity and a greater usefulness of the patient with hereditary bleeding anomalies and in the significant reduction of the incidence of hemorrhagic disease of the newborn.

The incidence of disorders of blood coagulation and hemostasis is not high, and these disorders may be classified generally as rare; nevertheless, the individual with a hemorrhagic crisis presents a special and acute problem in diagnosis and management. In this respect, the infant, because of its small size, presents a more critical problem than the adult. Statistics delineating the proportion of the afflicted population that is represented by the infant are not available; however, the infant is a frequent "case record" in the literature describing hereditary defects and is, of course, the central theme of hemorrhagic disease of the newborn.

A discussion of hemorrhagic disorders is best prefaced by at least a brief review of the mechanisms of blood coagulation and hemostasis, since their classification and etiology are based primarily on a knowledge of those mechanisms.

BLOOD COAGULATION MECHANISM

The classic blood coagulation mechanism based on the interaction of many individual factors is now conceived as a bimodal pathway to the conversion of prothrombin to an active and specific proteolytic enzyme, thrombin. Thrombin intitiates the transformation of fibrinogen to fibrin monomer which polymerizes to insoluble fibrin, the essence of the blood clot. Recent reviews summarize the extensive literature[19, 48, 54, 70, 73]. One way of depicting the mechanism involved is shown in Figure 1. Similar schemes are widely used by the clinician for the analysis of blood clotting disorders[21, 27, 43, 45, 64, 81, 90]. An alternative mechanism, the auto-prothrombin derivative theory[85], which invokes the direct activation of the prothrombin molecule without the intervention of a prothrombin activator, has been proposed and is substantiated on both biochemical and clinical grounds. A critical analysis of both theories has been presented[48, 85].

According to the classic concept, prothrombin activator is elaborated by either an intrinsic or extrinsic system. The intrinsic system is characterized by a sequence or cascade or enzymatic reactions initiated with the activation of Hageman factor (XII) by a foreign surface (damage endothelium, glass, etc.)[55, 73].* Activated Hageman factor then transforms plasma thromboplastin antecedent (Factor XI) to an activated Factor XI. The interaction product of these two factors is known as contact factor; the reaction does not require calcium. The subsequent reactions of Factors IX (plasma thromboplastin component), VIII (antihemophilic globulin) and X (Stuart factor) require calcium or calcium and phospholipid and result in the formation of an activated Factor X. Early in this sequence of activations, platelets undergo viscous metamorphosis releasing Platelet Factor 3. The latter is a lipoprotein or phospholipid complex[34, 46]. Phosphatidylserine and phosphatidylethanolamine, among other phospholipids, are known to accelerate the clotting reaction[7]. Platelet Factor 3 appears to be present in granules or in platelet membrane[58]. The interaction of activated Factor X, activated Factor V and calcium with Platelet Factor 3 produces a hypothetical intrinsic prothrombin activator (plasma thromboplastin) whose exact nature is yet to be established. The slowness of the intrinsic system is reflected in the relatively long clotting time of the whole blood.

The formation of extrinsic activator follows a different and more rapid pathway. Tissue thromboplastin (Factor III) reacts with Factor VII (proconvertin) in the presence of calcium and thereby activates Factor X, thus substituting for the activity of Factors XII, XI, VIII and IX. The contact phase is bypassed; the remaining sequence is similar to that of the intrinsic system. The hypothetical substance derived from this sequence of reactions is referred to as extrinsic prothrombin activator; this system rapidly generates thrombin in a matter of seconds depending on the source of thromboplastin (Factor III). The extrinsic system may represent an important component of the hemostatic mechanism[53].

---

*A description of clotting factors and their numerical designations may be found in Reference[45]. Factor XIII (fibrin stabilizing factor or fibrinase) has been added recently to the list of factors accepted by the International Committee for the Nomenclature of Blood Clotting Factors.[23]

The conversion of prothrombin to thrombin and of fibrinogen to fibrin needs little comment except to note the recent adoption as Factor XIII, an enzyme that forms the compact, urea-insoluble fibrin clot essential for good hemostasis[24].

THE HEMOSTATIC MECHANISM

Various schemes have been proposed for the mechanism of hemostasis[27, 43, 51, 72, 77, 80, 88]. Figure 2 illustrates an adaptation of a mechanism[72] based on recent investigations of platelet adhesiveness and aggregation. Shed blood may contribute to hemostasis in three ways, through the activation of its platelets and its intrinsic and extrinsic systems. Platelets contribute significantly to the control of bleeding from capillaries through the mechanism of white platelet plug formation[80], for which fibrin formation seems unessential. The participation of the intrinsic and extrinsic clotting systems produce the hemostatic or red platelet plug. The central role of platelets in hemostasis has become more evident in recent years; the many contributions are reviewed briefly elsewhere[43, 51, 61]. Platelets exposed to injured tissue become adhesive and, in contact with collagen fibers, release adenosine diphosphate (ADP) from platelet stores of adenosine triphosphate. ADP induces reversible aggregation of platelets; calcium ions are required for aggregation, and the reaction is intensified by a plasmatic factor

Fig. I

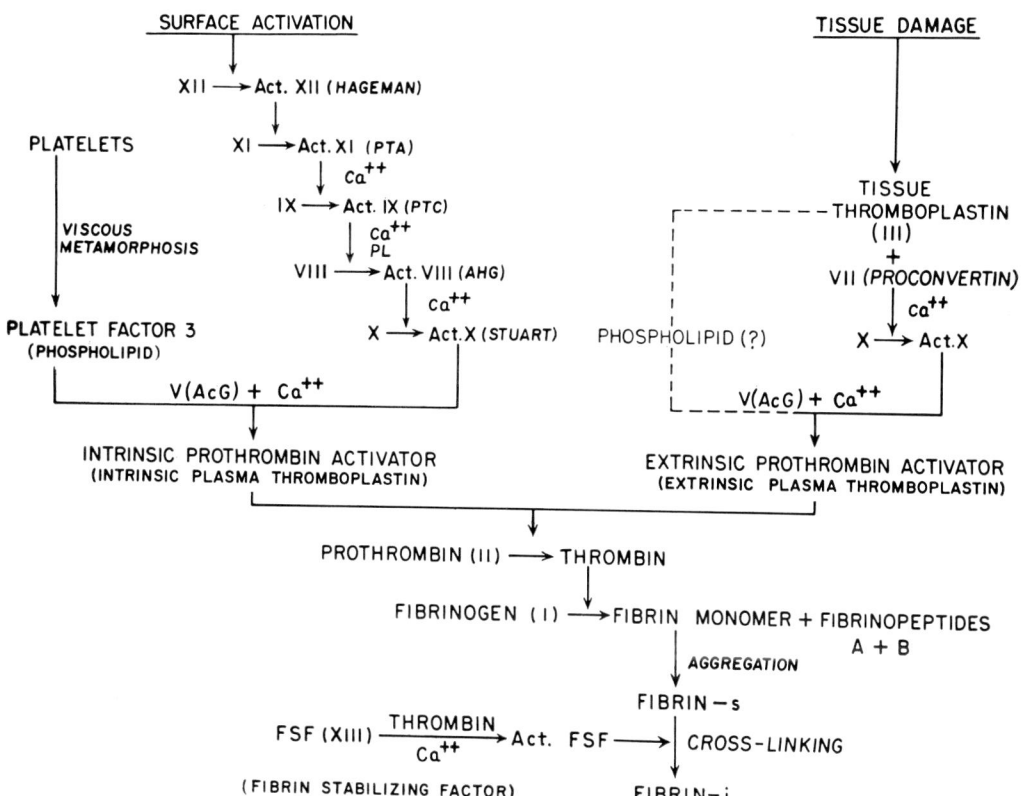

CURRENT CONCEPT OF MECHANISM OF BLOOD COAGULATION

Fig. 2

MECHANISM OF HEMOSTASIS

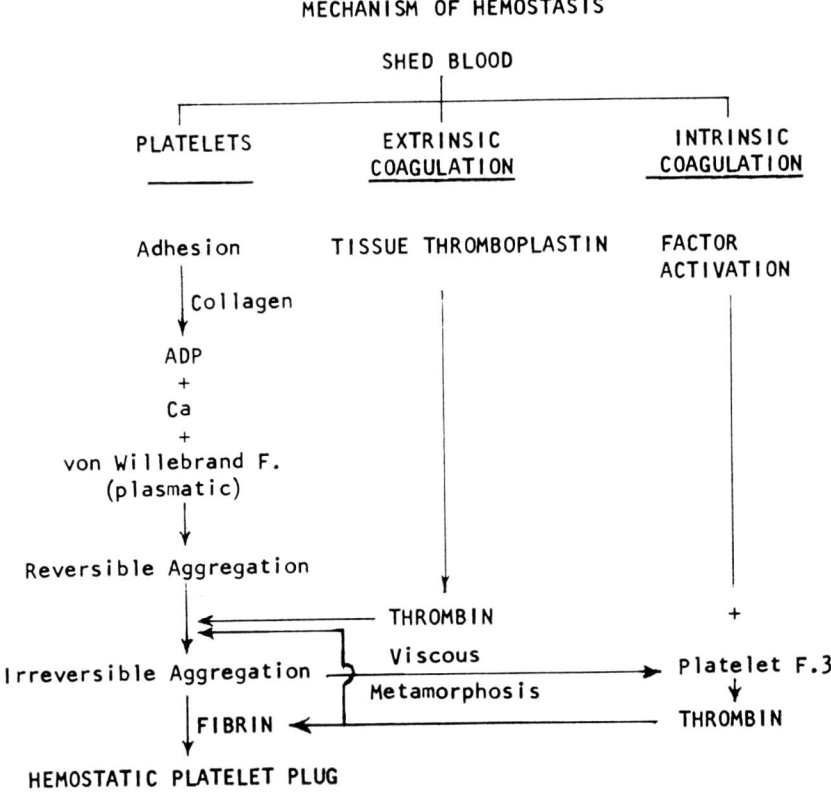

(anti-Willebrand factor). Thrombin is required for the formation of the irreversible-aggregated platelet plug. Thrombin theoretically may be derived from the rapidly acting extrinsic system[53] or from the action of the intrinsic system on the surface of the platelet, on which are adsorbed essential clotting factors such as fibrinogen, Factor V, XI and XII[38]. Irreversible aggregation is accompanied by viscous metamorphosis which releases adequate amounts of Platelet Factor 3 for the participation of the intrinsic system. Consolidation of the platelet plug follows through the action of thrombin and fibrin deposition. The anti-Willebrand factor is essential for the formation of the hemostatic platelet plug; it is a substance that is missing in the plasma of patients with von Willebrand's disease but which is present in normal plasma[68].

CLINICAL ASPECTS

Disorders of hemostasis and blood coagulation may be classified as acquired or temporary and as hereditary or permanent, and are briefly outlined in Figure 3. Although the skin bleeding time determination is considered inadequate for routine screening tests and is subject to much error and variation[3, 22], it does serve well to differentiate functionally the plasmatic from the hemostatic factor groups of hereditary diseases[43]. A hereditary deficiency of each factor has been described in which the bleeding time is *usually* normal (2 to 5 minutes). This group comprises the

Fig. 3

CONGENITAL DISORDERS OF BLOOD COAGULATION AND HEMOSTASIS IN INFANCY

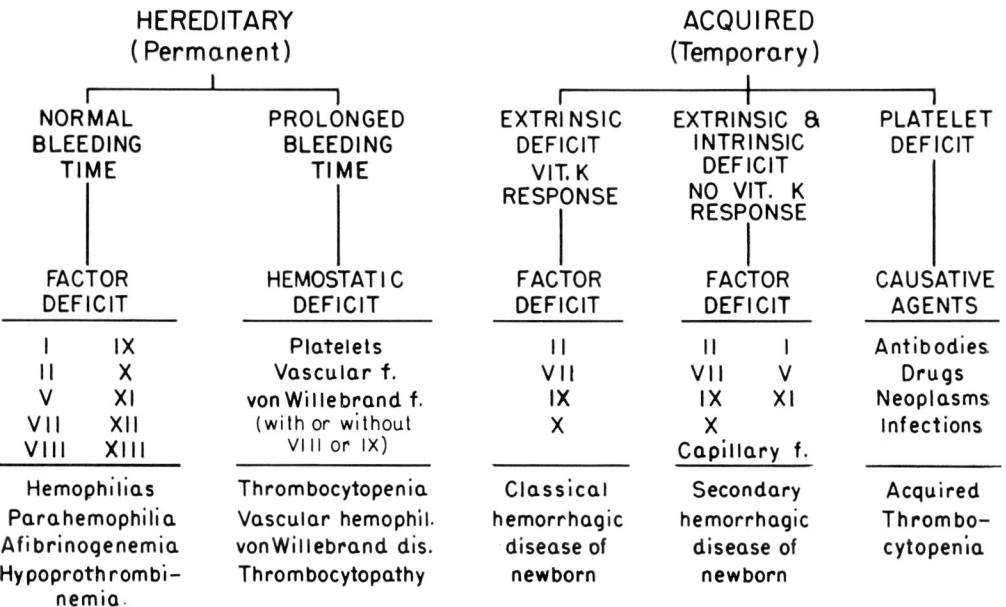

HEREDITARY (Permanent)		ACQUIRED (Temporary)		
NORMAL BLEEDING TIME	PROLONGED BLEEDING TIME	EXTRINSIC DEFICIT VIT. K RESPONSE	EXTRINSIC & INTRINSIC DEFICIT NO VIT. K RESPONSE	PLATELET DEFICIT
FACTOR DEFICIT	HEMOSTATIC DEFICIT	FACTOR DEFICIT	FACTOR DEFICIT	CAUSATIVE AGENTS
I IX II X V XI VII XII VIII XIII	Platelets Vascular f. von Willebrand f. (with or without VIII or IX)	II VII IX X	II I VII V IX XI X Capillary f.	Antibodies Drugs Neoplasms Infections
Hemophilias Parahemophilia Afibrinogenemia Hypoprothrombi- nemia.	Thrombocytopenia Vascular hemophil. von Willebrand dis. Thrombocytopathy	Classical hemorrhagic disease of newborn	Secondary hemorrhagic disease of newborn	Acquired Thrombo- cytopenia

hemophilias, parahemophilias, afibrino-genemia, deficiencies of the prothrombin complex and of fibrin stabilizing factor. An equally important group of hereditary disorders is characterized by a prolonged bleeding time. In this group the hemostatic deficit is centered about the quantitative (thrombocytopenic) or qualitative (thrombasthenic) deficiency of platelets, with or without an associated deficiency of certain plasmatic factors[5, 49, 51]. The acquired group of infant diseases are represented by thrombocytopenias, by disorders of the prothrombin complex (extrinsic system) as well as by thromboplastic deficiencies of the intrinsic system. Classical hemorrhagic disease of the newborn is associated with deficiencies of Factors II, VIII, IX and X. Secondary hemorrhagic disease of the newborn comprises a group of infants in which a deficiency may exist also among Factors I, V and XI as well as in hemostatic function[2,3, 37, 43, 63, 82, 83, 85a, 87].

HEREDITARY DISORDERS OF BLOOD CLOTTING FACTORS WITH NORMAL BLEEDING TIME

Hereditary disorders associated with a deficiency of the blood clotting factors are usually characterized by a normal bleeding time. The clotting factor deficiency may be partial or complete; clinically, the disease may be mild or severe. A deficiency of any of the clotting factors may result in a hemorrhagic diathesis[11, 17, 18, 24, 29, 30, 37, 43, 75, 77, 83, 90]. except for Factor XII, Hageman factor, for which only one or two cases with hemorrhagic symptoms are on record[78]. Tables I and II summarize some of the more important hereditary aspects and the laboratory data for this group of disorders. The incidence of each dis-

order in the general population is very low and varies considerably with the factor concerned[37]. Clinical surveys in many instances have provided an approximate listing of the actual number of cases on record. Hemophilia A and B are most common, followed by deficiencies of Factors VII and X. It is of interest that Factor XI deficiency has a regional distribution, some 200 cases having been described in New York City and Los Angeles[78]. Combined deficiencies of Factors V + VII, VIII + IX, and II, VII, IX and X have been observed but are rare[43].

Blood clotting factors are inherited as paired genes (alleles) on autosomal chromosomes, except for Factors VIII and IX which are sex-linked and in which, clinically, a single gene appears to determine their inheritance[17, 30]. In hemophilia A and B, the abnormal gene is carried by the female on the x-chromosome, and the disease appears almost exclusively in the male. The female is simply a symptomless carrier, unless she is homozygous for the abnormal gene, as is the case for the offspring of a female carrier and a male hemophiliac. Only a few authentic cases of Hemophilia A in a female have been reported[66]. A current hypothesis favors the sub-unit mode of inheritance for Factor VIII[30]; however, even the concept of sex-linkage has been recently challenged with the suggestion that Factor VIII inheritance is also under the control of autosomal genes as well[47]. Clinically, the sex-linked nature of Hemophilia A and B is obvious.

The hereditary deficiency of factors other than VIII or IX appears with equal frequency among male and female subjects, being characterized by an incompletely recessive or intermediate

TABLE 1 CONGENITAL DISORDERS OF CLOTTING FACTORS — HEREDITARY
ASPECTS

Blood Clotting Factor			Congenital Disorder	Hereditary Incidence	Mode of Transmission	Factor Level°
I	Fibrinogen[4, 29, 62, 40]		afibrinogenemia	(60 cases)	autosomal recessive	<5 mg per 100 ml
II	Prothrombin[20, 43, 44, 76]		hypo-prothrombinemia	(5 cases)	autosomal recessive	1%
V	Accelerator globulin[26, 29, 57]	AcG	parahemophilia	1:1,000,000 (32 cases)	autosomal recessive	0-10%
VII	Proconvertin stable factor[29, 33, 60, 71]	SPCA	hypopro-convertinemia	1:500,000 (52 cases)	autosomal recessive or intermediate	He = 50% Ho = 0-3%
VIII	Antihemophilic globulin[14, 29, 47, 67]	AHG	hemophilia A	1:25,000	sex-linked recessive	He = 2-30% Ho = 1%
IX	Plasma thromboplastin component[10, 29]	PTC	hemophilia B Christmas disease	1:100,000	sex-linked recessive	He = 5-20% Ho = 5%
X	Stuart-Prower factor[6, 29]		factor X deficiency	1:500,000 (60 cases)	autosomal recessive or intermediate	He = 50% Ho = 1-5%
XI	Plasma thromboplastin antecedent[78]	PTA	hemophilia C	(200 cases) regional	autosomal recessive	He = 30-60% Ho = 3-20%
XII	Hageman factor[16, 78]	HF	Hageman trait	81 cases	autosomal recessive	He = 20-50% Ho = 0-5%
XIII	Fibrin stabilizing factor fibrinase[9, 24, 52]	FSF	FSF deficiency	15 cases	autosomal intermediate	Ho = <2%

°He: heterozygous; Ho: homozygous.

autosomal mode of inheritance (Table I). In general, clinical abnormalities resulting from a deficiency of a given factor are expressed only when the individual is homozygous for the recessive characteristic. In the homozygote, plasma levels of the respective clotting factors are very low and the hemorrhagic manifestations are severe. The heterozygote, however, is not always unaffected, as might be anticipated for a purely recessive inherited characteristic. The reduction in the plasma level of the factor is variable, suggesting an intermediate autosomal mode of inheritance. Many heterozygotes experience mild bleeding problems that sometimes do not even require the attention of a physician and thus are missed in family studies of the disease and can only be detected by laboratory tests. The difference between recessive and intermediate gene expression and that of the dominant gene expression earlier suggested for many deficiencies appears to be one of quantitation[43]; however, the entire question of the mode of inheritance is far from settled and requires much more study. Nevertheless, the advances in this field have been significant, and the investigation of the hereditary aspects of blood clotting diseases promises a further elucidation of this complex field.

The laboratory tests differentiating the various factor deficiencies are de-

TABLE II CONGENITAL DISORDERS OF CLOTTING FACTORS — HEREDITARY ASPECTS COAGULATION TESTS

Factor Deficiency	Clinical Grade	Laboratory Data						Corrected by
		WBCT	PT	PC	PTT	TGT	BT	
I	mild	poor	P	N	P	N	N	plasma or fibrinogen
II	mild or severe	N or P	P		P	N	N	aged plasma
V	mild or severe	P	P	poor	P	Abn (plasma)	N	fresh BaSO$_4$ ads. plasma
VII	mild or severe	N	P†	N	N	N	N	serum or aged plasma
VIII	mild or severe	P	N	poor	P	Abn (plasma)	N	BaSO$_4$ ads. plasma
IX	mild or severe	P	N	poor	P	Abn (serum)	N	serum
X	mild	P	P°	poor	P	Abn (serum)	N	serum or aged plasma
XI	mild	P	N	poor	P	Abn (both)	N	serum or BaSO$_4$ ads. plasma
XII	normal	P	N	poor	P	Abn (both)	N	serum or BaSO$_4$ ads. plasma
XIII	severe	N	N	N	N	N	N	plasma

WBCT: whole blood clotting time; PT: prothrombin time one-stage;
PC: prothrombin consumption; PTT: partial thromboplastin time;
TGT: thromboplastin generation; BT: bleeding time; P: prolonged;
N: normal; ABN: abnormal.

†Normal with Russell's viper venom (RV).   °Not normalized with RVV.

scribed in Table II. It should be mentioned that the bleeding time in this group of diseases is usually normal; however, isolated exceptions exist. In general, the whole blood clotting times are considered not to be too reliable, but the remaining tests enable the coagulationist to characterize each deficiency more or less adequately. For a discussion of laboratory testing the reader is referred to the following references 2, 3, 12, 21, 25, 27, 28, 43, 49, 75, 82, 83, 86, 91.

HEREDITARY DISORDERS WITH PROLONGED BLEEDING TIME

The simplest malfunction in hemostasis is represented by thrombocytopenia, in which there is an insufficient number of platelets for the clotting mechanism to function normally. Infants with primary congenital (idiopathic) thrombocytopenic purpura of hereditary origin are extremely rare; in the few proven cases the thrombocytopenia is inherited as an autosomal dominant trait[13]. The platelet count is less than 50,000 per cu mm, an approximate critical point for effective hemostasis.

Congenital disorders with a normal platelet count but a prolonged bleeding time are a heterogeneous group, difficult to classify primarily because their etiology is not clearly understood. As a result, there is much confusion in regard to nomenclature. Since the blood coagulation mechanism is normal in many cases, the hemorrhagic manifestations of the diseases point to the importance of platelets for hemostatic function. Factor deficiencies, however, are involved, and these more recent findings are helpful for the clarification of some of the problems of nomenclature. Various classifications have been formulated[21, 37, 43, 81, 87, 89]. The following division of congenital hemorrhagic disorders based on laboratory tests is informative[51]:

1. Prolonged bleeding time without platelet anomaly;
2. Prolonged bleeding time with platelet abnormality;
3. Prolonged bleeding time with plasma factor deficiency.

VASCULAR DEFICIT

In the first group are patients with prolonged bleeding time, apparently normal platelets and normal coagulation factors. There are only a few patients in this group; a vascular factor deficit is suspect. The mechanism of the defect is not known, although platelet adhesiveness is abnormal[39].

THROMBOCYTOPATHY

The thrombopathies constitute the second group in which the bleeding time is prolonged and the platelet count is normal but in which platelet function is abnormal. The impairment of platelet hemostatic function is complex. A bleeding tendency is caused by abnormality of functional platelets in which a qualitative defect may exist in one or more of a number of platelet factor activities; twelve such activities have been described[43]. These deficits are a result of inborn errors of platelet metabolism and ultrastructure. Theoretically, a reduction in the activity of only one of these factors may affect the hemostatic mechanism. Platelet Factor 3 (thromboplasin), Platelet Factor 5 (fibrinogen) and Platelet Function 11 (clot retraction) seem to have greater importance, but the potential role of other platelet factors is not to be minimized; furthermore, deficiencies in metabolic platelet enzyme activity (dehydrogenases, pyruvate-kinase, glycolysis) are associated with abnormal platelet function[32]. The current investigations of platelet function and its disorders offers promise of much-needed clarification of this group of disorders of hemostasis.

VON WILLEBRAND'S DISEASE

The third and largest group of hereditary disorders with prolonged bleeding time is von Willebrand's disease (pseudohemophilia, vascular hemophilia) which is characterized by a deficit of Clotting Factor VIII (AHG) and another plasmatic factor, the vascular or anti-Willebrand factor[8, 15, 30, 51, 68]. As mentioned above, prolonged bleeding time also is found in a few cases of congenital afibrinogenemia, hypofibrinogenemia and of Factor IX, X and XI deficiencies, but the exact mechanisms involved are not clear[51].

Von Willebrand's disease is the best characterized of the diseases with prolonged bleeding time associated with a clotting factor deficiency. The chief laboratory findings are a reduced level of Factor VIII (50%) and an apparent impairment of adhesiveness of platelets.* Studies of platelet adhesiveness have clarified the etiology of this disorder to a great extent. Actually, platelets taken from patients with von Willebrand's disease and suspended in normal human platelet-free plasma behave like normal platelets, even with respect to the property of adhesiveness. Tests for normal adhesiveness and for the level of Factor VIII are essential for the diagnosis of this disease. Both the property of adhesiveness and the prolonged bleeding time are corrected *in vivo* in patients by the infusion of normal human platelet-free plasma or by plasma fractions which contain the anti-Willebrand factor[69]. This plasmatic factor can be separated from Cohn Fraction 1. It too will produce normal platelet adhesiveness and correct the prolonged bleeding time of von Willebrand's disease subjects; furthermore, it participates in the synthesis of Factor VIII.

A genetic relationship exists between anti-Willebrand factor and Factor VIII;

the functional relationship is illustrated by transfusion experiments. The plasma from a Hemophilia A patient (deficient in Factor VIII) will not correct *in vitro* the prolonged partial thromboplastin time of plasma from von Willebrand's disease patients. The infusion of Hemophilic A plasma into a patient with von Willebrand's disease, however, induces the new synthesis of Factor VIII in a period of twenty-four hours[30, 68]. Von Willebrand's disease is transmitted as an autosomal dominant gene[68, 69] and the evidence for transmission favors (but does not prove) the combining subunit model for AHG biosynthesis[8, 30]. The synthesis of Factor VIII appears to be under the control of both an autosomal gene and a sex-linked gene; in Hemophilia A, the mutant gene is located on the x-chromosome. Thus, two (normal) genes on different chromosomes appear to be necessary for the biosynthesis of Factor VIII. Failure of the platelet to function normally arises from the lack of the plasma factor (anti-Willebrand factor, pro-factor) in von Willebrand's disease subjects[69].

ACQUIRED CONGENITAL PLATELET DISORDERS

Acquired or secondary thrombocytopenia occurs in the newborn with a variable etiology[5, 49, 82, 85a]. Idiopathic thrombocytopenia may be maternal in origin, that is, caused by passive transfer of maternal antibodies[35, 41] or by blood platelet group incompatibility[89]. It may be non-maternal in origin, in which either a defect of the vascular wall or a megakaryocytic hypoplasia presumably are the cause of secondary thrombocytopenic purpura. The passive transfer of quinine from mother to infant associated with a platelet agglutinin has

---

*The reports of the apparent impairment of adhesiveness of platelets have been challenged by a recent investigation which showed that in 200 cases of von Willebrand's Disease in 88 Swedish families there was no defect in platelet adhesiveness to glass or any abnormal reaction to ADP or collagen (S. Cronberg, I. M. Nilsson and J. Silwer, Studies on the Platelet Adhesiveness in von Willebrand's Disease. Acta. Med. Scand. **180**:43-54, 1966.)

been described[35]. Drugs, neoplasms and infections sometimes account for the etiology[82]. With supportive therapy, the mild and some of the severe cases eventually overcome the effects of the thrombocytopenia, and the congenital disorder becomes self-limiting.

HEMORRHAGIC DISEASE OF THE NEWBORN

Hemorrhagic disease of the newborn is a hemorrhagic disorder appearing in the first days of life; it is caused by a deficiency of Vitamin K and is characterized by a deficiency of the prothrombin complex[79]. In recent years it has become evident that factors *other* than II, VII and X may be deficient at birth or shortly thereafter, and the term, *secondary hemorrhagic disease,* is used to describe the atypical form of the disease[2, 43, 63]. In classical hemorrhagic disease of the newborn, the concentration of prothrombin and Factor VII are sufficiently low to account for the disease; furthermore, the condition is aggravated by deficiencies of Factors X and IX, the latter producing a defect in the intrinsic clotting system as well[83].

With the advent of quantitative assays for the various clotting factors, it has become apparent that the so-called normal, full-term infant in many cases does not possess an adult coagulation system and has temporary deficiencies of certain clotting factors[2, 43, 63, 83]. Some of the complexities of the problem are illustrated in Table III. The full-term normal infant at birth usually has a normal concentration of blood clotting factors[2]; however, in two to five days, certain factors may be reduced to less

TABLE III CONGENITAL DISORDERS OF COAGULATION — NEONALIAL

Clotting Factor	Full-term Infant (2 to 5 days)			Secondary HDN†	Hemorrhagic Disease of Newborn*
	Level	Range	Normalcy		
Fibrinogen	normal	100-350 mg%		low normal	normal
Prothrombin	low	5-60%	2-12 months	very low	low
V (AcG)	high	75-300%		low	normal
VII (proconvertin)	low	5-50%	2-12 months	very low	very low
VIII (AHG)	normal	100%		low normal	normal
IX (PTC)	low to normal	19-90%	3-9 months	very low	very low
X (STUART)	low	10-50%	2-12 months	low	very low
XI (PTA)	low to normal	13-85%	2 months	very low	normal
XII (HF)	low to normal	25-100%	10-14 days		
Platelet count	normal	205,000 to 290,000		31,000 to 197,000	normal

*Response to vitamin K.   †No response to vitamin K.

than normal range. Fibrinogen, Factor V and Factor VIII are normal[2], as is the platelet count[65]. The prothrombin complex factors[1] (II, VII, IX and X, as well as Factors XI and XII) frequently are below average normal levels[1, 2, 36, 60]. The deficiencies are temporary, and the factors slowly approach normal adult concentration in two to twelve months, except for Factor XII, which reaches a normal level in ten to fourteen days[50]. Vitamin K usually does not correct the deficient state. In the infant with low levels of clotting factors there may be a tendency to hemorrhage, especially after circumcision, but the deficient state is not associated with a hemorrhagic diathesis. In these full-term deficiencies, the whole blood clotting time and bleeding time are normal. Vascular permeability is not altered and capillary resistance is even greater than that of the adult[2]. Factor V (accelerator globulin) is frequently found at higher-than-normal values, up to 300 per cent; its hyperactivity along with normal levels of fibrinogen, antihemophilic globulin and platelets may make up for deficiencies of the other factors and contribute to a functionally normal hemostatic mechanisms[2, 63].

The premature infant, on the other hand, may be afflicted with a more generalized deficiency state which is a result of developmental immaturity, especially of the liver[2, 43, 82]. In this group, hemorrhagic symptoms are more common. There may be an increased fragility, a prolonged bleeding time and abnormalities of platelets[65]. The thromboplastic activity of serum in the thromboplastin generation test is abnormal[3]. Apparently, the premature infant does not have the capacity to synthesize a full complement of factors. The response to Vitamin K in this group is poor and variable. The hemorrhagic diathesis encountered in this group, which occurs when the deficiencies are severe, has been classified as secondary hemorrhagic disease. The prognosis is not always good in secondary hemorrhagic disease[2].

Classical hemorrhagic disease of the newborn may be considered as a later stage in the development of the full-term neonate in which certain factors have already reached essentially hemostatic levels but in which the prothrombin complex is still poorly functional and the thromboplastin generating system may be abnormal. The one-stage prothrombin time is prolonged, and the levels of prothrombin and Factor VII, as well as Factor IX, are usually low. These infants respond clinically to vitamin K in a dramatic manner, sometimes in matter of hours[1, 2, 37, 43, 63].

COMMENT

Although the incidence of clotting disorders in infants may be considered quite low, since they represent only a small percentage of all patients suffering from hemorrhagic problems, they represent nevertheless, an important segment of hematologic practice. Because of the tender age of the subject, the infant presents special problems and requires special attention. In the acquired group of disorders the incidence has been reduced by the prophylactic use of vitamin K; however, this has not been a therapeutic panacea, and some clinical problems among full-term and premature infants alike persist. In this group, the short tenure of the disorder and modern diagnosis and therapy contributes to a successful prognosis. The individual with an inborn error of the coagulation or hemostatic mechanisms is not spared the threat to his life at any age; however, early detection of the disorder and proper measures or treatment have contributed significantly to an increased longevity and a more useful life.

REFERENCES

1. Aballi, A. J., Banus, V. L., de Lamerans, S., and Rozengvaig, S.: Coagulation studies in the newborn period. IV. Deficiency of Stuart-Prower factor as a part of the clotting defect in the newborn. Arch. Dis. Child., **97**:549-560, 1959.
2. Aballi, A. J., and de Lamerans, S.: Coagulation changes in the neonatal period and in early infancy. Pediat. Clin. N. Amer., **9**:785-818, 1962.
3. Abildgaard, C. F., Cornet, J. A., Johnson, H., and Schulman, I.: Screening tests for disorders of thromboplastin formation. Pediat. Clin. N. Amer., **9**:819-832, 1962.
4. Alexander, B., Goldstein, R., Rich, L., Le Bolloc'h, A. G., Diamond, L. K., and Borges, W.: Congenital afibrinogenemia. A study of some basic aspects of coagulation. Blood, **9**:843-865, 1954.
5. Anthony, B., and Krivit, W.: Neonatal thrombocytopenia purpura. Pediatrics, **30**:776-783, 1962.
6. Bachman, F.: Mode of inheritance of Factor X deficiency. Throm. Diath. Haemorrh. Suppl., **17**:191-199, 1965.
7. Barkhan, P., and Silver, M. J.: Biological activities of human platelets. Progr. Hemat., **3**:170-202, 1962.
8. Barrow, E. M., and Graham, J. B.: Von Willebrand's disease. Progr. Hemat., **4**:203-221, 1964.
9. Barry, A., and Delage, J. M.: Congenital deficiency of fibrin stabilizing factor. New Eng. J. Med., **272**:943-946, 1965.
10. Bergsagel, D. E., Setna, S. S., Cartwright, G. E., and Wintrobe, M. M.: Mild PTC (plasma thromboplastin component) deficiency occurring in two brothers. Blood, **9**:866-874, 1954.
11. Biggs, R., and MacFarlane, R. G.: Christmas disease. Postgrad. Med. J., **38**:3-12, 1962.
12. Biggs, R., and MacFarlane, R. G.: Human Blood Coagulation. Philadelphia, Davis, 3rd ed., 1962.
13. Bithell, T. C., Didisheim, P., Cartwright, G. E., and Wintrobe, M. M.: Thrombocytopenia inherited as an autosomal dominant trait. Blood, **25**:231-240, 1965.
14. Blattner, R. J.: Antihemophilic globulin levels in carriers of hemophilia A, J. Pediat., **58**:298-300, 1961.
15. Blombäck, M., Jorpes, E. J., and Nilsson, I. M.: Von Willebrand's disease. Amer. J. Med., **34**:236-241, 1963.
16. Bok, J., Veltkamp, J. J., and Loeliger, E. A.: Moderate factor XII deficiency. Thromb. Diath. Haemorrh., **13**:8-11, 1965.
17. Brinkhous, K. M.: The development of our knowledge of Hemophilia A and B. Xth Congr. Int. Soc. Hemat. Scand. J. Haemat. Series Haemat., **7**:1-13, 1965.
18. Brinkhous, K. M.: Hemophilia-Pathophysiologic studies and the evolution of transfusion therapy. Amer. J. Clin. Path., **41**:342-351, 1964.
19. Davie, E. W., and Ratnoff, O. D.: The proteins of blood coagulation. In Neurath, H. (ed.): The Proteins, Vol. 3, New York Academic Press, 1965, p. 360.
20. de Bastos, O., and Reno, R.: A study of three cases of congenital hypoprothrombinemia (Factor II deficiency). Thromb. Diath. Haemorrh., **11**:497-505, 1964.
21. De Gruchy, G. C.: Clinical Hematology. Philadelphia, Davis, 1964.
22. Den Ottolander, G. J. H., and Bleijinberg, A.: Factors which influence the bleeding time. Thromb. Diath. Haemorrh., **8**:511-523, 1963.
23. de Vreker, R. A.: Fibrin stabilizing factor. Thromb. Diath. Haemorrh. Suppl., **13**:411-418, 428, 1964.
24. Duckert, F.: The fibrin stabilizing factor. Xth Congr. Int. Soc. Hemat. Scand. J. Haemat. Series Haemat., **7**:58-69, 1965.
25. Erwin, J. C.: Interpretation of laboratory tests in diagnosis of hemorrhagic disorders. Med. Clin. N. Amer., **46**:63-78, 1962.
26. Fantl, P.: Parahemophilia (proaccelerin deficiency), occurrence and biochemistry. In Brinkhous, K. M. (ed.): Hemophilia and Hemophiloid Disease. Chapel Hill, Univ. N. Carolina Press, 1957, pp. 79-92.
27. Ferguson, J. H.: Blood and Body Functions. Philadelphia, Davis, 1965, pp. 81-128.
28. Gaston, L. W.: The blood clotting factors. New Eng. J. Med., **270**:236-242, 290-298, 1964.
29. Graham, J. B.: Genetic problems: Hemophilia and allied diseases. In Brinkhous, op. cit., pp. 137-162.

30. Graham, J. B.: The genetics of hemophilia. Xth Congr. Int. Soc. Haemat. Scand. J. Haemat. Series Haemat., 7:14-28, 1965.

31. Graham, J. B., Barrow, E. M., and Roberts, H. R.: Possible implications of the autosomal and X-linked hemophilia phenotypes. Thromb. Diath. Haemorrh. Suppl., 17:151-161, 1965.

32. Gross, R.: Metabolic aspects of normal and pathological platelets. In Johnson, S. A., Monto, R. W., Rebuck, J. W., and Horn, R. C. (eds.): Blood Platelets. Boston, Little, 1961, p. 407.

33. Hall, C. A., Rapaport, S. I., Ames, S. B., and deGroot, J. A.: A clinical and familial study of hereditary proconvertin (Factor VII) deficiency. Amer. J. Med., 37:172-181, 1964.

34. Hanahan, D. J., and Papahadjopoulos, D.: Interactions of phospholipids with coagulation factors. Thromb. Diath. Haemorrh. Suppl., 17:71-84, 1965.

35. Harrington, W. J., Minich, V., Hollingsworth, J. W., and Moore, C. V.: Demonstration of a thrombocytopenic factor in the blood of a patient with thrombocytopenic purpura. J. Lab. Clin. Med., 38:1-10, 1951.

36. Hilgartner, M. W., and Smith, C. H.: Plasma thromboplastin antecedent (Factor XI) in the neonate. J. Pediat., 66:747-52, 1965.

37. Hougie, C.: Fundamentals of Blood Coagulation in Clinical Medicine. New York, McGraw, 1963.

38. Iatridis, P. G., and Ferguson, J. H.: The plasmatic atmosphere of the blood platelets. Evidence that only fibrinogen, AcG, activated Hageman factor are present on the surface of the platelets. Thromb. Diath. Haemorrh., 13:114-125, 1965.

39. Inceman, S., Unügür, A., and Aran, M.: Essential athrombia. Thromb. Diath. Haemorrh., 8:502-510, 1962.

40. Jackson, D. P., Beck, E. A., and Cherache, P.: Congenital disorders of fibrinogen. Fed. Proc., 24:816-821, 1965.

41. Jackson, D. P., Schmid, H. J., Zieve, P. D., Levin, J., Conley, C. L.: Nature of a platelet-agglutinating factor in serum of patients with idiopathic thrombocytopenia purpura. J. Clin. Invest., 42:383-390, 1963.

42. Johnson, S. A., Zalboa, R. S., Pederson, H. J., and Buckley, M.: The ultra-structure of platelet participation in hemostasis. Thromb. Diath. Haemorrh., 13:65-83, 1965.

43. Johnson, S. A., and Greenwalt, T. J.: Coagulation and Transfusion in Clinical Medicine. Boston, Little, 1963.

44. Josso, F., Prou-Wartelle, O., and Soulier, J.: Etude d'un cas d'hypoprothrombinémia congénitale. Nouv. Rev. Franc. Hemat., 2:647-672, 1962.

45. Kazal, L. A.: Coagulation proteins. In Sunderman, F. W., and Sunderman, F. W., Jr. (eds.): Serum Proteins and the Dysproteinemias. Philadelphia, Lippincott, 1964, pp. 261-288.

46. Kazal, L. A.: Interactions of phospholipids with lipoproteins, with serum and its proteins, and with proteolytic and non-proteolytic enzymes in blood clotting. Trans. N.Y. Acad. Sci., 27:613-627, 1965.

47. Kerr, C. B., Preston, A. E., Barr, A., and Biggs, R.: Inheritance of Factor VIII. Thromb. Diath. Haemorrh. Suppl., 17:173-179, 1965.

48. Kline, D. L.: Blood coagulation: Reactions leading to prothrombin activation. Ann. Rev. Physiol., 27:285-306, 1965.

49. Krivit, W.: Purpuras: Diagnosis and treatment. Pediat. Clin. N. Amer., 9:833-850, 1962.

50. Kurkcouglu, M., and McElfresh, A. E.: The Hageman factor: Determination of its concentration during the neonatal period and presentation of a case of H.F. deficiency. J. Pediat., 57:61-65, 1960.

51. Larrieux, M. J.: Congenital hemorrhagic disorders with normal platelet count and prolonged bleeding time. Xth Congr. Int. Soc. Hemat. Scand. J. Haemat. Series Haemat., 7:39-57, 1965.

52. Lasowsky, M. S., Hall, R., and Goldie, W.: Congenital deficiency of fibrin-stabilizing factor. Lancet, 11:156, 1965.

53. Loeliger, E. A., Esch, B. V. D., Romeny-Wachter, C., and Booij, H. L.: Factor VII: Its turnover rate and its possible role in thrombogenesis. Thromb. Diath. Haemorrh., 4:196-200, 1960.

54. Lorand, L.: Physiological roles of fibrinogen and fibrin. Fed. Proc., 24:784-793, 1965.

55. MacFarlane, R. G.: An enzyme cascade in the blood clotting mechanism and its functions as a biochemical amplifier. Nature (London), 202:498-499, 1964.

56. MacFarlane, R. G.: A clotting scheme for 1964. Thromb. Diath. Haemorrh. Suppl., 17:45-51, 1965.

57. Mangel, M., Horder, M., and Hiemeyer, V.: Kongenitaler, Factor V. Med. Klin., 58:2042, 1963.

58. Marcus, A. T.: Some biological properties of human platelet granules and membranes. Thromb. Diath. Haemorrh. Suppl., 17:85-88, 1965.

59. Marcus, A. T., and Zucker, M. B.: The Physiology of Blood Platelets. New York, Grune, 1965, p. 13.

60. Marder, V., and Schulman, N.: Clinical aspects of congenital Factor VII deficiency. Amer. J. Med., 37:182-194, 1964.

61. Marr, J., Barboriak, J. J., and Johnson, S. A.: Relationship of appearance of adenosine diphosphate, fibrin formation, and platelet aggregation in the haemostatic plug *in vivo*. Nature (London), 205:259-262, 1965.

62. Maupen, B., Moullec, J., and Kherwman, R.: Trois cas d'afibrinogénémie congénitale dans une même fratrie. Hemostase, 2:229-238, 1962.

63. McElfresh, A. E.: Coagulation in the neonatal period. Amer. J. Med. Sci., 242:171-181, 1961.

64. McKay, D. G.: Disseminated Intravascular Coagulation. New York, Harper, 1965.

65. Medoff, H. S.: Platelet counts in premature infants. J. Pediat., 64:287-289, 1964.

66. Mellman, W. J., Wolman, I. J., Wurzel, H. A., Moorhead, P. S., and Qualls, D. H.: A chromosomal female with hemophilia A. Blood, 17:719-727, 1965.

67. Mulder, E., Machtar, I. A., van Creveld, S., Cardozo, E. P. L.: Factor VIII activity in carriers of hemophilia A. Brit. J. Haemat., 11:206-209, 1965.

68. Nilsson, I. M., Blombäck, M., Jorpes, E., Blombäck, B., and Johansson, S-A: Von Willebrand's Disease and its correction with human plasma fraction 1-o. Acta Med. Scand., 159:179-188, 1957.

69. Nilsson, I. M., and Blombäck, M.: Von Willebrand's disease in Sweden. Occurrence, pathogenesis and treatment. Thromb. Diath. Haemorrh., 9: Suppl. 2, 103-118, 1963.

70. Nossel, H. L.: The Contact Phase of Blood Coagulation. Oxford, Blackwell, 1964.

71. Owen, C. A., Jr., Admunsen, M. H., Thompson, J. H., Spittel, J. A., Bowie, E. J. W., Stillwell, G. G., Hoewlett, I. S., Mills, S. D., Lauer, W. B., and Gage, R. P.: Congenital deficiency of Factor VII (hypoconvertinemia). Amer. J. Med., 37:71-91, 1964.

72. Owren, P. A.: The haemostatic plug. Thromb. Diath. Haemorrh. Suppl., 13:325-333, 1964.

73. Pool, J. G.: Thromboplastin formation. Ann. Rev. Med., 15:215-232, 1964.

74. Preston, A. E.: The plasma concentration of Factor VIII in the normal population. I. Mother and babies at birth. Brit. J. Haemat., 10:110-114, 1964.

75. Quick, A. J., and Hussey, C. V.: Hemophilia B (PTC deficiency, or Christmas disease). Arch. Intern. Med., 103:762-775, 1959.

76. Quick, A. J., Pisciotta, A. V., and Hussey, C. V.: Congenital hypoprothrombinemia states. Arch. Intern. Med., 95:2-14, 1955.

77. Ratnoff, O. D.: Bleeding Syndromes. Springfield, Thomas, 1960, p. 111.

78. Ratnoff, O. D.: PTA deficiency and Hageman trait. Xth Congr. Int. Soc. Hemat. Scand. J. Haemat. Series Haemat., 7:29-38, 1965.

79. Report of Committee on Nutrition Vitamin K compounds and their water soluble analogs. Pediatrics, 28:501-507, 1961.

80. Roskam, J.: Arrest of Bleeding. Springfield, Thomas, 1954, p. 111.

81. Salzman, E. W., and Britten, A.: Hemorrhage and Thrombosis. Boston, Little, 1965.

82. Schaffer, A. J.: Diseases of the newborn. In Blood Coagulation Defects. Philadelphia, Saunders, 1965, Chapter 66.

83. Schulman, I.: Pediatric aspects of the mild hemophilas. Med. Clin. N. Amer., 46:93-105, 1962.

84. Schulz, J., and van Creveld, S.: Stuart-Prower factor in newborn infants. In Brinkhous, op. cit., pp. 167-175.

85. Seegers, W. H.: Basic enzymology of blood coagulation. Thromb. Diath. Haemorrh., 14:213-228, 1965.

85a. Smith, C. H.: Blood Diseases in Infancy and Childhood. Chapter 26, Blood Coagulation p. 625. Chapter 27, Purpuras, p. 695, 2nd Ed. St. Louis, Mo., Mosby, 1966.

86. Tocantins, L. M., and Kazal, L. A.: Blood Coagulation, Hemorrhage and Thrombosis. New York, Grune, 1964.

87. Tocantins, L. M., and Rodriguez, R.: Hemorrhagic disease in children. Notes on pathological physiology and clinical management. Med. Clin. N. Amer., 36;1693-1709, 1952.

88. Tocantins, L. M., Reid, W. O., Silver, M. J., and Kazal, L. A.: Current problems in hemostasis. Ann. N.Y. Acad. Sci., 115:21-30, 1964.

89. Vandenbroucke, J., and Verstraete, M.: Thrombocytopenia due to platelet agglutinins in the newborn. Lancet, 1:593-594, 1955.

90. Veltkamp, J. J., Hemker, H. C., and Loeliger, E. A.: Detection of heterozygotes for Factor VIII, IX and XII deficiency. Thromb. Diath. Haemorrh. Suppl., 17:181-189, 1965.

91. Whitby, L. E. H., and Britton, C. J. C.: Disorders of the Blood, New York, Grune, 1963.

Congenital Disorders of Amino Acid Metabolism

MARY L. EFRON, M.D.

Phenylketonuria (PKU) is the best-known disorder of amino acid metabolism, but it is by no means the only one, and it may not even be the most common. Homocystinuria, which was not even known until 1962, may prove to be more common than PKU. Cystinuria is almost certainly more common. Some of the less well-known amino acid disorders, and methods for detecting them are reviewed in this chapter.

Table I shows an incomplete list of some of the inherited disorders of amino acid metabolism in which one or more amino acids are elevated in concentration in the blood. In these disorders, one can best detect the amino acid abnormality in blood; urine is much less effective. In most of these disorders, there is a metabolic block, i.e., deficient enzyme activity, so that the amino acid is not degraded and consequently accumulates in the blood. The kidney tubule is very efficient in resorbing the amino acid so that very little of it is excreted into the urine. For example, in phenylketonuria, urine testing for screening programs has proved very ineffective in picking up the disease; screening must be done

with blood. That is true of all the "overflow" aminoacidurias.

A simple procedure for detecting "overflow" aminoacidurias is illustrated in Figure 1[1]. Figure 1 is a chromatogram of 10 μl of normal serum compared with 10 μl of serum from a patient with maple syrup urine disease. In the normal

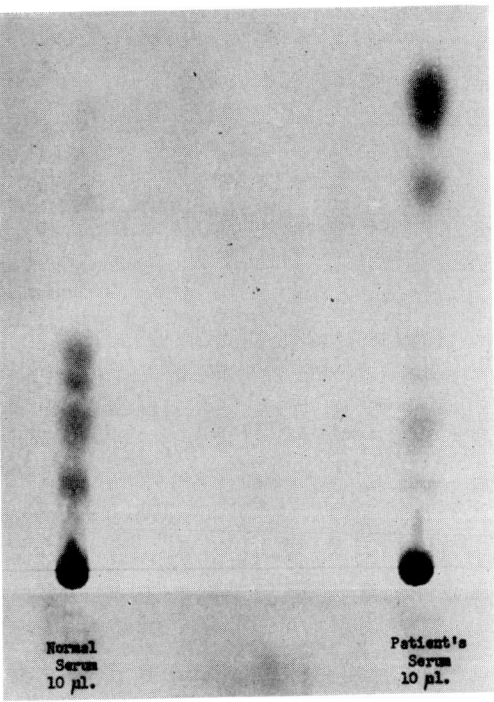

Fig. 1. One-dimensional chromatogram of amino acids in normal serum and in serum from a patient with maple syrup urine disease.

TABLE I PRIMARY OVERFLOW AMINOACIDURIAS

	Amino Acids Elevated in Blood	Deficient Enzyme If Known
Phenylketonuria	phenylalanine	phenylalanine hydroxylase
Tyrosinemia	tyrosine	p-Hydroxyphenylpyruvic acid oxidase
Histidinemia	histidine	histidase
Maple syrup urine disease	valine, leucine, isoleucine	branded chain keto acid decarboxylase
Hypervalinemia	valine	valine transaminase
Hyperglycinemia	glycine	unknown
Hyperprolinemia		
Type I	proline	proline oxidase
Type II	proline	Δ'pyrroline-5-carboxylate dehydrogenase
Hypermethionemia		
Type I	methionine	? methionine activating enzyme, ? secondary to tyrosinemia
Homocystinuria	methionine, homocystine	cystathionine synthetase
Citrullinemia	citrulline	argininosuccinic acid synthetase
Hyperlysinemia	lysine	unknown
Congenital lysine intolerance	lysine, arginine	unknown
Sarcosinemia	sarcosine	unknown
Hyperbeta-alaninemia	B alanine	probably B alanine transaminase
Ornithinemia†	ornithine, lysine	unknown

†Associated with ammonia intoxication. EFRON, M. L.: Unpublished data.

serum, there are no large spots at the top of the chromatogram, while in the patient's serum there are large spots in the position of leucine, isoleucine and valine. With this procedure, it took only a few hours to make the diagnosis. There is no need to deproteinize the serum or do any other elaborate preparation. One merely spots the serum on paper, chromatographs the paper and stains for amino acids.

On Figure 2 is illustrated a chromatogram from the same baby using dried blood in lieu of serum[1]. This chromatogram was made from blood spots collected on filter paper for the PKU screening program. The serum was taken from the patient when maple syrup urine disease was diagnosed at age thirty-nine days. The baby was already damaged neurologically. On Figure 2 is presented a comparison of the serum chromatographic pattern with the blood patterns of filter paper speci-

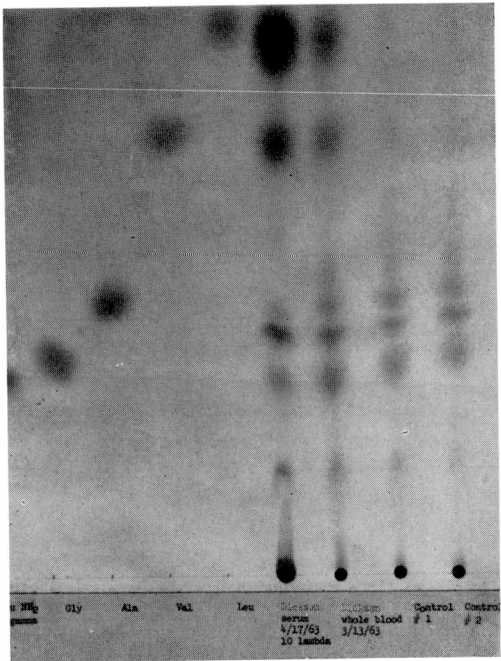

Fig. 2.   One-dimensional chromatogram of amino acids in serum and whole blood from a patient with maple syrup urine disease. (See text).

Renal (Transport) Aminoacidurias	Amino Acids Excreted in Excess
Cystinuria	cystine, lysine, arginine, ornithine
Hartnup disease	valine, leucine, isoleucine, tyrosine, phenylalanine, tryptophane, serine, threonine, alanine, glutamine, asparagine, citrulline, histidine
Joseph's syndrome	proline, hydroxyproline, glycine
Methionine malabsorption syndrome	methionine, smaller amounts of valine, leucine, isoleucine, tyrosine and phenylalanine
Glycinuria with renal stones	glycine
"No Threshold" Aminoacidurias	
Argininosuccinic aciduria	argininosuccinic acid
Cystathioninuria	cystathionine
Homocystinuria	homocystine
Hypophosphatasia	phospho-ethanolamine
B aminoisobutyric aciduria	B aminoisobutyric acid
Juvenile form of familial amaurotic idiocy	histidine, methyl-histidine, carnosine anserine

mens which were collected from the same infant at age five days, and from several normal infants born at the same time. These specimens had been stored in a filing cabinet in the state laboratory of Massachusetts for five months. It is obvious that the disease could have been diagnosed at age five days.

The renal aminoacidurias which are listed in Table II are diagnosed by the examination of amino acids in urine. The abnormalities are difficult or impossible to detect in blood. There are two sub-categories of renal aminoacidurias. (a) The first is "transport" diseases in which the defect is in the kidney. For instance in cystinuria, the best-known renal aminaciduria, the kidney tubule has a defect so that it cannot re-absorb cystine, lysine, arginine and ornithine into the blood[2]. These amino acids, therefore, leak into the urine while the blood levels are normal or even low. Any program designed for screening for cystinuria would have to employ urine screening and not blood tests. (b) The second subgroup is the "no-threshold" aminoacidurias. These substances normally are intracellular. The kidney has no mechanism for handling them, so when they accumulate and leak out into the blood, they are rapidly excreted into the urine. In the "no-threshold" aminoacidurias, the blood levels are elevated, but only very little, so that screening must be by examination of urine.

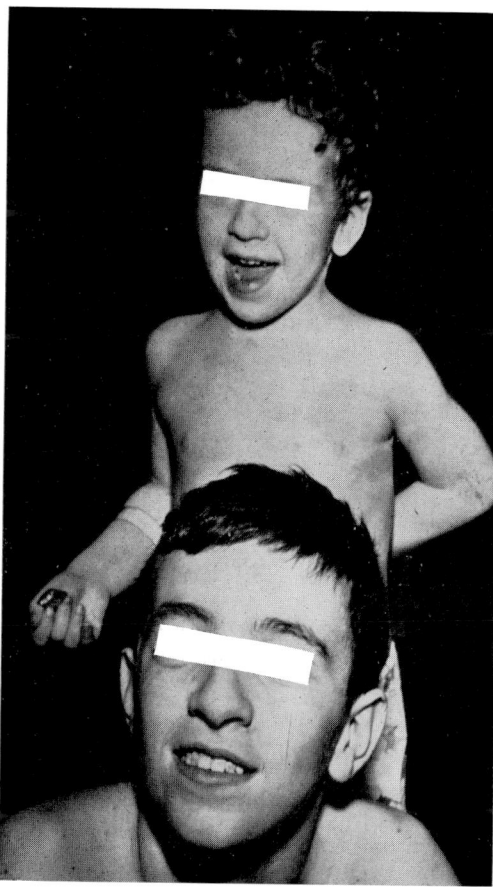

Fig. 3.   Photograph of two mentally retarded children with argininosuccinic aciduria.

Figure 3 is a photograph of two retarded children with curly hair. Both of these children have argininosuccinic aciduria[3]. The curliness of the hair is important because, in the original reports of this disease[4, 5], hair which never had to be cut and which fell out was thought to be a cardinal diagnostic feature. In these children, the disease

was diagnosed from an electrophoretic separation of the urine amino acids (Fig. 4). Amounts of argininosuccinic acid, up to 9 gms a day, were excreted in the urine. Since argininosuccinic acid is a "no-threshold" substance, and since the blood level of argininosuccinic acid rises only to about 4 mg per 100 ml, this disease could not be diagnosed easily from blood.

The enzyme defect in arginosuccinic aciduria is illustrated in Figure 5. This is the urea cycle which converts ammonia to urea. Argininosuccinic acid accumulates because of a block in step 4 of this cycle. Human diseases are known which affect four of the five enzymes in the urea cycle. It is not surprising that patients with argininosuccinic aciduria have ammonia intoxication. There is marked clinical improvement when measures are taken to decrease the production of ammonia, e.g., frequent small meals and a low-protein diet[3, 6].

Another "no-threshold" disease, homocystinuria, has raised interesting questions. On Figure 6 is illustrated the enzymatic block in homocystinuria. Homocystine is an intermediate between methionine and cystine[7]. There are known to be three human diseases in the methionine pathway. Cystathioninuria is caused by a defective enzyme in Step 5[8]. Homocystinuria is due to a deficiency of the enzyme mediating Step 4[7]. As a result, homocystine accumulates in the blood, but the blood level never gets very high, since it is a "no-threshold" substance which is cleared like inulin, and is therefore excreted in quantity in the urine. This disease is very easy to diagnose by means of the nitroprusside test[9]. One of the

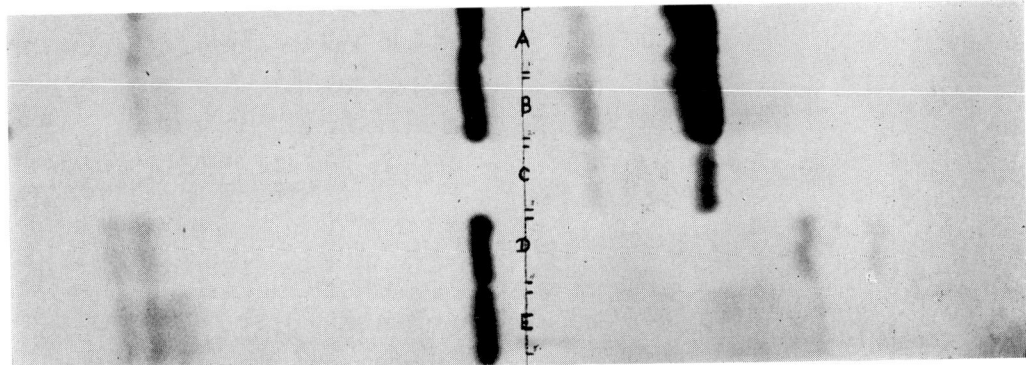

Fig. 4.   Electrophoretic separation of urinary amino acids in argininosuccinic aciduria. Positions A and B indicate the patterns obtained with 10 μl of urine from the two patients with argininosuccinic acidurias. Position C indicates a pattern obtained with argininosuccinic acid from the first patient described with this disease. At Positions D and E are given patterns of a standard mixture of amino acids and a normal urine.

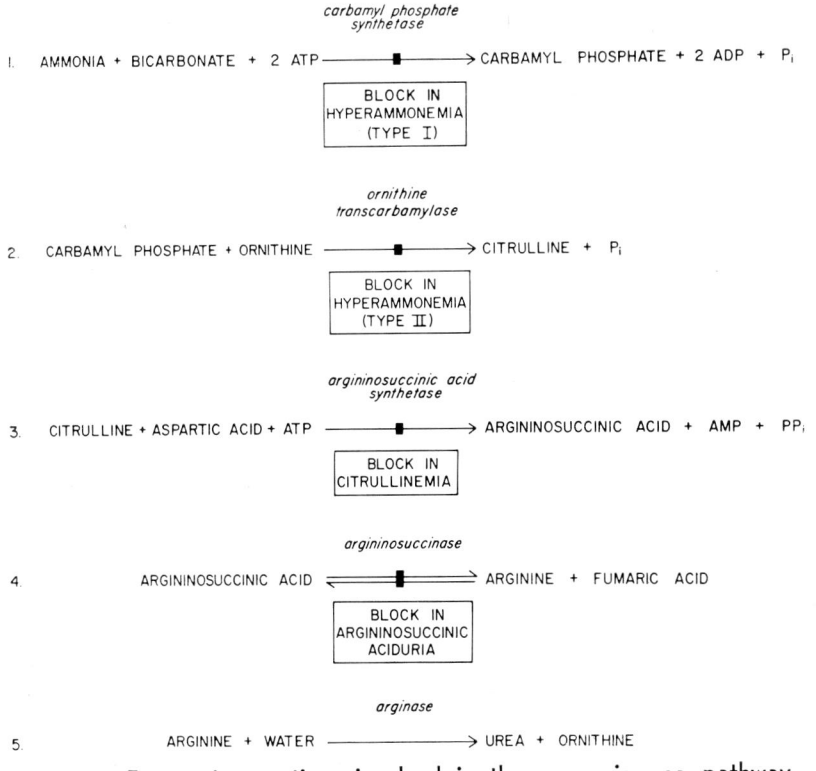

Fig. 5.   Enzymatic reactions involved in the ammonia-urea pathway.

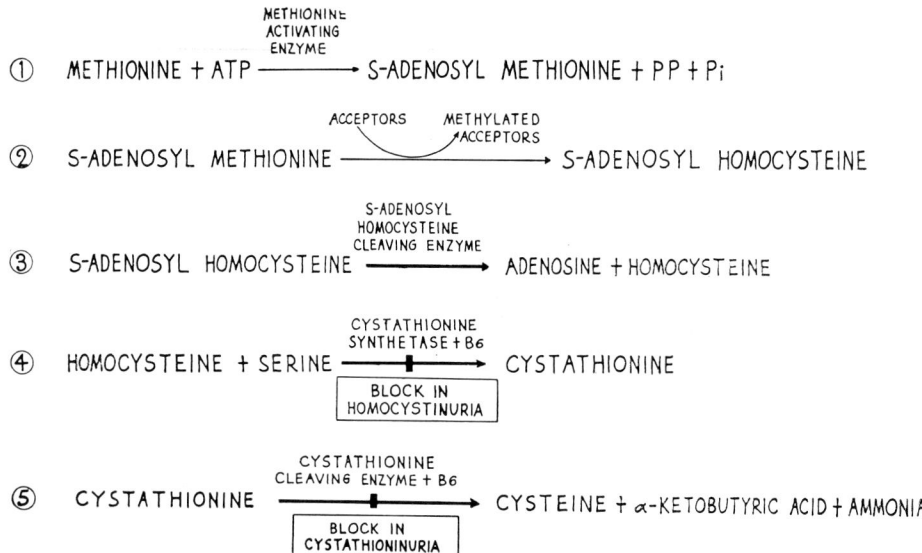

Fig. 6. Enzymatic reactions involved in the methionine-cysteine pathway.

original inborn errors that Garrod studied was cystinuria. Using the nitroprusside test, Garrod found that a few people with cystinuria excreted much more cystine than normal. Homocystine is equally well detected by the nitroprusside test. This disorder was first found by screening a retarded population in northern Ireland. Ten cases were detected in 3,000 tests, so it appeared that this disease might be common in institutions for the retarded[10]. Since 1962, many institutions all over the world have been screened; however, few cases have been found in institutions, even in Massachusetts, with its large Irish population. Nitroprusside tests have been made on over 2,000 retarded patients in one institution in Massachusetts without finding any homocystinuria. McKusick noted that these patients resembled patients with Marfan's syndrome. He instituted a program to screen patients with Marfan's syndrome and dislocated lenses by means of the nitroprusside test[11]. A number of cases were found in this way, and hundreds of patients with this disease are now known. The reason that homocystinuria is not often found in institutions for the retarded is that they are not often severely retarded. The definition of retardation for most institutions is an IQ below 70. Homocystinurics often have an IQ between 70 and 100, so they are not formally retarded, although their IQ's are frequently lower than those of their siblings and parents. The clinical picture is quite characteristic. All patients with homocystinuria detected so far have had dislocated lenses. They have a Marfan's-like picture with long fingers and toes. They have emboli and thrombi, and may have cerebrovascular accidents at an early age. It would seem advisable to undertake nitroprusside tests on mildly retarded people, patients with thromboembolic diseases and on patients with dislocated lenses. McKusick estimates that 5 per cent of all patients with dislocated lenses have this disorder[11].

No reliable statistics regarding the incidence of various aminoacidurias are available. For instance, there is much written about maple syrup urine disease, yet an actual screening program, now being conducted throughout the country, has detected only two patients in over 300,000 tests. Perhaps this incidence is too low to make it worthwhile to support a massive screening program for this disease, unless the test can be combined with screening for more common disorders, such as phenylketonuria. Pilot studies are needed to find out which tests are worthwhile.

Disorders of amino acid metabolism present in many different ways because the enzyme abnormalities may be involved in many different metabolic reactions. Inborn errors often are associated with mental retardation; since many biochemical defects damage the brain. Not all of the aminoacidurias produce retardation. For example, two new disorders, tyrosinosis[12] and hypermethioninemia[13] are associated with cirrhosis. These patients are not retarded mentally; they present with liver disease.

Much interesting clinical research is underway regarding the treatment of patients with these inborn errors of aminoacid metabolism. The first step is to find a number of cases in the newborn period when treatment might still be possible. Each year, several new inborn errors of amino acid metabolism are described. Each disorder adds much to our knowledge of normal human biochemistry and of biochemical pathology-physiology. It is an exciting field, and we can look forward to many unexpected developments.

REFERENCES

1. Efron, M. L., Young, D., Moser, H. W., MacCready, R. A.: A simple chromatographic screening test for the detection of disorders of amino acid metabolism. New Eng. J. Med., **270**:1378-1383, 1964.

2. Knox, W. E.: Phenylketonuria. In Stanbury, J. D., Wyngaarden, J. D., Fredrickson, D. S. (eds.): The Metabolic Basis of Inherited Disease. New York, McGraw 2nd ed., 1966, pp. 258-294.

3. Moser, H. W., Efron, M. L., Brown, H., Diamond, R., Neumann, C. G.: Argininosuccinicaciduria. Report of two new cases and demonstration of intermittent elevations of blood ammonia. Amer. J. Med. in press.

4. Allen, J. D., Cusworth, D. C., Dent, C. E. and Wilson, V. K.: A disease, probably hereditary, characterized by severe mental deficiency and constant gross abnormality of aminoacid metabolism. Lancet, **1**:182-187, 1958.

5. Levin, B., Mackay, H. M. M., and Oberholzer, V. G.: Argininosuccinicaciduria: an inborn error of amino acid metabolism. Arch. Dis. Child., **36**:622, 1961.

6. Efron, M. L. Diseases of the urea cycle. In Stanbury et al., op. cit., pp. 393-408.

7. Finkelstein, J. D., Mudd, S. H., Irreverre, F., and Laster, L.: Homocystinuria due to cystathionine synthetase deficiency; Mode of inheritance. Science, **146**:785-787, 1964.

8. Frimpter, G. W.: Cystathioninuria. Nature of the defect. Science, **149**:1095-1096, 1965.

9. Brand, E., Harris, M., and Biloon, S.: Cystinuria: Excretion of cystine complex which decomposes in urine with liberation of free cystine. J. Biol. Chem., **86**:315-331, 1930.

10. Carson, N. A. J., et al.: Homocystinuria: New inborn error of metabolism associated with mental deficiency. Arch. Dis. Child., **38**:425-436, 1963.

11. Schimke, R. T.: Adaptive characteristics of urea cycle enzymes in the rat. J. Biol. Chem., **237**:459, 1962.

12. Halvorsen, S., and Gjessing, L. R.: Studies on tyrosinosis. 1. Effect of low-tyrosine and low phenylalanine diet. Brit. Med. J., ii:1171-1173, 1964.

13. Perry, T. L., Hardwick, D. F., Dixon, G. H., Dolman, C. L., Hansen, S.: Hypermethioninemia: A metabolic disorder associated with cirrhosis, islet cell hyperplasia, and renal tubular degeneration. Pediatrics, **36**:236-250, 1965.

Phenylketonuria and Phenylalaninemia

MARY L. EFRON, M.D.

It is now more than three years since the phenylketonuria (PKU) screening program was instituted in Massachusetts. Since 1963, almost all new-born infants in Massachusetts have been tested by means of the Guthrie test. More than thirty-five patients with persistent blood phenylalanine concentrations over 20 mg per 100 ml have been detected and treated with a low phenylalanine diet[1, 2]. It would be appropriate at this time to discuss the conclusions which seem warranted.*

It is now obvious that there are at least two different and distinct types of patients, detected by the Guthrie bacterial inhibition assay for blood phenylalanine[3]. About three quarters of these infants seem to have "classical" PKU based upon observations of institutionalized untreated patients and of newborn PKU siblings of PKU patients. This group has the following characteristics:

1. There is often a positive family history. One quarter of the patients in

this group have siblings with phenylketonuria.

2. The initial blood phenylalanine at age four to five days as measured by the Guthrie inhibition assay is near or over 20 mg per 100 ml. By the confirmatory La Du test, usually performed about one to four weeks of age, the concentration of plasma phenylalanine has been near or over 40 mg per 100 ml.

3. The ferric chloride test is positive, often not in the first few weeks of life, but later, when the blood phenylalanine rises during infection, etc. Since these patients are treated early, they do not often have a positive ferric chloride test, but all but one of the patients in this group have had a positive test on at least one occasion.

4. The phenylalanine tolerance is low. These newborns cannot take much more than the minimum daily requirement as established for normal newborn infants. If more phenylalanine is fed, the blood phenylalanine concentration rises to high levels. If the blood concentration is to be kept near normal, these infants must have a markedly restricted phenylalanine intake.

In contrast, about one quarter of the infants with hyperphenylalaninemia in Massachusetts fall into another distinct

---

*Most of these patients are now being treated by Dr. Joseph L. Kennedy, Jr., at the PKU Clinic of the Children's Hospital Medical Center. I am very grateful to Dr. Kennedy for many helpful suggestions and for allowing me to comment on his patients.

category with the following characteristics.

1. Few have had siblings or other relatives with phenylalaninemia or retardation.

2. The initial blood phenylalanine concentration at age four to five days is below 20 mg per 100 ml although it rises above 20 mg per 100 ml later. There seems to be a slow rise of plasma phenylalanine after birth. One infant in this group had a plasma phenylalanine concentration of only 4 mg per 100 ml on the fourth day of life. The policy in the State Diagnostic Laboratory in such cases is to send a notice to the baby's doctor requesting a follow-up measurement of blood phenylalanine when the baby is four to six weeks of age. In this group of patients, the blood phenylalanine concentration by confirmatory La Du test[7] has been under 40 mg per 100 ml in most cases.

3. The ferric chloride test has never been spontaneously positive in any of these treated infants, even when they have illnesses, but it does become weakly positive after feeding high-protein diets for several weeks.

4. The phenylalanine tolerance increases with age. Older infants can take much more phenylalanine than can a phenlyketonuric, without a marked rise in blood phenylalanine concentration. Kennedy has recently followed the older patients while raising their intake of phenylalanine at weekly intervals. He has found that these infants can take an amount of phenylalanine many times the minimal daily requirement (e.g., 2 gm/kg/day of protein) without increasing the plasma phenylalanine concentration above about 15 to 20 mg per 100 ml. When the blood concentration rises to about 18 to 20 mg per 100 ml., the ferric chloride test may become weakly positive. Obviously, these infants have a greater ability to degrade phenylalanine than do the "classical" phenylketonurics. Some of these infants may do well on formulae resembling breast milk; they may not need Lofenalac®, especially after the first few weeks or months.

It seems likely that this second group represents some condition other than "classical" PKU. Perhaps these are the infants with only a partial block in phenylalanine hydroxylase activity. Since, however, there is no family history to suggest phenylketonuria, and since this condition has not been observed in infant siblings of patients with "classical PKU," it may be that the genetic defect is distinct from that in phenylketonuria.

Could this disorder represent a different disease? This question might be resolved by liver biopsy and assay of phenylalanine hydroxylase and phenylalanine transaminase, the main enzymes concerned with phenylalanine metabolism, and by study of the coenzyme which is needed for the conversion of phenylalanine to tyrosine. Too few patients have been studied thus far; more experience is needed with these infants before it can be decided that they are or are not phenylketonuric.

Auerbach and colleagues reported the case of an infant whom they believe to have a disorder which differed from phenylketonuria[4]. They called this disorder "phenylalaninemia." The infant was premature and had a high plasma tyrosine as well as an elevated phenylalanine concentration. The phenylalanine concentration rose slowly to 40 mg per 100 ml and fell rapidly to normal when the infant was treated either with Lofenalac or with a formula that resembled breast milk. The infant developed an elevated concentration of plasma phenylalanine on cow's milk[4]. It was suggested that this child had a deficiency of phenylalanine transaminase but normal phenylalanine hydroxylase. This was not proven. This patient never had a positive ferric chloride test.

It is not clear whether Kennedy's second group is the same entity as that reported by Auerbach *et al.* Infants in Kennedy's second group on normal protein diets have had a positive ferric chloride test. Auerbach's case may be an example of still a third disorder with phenylalaninemia and tyrosinemia, or the tyrosinemia might have been merely an incidental finding due to prematurity. There is much still to be learned about the various conditions which constitute the entity "phenylalaninemia."

Meanwhile there is an obvious conclusion that can be drawn. The treatment of infants with phenylalaninemia detected in screening programs is not a simple matter. It is at least as difficult as the treatment of infantile diabetes and should not be undertaken by anyone who is not specially trained in infant nutrition. It is very easy to produce an abnormally low concentration of plasma phenylalanine. This is potentially a very dangerous situation, because the infant cannot make proteins if the supply of phenylalanine is deficient. Deficient body phenylalanine can lead to severe complications; anemia[5]; hypoglycemia[6]; kwashiorkor-like symptoms; and even death[1].

Two infants who had phenylketonuria detected in the first months of the Massachusetts screening program died while on Lofenalac[1]. Neither was ever seen at the Children's Hospital PKU Clinic. In both cases, the blood phenylalanine concentration was not monitored frequently, and it may be that these infants died of some complication of phenylalanine depletion.

Since the danger of phenylalanine depletion exists, it would seem wise to study all infants very frequently during the first weeks of treatment. Blood phenylalanine should be monitored at least every few days so that the phenylalanine intake which is optimal for growth and maintenance of normal or slightly elevated blood phenylalanine concentration can be determined for each infant.

The blood phenylalanine must be monitored at very frequent intervals during the entire course of therapy. There is no reason that the Guthrie bacterial inhibition assay[5] cannot be used for this purpose. The test has proved to be remarkably quantitative when the concentration is below 20 mg per 100 ml. The blood phenylalanine can also be estimated by means of blood spots on paper, using a chromatographic method[8]. This is cheap and simple and easier than the chemical method. The mother or a visiting nurse can prick the baby's heel, put a drop of whole blood on filter paper and send it through the mail to the laboratory. The blood phenylalanine concentration can be estimated chromatographically or with the Guthrie test[3]; either method is sufficiently accurate for following blood levels in these patients. The simplicity of collection of blood spots makes frequent testing possible. The babies followed in this manner cannot be out of control, either too high or too low, for many days without the physician knowing about it and changing the diet.

When a phenylalaninemic infant of either type is detected, a package of special filter paper could be mailed by the laboratory to the baby's doctor. The physician could be instructed to send in a blood sample at least once a week. The screening laboratory could easily serve as the monitoring laboratory as well.

In Massachusetts, the incidence of phenylketonuria and other forms of phenylalaninemia with blood phenylalanine over 20 mg per 100 ml has been about 1 in 10,000. In addition, 1 infant in 850 has had some elevation, over 2 mg per 100 ml. About one third of these infants are premature, and most of them have tyrosinemia. Apparently, there is an accumulation of phenylalanine as well as tyrosine behind the "block" in p-hydroxy phenylpyruric acid oxidase. Two thirds are term babies, many of whom also have tyrosinemia[9].

Hsia[10] reported that infants with more than the usual jaundice, i.e., the more immature infants, are more likely to have neonatal tyrosinemia. It has been established that 40 per cent of all premature infants who are fed more than 5 gm per kg per day of protein have an elevated blood tyrosine[11]; many of these infants also have transient phenylalaninemia.

In other infants with elevated phenylalanine, there is no tyrosinemia. Many of these infants appear to have a transient immaturity of phenylalanine hydroxylase. Often these are considered to be PKU[12]; some may be just immature infants with delayed production of phenylalanine hydroxylase; still others may be examples of a different disease.

The label "PKU heterozygote" should not be given to an infant on the basis only of a transient elevation of blood phenylalanine.

Most infants with only moderate elevation of the plasma phenylalanine concentration lose their phenylalaninemia, often at about three to six months. Several infants have had more persistent elevations. It is not known whether these few infants have phenylketonuria with only a partial deficiency of phenylalanine hydroxylase, or whether they have a different disorder. One such infant in Massachusetts was followed for one and one half years without a diagnosis. A sibling was then born and appeared to have phenylketonuria (blood phenylalanine 60 mg per 100 ml., positive ferric chloride test) which however is somewhat atypical (relatively high phenylalanine tolerance and tendency for the blood level to fall quickly to subnormal levels on diet[13]).

In our opinion, it is not wise to attempt to achieve a "normal" blood phenylalanine level on therapy. Rather, it seems reasonable to try to keep the blood level no lower than 3 and preferably closer to 8 mg per 100 ml. This avoids any possible danger of phenylalanine starvation, while preventing the very high phenylalanine concentrations which cause amino acid imbalance. There is no good evidence that such levels (3 to 8 mg per 100 ml.) lead to retardation, and with subnormal blood phenylalanine concentrations, there is a possibility of damage to the infant by phenylalanine depletion.

More than 5000 institutionalized, mentally retarded patients in Massachusetts have been screened by means of the Guthrie test[14, 15]. None were found to have a plasma phenylalanine concentration in the range of 2 to 20 mg per 100 ml. The "classical" phenylketonurics all had a concentration of blood phenylalanine of 20 mg per 100 ml. or more. One untreated child, however, whose blood phenylalanine concentration was normal by the Guthrie test, is known to have had a markedly, elevated blood phenylalanine concentration in the first 2 years of life. Since this child is severely retarded, it must be concluded that all infants with marked phenylalaninemia, should have treatment even though not all will prove to have "classical" PKU.

How are the treated phenylketonuric babies doing? In the Massachusetts group, none are obviously retarded, although they are not yet old enough for a final statement in this regard. It is planned to compare them with non-phenylketonuric siblings. It appears at this writing that the average IQ will be near average for the population, although it may not match that of the non-phenylketonuric siblings[1]. All of the "phenylalaninemic" patients appear normal.

It is not known: (a) how many of these children would have had a normal IQ without treatment; (b) whether any damage is done by the diet, if the blood phenylalanine has been kept too low for any prolonged period; or (c) how many of the treated female phenylketonuric infants will grow up to have retarded children because of exposure of the fetus to high phenylalanine concentration in utero[16]. It is not surprising that detection of all cases of phenylalaninemia has raised problems that were not known to exist before mass screening tests.

REFERENCES

1. MacCready, R. A., and Hussey, M. G.: New-born phenylketonuria detection program in Massachusetts. Amer. J. Public Health, **54**: 2075-2081, 1964.
2. Kang, E. S., Kennedy, J. L., Jr., Gates, L., Burwash, I., and McKinnon, A.: Clinical observations in phenylketonuria. Pediatrics, **35**:932-943, 1965.
3. Guthrie, R., and Susi, A. Simple phenylalanine method for detecting phenylketonuria in large populations of newborn infants. Pediatrics, **32**:338-343, 1963.
4. Auerbach, V. H., DiGeorge, A. M., Carpenter, G. C., and Dobes, J. M.: Phenylalaninemia. Abstract Soc. Ped. Res., Philadelphia, May, 1965.
5. Sherman, J. D., Greenfield, J. B., and Ingall, D.: Reversible bone-marrow vacuolizations in phenylketonuria. New Eng. J. Med., **270**:810-814, 1964.
6. Dodge, P. R., Mancall, E. L., Crawford, J. D., Knapp, J., and Paine, R. S.: Hypoglycemia complicating treatment of phenylketonuria with a phenylalanine deficient diet. New Eng. J. Med., **260**:1104-1111, 1959.
7. La Du, B. N., and Michael, P. J.: Enzymatic spectrophotometric method for determination of phenylalanine in blood. J. Lab. Clin. Med., **55**:491-496, 1960.
8. Efron, M. L., Young, D., Moser, H. W., and MacCready, R. A.: A simple chromatographic screening test for the detection of disorders of amino acid metabolism. New Eng. J. Med., **270**:1378-1383, 1964.
9. Kennedy, J. L., Jr.: To be published.
10. Hsia, D. Y., Litwack, M., O'Flynn, M., and Jakovcic, S.: Serum phenylalanine and tyrosine levels in the newborn infant. New Eng. J. Med., **267**:1067-1070, 1962.
11. Mathews, J., and Partington, M. W.: Plasma tyrosine levels of premature babies. Arch. Dis. Child., **39**:371-378, 1964.
12. Allen, R. J., Heffelfinger, J. C., Masotti, R. E., and Tsau, M. U.: Phenylalanine hydroxylase activity in new-born infants. Pediatrics, 512-525, April 1964.
13. Connelly, J. P.: Personal communication. To be published.
14. Bixby, E. M., Pallatao, L. G., and Pryles, C. V.: Evaluation of the bacillus subtilis inhibition-assay technic as a screening procedure for the detection of phenylketonuria. New Eng. J. Med., **268**:648-651, 1963.
15. MacCready, R. A.: Unpublished data.
16. Mabry, C. C., Denniston, J. C., Nelson, T. L., and Son, C. D.: Maternal phenylketonuria. A cause of mental retardation in children without the metabolic defect. New Eng. J. Med., **268**:648-651, 1963.

Measurement of Amino Acids in Blood by Paper Chromatography

MARY L. EFRON, M.D.

METHOD

Blood is collected in the same manner as in the bacterial inhibition assay of Guthrie[1]. The concentrations of amino acid in blood are estimated by direct paper chromatography of blood spots. Estimations of concentrations are made on the basis of size and color of the amino acid spots.

MATERIALS AND EQUIPMENT

1. *Filter paper cards* may be obtained from Schleicher and Schuell. Paper 903C is used; this paper is highly absorbant. Cards made of this paper, approximately 4 x 5 in, are in common use in most states for the Guthrie assay for phenylalanine. These cards are designed with space for writing in the name and address of the patient, along with other required information.

2. *Chromatography tanks* and *large sheets of paper* of approprite dimensions for ascending or descending chromatography in the tank. Schleicher and Schuell 593C or Whatman 3MM paper is suitable. A paper 24 x 10½ in will hold twenty-five blood spots and two disks soaked in standard solutions of amino acids for ascending chromatography.

3. *A paper punch.* 3/16 in in diameter.

4. *A wallpaper roller.*

5. *An autoclave.*

REAGENTS

1. *Butanol-acetic acid-water* (12:3:5).

2. *Ninhydrin*, 0.2 per cent, in acetone.

3. *Ehrlich's reagent*: p-dimethylaminobenzaldehyde, 10 per cent in concentrated hydrochloric acid (diluted with four volumes of acetone just before use).

4. *Isatin*, 0.2 per cent, in butanol containing 5 per cent acetic acid.

5. *Diazotized sulfanilic acid reagent;* sulfanilic acid (9 gm in 90 ml of concentrated hydrochloric acid and 900 ml of water), one volume; sodium nitrite (5 per cent in water), one volume; sodium carbonate (10 per cent in water), two volumes. Just before use, the first two reagents are mixed and allowed to stand for four or five minutes in the refrigerator. The last reagent is added slowly, since it effervesces. The mixture is used immediately.

COLLECTION OF BLOOD AND PREPARATION FOR CHROMATOGRAPHY

Two or three spots of blood, each about 1 cm in diameter, are obtained by heel or finger puncture on a filter paper card. Care should be taken to obtain sufficient blood so that the paper is soaked through to the opposite side. The sample is then mailed to the laboratory.

The paper is autoclaved for one to three minutes at 250 F. The papers must come into contact with the steam and become wet. Autoclaving is necessary to prevent diffusion of blood during subsequent chromatography; is also necessary for the Guthrie test.

The Chromatography

Duplicate paper chromatograms are prepared by taking two sheets of chromatography paper and punching 3/16 in holes along the bottom of each sheet. With the same punch, two circles of filter paper are cut from the center of the blood spots and are inserted into a hole in each paper. Pressure is applied so that the edges of the inserted discs and of the holes are exactly approximated; a wallpaper roller is useful for this purpose. Both sheets are chromatographed, ascending or descending, using butanol-acetic and water as the solvent. The papers are dried in air or at 60° and are then ready for staining.

Staining the Chromatograms

One of the duplicate chromatograms is dipped in the ninhydrin reagent, and the other in isatin. On the isatin-stained chromatogram, proline gives a blue color, stable to washing in one normal hydrochloric acid. Hydroxyproline is then detected by staining with Ehrlich's reagent over the isatin.

The ninhydrin-stained chromatogram is inspected for increased amino acids. Following this, the histidine spot is counter-stained with the sulfanilic acid reagent and the rest of the paper is stained with Ehrlich's reagent to detect citrullinemia or increased tryptophane.

Standards

This method will easily detect even small increases in concentration of most blood amino acids. Solutions containing 5 and 10 mg per 100 ml of each amino acid are suitable for standards. These solutions are spotted on filter paper and autoclaved exactly like blood. Standard disks soaked with each of the two standard solutions are chromatographed on the same sheet along with twenty-five blood samples. There is one area of the chromatogram which has several overlapping amino acids including glycine. Blood glycine in a concentration of 10 mg per 100 ml can however be detected by this technique. Very small increases in amino acids might be missed by this procedure, i.e., 5 mg per 100 ml of glycine. Above 10 mg per 100 ml, however, the amino acid spot appears large even in the crowded area of the chromatogram. By comparison with the color of the standard amino acid spots, an estimate of the concentration of each amino acid is obtained.

REFERENCES

1. Guthrie, R., and Susi, A.: Simple phenylalanine method for detecting phenylketonuria in large populations of newborn infants. Pediatrics, 32: 338-343, 1963.
2. Efron, M. L., et al.: A simple chromatographic screening test for the detection of disorders of amino acid metabolism. New Eng. J. Med., 270:1378-1383, 1964.
3. Culley, W. J., et al.: Paper chromatographic estimation of phenylalanine and tyrosine using finger-tip blood. Its application to phenylketonuria. Clin. Chem., 8:266-269, 1962.
4. Scriver, C. R., Davies, E., and Cullen, A. M.: Application of a simple micromethod to the screening of plasma for a variety of aminoacidopathies. Lancet, 2:230-232, 1964.

Chapter 10

Measurements of Alpha Amino Acid Nitrogen in Urine and Plasma

BYRON RUSKIN, M.D., AND F. WILLIAM SUNDERMAN, JR., M.D.

The principal methods for the determination of amino acid nitrogen in plasma and urine involve the reactions listed in Table I. In the *formol titration procedures,* carboxyl groups of the amino acids are titrated in the presence of formalin[40, 58, 61]. The *nitrous acid procedures* are based upon gasometry of N_2 liberated from amino groups by nitrous acid[33, 45]. The *naphthoquinone procedures* depend upon colorimetry of brown complexes which are formed by reaction of amino acids with β-naphthoquinone-4-sulfonate[9, 17, 20, 21, 23, 24, 48]. The *copper procedures* involve titration, colorimetry or flame photometry of amino acid-copper complexes[1, 2, 30, 31, 46, 52, 53]. The *ninhydrin procedures* are based either upon gasometry of CO_2 evolved by decarboxylation of α-amino acids with ninhydrin[16, 25, 26, 35, 38, 50, 55, 56, 59], or upon colorimetry of the amino acid-ninhydrin complexes[15, 18, 28, 29, 32, 39, 47, 49, 54]. The *bromosuccinimide procedures* involve gasometry of CO_2 following decarboxylation of α-amino acids with n-bromosuccinimide[10, 34].

Although the gasometric ninhydrin and bromosuccinimide procedures are technically difficult, they are generally accepted as the reference procedures for measurements of α-amino acids in biological fluids. Because these methods are laborious and require special apparatus, they have not proven to be convenient for routine use in clinical laboratories. The formol, naphthoquinone, copper and colorimetric ninhydrin reactions are less troublesome, but are subject to varying degrees of interference from other amines and from urea, uric acid and ammonia[12, 44]. For determinations of amino acid nitrogen in urine, the colorimetric procedure of Sobel and associates[52] has been selected by our laboratory for routine use. Results obtained by this procedure agree closely with those obtained by the gasometric ninhydrin technique. Moreover, the method can be performed with relative ease and lends itself to multiple determinations. Because of its

TABLE I REACTIONS FOR DETERMINATION OF TOTAL AMINO ACID NITROGEN IN BIOLOGICAL FLUIDS

I. Formol reaction
II. Nitrous acid reaction
III. Naphthoquinone reaction
IV. Copper reaction
V. Ninhydrin reactions
VI. Bromosuccinimide reaction

simplicity and dependability, the colorimetric naphthoquinone procedure of Frame and associates[22, 48] has been selected by our laboratory as the routine method for determinations of amino acid nitrogen in plasma. In the absence of azotemia, this procedure affords good correlation with measurements by the gasometric ninhydrin technique.

Measurement of Alpha Amino Acid Nitrogen in Urine

MODIFICATION OF THE METHOD OF SOBEL ET AL.[52]

INTRODUCTION

In 1939, Pope and Stevens[46] described a method in which a suspension of copper phosphate was used to form a copper complex with α-amino acids. The copper present in the complex was determined quantitatively by iodometric titration. Albanese and Irby[1], in 1944, adapted this procedure to the determination of α-amino acid nitrogen in urine. In 1957, Sobel and co-workers[52] increased the accuracy of the procedure of Albanese and Irby[1] by use of a chromatographic column of ion exchange resin to isolate the amino acids, and by colorimetric determination of the amino acid-copper complex with sodium diethyldithiocarbamate.

METHOD

After preliminary isolation of amino acids on an ion exchange resin, the acids are eluted and complexed with divalent copper. The copper is determined photometrically with sodium diethyldithiocarbamate. The chemical reactions are given in Figure 1.

REAGENTS

1. *Dowex ion exchange resin (50 x 8),* 200 to 400 mesh, A. R. grade, hydrogen form (A. R. Baker Co.).

2. *Cupric chloride,* 2.80 per cent (w/v) solution of $CuCl_2 \cdot 2H_2O$. This solution is filtered and stored at room temperature.

3. *Sodium phosphate,* 6.85 per cent (w/v) solution of $Na_3PO_4 \cdot 12H_2O$. This solution is filtered and stored at room temperature.

4. *Borax,* 1.90 per cent (w/v) solution of $Na_2BO_7 \cdot 10H_2O$. This solution is filtered and stored at room temperature.

5. *Copper phosphate suspension.* Thirty ml of sodium phosphate solution are transferred to a 50 ml centrifuge tube. Twenty ml of the cupric chloride solution are slowly added to the centrifuge tube with shaking. The solution is centrifuged and the supernatant discarded. The precipitate is suspended

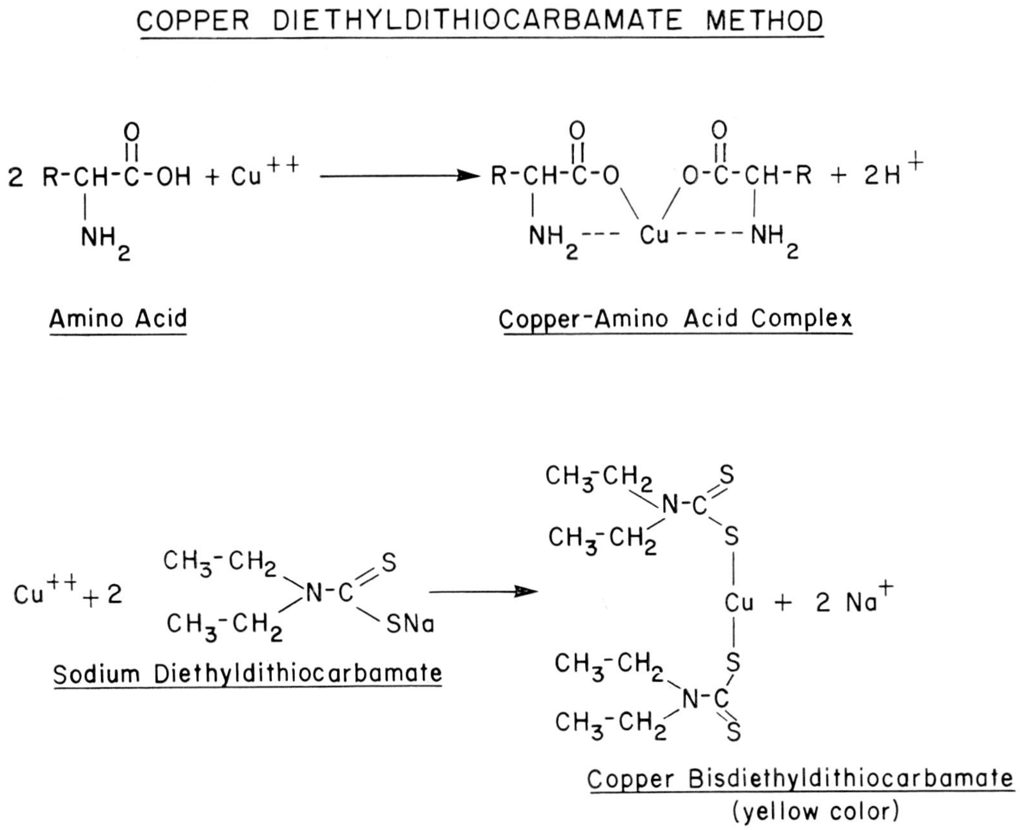

COPPER DIETHYLDITHIOCARBAMATE METHOD

Fig. I.   Chemical reactions for the determination of amino acids with diethyldithiocarbamate.

in 15 ml of borax solution with the aid of a glass rod. An additional 35 ml of borax solution are added, mixed and centrifuged. The supernatant is discarded and the washing procedure repeated. Finally, the precipitate is suspended in 75 ml of borax solution, to which 2.25 gm of sodium chloride has been added. This reagent is stable for several weeks at room temperature.

6. *Sodium diethyldithiocarbamate solution.* One half gm of sodium diethyldithiocarbamate is dissolved in 25 ml of distilled water and filtered. The solution must be prepared immediately before use.

7. *Standard solution of α-amino acid nitrogen (1 ml = 0.2 mg α-amino acid nitrogen.)* Exactly 0.268 gm of glycine, 0.525 gm of glutamic acid, and 1.0 gm of sodium benzoate are transferred to a 500 ml volumetric flask. Three hundred ml of distilled water are added and the solids are dissolved. Four ml of concentrated hydrochloric acid are added and the solution is diluted to the mark with distilled water.

8. *Sodium hydroxide, 1 N.*

9. *Sodium hydroxide, 0.1 N.*

10. *Hydrochloric acid, 6 N.*

11. *Hydrochloric acid, 1 N.*

12. *Hydrochloric acid,* 0.01 N.

13. *Thymolphthalein indicator solution*

Special Apparatus

1. *Chromatography columns* (10 cm long, inner diameter 7.5 mm). These columns are prepared by removing the tips from 10 ml Mohr pipettes.

2. *Boekel filter pump.**

3. *Leffler aeration manifold*[36].

PROCEDURE

A. Isolation of Amino Acids by Ion Exchange Column

1. Glass wool plugs are placed in the bottoms of the chromatographic columns. The columns are filled with a slurry of Dowex resin suspended in water. The slurry is allowed to pass through the columns until the resin beds measure 5 cm. The tops of the resin beds are never allowed to become dry. A sufficient number of columns is prepared so that the standard, blank and urine samples may be determined in duplicate.

2. Ten ml of urine, 10 ml of the standard, and 10 ml of water are adjusted to pH 1 to 2 with 1 N HCl, using pH paper as an external indicator.

3. A column is partially inserted into a 1000 ml side-arm filter flask through a rubber stopper. The vacuum in the filter flask is adjusted to 18 cm of mercury with a Boeckel filter pump.

4. The acidified sample of urine is

poured onto a column and washed with 5 ml of 0.01 N HCl and then with 15 to 20 ml of water until the eluate is approximately pH 5. This eluate is discarded. The standards and blanks are treated in the same manner as the urine samples and carried through the entire procedure.

5. Twelve ml of 1 N sodium hydroxide are added to each column. When the sodium hydroxide front has descended to the middle of the resin bed, (detected as a change from a light brown to a dark brown), the collection of the eluate is begun. A 10 ml eluate from each column is collected in a 25 ml test tube graduated at 10 ml.

6. The eluate is aerated vigorously for 30 minutes by bubbling room air through the solution by means of the Leffler manifold. The volume of the eluate is adjusted to 10 ml with distilled water.

B. Determination of Alpha Amino Acid Nitrogen in the Eluate

1. Two and one half ml of each eluate are transferred to a 50 ml glass-stoppered centrifuge tube. Two and one half ml of distilled water are added and a drop of thymolphthalein. Hydrochloric acid (6 N) is added by drop by drop until the indicator is colorless. Then 1 N sodium hydroxide is added drop by drop until the indicator just turns blue.

2. Five ml of copper phosphate suspension are added to each tube. The tubes are stoppered and shaken for five minutes.

---

*L. K. B. Instruments, 4840 Rugby Avenue, Washington, D.C., Catalog No. W-1720.

3. The tubes are centrifuged at 2,000 rpm for five minutes and the supernatants are filtered through Whatman No. 1 filter paper.

4. One ml of each filtrate is diluted in a volumetric flask of 25 ml with distilled water.

5. Four ml of each diluted filtrate are transferred to properly labelled 19 mm Coleman cuvettes.

6. Two tenth ml of diethyldithiocarbamate reagent and 6.0 ml of isopropyl alcohol are added to each cuvette. The contents are mixed.

7. The spectrophotometer is adjusted to zero optical density at 435 mμ. The optical densities of the unknown, standard and blanks are recorded.

CALCULATIONS

Urinary α-amino acid N (mg per 24 hours) =

$$\frac{\text{O.D. unknown} - \text{O.D. blank}}{\text{O.D. standard} - \text{O.D. blank}} \times 20 \times \frac{\text{ml of urine/24 hours}}{10}$$

PROCEDURAL NOTES

Thirty ml of 6 N HCl plus 1 ml of 10 per cent alcoholic thymol may be added to the urine samples as a preservative. Urine stored at 4 C is stable for at least one month. Uric acid is removed from the urine by the ion exchange resin and ammonia is removed by aeration. The final color is stable for two hours and obeys Beer's law. It may be noted that taurine is not measured in this method, nor in the gasometric ninhydrin method. Taurine is measured in the β-naphthoquinone-4-sulfonate method. In our laboratory, the recovery of α-amino acids from urine averages 87 per cent.

NORMAL VALUES FOR AMINO ACID NITROGEN IN URINE

Measurements of α-amino acid nitrogen were performed in our laboratory upon urine collections from seventeen normal adults. These measurements yielded a mean excretion of 105 (SD $\pm$ 37) mg per twenty-four hours, with a range from 55 to 178 mg per twenty-four hours. In Table II these values are contrasted with those obtained by other investigators, employing a variety of analytical procedures. As shown in Table II, higher values were obtained by Zandrey[61], using the formol titration, and by Albanese and Irby[1] and by Kekki[30] using the direct copper reaction, than were reported by investigators who employed gasometric or colorimetric ninhydrin procedures. The values obtained in our laboratory by the modified method of Sobel and associates[52] were comparable to measurements by the various ninhydrin techniques.

Normal values for the excretion of amino acid nitrogen in urine of infants and children are listed in Table III. There is controversy regarding the best method for expressing the results of these analyses[6, 28, 41, 42, 51]. Reporting the results as mg per kg per day may lead to spurious elevations in children with malnutrition or muscular dystrophy.

TABLE II AMINO ACID NITROGEN IN URINE OF NORMAL ADULTS

Authors		No. of Subjects	Method	Mean ± SD (mg per 24 hours)		Range
Zandrey[61]	1922	6	formol titration	292	—	252-403
Albanese and Irby[1]	1944	15	copper reaction	—	—	221-694
Eckhardt and Davidson[19]	1948	8	gasometric ninhydrin	158	—	120-199
Thompson and Abdulnabi[55]	1950	13♂	gasometric ninhydrin	101	± 39	—
		11♀	gasometric ninhydrin	126	± 67	—
Loffler and Gerok[37]	1955	8♂	titrimetric ninhydrin	127	—	55-200
Kekki[30]	1959	7	copper reaction	257	—	110-358
Jagenburg[28]	1959	26♂	colorimetric ninhydrin	124	—	60-183
		11♀	colorimetric ninhydrin	105	—	69-165
Khachadurian et al.[32]	1960	18♂	colorimetric ninhydrin	117	± 48	60-264
Matthews et al.[39]	1964	10	colorimetric ninhydrin	129	± 82	47-293
Ruskin and Sunderman	1967	17	ion exchange; copper reaction	105	± 37	55-178

TABLE III AMINO ACID NITROGEN IN URINE OF INFANTS AND CHILDREN

Authors		No. of Subjects	mg/kg/day	% Total N	mg/100 mg Creatinine
Infants (3 days to 3 months)					
Childs[11]	1952	14 (premature + full-term)	8.5 (1.8-32)		
Jagenburg[28]	1959	21 (full-term)		1.4 (0.9-2.6)	24 (17-35)
		28 (premature)		1.9 (0.8-3.1)	32 (19-52)
O'Brien et al.[41]	1960	11 (premature)	12.5 (5.2-16)		
Children (6 months to 13 years)					
Childs[11]	1952	34	2.5 (1.6-4.3)		
Berger[5]	1956	40	3.0 (1.0-5.0)	1.2 (0.4-2.0)	
Huisman[27]	1957	72	2.5 ± 1.0	1.1 ± 0.3	
Khachadurian et al.[32]	1960	8			17 ± 6
Andrews et al.[4]	1961	8	3.1 (1.9-4.5)		
Constantsas et al.[15]	1964	10			18 ± 3
Van Gelderen and Dooren[56]	1964	42	2.9 ± 1.0	1.2 ± 0.3	
Ruskin and Sunderman	1967	12	3.1 (1.5-4.0)		16 ± 3

Reporting amino acid nitrogen excretion as a percentage of total urinary nitrogen may be misleading if the child receives a high-protein diet. Reporting the results in relationship to the excretion of creatinine is influenced by the variability of creatinine excretion in infants and young children[6]. It is probably best to interpret the excretion of amino acid nitrogen in infants and children on the basis of two or more indices. By all of the indices, the excretion of amino acids is proportionately greater in infants than in children, and greater in premature infants than in full-term infants.

Determination of Alpha Amino Acid Nitrogen in Plasma

(METHOD OF FRAME ET AL.[22, 48])

METHOD

In this method, measurements are made of the brown color which develops when α-amino acids react with β-naphthoquinone-4-sulfonate in alkaline solution. The chemical reaction is given in Figure 2.

REAGENTS

1. *Sulfuric acid*, 2/3 N.

2. *Sodium tungstate*, 10 per cent (w/v) solution.

3. *Sodium β-naphthoquinone-4-sulfonate*, 0.5 per cent (w/v) solution. This solution is prepared within an hour before use.

4. *Borax*: 2 per cent (w/v) solution of $Na_2B_4O_7 \cdot 10H_2O$. This solution is stable indefinitely.

5. *Sodium hydroxide*, 0.1 N.

6. *Phenolphthalein*, 0.25 per cent (w/v) ethanolic solution.

7. *Acid formaldehyde reagent*: 0.3 N HCl containing 3 ml of 40 per cent formaldehyde per liter.

8. *Sodium thiosulfate*, 0.05 M solution. Exactly 12.4 gm of $Na_2S_2O_3 \cdot H_2O$ are dissolved in one liter of distilled water. This solution is stable at 4° C.

9. *Stock standard α-amino acid solution*. This solution is the same as for the determination of urinary α-amino acid nitrogen.

10. *Working standard α-amino acid solution*. A 1:10 dilution of the stock standard is made with distilled water.

PROCEDURE

1. A protein-free filtrate is prepared by transferring 1.0 ml of plasma, 8.0 ml of distilled water, 0.5 ml of 2/3 N H_2

NAPHTHOQUINONESULFONATE METHOD

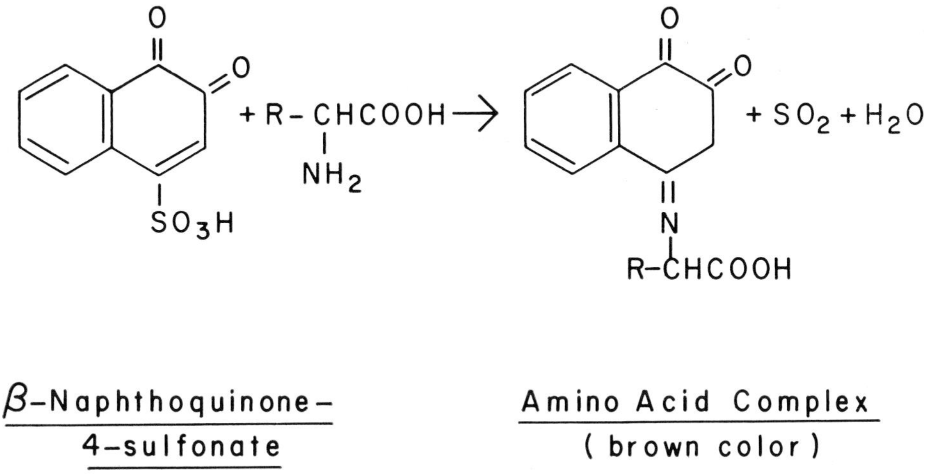

β-Naphthoquinone-4-sulfonate + R-CHCOOH(NH₂) → Amino Acid Complex + SO₂ + H₂O

β-Naphthoquinone-
4-sulfonate

Amino Acid Complex
(brown color)

Fig. 2. Chemical reactions for the determination of amino acids with
β-naphthoquinone-4-sulfonate.

SO_4 and 0.5 ml of 10 per cent sodium tungstate into a 13 x 125 mm test tube. The contents are mixed and filtered through Whatman No. 1 filter paper.

2. Five ml of the filtrate are transferred to a graduated 15 ml centrifuge tube.

3. A standard is prepared by transferring 1.5 ml of the working standard solution into a 15 ml graduated centrifuge tube and adding 3.5 ml of distilled water.

4. A reagent blank is prepared by transferring 5.0 ml of distilled water to a 15 ml graduated centrifuge tube.

5. One drop of phenolphthalein is added to each tube. One tenth normal sodium hydroxide is added drop by drop until a permanent pink color is produced.

6. One ml of the borax solution is added to each tube.

7. One ml of naphthoquinone reagent is added to each tube and mixed.

8. The tubes are then placed in cold water for five minutes.

9. One ml of the acid formaldehyde reagent is added and mixed.

10. One ml of the sodium thiosulfate solution is added and mixed.

11. The solution is diluted to the 15 ml mark with distilled water and mixed. The tubes are allowed to stand for ten minutes and spectrophotometer readings are made within thirty minutes.

12. The spectrophotometer galvanometer is adjusted to zero optical density at 470 mμ with the reagent blank. The optical densities of the standard and plasma samples are recorded.

CALCULATION OF RESULTS

The final value must be calculated from a standard curve since the final

CONSTRUCTION OF CALIBRATION CURVE

	Amino Acid Nitrogen (mg/100 ml)						
	0	2.0	4.0	6.0	8.0	10.0	12.0
Working standard solution (ml): (1 ml = 20 mg)	0	0.5	1.0	1.5	2.0	2.5	3.0
Distilled water (ml):	5.0	4.5	4.0	3.5	3.0	2.5	2.0

color does not obey Beer's law. The calibration curve is checked by the standard included in the analysis.

PROCEDURAL NOTES

Measurements of amino acids should be performed upon plasma rather than serum, inasmuch as several amino acids are released into serum during the process of coagulation[13, 14, 38]. Oxalate or heparin are used as the anticoagulant. Plasma is stable for several days when frozen. Ammonia and uric acid lead to erroneous results, but the concentrations of these substances in plasma are usually not of the magnitude to introduce serious errors. One mg of uric acid per 100 ml gives a color equivalent to 0.1 mg per 100 ml of amino acid nitrogen. In hyperuricemia, this correction factor may be applied. Sulfonamides also may lead to increased values. Deproteinization of plasma with tungstic or trichloroacetic acids is satisfactory for routine use, but, for most precise measurements, ultrafiltration is preferable[43].

TABLE IV AMINO ACID NITROGEN IN PLASMA OF NORMAL ADULTS

Authors		No. of Subjects	Method	Mean ± SD (mg per 100 ml)	Range
Kirk[33]	1933	6	gasometric nitrous acid	— —	4.0-6.5
Danielson[17]	1933	37	naphthoquinone reaction	4.8 —	3.9-5.7
Hamilton and Van Slyke[26]	1943	10	gasometric ninhydrin	4.1 ± 0.8	3.4-5.5
Cramer and Winnick[16]	1943	20	gasometric ninhydrin	4.2 ± 1.1	2.3-7.3
Woodruff and Man[60]	1945	21♂	gasometric ninhydrin	4.3 —	3.4-4.8
		16♀	gasometric ninhydrin	4.1 —	3.4-5.0
Albanese and Irby[2]	1945	13	copper reaction	7.9 ± 0.5	5.8-8.5
Brewer et al.[8]	1947	17	gasometric ninhydrin	4.2 ± 0.3	3.7-4.8
Kekki[30]	1959	12	copper reaction	4.4 —	3.7-5.3
Rosenblum et al.[47]	1959	23	colorimetric ninhydrin	3.7 ± 0.5	2.1-4.6
Saifer et al.[49]	1960	31	colorimetric ninhydrin	5.2 ± 0.5	—
Bjornesjo[7]	1963	53♂	colorimetric ninhydrin	4.2 ± 0.4	—
		53♀	colorimetric ninhydrin	3.9 ± 0.6	—
Matthews et al.[39]	1964	20	colorimetric ninhydrin	4.0 ± 0.4	3.7-5.4
Lacy and Crofford[35]	1964	11♂	gasometric ninhydrin	4.5 ± 0.3	4.1-5.0
		10♀	gasometric ninhydrin	4.1 ± 0.5	3.1-4.7
Ruskin and Sunderman	1967	14	naphthoquinone reaction	4.7 ± 0.4	3.9-5.5

NORMAL VALUES FOR AMINO ACID NITROGEN IN PLASMA

Normal values for the concentration of free amino acid nitrogen in plasma from adults are listed in Table IV. Excepting for the method of Albanese and Irby, which yields much higher values[2], the mean concentrations of amino acid nitrogen reported in plasma have ranged from 3.7 to 5.2 mg per 100 ml. As shown on the table, the mean concentration of plasma amino acid nitrogen obtained in our laboratory by the naphthoquinone technique of Frame and co-workers[22, 48] was 4.7 mg per 100 ml with a range from 3.9 to 5.5.

Excepting for the neonatal period, the concentrations of free amino acid nitrogen in plasma of infants and children do not differ significantly from those of adults, (Table V). Sereni and co-workers[51] observed increased concentrations of amino acid nitrogen in plasmas from premature infants who were less than seventeen days of age. Andrews and co-workers[3] reported higher concentrations of amino acids in serum from the umbilical veins of full-term infants than in serum from infants and children who were more than six weeks of age.

SUMMARY

A resume is presented of the biochemical methods for the determination of α-amino acid nitrogen in biological fluids. The procedures which are currently in routine use in the authors' laboratories are described in detail. The literature pertaining to the normal values for amino acid nitrogen in urine and plasma is reviewed, with emphasis upon the normal findings in infancy and childhood.

TABLE V   AMINO ACID NITROGEN IN PLASMA AND SERUM OF INFANTS

Group	Age	No. of Subjects	Mean ± SD (mgper100ml)		Range
Sereni *et al.*[51], 1955 (gasometric ninhydrin, plasma)					
Premature infants	(< 17 days)	5	5.6	—	4.5-7.0
Premature infants	(28-51 days)	7	4.2	—	3.4-4.9
Full-term infants	(9 days-17 mo)	7	3.4	—	2.7-4.5
Children and adults	(4-40 yr)	9	3.9	—	2.4-5.3
Andrews *et al.*[3], 1962 (colorimetric ninhydrin, serum)					
Full-term infants	(cord blood)	25	7.7 ± 2.0		2.3-12.0
Infants and children	(6 weeks-11 years)	32	5.0 ± 1.3		3.0-7.5
O'Brien and Butterfield[42], 1963 (ion-exchange chromatography, plasma)					
Premature infants	(30-60 days)	4	3 8	—	3.1-4.6
Full-term infants	(30-60 days)	3	4.5	—	3.8-5 3

BIBLIOGRAPHY

1. Albanese, A. A., and Irby, V.: Determination of urinary amino nitrogen by the copper method. J. Biol. Chem., 153:583-588, 1944.

2. Albanese, A. A., and Irby, V.: Determination of amino nitrogen of blood filtrates by the copper method. J. Lab. Clin. Med., 30:718-721, 1945.

3. Andrews, B. F., Bruton, O. C., and DeBaare, L.: Serum amino acid nitrogen in infancy and childhood. J. Pediat., 60:201-205, 1962.

4. Andrews, B. F., Bruton, O. C., and Knoblock, E. C.: Aminoaciduria in salicylate intoxication. Amer. J. Med. Sci., 242:411-414, 1961.

5. Berger, H.: The urinary amino nitrogen excretion at various ages. Ann. Paediat., 186:338-361, 1956.

6. Bergstedt, J., O'Brien, D., and Lubchenco, L. O.: Interrelationships in the urinary excretion of creatine, creatinine, free alpha amino acid nitrogen and total nitrogen in premature infants. J. Pediat., 56:635-638, 1960.

7. Bjornesjo, K. B.: The distribution of alpha amino nitrogen, urea nitrogen and non-protein nitrogen between erythrocytes and plasma in healthy males and females. Scand. J. Clin. Lab. Invest., 15 (Suppl. 69):25-37, 1963.

8. Brewer, G. E. F., Brown, W. S., Harvey, C. C., and Horwitt, M. K.: Variations of the individual blood plasma amino acid nitrogen level. J. Biol. Chem., 168:145-150, 1947.

9. Cagan, R. N., Goldberg, M., and Loewe, L.: A simple method for the determination of urinary amino nitrogen. Proc. Soc. Exp. Biol. Med., 78:713-716, 1951.

10. Chapelle, E. W., and Luck, J. M.: The decarboxylation of amino acids, proteins and peptides by n-bromosuccinimide. J. Biol. Chem., 229:171-179, 1957.

11. Childs, B.: Urinary excretion of free alpha-amino acid nitrogen in normal infants and children. Proc. Soc. Exp. Biol. Med., 81:225-228, 1952.

12. Chinard, F. P., and van Slyke, D. D.: Comparison of a modified Folin photometric procedure and the ninhydrin manometric method for the determination of amino-acid nitrogen in plasma. J. Biol. Chem., 169:571-581, 1947.

13. Christensen, H. N., and Lynch, E. I.: The conjugated non-protein amino acids of plasma. I. Post-absorptive concentrations of human plasma, serum and erythrocytes. J. Biol. Chem., 163:741-751, 1946.

14. Cohen, S. E.: The free amino acid changes in plasma following coagulation and plasminogen activation. Blood, 14:1345-1349, 1959.

15. Constantsas, N. S., and Danelatou-Athanassiadou, C.: Excretion of amino acids in childhood. A reliable method for the determination of amino acid nitrogen in urine. Clin. Chim. Acta, 9:1-12, 1964.

16. Cramer, F. B., Jr., and Winnick, T.: Amino acid nitrogen of normal human plasma. J. Biol. Chem., 150:259-260, 1943.

17. Danielson, I. S.: Amino acid nitrogen in blood and its determination. J. Biol. Chem., 101:505-522, 1933.

18. Delarue, J. C.: Determination of total amino acids by the Yemm-Cocking method. Its application to plasma free amino acids. Rev. Franc. Etud. Clin. Biol., 9:459-460, 1964.

19. Eckhardt, R. O., and Davidson, C. S.: Urinary excretion of amino acids following the rapid injection of a solution of amino acids in man. J. Clin. Invest., 27:727-736, 1948.

20. Folin, O.: A new colorimetric method for the determination of the amino acid nitrogen in blood. J. Biol. Chem., 51:377-391, 1922.

21. Folin, O.: A colorimetric determination of the amino acid nitrogen in normal urine. J. Biol. Chem., 51:393-418, 1922.

22. Frame, E., Russell, J. A., and Wilhelmi, A. E.: The colorimetric estimation of amino nitrogen in blood. J. Biol. Chem., 149:255-270, 1943.

23. Furman, M., Morrison, G., and Wagner, A.: Folin colorimetric procedure for amino acids. Anal. Chem., 22:1561-1562, 1950.

24. Greene, C. H., Sandiford, K., and Ross, H.: The amino acid content of the blood in normal and pathologic conditions. J. Biol. Chem., 58:845-855, 1924.

25. Gruendig, E., and Stur, O.: Manometric determination of α-amino acid N in blood plasma and urine with the aid of the Kopp-Natelson microgasometer. Clin. Chim. Acta, 6:801-804, 1961.

26. Hamilton, P. B., and Van Slyke, D. D.: The gasometric determination of free amino acids in blood filtrates by the ninhydrin-carbon dioxide method. J. Biol. Chem., 150:231-250, 1943.

27. Huisman, T. H. J.: Excretion of amino acids in normal infants of different ages. Arch. Franc. Pediat., 14:166-180, 1957.

28. Jagenburg, O. R.: The urinary excretion of free amino acids and other amino compounds by the human. Scand. J. Clin. Lab. Invest., **11** (Suppl. 43):1-183, 1959.

29. Kalant, H.: Colorimetric ninhydrin reaction for measurement of alpha-amino nitrogen. Anal. Chem., **28**:265-266, 1956.

30. Kekki, M.: Micro determination of amino nitrogen as copper complexes. A modification for plasma and urine. Scand. J. Clin. Lab. Invest., **11**:311-321, 1959.

31. Kekki, M., and Halonen, P. I.: Studies on plasma and urinary amino nitrogen in myocardial infarction. Acta Med. Scand., **168**: 133-139, 1960.

32. Khachadurian, A., Knox, W. E., and Cullen, A. M.: Colorimetric ninhydrin method for total alpha amino acids of urine. J. Lab. Clin. Med., **56**:321-332, 1960.

33. Kirk, E.: Amino nitrogen changes of the blood in nephritis. J. Clin. Invest., **12**:1091-1102, 1933.

34. Knauff, H. G., and Selmair, H.: Determination of free α-amino acids in urine with the aid of a new manometric method. Hoppe Seyler. Z. Physiol. Chem., **317**:108-115, 1959.

35. Lacy, W. W., and Crofford, O. B.: Automated determination of free plasma alpha amino acids by the ninhydrin carbon dioxide method. Normal sex difference in human plasma. J. Lab. Clin. Med., **64**:828-836, 1964.

36. Leffler, H. H.: Method for cholesterol and cholesterol esters in serum In Sunderman, F. W., and Sunderman, F. W., Jr. (eds.): Lipids and Steroid Hormones in Clinical Medicine. Philadelphia, Lippincott, 1960, pp 18-22.

37. Loffler, W., and Gerok, W.: The amino acid excretion in the urine in patients with liver disease and healthy persons on normal and high-protein diets. Arzneimittelforschung, **9**: 403, 1955.

38. MacFadyen, D. A.: Determination of amino acids in plasma by the ninhydrin-carbon dioxide reaction without removal of proteins. J. Biol. Chem., **145**:387-403, 1947.

39. Matthews, D. M., Muir, G. G., and Baron, D. N.: Estimation of alpha-amino nitrogen in plasma and urine by the colorimetric ninhydrin reaction. J. Clin. Path., **17**:150-153, 1964.

40. Northrop, J. H.: A convenient method for the formol titration. J. Gen. Physiol., **9**:767-769, 1926.

41. O'Brien, D., Bergstedt, J., Butterfield, J., Ibbott, F., and Lubchenco, L.: Observations on the urinary excretion of free amino acids by the premature infant. Acta Paediat., **49**: 258-264, 1960.

42. O'Brien, D., and Butterfield, L. J.: Further studies on renal tubular conservation of free amino acids in early infancy. Arch. Dis. Child., **38**:437-442, 1963.

43. Oepen, H., and Oepen, I.: Comparison of amino acid spectra of differently deproteinized blood serum. Klin. Wschr., **41**:921-926, 1963.

44. Opienska-Blanth, J.: Critical evaluation of methods used in aminoaciduria investigation. Clin. Chim. Acta, **4**:841-860, 1959.

45. Peters, J. P., and Van Slyke, D. D.: Quantitative Clinical Chemistry Vol. 2 (Methods). Baltimore, Williams & Wilkins, 1932, pp. 385-400.

46. Pope, C. G., and Stevens, M. F.: The determination of amino nitrogen using a copper method. Biochem. J., **33**:1070-1077, 1939.

47. Rosenblum, R., Wolfman, W., and Leiter, L.: A correction for the interference of urea in the determination of total alpha amino acid nitrogen in plasma by the ninhydrin photometric method. J. Lab. Clin. Med., **54**:132-135, 1959.

48. Russell, J. A.: Note on the colorimetric determination of amino nitrogen. J. Biol. Chem., **156**:467-468, 1944.

49. Saifer, A., Gerstenfeld, S., and Harris, A. F.: Photometric micro determination of amino acids in biological fluids with the ninhydrin reaction. Clin. Chim. Acta, **5**:131-140, 1960.

50. Schaefer, H.: Experience with the Van Slyke appartus simplified by Zuwerkalow for the volumetric determination of amino nitrogen. Clin. Chim. Acta, **8**:476-478, 1963.

51. Sereni, F., McNamara, H., Shibuya, M., Kretchmer, N., and Barnett, H. L.: Concentration in plasma and rate of urinary excretion of amino acids in premature infants. Pediatrics, **15**:575-585, 1955.

52. Sobel, C., Henry, R. J., Chiamori, N., and Segalove, M.: Determination of α-amino acid nitrogen in urine. Proc. Soc. Exp. Biol. Med., **95**:808-813, 1957.

53. Spier, H. W., and Pascher, G.: The quantitative micro determination of free amino acids with a simple copper complex method. Hoppe Seyler Z. Physiol. Chem., **296**:147-154, 1954.

54. Szentirmar, A., Braun, P., Horvath, I., and Hauk, M.: A rapid screening test for determination of total α-amino acids in urine and serum. Clin. Chim. Acta, 7:459-462, 1962.

55. Thompson, R. C., and Abdulnabi, M.: A study of the urinary excretion of α-amino nitrogen and lysine by humans. J. Biol. Chem., 185:625-628, 1950.

56. Van Gelderen, H. H., and Dooren, L. J.: The excretion of free α-amino acids in children. Arch. Dis. Child., 39:261-264, 1964.

57. Van Slyke, D. D., Dillon, R. T., MacFayden, D. A., and Hamilton, P.: Gasometric determination of carbonyl groups in free amino acids. J. Biol. Chem., 141:627-669, 1941.

58. Van Slyke, D. D., and Kirk, E.: Comparison of gasometric colorimetric and titrimetric determination of amino nitrogen in blood and urine. J. Biol. Chem., 102:651-682, 1933.

59. Van Slyke, D. D., MacFadyen, D. A., and Hamilton, P. B.: The gasometric determination of amino acids in urine by the ninhydrin carbon dioxide method. J. Biol. Chem., 150:251-258, 1943.

60. Woodruff, C. W., and Man, E. B.: Concentration of alpha-amino acid nitrogen in plasma of normal subjects. J. Biol. Chem., 157:93-97, 1945.

61. Zandrey, S.: A study of the question of the significance of pathological amino aciduria. Klin. Med., 94:101-139, 1922.

Chapter 11

Fractionations of Amino Acids in Biological Fluids by Thin-Layer Chromatography

F. WILLIAM SUNDERMAN, JR., M.D.

In 1945, Sanger[67] reported that dinitrofluorobenzene in alkaline solution reacts with the α-amino groups of amino acids and peptides to yield yellow dinitrophenyl (DNP) derivatives (Fig. 1). In addition to binding with the α-amino groups, Sanger[67] noted that a second dinitrophenyl radical becomes coupled to the ω-amino groups of the diamino acids, to the imidazole nucleus of histidine, to the phenol group of tyrosine and to the thiol group of cysteine. Based upon his observation that the various DNP-amino acids have differing solubilities in organic solvents, Sanger[67] developed a paper chromatographic technique for the separation

and identification of amino acids.

During the past twenty years, fractionations of DNP-amino acids have been accomplished by numerous techniques, including filter-paper[7, 8, 49], glass-paper[20], thin-layer[23, 44, 83], column[43, 46, 50, 51] and gas chromatography[58] and filter-paper electrophoresis[9, 52]. Methods for the separation of DNP-amino acids have been extensively used for the analysis of protein hydrolysates[7, 8, 56, 77], but have had little application to the identification of amino acids in biological fluids[34, 59].

In 1963, Walz and co-workers[83] published a technique for dinitrophenylation of urinary amino acids and

DINITROPHENYLATION OF AMINO ACIDS

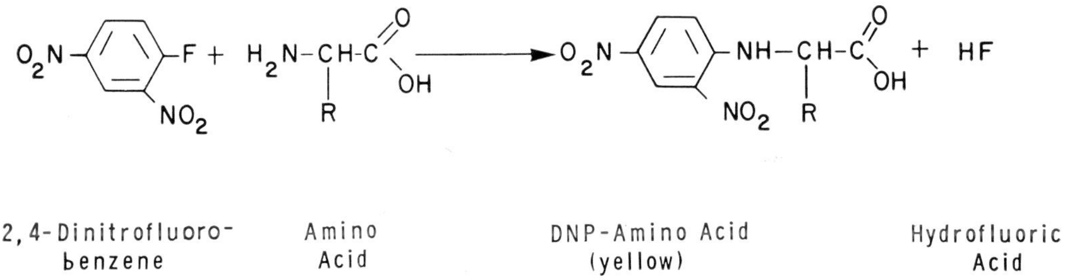

2,4-Dinitrofluoro-
benzene   Amino
Acid   DNP-Amino Acid
(yellow)   Hydrofluoric
Acid

Fig. 1. Dinitrophenylation reaction.

fractionation of the DNP-derivatives by thin-layer chromatography. This procedure permits the detection of low concentrations of amino acids in urine, inasmuch as the DNP-derivatives are extracted into organic solvents and subsequently are concentrated by evaporation of the solvents. The solvent extraction eliminates organic salts which cause interference in thin-layer chromatography of amino acids[4, 21, 62]. The DNP-amino acids possess intense yellow colors and ultraviolet fluorescence which permit their detection without staining the chromatograms. Moreover, the separated DNP-amino acids may be eluted from the thin-layer chromatograms and estimated semi-quantitatively by measurements of their ultraviolet absorption[34, 46].

Our laboratory has evaluated several recently published methods for fractionation of amino acids which employed thin-layer chromatography[3, 13, 28, 55], thin-layer electrophoresis[39] or glass-paper chromatography[20]. In our hands, the method of Walz and co-workers[83] produced the best resolution of amino acids, and was more dependable for routine use than the paper chromatographic procedure which was used previously[84]. The method of Walz and co-workers[83] has been modified in our laboratory to permit fractionations of amino acids in plasma and in urine which contains protein. The procedure for dinitrophenylation has been made more convenient, and the chromatographic technique for fractionation of "acid-soluble" DNP-amino acids has been improved. Fractionations have been performed by this technique upon approximately 400 specimens of urine or plasma from normal persons and from patients who were suspected of suffering from disorders of amino acid metabolism. These fractionations have lead to the diagnosis of subjects with phenylketonuria, histidinuria, cystinuria, homocystinuria, cystinosis and β-amino-isobutyric aciduria.

METHOD

PRINCIPLE

A flow-diagram for the preparation of DNP-amino acids is illustrated in Figure 2. An aliquot of urine or protein-free filtrate of plasma is adjusted to pH 8.3. Dinitrofluorobenzene and carbonate buffer are added, and the reaction mixture is incubated in the dark[65] at 37 C for one hour. Excess dinitrofluorobenzene is extracted into ether and discarded. The reaction mixture is acidified to pH 3 with hydrochloric acid and re-extracted with ether in order to separate the "ether-soluble" DNP-amino acids. The "ether-soluble" fraction includes the DNP-derivatives of virtually all of the amino acids found in biological fluids, except DNP-taurine, DNP-citrulline, DNP-arginine, DNP-cysteic acid and a portion of di-DNP-histidine, which is only slightly soluble in ether. These residual DNP-amino acids, which comprise the "acid-soluble" fraction, are extracted into a mixture of ethyl acetate and butanol. The solvent extracts containing the "ether-soluble" and "acid-soluble" fractions are concentrated by evaporation and are subjected to two-dimensional chromatography on silica gel, as described by Brenner et al.[15, 16]. The separated DNP-amino acids are identified by their chromatographic mobilities.

FLOW DIAGRAM FOR PREPARATION OF DINITROPHENYL-AMINO ACIDS

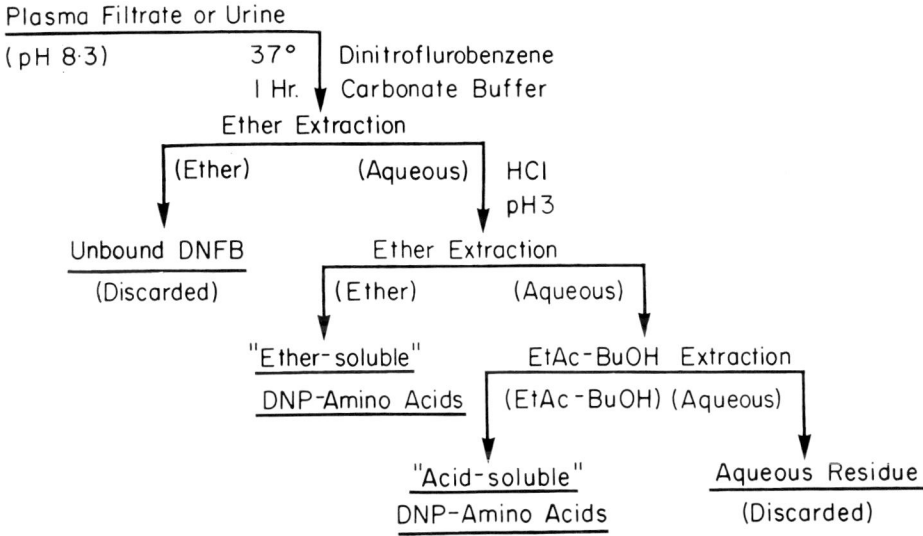

Fig. 2.   Outline of dinitrophenylation procedure.

REAGENTS

1. *Sodium hydroxide*, 5.0 N and 0.5 N.
2. *Hydrochloric acid*, 6.0 N and 0.5 N.
3. *Sodium sulfate*, anhydrous crystals.
4. *Ethanol*, absolute.
5. *Ethyl ether*, anhydrous, peroxide-free.
6. *Acetone*, absolute.
7. *Carbonate buffer.* Exactly 8.40 gm of $NaHCO_3$ are dissolved in cold water in a 100 ml volumetric flask. Two and one half ml of 5.0 N NaOH are added, and the solution is diluted to approximately 80 ml with distilled water. The solution is adjusted to pH 8.8 by appropriate additions of NaOH or $NaHCO_3$, and is diluted to the mark with distilled water.
8. *Dinitrofluorobenzene solution.* A 10 per cent (w/v) solution of 2,4-dinitrofluorobenzene in absolute ethanol is prepared immediately before use.

9. *Ethyl acetate: n-butanol mixture* (1:1, v/v).
10. *Composite amino acid standard.* Ten mg samples of alanine, citrulline, glycine, histidine, phenylalanine, proline, serine, taurine, tryptophan, tyrosine and valine are transferred to a 250 ml volumetric flask. The contents of the flask are dissolved in distilled water and diluted to the mark.
11. *Individual DNP-amino acid standards.* Five mg samples of purified DNP-derivatives of the amino acids[*] are dissolved in 5 ml of acetone. These standard solutions should be tightly stoppered, shielded from light and stored in the refrigerator. Under these conditions they are stable for one to two weeks.
12. *Silica gel G,* "according to Stahl,"

---

[*]DNP-amino acids may be obtained from Sigma Chemical Company, St. Louis, Missouri.

containing approximately 13 per cent CaSO$_4$ as a binder.[*]

13. *Tungsten-molybdenum phosphor.*[†]

14. *Solvent System "A"*[‡], (toluene: pyridine: ethylenechlorohydrin: 0.8 N. ammonia, 100:30:60:60, (v/v). The upper phase of this mixture serves as the initial solvent for chromatography of "ether-soluble" DNP-amino acids. The lower phase of this mixture is used for pre-treatment of thin-layer plates prior to chromatography of the "ether-soluble" fraction.

15. *Solvent System "B"*[‡] (chloroform: benzyl alcohol: glacial acetic acid, 70:30:3, v/v).

16. *Solvent System "C"*[‡] (n-propanol: 34 per cent ammonia, 70:30, v/v).

17. *Solvent System "D"*[‡] (n-butanol: 34 per cent ammonia, 80:20, v/v).

18. *Preservative spray, "Neatan."*[*]

Special Apparatus

1. *Water bath,* 37 C, adapted for shaking 10 ml flasks.

2. *Thin-layer chromatography apparatus* ("Desaga"), including five tanks for two-dimensional ascending chromatography.[*]

3. *Hair dryer,* with dual control for blowing and heating.[§]

4. *Hamilton microsyringes,* 5 and 10 μl capacity.[¶]

[*]Brinkmann Instruments Company, Westbury, New York.

[†]Phosphor Type 118-2-7, Lamp Metals and Components Department, General Electric Company, 1099 Ivanhoe Road, Cleveland 10, Ohio.

[‡]All solvents for chromatography should be of high purity. Fisher "spectranalyzed" or "certified" solvents have been employed in the author's laboratory.

[§]Airjet hair dryer, Model 202, Oster Manufacturing Co., Milwaukee, Wisconsin.

[¶]Hamilton Company, Whittier, California.

Procedure

A. Dinitrophenylation of Urine Amino Acids

1. Ten ml of fresh urine are adjusted to pH 8.3 by dropwise addition of 5.0 N and 0.5 N NaOH. The pH is measured with a pH meter. The alkalinized urine is filtered through Whatman #40 filter paper.

2. Four ml of urine filtrate, 0.4 ml of dinitrofluorobenzene solution and 1 ml of carbonate buffer are transferred to a 10 ml glass-stoppered flask. The flask is stoppered tightly and wrapped with aluminum foil to shield the contents from light.

3. The flask is placed in a water bath at 37 C and shaken vigorously for one hour. The flask is then cooled to room temperature.

4. The contents of the flask are transferred to a 50 ml teflon-stoppered centrifuge tube, together with a 5 ml washing of water and a 15 ml washing of ether. The centrifuge tube is stoppered and shaken vigorously, with care to release the ether vapor.

5. The ether and aqueous phases are separated by brief centrifugation at 1500 rpm. The ether phase is aspirated and discarded using a fine-tipped Pasteur pipette connected to suction via a trap bottle.

6. In this manner the aqueous phase is washed repetitively with 15 ml portions of ether until the ether washings are colorless. Three additional washings are usually required.

7. The aqueous phase is adjusted to pH 3 by dropwise addition of 6 N and 0.5 N HCl. Indicator paper is used to estimate the pH. The HCl should be added cautiously with constant mixing,

since CO_2 is evolved. After acidification the aqueous phase usually becomes cloudy.

8. Fifteen ml of ether are added and the tube is stoppered and shaken vigorously, with care to release the ether vapor. The stoppered tube is centrifuged briefly at 1500 rpm to separate the ether and aqueous phases. By use of a Pasteur pipette, the ether phase is transferred to a 125 ml glass-stoppered Erlenmeyer flask.

9. In this manner, the acidified aqueous phase is extracted repetitively with 15 ml portions of ether until the ether washings are colorless. Three additional extractions are usually required.

10. Five gm of anhydrous Na_2SO_4 crystals are added to the combined ether extracts. The Erlenmeyer flask is tightly stoppered, wrapped with aluminum foil and allowed to stand for several hours or overnight in the refrigerator. This ether extract contains the "ether-soluble" fraction.

11. The residual aqueous phase is extracted three times with 15 ml of ethyl acetate-butanol mixture. The ethyl acetate-butanol extracts are transferred to a 125 ml glass-stoppered Erlenmeyer flask, and the aqueous phase is discarded.

12. Five gm of anhydrous Na_2SO_4 crystals are added to the combined ethyl acetate-butanol extracts. The Erlenmeyer flask is tightly stoppered, wrapped with aluminum foil and allowed to stand for several hours or overnight in the refrigerator. This ethyl acetate-butanol extract contains the "acid-soluble" fraction.

13. The "ether soluble" fraction is filtered through cotton wool into a clean Erlenmeyer flask. The $Na SO_4$ crystals are washed with fresh ether until colorless, and the washings are added to the ether extract.

14. In similar manner, the "acid-soluble" fraction is filtered through cotton wool into a clean Erlenmeyer flask, and the Na_2SO_4 crystals are washed with ethyl acetate-butanol mixture until colorless.

15. Approximately 40 ml of the ether extract (Step 13) are decanted into a 50 ml centrifuge tube. The tube is placed in a beaker of water at 30 C and the contents of the tube are evaporated in a gentle stream of nitrogen. When the volume has decreased sufficiently, the remainder of the ether extract is decanted into the centrifuge tube. The ether extract is completely evaporated to dryness, and the residue is dissolved in 0.2 ml of acetone. The tube is stoppered tightly and centrifuged for fifteen minutes to pack any insoluble material in the tip. The final "ether-soluble" extract is transferred with a Pasteur pipette to a small (1.0 ml) glass-stoppered tube, which is stored in the refrigerator in the dark.

16. Approximately 40 ml of the ethyl acetate-butanol extract (Step 14) are decanted into a 50 ml centrifuge tube. The tube is placed in a water bath at 65 C, and the contents of the tube are evaporated in a gentle stream of nitrogen. As described in Step 15, the entire ethyl acetate-butanol extract is progressively decanted into the tube and evaporated to dryness. The residue is dissolved in 0.2 ml of ethyl acetate-butanol. The tube is stoppered tightly and centrifuged for fifteen minutes. The final "acid-soluble" extract is removed and stored in the same manner as the "ether-soluble" extract.

B. Deproteinization of Plasma and Urine

1. Sixteen ml of absolute ethanol are transferred to a 50 ml centrifuge tube in an ice bath. When the ethanol has reached 0 C, 4 ml of plasma or urine which contains protein are added. The contents of the tube are mixed with a "Vortex" rotary mixer and are allowed to stand in the bath for twenty minutes. The tube is centrifuged at 2000 rpm for thirty minutes in a refrigerated centrifuge at 0 C.

2. The supernatant is filtered through Whatman #40 filter paper into a clean 50 ml graduated centrifuge tube. The protein-free filtrate is evaporated to dryness in a water bath at 60 C under a gentle stream of nitrogen.

3. The residue is dissolved in 2 ml of distilled water and adjusted to pH 8.3 by dropwise addition of 0.5 N NaOH. The contents of the tube are diluted to 4 ml with distilled water, and transferred with a Pasteur pipette to a 10 ml glass-stoppered flask.

4. One ml of carbonate buffer and 0.4 ml of dinitrofluorobenzene solution are added, and the procedure for dinitrophenylation is continued as described in Step 2 of Section A.

C. Preparation of Thin-Layer Plates and General Technique for Chromatography

The preparation of chromatography plates and the general procedure for thin-layer chromatography is described in detail by Stahl[74]. The following specific instructions should be followed.

1. Thirty gm of silica gel G are transferred to a Waring blendor. Six tenths gm of tugnsten-molybdenum phosphor is added, and the dry powders are gently mixed with a stirring rod, with care to avoid inhalation.

2. Sixty ml of distilled water are added to the blendor and the mixture is homogenized. Within one minute the slurry is poured into the Desaga applicator. The slurry is immediately spread over the chromatography plates in a layer 0.25 mm thick. The quantity of slurry is sufficient for preparation of five plates measuring 20 x 20 cm.

3. The thin-layer chromatography plates are allowed to dry without disturbance for at least twenty minutes. They are then transferred to a desiccator cabinet for drying overnight. The plates may be stored in the desiccator cabinet for several weeks prior to use.

4. Five chromatography tanks are lined with chromatography paper. The tanks are labelled "A-LP," "A-UP," "B," "C" and "D," corresponding to Solvents A-lower phase, A-upper phase, B, C and D, respectively.

5. A glass rack is placed on the bottom of Tank A-LP to permit pre-equilibration of chromatography plates without direct contact with the lower phase of Solvent System A.

6. One hundred twenty ml of the approprite solvents are poured down the walls of each tank, saturating the filter paper liners. The depth of the solvent in the tank should be 1 cm. The glass tops of the tanks are sealed with a thin coating of silicone grease. At least one hour is allowed for equilibration of the tanks before chromatographic fractionations.

7. Two chromatographic plates are developed simultaneously. During pre-equilibration with the lower phase of Solvent System A, the coated sides of the plates are placed facing the filter paper liners, with the top edges resting upon the liners. To keep the solvent

from siphoning from the filter paper liners onto the layers of silica gel, a thick line is scribed in the silica gel, 1.5 cm from the top edge of each plate. During the chromatographic fractionations, the coated sides of the plates are placed facing each other.

8. The chromatographic solvents in each tank are renewed after three sets of fractionations have been performed. The filter paper liners should be saturated with the solvent before each chromatographic fractionation.

D. *Fractionations of "Ether-Soluble" DNP-Amino Acids*

1. Chromatography plates are equilibrated overnight in Tank A-LP containing the lower phase of Solvent System A. During this pre-treatment the plates absorb moisture from the vapors of the lower phase. To achieve constant R_f values, it is essential that the absorbed moisture not be permitted to evaporate during application of the sample. After the plates are removed from Tank A-LP, each plate is immediately covered with a plastic spotting template, leaving a margin of 2.2 cm for spotting.

2. Using a Hamilton microsyringe, 5 μl of the "ether-soluble" extracts are spotted onto the left lower corner of each plate, at a point 2 cm from each edge.

3. The chromatography plates are immediately placed in Tank A-UP. No more than five minutes should elapse in transferring the plates from Tank A-LP to Tank A-UP.

4. In Tank A-UP, sixty to seventy-five minutes are required for the solvent front to reach the line which was scribed 1.5 cm from the top edge of each plate.

5. The plates are removed from the tank and dried for ten minutes in an unheated draft of air from the hair dryer.

6. The plates are placed in a drying oven at 60 C for ten minutes.

7. The plates are cooled to room temperature for ten minutes in an unheated draft of air from the hair dryer.

8. The plates are immediately placed in Tank B, with the original application spots positioned at the right lower corner of each plate. One hundred twenty to 135 minutes are required for the solvent fronts to reach the top edges of the plates.

9. The plates are removed from Tank B and are allowed to dry in an unheated draft of air from the hair dryer.

E. *Fractionations of "Acid-Soluble" DNP-Amino Acids*

1. No pre-treatment of plates is required for the fractionation of the "acid-soluble" extract. Using a Hamilton microsyringe, 10 μl of "acid-soluble" extracts are spotted onto the left lower corners of two chromatography plates at points similar to those used for the "ether-soluble" extract. The spotting procedure is performed under a heated draft of air from the hair dryer.

2. The chromatography plates are placed in Tank C, with the application spots positioned at the left lower corner of each plate. Ascending chromatography in this solvent system requires approximately two hours. At the end of this time the solvent fronts should be approximately 3 cm from the top edges of the plates.

3. The plates are dried in air for ten minutes, transferred to the oven at 60 C for ten minutes, and then cooled to

room temperature for ten minutes.

4. The plates are placed in Tank D with the original application spot positioned at the right lower corner of each plate. Approximately three hours are required for the solvent fronts to reach the top edges of the plates.

5. The plates are removed from Tank D and are dried under an unheated draft of air from the hair dryer.

F. Identification of Amino Acids

1. The chromatography plates are examined under incandescent and ultraviolet lights. Under incandescent light, the DNP-amino acids appear as bright yellow spots. Under ultraviolet light, the DNP-amino acids appear as dark magenta spots.

2. For standardization of the technique, 5 ml of the composite amino

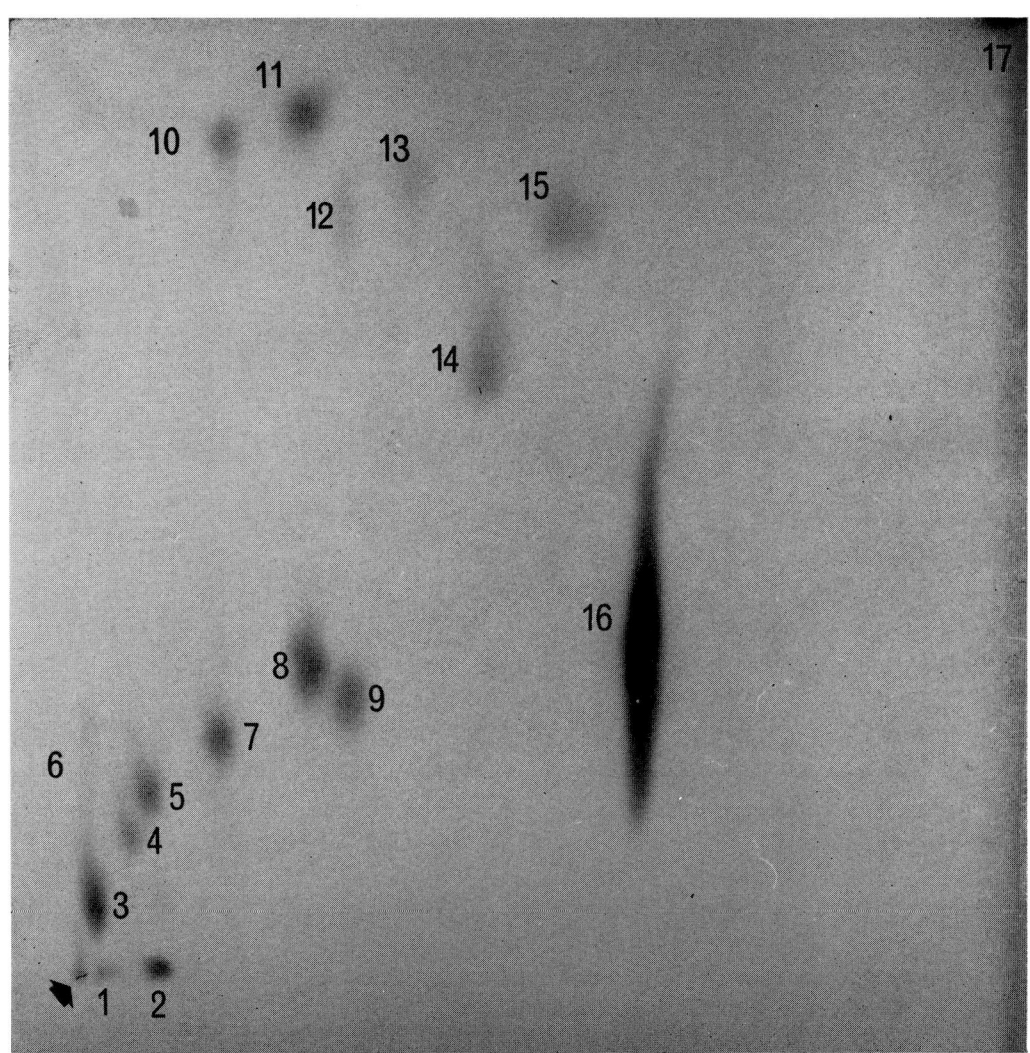

Fig. 3. Chromatographic fractionation of "ether soluble" DNP-amino acids from normal plasma. (1) Asp, (2) Glu, (3) Glu-N and Asp-N, (4) Ser, (5) Thr, (6) Cys, (7) Gly, (8) Ala, (9) Pro, (10) Orn, (11) Tyr and Lys, (12) Try, (13) Phe, (14) Val and Norval, (15) Leu and Ileu, (16) DNP-OH, (17) 2,4-DNA.

acid standard are treated similarly to the urine samples and are carried through the entire procedure. If there is doubt regarding the identity of an unusual amino acid, the amino acid extract is spotted simultaneously upon two chromatographic plates. To one of the starting points is added 5 μl of a standard solution of the purified DNP-derivative of the suspected amino acid. Coincidence of the standard spot with the unknown spot provides presumptive identification of the abnormal amino acid. Definitive identification is obtained by eluting the DNP-amino acids in acetone, evaporating the extracts to dryness and measuring the infrared absorption spectrums of the residues. Coin-

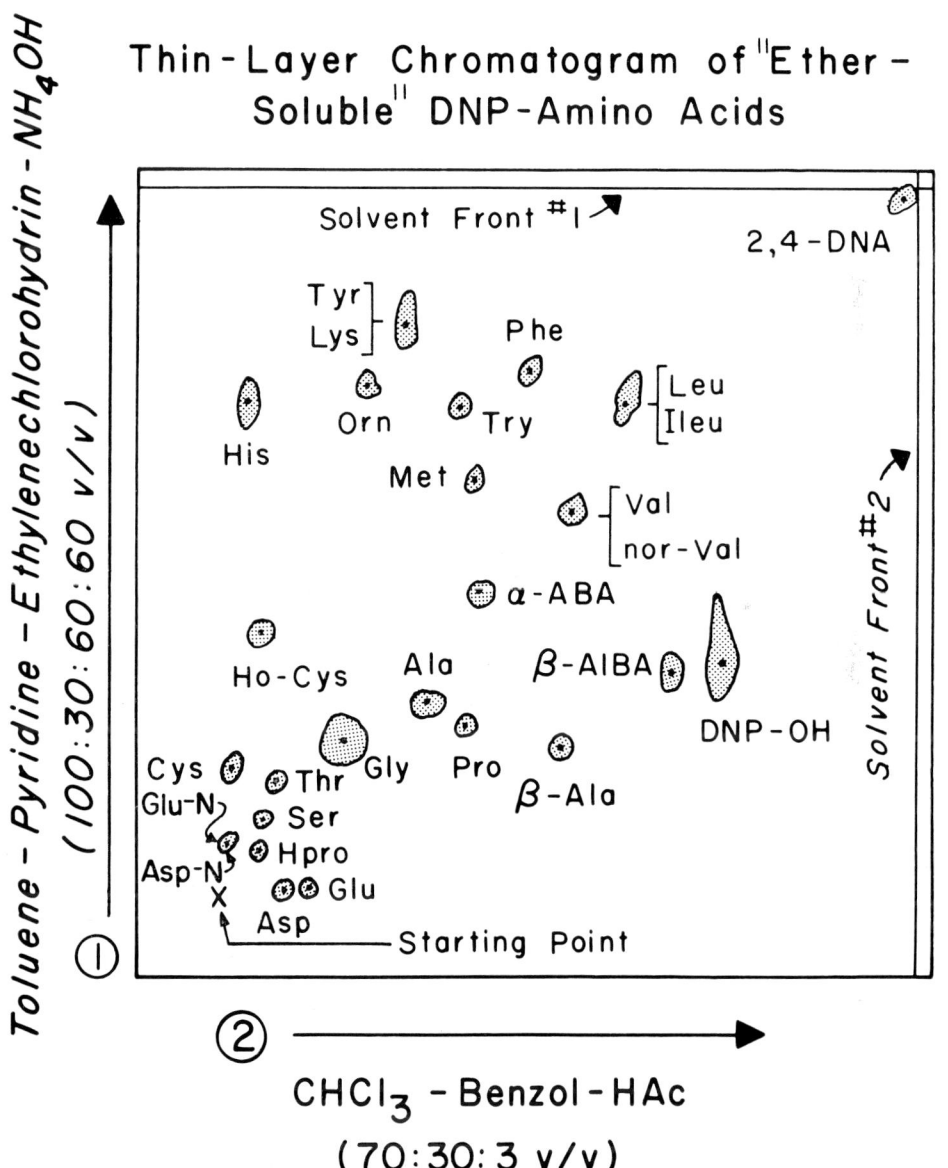

Fig. 4.   Fractionation of "ether-soluble" DNP-amino acids.

cidence of the absorption spectrums of the two samples establishes the identity of the amino acid[44].

3. The reproducibility of the chromatographic mobilities of DNP-amino acids permits immediate identification, usually without the necessity of computing R_f values. The analyst soon recognizes the relative intensities of the amino acid spots which are observed with normal urine or plasma. With a little practice, abnormal amino acid patterns are readily detected by visual inspection of the chromatograms, provided, of course, that quantitative measurements have been made of total free amino acid nitrogen in the urine or plasma.

4. For preservation of the chromatograms, "Neatan" preservative is sprayed

Thin-Layer Chromatogram of "Acid-Soluble" DNP-Amino Acids

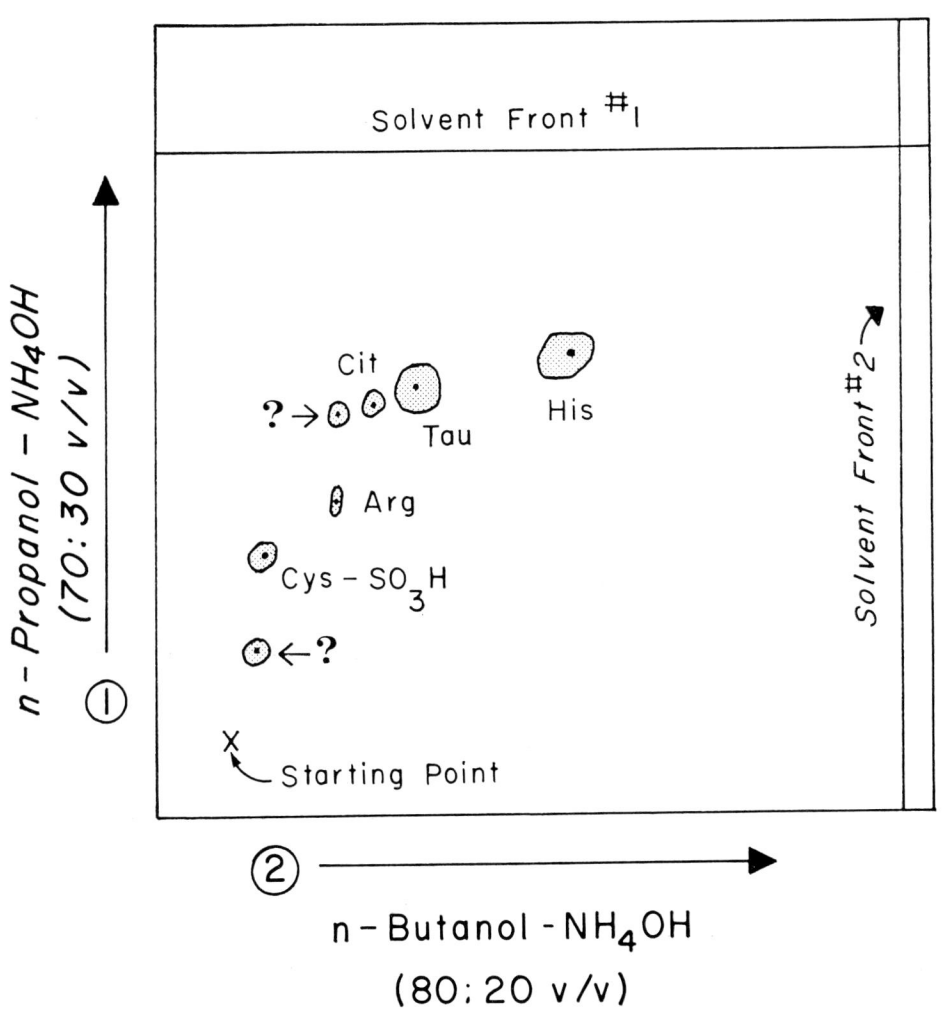

Fig. 5. Fractionation of "acid-soluble" DNP-amino acids.

as a thin coating over the silica gel. The chromatograms may then be copied photographically or with a Xerox copying machine.

Results and Discussion

Typical chromatographic patterns of "ether-soluble" DNP-amino acids observed with extracts of normal plasma are illustrated in Figure 3. The chromatographic mobilities of "ether-soluble" and "acid-soluble" DNP-amino acids are portrayed graphically in Figures 4 and 5. The R_f values for each of these amino acids were determined in our laboratory for pure standards and for amino acids added to normal urine and protein-free filtrates of plasma (Tables I and II).

It may be noted from Figure 4 and Table I that the DNP-derivatives of norvaline and valine, and of leucine and isoleucine are not separated by chromatography in Solvent Systems A and B. In those uncommon instances in which it is necessary to separate these amino acids, a solvent system containing benzene, pyridine and glacial acetic acid (80:20:2, v/v) is substituted for Solvent System B. Fractionations in this system are performed by continuous-flow chromatography, as described by Brenner and Niederwieser[14, 16]. DNP-derivatives of tyrosine and lysine similarly are not separated in Solvent Systems A and B. To achieve separation of these amino acids, a solvent system containing chloroform, methanol and glacial acetic acid (95:5:1 v/v) is substituted for Solvent System B. Chromatographic separations in this system are likewise performed by the continuous-flow technique[14, 16].

In approximate order of decreasing concentrations, the following amino acids were detected by thin-layer chro-

TABLE I R_f VALUES OF "ETHER-SOLUBLE" DNP-AMINO ACIDS

Amino Acid	Solvent A[°]	Solvent B[†]
DNP-glutamic acid	0.4	13.
DNP-aspartic acid	0.8	9.3
DNP-hydroxyproline	6.8	6.8
DNP-asparagine + DNP-glutamine	7.2	1.7
DNP-serine	12.	7.1
DNP-threonine	17.	8.6
Di-DNP-cystine	18.	2.0
DNP-β-alanine	21.	50.
DNP-glycine	22.	18.
DNP-proline	25.	38.
DNP-alanine	29.	31.
DNP-β-aminoisobutyric acid	34.	67.
Di-DNP-homocystine	39.	6.2
DNP-α-aminobutyric acid	44.	39.
DNP-valine + DNP-norvaline	56.	53.
DNP-methionine	61.	38.
Di-DNP-histidine	71.	3.9
DNP-tryptophan	72.	36.
DNP-leucine + DNP-isoleucine	73.	61.
Di-DNP-ornithine	68.	20.
DNP-phenylalanine	77.	47.
Di-DNP-tyrosine + Di-DNP-lycine	82.	28.
(2,4-dinitrophenol)	35.	74.
(2,4-dinitroaniline)	98.	98.

[°]Solvent A: Upper phase of toluene-pyridine-ethylenechlorohydrin-ammonia (100:30:60:60, v/v).

[†]Solvent B: Cholorform-benzol-glacial acetic acid (70:30:3, v/v).

TABLE II R_f VALUES OF "ACID-SOLUBLE" DNP-AMINO ACIDS

Amino Acid	Solvent C[°]	Solvent D[†]
DNP-cysteic acid	33.	5.0
α-DNP-arginine	41.	16.
DNP-citrulline	58.	20.
DNP-taurine	62.	28.
Di-DNP-histidine	66.	51.

[°]Solvent C: propanol-ammonia (70:30, v/v).

[†]Solvent D: n-butanol-ammonia (80:20, v/v).

matography in plasmas from normal adults: glycine; alanine; glutamine and asparagine; valine and norvaline; proline; threonine; lysine and tyrosine; leucine and isoleucine; serine; histidine; arginine; cystine; phenylalanine; ornithine; taurine; tryptophan; glutamic acid; methionine; α-aminobutyric acid; and aspartic acid. As shown in Figure 6, this sequence corresponds to the order of decreasing concentrations of amino acids in plasmas of normal adults, based upon the paper chromatographic fractionations of Knauff et al.[45], and the ion-exchange chromatographic fractionations of Iob and co-workers[42] and of Ackerman and Kheim[1]. In Figure 6, the mean concentration of each amino acid in μM per liter is indicated by the height of each column, and the range

of ± 1 standard deviation is indicated by the dots above and below the mean. Measurements of glutamine are unreliable by the ion-exchange technique and were not reported by Iob and associates or by Ackerman and Kheim[1].

In approximate order of decreasing concentrations, the following amino acids were detected by thin-layer chromatography in twenty-four-hour collections of urine from twenty normal adults: glycine; taurine; glutamine and asparagine; serine; alanine; β-aminoisobutyric acid; histidine; threonine; tyrosine and lysine; phenylalanine; leucine and isoleucine; cystine; valine and norvaline; methionine; aspartic acid; glutamic acid; arginine; β-alanine; tryptophan; cysteic acid; and hydroxy proline. In the thin-layer technique,

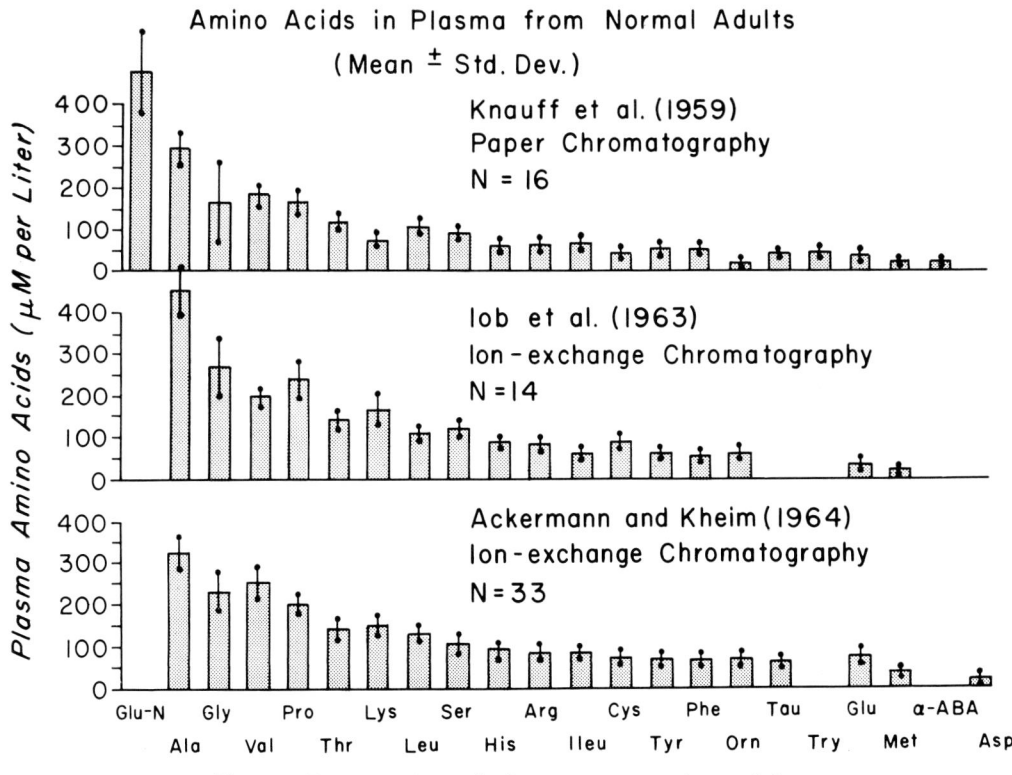

Fig. 6.   Fractionations of plasma amino acids in adults.

1-methylhistidine and 3-methylhistidine are apparently not detected, and the relative excretion of histidine is less than observed by ion-exchange chromatography. With these exceptions, the sequence of amino acids observed by thin-layer chromatography conforms, in general, to the order of decreasing concentrations of amino acids in urine from normal adults, as reported by Soupart[71], Stein[75], and Evered[27], using ion-exchange chromatography (Fig. 7).

Fractionations of amino acids by the thin-layer technique were performed in our laboratory upon five specimens of plasma and ten collections of urine from normal children. These fractionations followed the same general pattern that was observed in adults. These findings are in agreement with fractiona-

tions of amino acids in specimens of plasma and urine from normal infants and children by ion-exchange chromatography, as shown in Figure 8 and Figure 9. The fractionations in Figures 9 and 10 are based upon the investigations of Vis[78], Holt and co-workers[38], Ghadimi and Pecora[32], Armstrong and co-workers[2], Huisman[40] and Carver and Paska[18].

At the top of the Figure 9 are illustrated measurements reported by Armstrong and co-workers of the urinary excretion of amino acids during the first twenty-four hours of life[2]. These fractionations attest to the relatively great excretion of taurine which occurs during the first few days of life. Fractionations of amino acids in urine of older infants and children, as reported

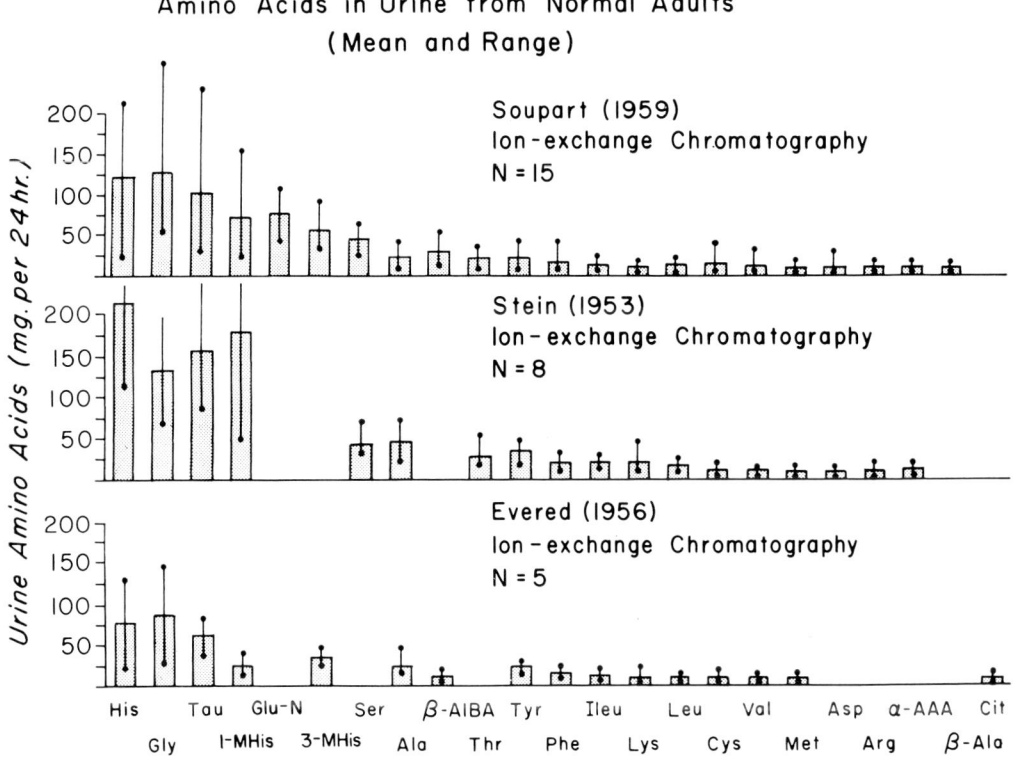

Fig. 7.   Fractionations of urine amino acids in adults.

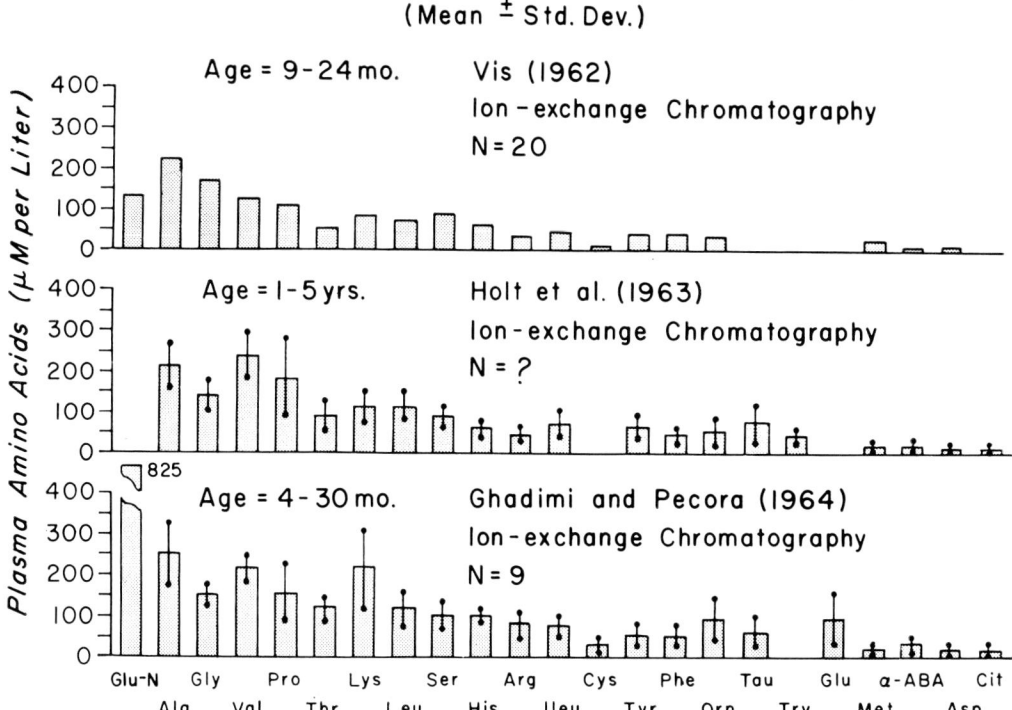

Fig. 8.   Fractionations of plasma amino acids in children.

by Huisman[40] and by Carver and Paska[18], did not differ strikingly from the fractionations obtained with urine collections from normal adults.

Our experience indicates that the diagnostic applications of the thin-layer chromatographic procedure for fractions of amino acids are comparable to those of high-voltage electrophoresis[10, 12, 29, 35, 47, 48, 53, 66, 79, 80], two-dimensional paper chromatography[5, 6, 11, 33, 54, 68, 70, 81, 85], or the combination of electrophoresis and chromatography[22, 25, 30, 60, 61, 64, 72, 82]. It should be emphasized that the procedure is *not* intended as a substitute for quantitative determinations of individual amino acids by the ion-exchange chromatographic methods[17, 19, 24, 31, 36, 37, 41, 57, 63, 72, 73, 76]. Neither is it intended as a substitute for the rapid screening

procedures used in population surveys, such as the various one-dimensional chromatographic techniques[26, 69, 86]. Rather, the thin-layer chromatographic procedure is designed to fulfill the need of clinical laboratories for a practical and reliable method for the study of patients who are suspected of suffering from one of the aminoacidopathies.

SUMMARY

The technique of Walz and co-workers[83] for thin-layer chromatography has been modified in our laboratory for routine use as a diagnostic procedure for the detection of the specific aminoacidopathies. Unlike most methods for fractionations of amino acids in biological fluids, this technique involves preliminary dinitrophenylation

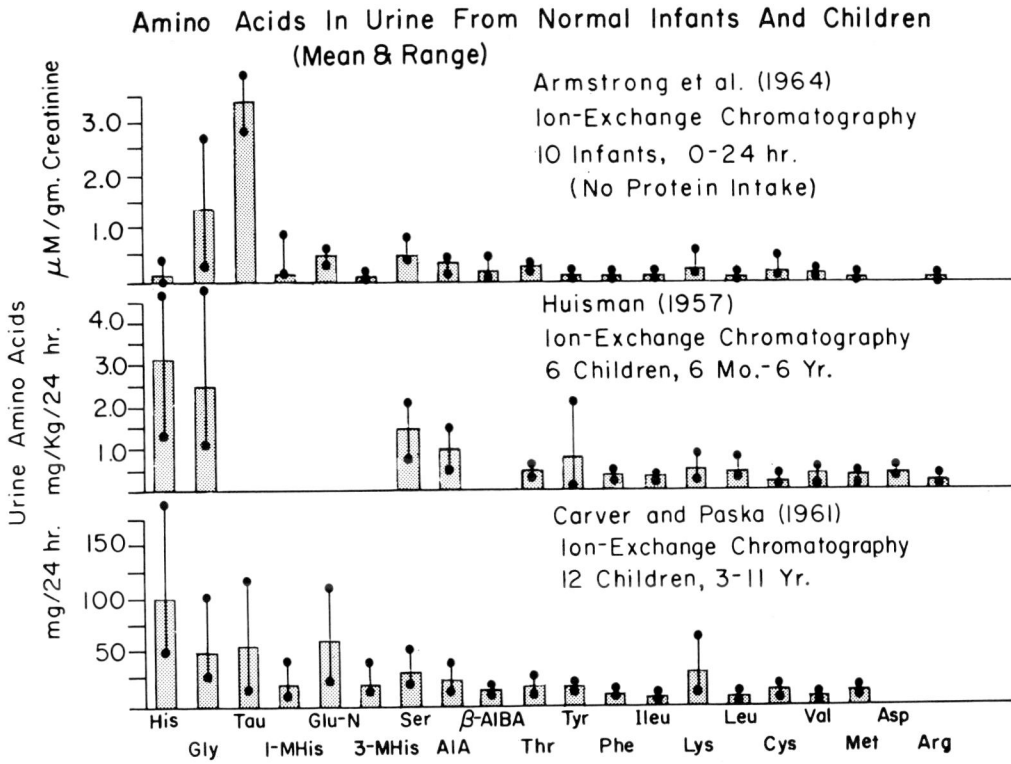

Fig. 9.   Fractionations of urine amino acids in children.

of the amino acids. A major advantage of this procedure is that the dinitrophenyl (DNP) amino acids are extractable into organic solvents and are readily concentrated by evaporation of the solvents. Thin-layer chromatography of the DNP-amino acids is free from interference owing to inorganic salts and other constituents of urine. The DNP-amino acids possess intense yellow colors and ultraviolet fluorescence which permit their detection without staining the chromatograms. Morevore, the resolution of the amino acids is superior to that which is commonly achieved by paper chromatography or electrophoresis. The method has proved to be practical and reliable, and is recommended for use in clinical laboratories.

REFERENCES

1. Ackermann, P. G., and Kheim, T.: Plasma amino acids in young and older adult human subjects. Clin. Chem., **10**:32-40, 1964.

2. Armstrong, M. D., Yates, K. N., and Connelly, J. P.: Amino acid excretion of newborn infants during the first 24 hours of life. Pediatrics, **33**:975-978, 1964.

3. Arx, E. von, and Neher, R.: A multidimensional technique for chromatographic identification of amino acids. J. Chromatogr., **12**: 329-341, 1963.

4. Baron, D. N., and Economidis, J.: Thin-layer chromatography for amino acids and sugars. J. Clin. Path., **16**:484-486, 1963.

5. Berry, H. K.: Amino acid excretion in urine of normal infants and children. Paper chromatographic methods for amino acid analyses. Pediatrics, **25**:983-996, 1960.

6. Berry, H. K.: Individual metabolic patterns: I. Amino acid excretion studies in 700 children. Metabolism, **9**:363-372, 1960.

7. Biserte, G., Holleman, J. W., Holleman-Dehove, J., and Sautiere, P.: Chromatography upon paper of dinitrophenylamino acids. J. Chromatogr., 2:225-271, 1959.

8. Biserte, G., Holleman, J. W., Holleman-Dehove, J., and Sautiere, P.: Paper chromatography of dinitrophenylamino acids. Chromatogr. Rev., 2:59-104, 1960.

9. Biserte, G., Holleman, J. W., Holleman-Dehove, J., and Sautiere, P.: Chromatography of dinitrophenylamino acids on paper. J. Chromatogr., 3:85-86, 1960.

10. Blackburn, S.: The determination of amino acids by high-voltage paper electrophoresis. In Glick, D. (ed.): Methods of Biochemical Analysis. New York, Interscience, 1965, pp. 1-46.

11. Bowden, C. H.: An improved solvent combination for amino acid chromatography. Clin. Chim. Acta, 4:539-544, 1959.

12. Braun, L.: On the quantitative determination of amino acids using high voltage electrophoresis. Biochem. Z., 339:8-12, 1963.

13. Brenner, M., and Niederwieser, A.: Thin-layer chromatography of amino acids. Experientia, 16:378-383, 1960.

14. Brenner, M., and Niederwieser, A.: Continuous-flow thin-layer chromatography. Experientia, 17:237-238, 1961.

15. Brenner, M., Niederwieser, A., and Pataki, G.: Thin-layer chromatography of amino acid derivatives on Kieselgel G. N-(2,4-dinitrophenyl)-amino acids and 3-phenyl-2-thiohydantoine. Experientia, 17:145-153, 1961.

16. Brenner, M., Niederwieser, A., and Pataki, G.: Amino acids and derivatives. In Stahl, E. (ed.): Thin Layer Chromatography. New York, Academic Press, 1965, pp. 391-441.

17. Cadavid, N. G., and Paladini, A. C.: Automatic amino acid analysis: Reagent and instrumental improvements. Anal. Biochem., 9:170-174, 1964.

18. Carver, M. J., and Paska, R.: Ion-exchange chromatography of urinary amino acids. I. Normal children. Clin. Chim. Acta, 6:721-724, 1961.

19. Corfield, M. C., and Robson, A.: Automatic analyses of amino acids by polarographic estimation of their copper complexes. Biochem. J., 84-146-151, 1962.

20. Dessauer, H. C., Hamilton, J. G., and Calvet, J. K.: Chromatography of dinitrophenylamino acids on silica gel-impregnated glass paper. J. Chromatogr., 18:192-194, 1965.

21. Dimililier, I., and Trout, R. G.: Changes in blood amino acids during cardiopulmonary bypass as determined by thin-layer chromatography. A preliminary report. J. Thorac. Cardiov. Surg., 48:822-827, 1964.

22. Dixon, G. H., Kauffman, D. L., and Neurath, H.: Amino acid sequence in the region of diisopropylphosphoryl binding in diisopropylphosphoryltrypsin. J. Biol. Chem., 233:1373-1381, 1958.

23. Drawert, F., Backmann, O., and Reuther, K. H.: Thin-layer chromatography of C^{14}-dinitrophenylamino acids. J. Chromatogr., 9:376-378, 1962.

24. Eastoe, J. E.: A semi-micro method for the determination of amino acids by ion-exchange chromatography. Biochem. J., 29:652-656, 1961.

25. Efron, M. L.: Two way separation of amino acids and other ninhydrin-reacting substances by high voltage electrophoresis followed by paper chromatography. Biochem. J., 72:691-694, 1959.

26. Efron, M. L.: A simple chromatographic screening test for the detection of disorders of amino acid metabolism. A technique using whole blood or urine collected on filter paper. New Eng. J. Med., 270:1378-1383, 1964.

27. Evered, D. F.: The excretion of amino acids by the human. A quantitative study with ion-exchange chromatography. Biochem. J., 62:416-427, 1956.

28. Fahmy, A. R., Niederwieser, A., Pataki, G., and Brenner, M.: Thin-layer chromatography of amino acids on Kieselgel G. A rapid method for separation and qualitative identification of 22 amino acids. Helv. Chim. Acta, 44:2022-2026, 1961.

29. Fischl, J., and Segal, S.: "Small-volume" electrophoresis: separation of amino acids. Clin. Chim. Acta, 8:399-405, 1963.

30. Fischl, J., and Segal, S.: "Small-volume" electrophoresis. II. Electro-chromatography. Clin. Chim. Acta, 8:479-481, 1963.

31. Frame, E. G.: The levels of individual free amino acids in the plasma of normal man at various intervals after a high-protein meal. J. Clin. Invest., 37:1710-1723, 1958.

32. Ghadimi, H., and Pecora, P.: Plasma amino acids after birth. Pediatrics, 34:182-191, 1964.

33. Ghadimi, H., and Shwachman, H.: Evaluation of aminoaciduria in infancy and childhood. J. Dis. Child., 99:457-475, 1960.

34. Goedde, H. W., and Brunschede, H.: β-aminoisobutyric acid: a thin layer chromatographic method for the quantitative estimation in human urine. Clin. Chim. Acta, 11:485-490, 1965.

35. Gross, D.: Two dimensional high-voltage paper electrophoresis of amino and other

organic acids. Nature (London), **184**:1298-1301, 1959.

36. Hamilton, P. B.: Ion-exchange chromatography of amino acids. Micro-determination of free amino acids in serum. Ann. N.Y. Acad. Sci., **102**:55-75, 1962.

37. Hannig, K.: Experiences with quantitative amino acid determinations on ion-exchange columns and automatic recording of the results. Clin. Chim. Acta, **4**:51-57, 1959.

38. Holt, L. E. Jr., Snyderman, S. E., Norton, P. M., Roitman, E., and Finch, J.: The plasma amino-gram in kwashiorkor. Lancet, **2**:1342-1348, 1963.

39. Honegger, C. G.: Thin-layer electrophoresis and thin-layer electrophoresis-chromatography. Helv. Chim. Acta, **44**:173-179, 1961.

40. Huisman, T. H. J.: The excretion of amino acids in normal infants of different ages. Arch. Franc. Pediat., **14**:166-180, 1957.

41. Inglis, A. S.: An improved amino acid analyzer. Anal. Biochem., **7**:168-177, 1964.

42. Iob, V., McMath, M., and Coon, W. W.: Intra-individual and inter-individual variations in plasma free amino acids in normal adults. J. Surg. Res., **3**:85-89, 1963.

43. Kesner, L., Muntwyler, E., Griffin, G. E., and Abrams, J.: Automatic column chromatography of ether and water soluble 2,4-dinitrophenyl-derivatives of amino acids, peptides and amines. Anal. Chem., **35**:83-89, 1963.

44. Kimmel, H. S., and Saifer, A.: Infra-red spectra of the biologically important DNP and PTH amino acids. Anal. Biochem., **9**: 316-342, 1964.

45. Knauff, H. G., Dieterle, P., and Zickgraf, H.: Quantitative determination of 21 free amino acids in the blood of healthy subjects. Hoppe Seyler. Z. Physiol. Chem., **316**:186-198, 1959.

46. Lucas, F., Shaw, J. T. B., and Smith, S. G.: Amino acid analysis with fluordinitrobenzene. Anal. Biochem., **6**:335-351, 1963.

47. Mabry, C. C., and Karam, E. A.: Measurement of free amino acids in plasma and serum by means of high voltage paper electrophoresis. Amer. J. Clin. Path., **42**:421-430, 1964.

48. Mabry, C. C., and Todd, W. R.: Quantitative measurement of individual and total free amino acids in urine. Rapid method employing high-voltage paper electrophoresis and direct densitometry and its application to the urinary excretions of amino acids in normal subjects. J. Lab. Clin. Med., **61**:146-157, 1963.

49. Maddy, A. H.: Detection of 2,4-dinitrophenyl-amino acids on paper chromatogram. Nature (London), **184** (Suppl. 18): 1397-1398, 1959.

50. Mathieson, N. A.: An improved method of separating amino acids as N,-2,4-dinitrophenyl derivatives. Biochem. J., **88**:146-151, 1963.

51. Mills, G. L.: Observations on the application of fluorodenitrobenzene to the quantitative analysis of proteins. Biochem. J., **50**:707-712, 1952.

52. Munier, R. L., and Sarrazin, G.: Chromato-electrophoresis procedure permitting the separation of water soluble dinitrophenyl-amino acids. J. Chromatogr., **12**:542-544, 1963.

53. Naughton, M. A., and Hagopian, H.: Some applications of two-dimensional iontophoresis. Anal. Biochem., **3**:276-284, 1962.

54. Nettelbladt, E., and Sandell, B. M.: Amino acid content of serum in rheumatoid arthritis. Ann. Rheum. Dis., **22**:269-272, 1963.

55. Opienska-Blauth, J., Kraczkowski, H., and Brzuskiewicz, H.: Adaptation of the technique of thin-layer chromatography to amino-acid-uria investigation. In Martini-Bettolo, G. B. (ed.): Thin-Layer Chromatography. Amsterdam, Elsevier, 1964, pp. 165-173.

56. Pataki, G.: Application of thin-layer chromatography to sequence analysis of peptides. Nondestructive detection of amino acids on the thin-layer chromatogram. J. Chromatogr., **16**:541-543, 1964.

57. Pietz, K. A., and Morris, L.: A modified procedure for the automatic analysis of amino acids. Anal. Biochem., **1**:187-201, 1960.

58. Pisano, J. J., Vandenheuvel, W. J., and Horning, E. C.: Gas chromatography of phenylthiohydantoin and dinitrophenyl derivatives of amino acids. Biochem. Biophys. Res. Commun., **7**:82-86, 1962.

59. Rapp, R. D.: Determination of serum amino acids. Clin. Chem., **9**:27-30, 1963.

60. Relvas, M. E., and Ferraz, F. G. P.: Amino-acidemia in the normal state and in various pathological cases. Clin. Chim. Acta, **8**:533-537, 1963.

61. Rey, J., Mayer, M. A., Deysson, A., Reezal, J., and Lamy, M.: Bidimensional separation of amino acids by means of high voltage electrophoresis and paper chromatography. Rev. Franc. Etud. Clin. Biol., **7**:877-882, 1962.

62. Rokkones, T.: Thin-layer chromatography of amino acids in urine. Scand. J. Clin. Lab. Invest., **16**:149-152, 1964.

63. Rosen, H., Berard, C. W., and Levenson, S. M.: A simplified procedure for automatic amino acid analysis. Anal. Biochem., **4**:213-221, 1962.

64. Rothman, F., and Higa, A.: A new two-dimensional system for the separation of amino acids on paper. Anal. Biochem., 3: 173-177, 1962.

65. Russell, D. W.: Studies on the photochemical behavior of 2,4-dinitrophenyl derivatives of some amino acids and peptides. Biochem. J., 87:1-4, 1963.

66. Sackett, D. L.: Adaptation of monodirectional high-voltage electrophoresis on long papers to the rapid qualitative identification urinary amino acids. J. Lab. Clin. Med., 63:306-314, 1964.

67. Sanger, F.: The free amino groups of insulin. Biochem. J., 39:507-515, 1945.

68. Saxena, K. N., and Gandhi, J. R.: Separation and identification of amino acids by two-dimensional chromatography. J. Chromatogr., 8:546-550, 1962.

69. Scriver, C. R., Davies, E., and Cullen, A. M.: Adaptation of a simple micromethod to the screening of plasma for a variety of amino-acidopathies. Lancet, 2:230-232, 1964.

70. Sereni, F., McNamara, H., Shibuya, M., Kretchmer, N., and Barnett, H. L.: Concentration in plasma and rate of urinary excretion of amino acids in premature infants. Pediatrics, 15:575-585, 1955.

71. Soupart, P.: Urinary excretion of free amino acids in normal adult men and women. Clin. Chim. Acta, 4:265-271, 1959.

72. Spackman, D. H.: Ion-exchange chromatography of protein hydrolysates. In Sunderman, F. W., and Sunderman, F. W., Jr. (eds.): Serum Proteins and the Dysproteinemias. Philadelphia, Lippincott, 1964, pp. 166-181.

73. Spackman, D., Stein, W. H., and Moore, S.: Automatic recording apparatus for use in the chromatography of amino acids. Anal. Chem., 30:1190-1206, 1958.

74. Stahl, E.: Instruments used in thin-layer chromatography and their operation. In Stahl, *op cit.*, pp. 5-28.

75. Stein, W. H.: A chromatographic investiga-tion of the amino acid constituents of normal urine. J. Biol. Chem., 201:45-58, 1953.

76. Stein, W. H., and Moore, S.: The free amino acids of human blood plasma. J. Biol. Chem., 211:915-926, 1954.

77. Tonge, B. L.: Reaction of fluoro-2,4,dinitrobenzene with amino acids and peptides. Nature (London), 195:491, 1962.

78. Vis, H., cited by Soupart, P.: Free amino acids of blood and urine in the human. In Holden, J. T. (ed.): Amino Acid Pools. Amsterdam, Elsevier, 1962, pp. 220-232.

79. Visakorpi, J. K., and Puranen, A. L.: High voltage paper electrophoresis. A rapid method for determination of urinary amino acids. Scand. J. Clin. Lab. Invest., 10:196-202, 1958.

80. Visakorpi, J. K., Puranen, J., and Puraven, A. L.: The analysis of amino acids by high voltage paper electrophoresis. Acta Paediat., 48 (Suppl. 118):124-125, 1959.

81. Wade, E. H. M., Matheson, A. T., and Hanes, C. S.: Quantitative chromatographic methods. Factors controlling the patterns of separation of amino acids on paper chromatograms. Canad. J. Biochem., 39:141-162, 1961.

82. Walker, D. G., Prasad, A. S., and Sadrieh, J.: Free amino acid levels in ultrafiltrates of human blood plasma. J. Lab. Clin. Med., 59:110-117, 1962.

83. Walz, D. Fahmy, A. R., Pataki, G., Niederwieser, A., and Brenner, M.: Thin-layer chromatographic separation of urinary amino acids. Experientia, 19:213-217, 1963.

84. Wheeler, T. E.: Paper chromatography of protein hydrolysates. In Sunderman and Sunderman, *op. cit.*, pp. 159-165.

85. Whitehead, R. G., and Dean, R. F. A.: Serum amino acids in kwashiorkor. I. Relationship to clinical condition. Amer. J. Clin. Nutr., 14:313-319, 1964.

86. Whitehead, R. G., and Dean, R. F. A.: Serum amino acids in kwashiorkor. II. An abreviated method of estimation and its application. Amer. J. Clin. Nutr., 14:320-330, 1964.

Chapter 12

The Biochemistry of Branched-chain Ketoaciduria

(Maple Syrup Urine Disease)

MANFORD D. MORRIS, Ph.D.

INTRODUCTION

Branched-chain ketoaciduria (maple syrup urine disease [MSUD]) is usually manifest as a rapidly fatal disorder in which affected, apparently normal, neonates undergo rapid deterioration and early death. The early symptoms include the absence of a Moro's reflex, respiratory irregularities, progressively increasing rigidity, opisthotonus and marked mental retardation. Coincident with the appearance of the clinical symptoms there occurs the excretion of a pleasant-smelling urine with an odor similar to maple syrup. Analysis of blood and urine from such patients reveals increased amounts of the branched-chain amino acids leucine, isoleucine and valine as well as their respective α-keto acids[4, 7, 10, 11, 19, 20].

A variant of the classical type of branched-chain ketoaciduria has been reported in infants and children whose growth and development, both physical and mental, are not impaired[6, 12, 13].

Early diagnosis of branched-chain ketoaciduria is mandatory since recent reports suggest that early dietary management of such infants, by institution of diets low in leucine, isoleucine and valine, may allow normal physical and mental development[18].

METABOLISM OF LEUCINE, ISOLEUCINE AND VALINE

Leucine, isoleucine and valine are branched-chain essential amino acids which contain an aliphatic residue. The major metabolic pathways of these three amino acids are either incorporation into proteins or conversion to simple acyl derivatives. The catabolism of these three closely related compounds is believed to be similar, particularly in the early degradation steps. Since the defect in branched-chain ketoaciduria is restricted to the catabolic pathway, only the degradative steps of the branched-chain amino acids will be considered.

An abbreviated scheme for the degradation of leucine, isoleucine and valine is shown in Figure 1. The initial step in the degradation is a transamination reaction catalyzed by a transaminase enzyme which converts the amino acid to the corresponding α-keto acid. This enzyme, which apparently

Fig. I

Metabolism of Branched-Chain Amino Acids - Metabolic Block in Branched-Chain Ketoaciduria

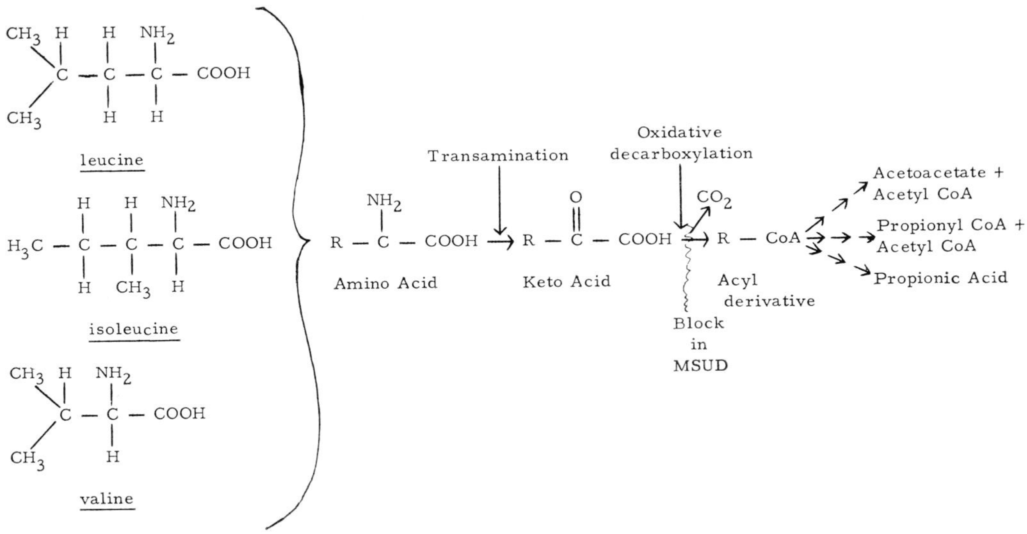

acts on all three amino acids, is widely distributed in animal tissue and is presumably a typical glutamate transaminase[8]. The α-keto acid is converted to an acyl-coenzyme A derivative by oxidative decarboxylation. This complex reaction involves at least five coenzymes or cofactors, i.e., thiamine pyrophosphate, lipoic acid, coenzyme A, FAD, and NAD and perhaps four separate enzymes.

Detailed studies have been carried out on the pyruvate and α-ketoglutarate decarboxylases and have been reviewed by Sanadi[15]. Using classical methods of protein fractionation it has not been possible to resolve the highly associated complex into individual components, but the overall sequence of reactions in the oxidative decarboxylation of α-keto acids is believed to take place as shown in Figure 2 adapted from Sanadi[15]. This scheme shows the release of CO_2 and the formation of an acyl derivative (Reaction 1) which is transferred sequentially from thiamine pyrophos-

phate (TPP) to lipoate (lip S_2) to coenzyme A (CoA) (Reactions 2 and 3). Reactions 4 to 6 involve dehydrogenation reactions necessary to restore the decarboxylation complex to its initial form such that another molecule of α-keto acid can be accepted. The hydrogens transferred to the $NADH_2$ travel the cytochrome electron transport system. Although the enzyme system responsible for the oxidative decarboxylation of the branched-chain α-keto acids is widespread in tissues[2], no detailed studies have appeared regarding the mechanism of this reaction. In the present schema, it is only by analogy to the α-ketoglutarate and pyruvate systems that these same reactions are presumed to take place. At the present time it is not definitely known whether one enzyme is responsible for all three keto acids or whether there are three closely related enzymes. In view of the accumulation of the three keto acids derived from leucine, isoleucine and valine, it is probable that

Fig. 2

Oxidative Decarboxylation of Alpha-Keto Acids

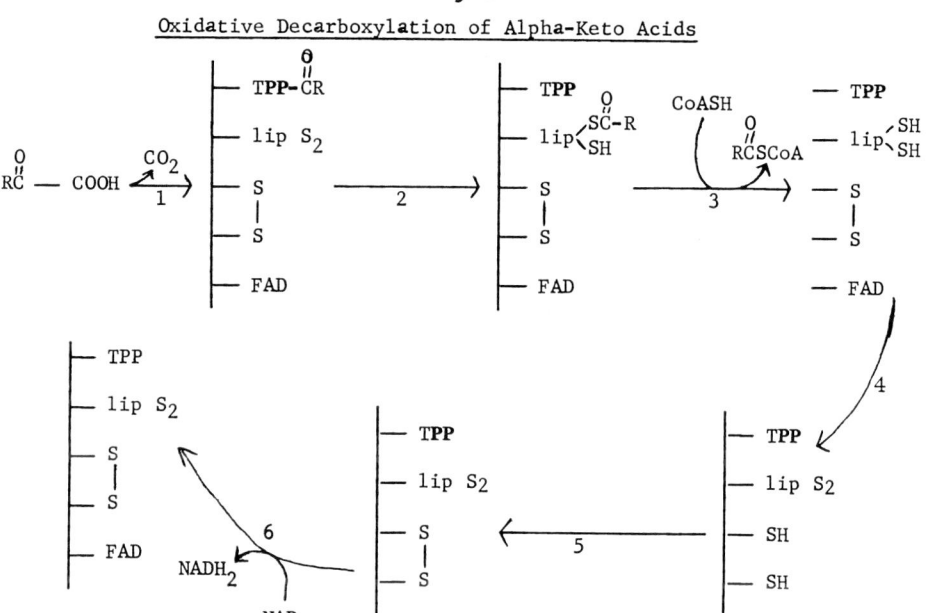

TPP = thiamine pyrophosphate; lip S_2 = oxidized lipoate;
-S-S- = flavoprotein thiol; FAD = flavin adenine nucleotide;
NAD = nicotinamide adenine nucleotide.

a single enzyme complex is responsible for their conversion to the acyl coenzyme A derivatives.

The remaining oxidative degradation of the acyl CoA derivatives proceeds in a manner similar to that for the oxidation of fatty acids. The final products are acetoacetic acid and acetyl coenzyme A (leucine), propionyl coenzyme A and acetylcoenzyme A (isoleucine) and propionyl coenzyme A (valine).

NATURE OF THE ENZYMATIC DEFECT IN BRANCHED-CHAIN KETOACIDURIA

Westall, Dancis and Miller[19] first showed that, in a patient with MSUD, plasma and urinary concentrations of leucine, isoleucine and valine were greatly elevated. Later studies by MacKenzie and Woolf[7] and by Dancis and co-workers[4] confirmed the presence of large excesses of branched-chain keto and amino acids in the blood and urine obtained from patients with MSUD. Menkes[10] identified the urinary keto acids as those corresponding to leucine, isoleucine and valine, and, in a later study, this same investigator[9] was unable to detect any of the expected metabolites of the acyl coenzyme A derivatives of the branched-chain keto acids. The presence of normal transaminase activity and the deficiency or lack of oxidative decarboxylase activity toward the branched-chain keto acids in both leukocytes and skin fibroblasts, has localized the defect in MSUD to the level of oxidative decarboxylation.

The inability to catabolize properly the α-keto acids results in the most outstanding biochemical characteristic of branched-chain ketoaciduria, namely, the accumulation in blood and other body fluids of branched amino acids and the keto acids derived from them by transamination.

Other less notable biochemical features of this disease include hypoglycemia, indolyl uria, elevated plasma and urinary alloisoleucine, elevated urinary α-hydroxy acids and decreased levels of some plasma amino acids. The significance of these later changes are not clear, but it can be assumed that they are secondary to the primary inability to metabolize properly the α-keto acids.

DIAGNOSIS

Since irreversible brain damage may occur very early in branched-chain ketoaciduria and since apparently successful treatment has been achieved, an early diagnosis is mandatory[18]. Increased urinary keto acid excretion can be detected by addition of 2,4-dinitrophenyl hydrazine to a sample of urine. A precipitate indicates increased keto acids. The chromatography of the acidic hyrazones on thin layer plates of silica gel G shows qualitative distribution of the α-keto acids. Qualitative single-dimensional paper chromatography of plasma and urine is suitable for detecting the presence of excessive quantities of branched-chain amino acids. The presence of leucine (isoleucine) and valine bands without generalized aminoaciduria is diagnostic of branched-chain ketoaciduria. A typical maple syrup urine odor is also a common, though not absolute, finding.

DISCUSSION

The most prominent biochemical feature of branched-chain ketoaciduria is the marked increase in blood and urinary branched-chain amino and α-keto acids. Tissue transaminase activity, responsible for keto acid formation, is normal in patients with this disease. Neither leukocytes nor skin fibroblasts[1,3] from affected patients can decarboxylate exogenous branched-chain keto acid substrates or similar substrates generated by the transaminase reaction. No other simple metabolites of the branched-chain keto acids have been detected. Thus, all evidence suggests that the biochemical defect in branched-chain ketoaciduria occurs at the oxidative decarboxylation step in the catabolism of the α-keto acids.

The branched-chain keto acid decarboxylase may have a broad specificity, since α-ketobutyrate metabolism, in addition to that of the branched-chain keto acids, is altered, but there is no evidence for a greatly changed pyruvate or α-ketoglutarate metabolism in these patients. No studies have been reported on the nature of the branched-chain decarboxylase, but it appears to be widely spread. Skeletal muscle appears to lack branched-chain keto acid decarboxylase activity. Investigations of the intracellular distribution have shown a mitochondrial origin for the enzymatic activity in guinea pig liver[2].

The finding of other secondary metabolic alterations in patients with branched-chain ketoaciduria is not surprising. The earlier observation of plasma and urinary methionine lead to the discovery of L-alloisoleucine as a metabolite of isoleucine in these patients. Snyderman and associates observed[16], in an infant with MSUD fed a known amino acid mixture, elevated plasma "methionine," even when the methionine intake was restricted or omitted from the diet altogether. Dent and Westall[5] observed elevated "methionine" in plasma after their patient was given an isoleucine load. The anomalous occurrence of "methionine" was resolved when a different system of chromatography was used, and these studies eventually lead to the isolation and characterization of L-alloisoleucine as the true metabolite of isoleucine.

The finding of increased α-hydroxy acids[14] is probably due to a nonspecific reduction of the α-keto acids which are present in such high concentration.

Although reports of hypoglycemia have appeared in some of these infants, there is some question with regard to its role in the eventual course of the disease. There is little question that the outstanding clinical features of branched-chain ketoaciduria are those changes associated with the central nervous system. The neurologic damage observed in early onset type branched-chain ketoaciduria occurs much earlier than in phenylketonuria. Snyderman and co-workers[16] have treated a patient with neonatal MSUD, from seventeen days of age, with a diet low in leucine, isoleucine and valine. Although the treatment was complicated by periods of deprivation of methionine, these authors suggest that, among other possibilities, the diet was started too late to prevent irreversible brain damage.

Westall[18] has apparently successfully treated a patient with MSUD; at the age of about fifteen months this infant appeared normal. Cord blood obtained at birth showed normal branched-chain amino and keto acids. A normal pattern of amino and keto acids was observed during the first three days of life. On the fourth to sixth days, the urinary excretion of the branched-chain keto acids rose dramatically. On the fourth day, paper chromatography of plasma amino acids revealed an abnormally high level of leucine, isoleucine and valine. By the fifth day, she showed a reluctance to feed, and a urine sample collected on the sixth day had the characteristic smell of maple syrup. Dietotherapy, in which branched-chain amino acid intake was limited, corrected all the major biochemical abnormalities to near-normal levels in about a week. This patient has continued to develop normally both physically and mentally on the artificial diet, but is sensitive to intercurrent infections. These excellent studies lend further support to the notion that there is but a single biochemical defect in branched-chain ketoaciduria and that other changes are secondary to the absence of branched-chain α-keto acid decarboxylase. These observations again emphasize the complete reversal of otherwise hopeless clinical disease and the necessity for feeding diets low in branched-chain amino acid at the earliest possible time.

A variant of the classical type branched-chain ketoaciduria has been described in which clinical symptoms related to MSUD may be delayed for as long as eight years[6]. Two siblings in each of two families have been shown to have the major biochemical abnormalities of branched-chain ketoaciduria during acute exacerbations, but these factors return to normal following remission. These patients apparently have no early abnormalities relative to amino and keto acid metabolism, although during the clinical stages of the disease prolonged elevations of keto acids may exist. In spite of the periodic high levels of blood and urine α-amino and keto acids, the mental and physical development in these children has been normal.

Reasons for this sensitivity to abnormal branched-chain amino acid metabolism during the newborn period are not apparent, and attempts to induce alterations of acetate, alanine and glutamate metabolism, by injecting newborn rats and rabbits with large amounts of the leucine keto acid, have been unsuccessful.

Patients with late-onset-type disease probably have a partial decarboxylase deficiency, and, because of this, the metabolic aberrations attributable to the defect become manifest only when the patient is severely catabolic.

Thus, it would appear that the neonatal brain is particularly sensitive to increased quantities of branched-chain amino acids and/or their metabolites. The reasons for this particular sensitivity are not known. Brain glutamic acid decarboxylase activity[17], however, is inhibited by branched-chain keto acids, although the significance of these studies cannot presently be assessed.

REFERENCES

1. Dancis, J., Hutzler, J., and Levitz, M.: Metabolism of white blood cells in maple syrup urine disease Biochim. Biophys. Acta, 43: 342, 1960.
2. Dancis, J., Hutzler, J., and Levitz, M.: Tissue distribution of branched-chain keto acid decarboxylase. Biochim. Biophys. Acta, 52: 60, 1961.
3. Dancis, J., Jansen, V., Hutzler, J., and Levitz, M.: The metabolism of leucine in tissue culture of skin fibroblasts of maple-syrup-urine disease. Biochim. Biophys. Acta, 77: 523, 1963.
4. Dancis, J., Levitz, M., Miller, S., and Westall, R. G.: "Maple syrup urine disease." Brit. Med. J., 5114:91, 1959.
5. Dent, C. E., and Westall, R. J.: Studies in maple syrup urine disease. Arch. Dis. Child., 36:259, 1961.
6. Kiil, R., and Rokkones, T.: Late manifesting variant of branched-chain ketoaciduria (maple syrup urine disease). Acta Paediat., 53:356, 1964.
7. MacKenzie, D. Y., and Woolf, L. I.: "Maple syrup urine disease." An inborn error of the metabolism of valine, leucine, and isoleucine associated with gross mental deficiency. Brit. Med. J., 1:90, 1959.
8. Meister, Alton: Biochemistry of the Amino Acids. New York, Academic Press, 2nd ed., 1965.
9. Menkes, J. H.: Maple syrup disease. Investigations into the metabolic defect. Neurology, (Minneap.), 9:826, 1959.
10. Menkes, J. H.: Maple syrup disease; Isolation and identification of organic acids in the urine. Pediatrics, 23:348, 1959.
11. Menkes, J. H., Hurst, P. L., and Craig, J. M.: A new syndrome: progressive familial infantile cerebral dysfunction associated with an unusual urinary substance. Pediatrics, 14:462, 1954.
12. Morris, M. D., Fisher, D. A., and Fiser, R.: Late onset branched-chain ketoaciduria (maple syrup urine disease). J. Lancet, in press.
13. Morris, M. D., Lewis, B. D., Doolan, P. D., and Harper, H. A.: Clinical and biochemical observations on an apparently nonfatal variant of branched-chain ketoaciduria (maple syrup urine disease). Pediatrics, 28:918, 1961.
14. Patrick, A. D.: Maple syrup urine disease. Arch. Dis. Child., 36:269, 1961.
15. Sanadi, D. R.: Pyruvate and -ketoglutarate oxidation enzymes. In Boyer, P. D., Lardy, H., and Myrbäck, K. (eds): The Enzymes, Vol. 7, New York, Academic Press, 2nd ed., 1963, pp. 307-344.
16. Snyderman, S. E., Norton, P. M., Roitman, E., and Holt, L. E., Jr.: Maple syrup urine disease, with particular reference to dietotherapy. Pediatrics, 34:454, 1964.
17. Tashian, R. E.: Inhibition of brain glutamic acid decarboxylase by phenylalanine, valine, and leucine derivatives: A suggestion concerning the etiology of the neurological defect in phenylketonuria and branched-chain ketonuria. Metabolism, 10:393, 1961.
18. Westall, R. G.: Dietary treatment of a child with maple syrup urine disease (branched-chain ketoaciduria). Arch. Dis. Child., 38: 485, 1963.
19. Westall, R. G., Dancis, J., and Miller, S.: Maple syrup urine disease. A.M.A. J. Dis. Child. 94:571, 1957.
20. Westall, R. G., Dancis, J., Miller, S., and Levitz, M.: Maple syrup urine disease. Fed. Proc., 17:334, 1958.

Fluorimetric Measurement of Phenylalanine in Serum

ALFRED H. FREE, Ph.D., AND HELEN M. FREE, B.S.

INTRODUCTION

Many methods are available for the determination of phenylalanine in serum or for the detection of elevated levels. These include: estimation by comparison with standards after paper chromatography of serum or blood filtrate [1, 2]; enzymatic decarboxylation with subsequent colorimetric measurement of the resulting phenylethylamine[12]; oxidation by snake venom L-amino acid oxidase to phenylpyruvic acid with subsequent measurement of a borate-enol complex of phenylpyruvic acid by its absorption in the ultraviolet[8]; oxidation to benzoic acid with colorimetric determination of the nitrated derivative[6]; ion exchange chromatography for separation from other amino acids and subsequent spectrophotometric measurement of the ninhydrin reaction[11]; microbiological inhibition assay in which increasing quantities of phenylalanine produce increasing growth of spores of *B. subtilis* in media containing β-2-thienylalanine[4]; fluorimetric determination of the ninhydrin-phenylalanine product in the presence of a peptide[3, 9].

This paper reviews a fluorimetric method, essentially that of McCaman and Robins[9], which appears to satisfy the requirements of accuracy, precision, reliability and adaptability to relatively large numbers of samples without use of highly specialized equipment and employing the ultramicroquantities of serum necessary for its use on infants.

METHOD

The method depends on the fluorescence of a phenylalanine-ninhydrin reaction product. Its sensitivity is due to the presence of the peptide, leucylalanine, which enhances the reaction between phenylalanine and ninhydrin. Its specificity is due to the reaction pH of 5.8, at which other amino acids will not react with ninhydrin.

REAGENTS

1. *0.6 N trichloroacetic acid.* 98.0 gm of trichloroacetic acid are dissolved in water and diluted to a volume of 1 liter. To obtain 0.3 N trichloroacetic acid for the blank and for making up standards, 0.6 N trichloroacetic acid is diluted with an equal volume of water.

2. *0.3 M succinate buffer, pH 5.8.* 5.94 gm of sodium succinate ($Na_2C_4H_4O_4 \cdot 2H_2O$) (or 8.1 gm of $Na_2C_4H_4O_4 \cdot 6H_2O$) are dissolved in water, and 4 ml of 1 N HCl are added. The volume is

made to 100 ml with water, and the pH is adjusted to 5.8 ($\pm$ 0.1) with 1 N HCl or 1 N NaOH. The buffer should be stored in the refrigerator.

3. *30 mM ninhydrin.* 0.534 gm of ninhydrin (1, 2, 3-indantrione — $C_9H_4O_3 \cdot H_2O$) is dissolved in water and diluted to 100 ml. The reagent is stored in a brown bottle at room temperature.

4. *5 mM L-leucyl-L-alanine.* 0.1011 gm of L-leucyl-L-alanine is dissolved in water and diluted to 100 ml. This reagent should be dispensed into small vials or tubes in approximately 1 ml aliquots and stored in the deep freeze.

5. *Copper reagent.* Dissolved separately in about 300 ml of water each are 1.6 gm sodium carbonate (Na_2CO_3), 100 mg potassium sodium tartrate ($KNaC_4H_4O_6 \cdot 4H_2O$) and 60 mg copper sulfate ($CuSO_4 \cdot 5H_2O$). The sodium carbonate and tartrate solutions are mixed together, and the copper sulfate is then added and the volume made to 1 liter. This prevents precipitation of the cupric ions in alkaline medium. This reagent is kept at room temperature.

All reagents may be prepared or may be purchased from commercial sources.

STANDARD SOLUTIONS

Standard solutions are prepared by dissolving L-phenylalanine in 0.3 N trichloroacetic acid. A suitable method is to dissolve 100 mg of L-phenylalanine in acid and dilute to 100 ml to obtain a stock solution. Appropriate dilutions are made in 0.3 N trichloroacetic acid to give working standards ranging from 0.5 to 10 mg phenylalanine per 100 ml. These are equivalent to 1 to 20 mg phenylalanine per 100 ml serum or plasma since deproteinization produces a 1:2 dilution. Both stock solution and working standards are stored in the refrigerator.

SPECIAL APPARATUS

A suitable fluorometer with proper cuvettes and filters, a water bath at 60 C and a microcentrifuge are required. Satisfactory instruments and filter combinations as tabulated by Faulkner[3] are shown in Table I below:

TABLE I FLUOROMETERS AND FILTER COMBINATIONS

Instrument	Primary	Secondary
Farrand model A	Corning glass filter No. 5860 (365 Mμ)	No. 4304 and 3384 (505 to 530 mμ)
Turner model 110	Corning No. 7-51 (365 mμ) or Corning No. 7-60 (350 mμ)	Wratten No. 8 plus Wratten No. 65A (510 mμ)
Coleman fluorometer model 12C	Narrow-pass filter with peak transmission at 405 mμ	Sharp-cut filter starting transmission at 485 mμ

PROCEDURE

1. Serum or heparinized plasma is deproteinized by mixing equal quantities (0.05 ml or more) of sample and 0.6 N trichloroacetic acid. The mixture is allowed to stand for approximately ten minutes and centrifuged (about 2000 rpm) for ten minutes.

2. While samples are centrifuging, mixed reagent is prepared by adding together succinate buffer, ninhydrin and leucylalanine in the volume ratio of 10:4:2. (0.8 ml of the mixture is required for each sample, blank or standard.)

3. In small tubes, 0.80 ml mixed reagent is mixed with 0.05 ml supernatant (from deproteinization of sample), or standard working solution, or 0.3 N trichloroacetic acid (for the blank).

4. After thorough mixing, the tubes are incubated in a water bath at 60 C for two hours.

5. Tubes are cooled in an ice bath, and 5 ml of copper reagent are added to each. Tube contents are mixed thoroughly and allowed to stand at room temperature for ten to fifteen minutes.

6. The fluorescence of the standards and samples is measured setting the blank at zero fluorescence. Primary (activating) wavelength used is 390 mμ, and the secondary (fluorescing) wavelength used is 485 mμ (or filters closest to these wavelengths).

7. Phenylalanine concentration of samples is calculated from a standard curve plotting fluorescence against phenylalanine concentration of the standards.

DISCUSSION

The method requires a fluorometer, which is a special type of equipment. Such an instrument is relatively simple to manipulate and gives reliable results. The method has no unstable enzymes as reagents, and it is much faster than many methods such as chromatography, except for a recent chromatographic screening method[5]. It yields quantitative results, is adaptable to use with many samples, requires only a drop of sample and appears extremely suitable for confirmation of positive urine screening tests or presumptive positives with the microbiological inhibition method. The method has been adapted to automation[7].

SOURCES OF ERROR

Potential sources of error of this method include:

1. Obtaining blood at the wrong time (postprandial bloods are most likely to show elevation of serum phenylalanine);

2. Inaccurate measurements of sample or reagents;

3. Disregarding directions (prolonged heating or cooling time);

4. Use of unstable reagents (leucylalanine must be discarded at the end of the day's run and should not be refrozen).

RANGE OF VALUES

Phenylalanine values for normal infants and children as measured by this method are less than 2 mg per 100 ml. In the following tabulation compiled by Faulkner[3], normal values differ markedly from the extreme elevations shown in two series of known phenylketonurics.

TABLE II PHENYLALNINE CONCENTRATIONS
IN HUMAN SERUM

No. of Patients	Age Range	Type of Patient	Reported by	mg per 100 ml	
				Mean	SD
4	newborn	normal	McCaman	1.67	0.77
15	1 mo to 14 yr	normal	McCaman	1.42	0.58
6		phenyl-ketonuric	McCaman	33.0	2.04
30	1 mo to 16 yr	normal	Smith	1.94	0.53
3	newborn	normal	Faulkner	1.51	0.82
13	8 mo to 13 yr	normal	Faulkner	1.83	0.94
5	9 mo to 8 yr	phenyl-ketonuric	Faulkner	26.0	10.0

RÉSUMÉ OF CLINICAL INTERPRETATIONS

Phenylalanine is an essential amino acid which is present in most natural proteins. The proteins of milk have relatively high concentration in comparison with many other proteins of the diet[13].

Elevation of blood phenylalanine may be due to either excessive ingestion or inadequate metabolism. Excessive ingestion is not readily achieved with any type of diet, though it is possible with feeding of the amino acid itself in high quantities. Inadequate metabolism therefore is the chief cause of high levels of serum phenylalanine. High values occur in phenylketonuria (PKU). High values also may be noted in infants with no recognizable disease, particularly premature infants. An elevated blood phenylalanine level in a newborn infant requires follow-up repeat testing no matter what method was used for phenylalanine determination. A single high serum phenylalanine determination is not an unequivocal indication of PKU. Usually, in non-PKU infants, the extent of the elevation is not as great, and the trend is for serial phenylalanine determinations to show lower and lower values. However, in cases of PKU, progressively higher blood phenylalanine levels are reached, and positive urine reactions for phenylpyruvic acid are obtained (positive PHENISTIX)[10].

REFERENCES

1. Berry, H. K.: Paper chromatographic method for estimation of phenylalanine. Proc. Soc. Exp. Biol. Med., **95**:71-73, 1957.
2. Culley, W. J., Mertz, E. T., Luce, M. W., Calandro, J. M., and Jolly, D. H.: Paper chromatographic estimation of phenylalanine and tyrosine using finger-tip blood. Its application to phenylketonuria. Clin. Chem., **9**: 266-269, 1962.
3. Faulkner, W. A.: Phenylalanine. In Meites, S. (ed.): Standard Methods of Clinical Chemistry, **5**:199-209, 1965.
4. Guthrie, R., and Susi, A.: A simple phenylalanine method for detecting phenylketonuria in large populations of newborn infants. Pediatrics, **32**:1185-1190, 1958.

5. Hanson, D. J.: Rapid screening test for serum phenylalanine. Amer. J. Med. Sci., **249**:682-684, 1965.

6. Henry, R. J., Sobel, C., and Chiamori, N.: Method for determination of serum phenylalanine with use of the Kapeller-Adler reaction. Amer. J. Dis. Child., **94**:604-608, 1957.

7. Hill, J. B., Summer, G. K., Pender, M. W., and Rozel, N. O.: An automated procedure for blood phenylalanine. Clin. Chem., **11**: 541-546, 1965.

8. LaDu, B. N., and Michael, P. J.: An enzymatic spectrophotometric method for the determination of phenylalanine in blood. J. Lab. Clin. Med., **55**:491-496, 1960.

9. McCaman, M. W., and Robins, E.: Fluorimetric method for the determination of phenylalanine in serum. J. Lab. Clin. Med., **59**: 885-890, 1962.

10. McCready, R. A. and Hussey, M. G.: Newborn phenylketonuria detection program in Massachusetts. Amer. J. Public Health, **54**: 2075-2081, 1964.

11. Moore, S., Spochman, D. H., and Stein, W. H.: Chromatography of amino acids on sulfonated polystyrene resins. An improved system. Anal. Chem., **30**:1185-1190, 1958.

12. Udenfriend, S., and Cooper, J. R.: Assay of L-phenylalanine as phenylethylamine after enzymatic decarboxylation; application to isotopic studies. J. Biol. Chem., **203**:953-960, 1953.

13. Webb, B. H.: Dairy products. In Blank, F. (ed.): Handbook of Food and Agriculture. New York, Rheinhold, 1955, pp. 453-476.

Inhibition Assay for Measurement of Blood Phenylalanine

ALFRED H. FREE, Ph.D., AND HELEN M. FREE, B.S.

INTRODUCTION

Screening of newborn infants for phenylketonuria is being carried out in many parts of the world at the present time. The number of positive findings is not great, but the importance of being able to avert the serious mental injury which ensues in the untreated case is the basis for the popularity of such programs.

Two types of screening test are currently employed. One of these involves tests on the urine for phenylpyruvic acid, and the other involves measurement of phenylalanine in the blood. An advantage of the blood measurement is that it can be carried out during the first three to five days of life prior to discharge of the infant from the hospital.

Guthrie[5] has described a microbiological inhibition assay for measurement of blood phenylalanine. This method involves collection of blood on a piece of filter paper and subsequent measurement of the growth response the phenylalanine in the sample produces with *B. subtilis* contained in medium with a growth antagonist β-2-thienylalanine.

This report describes the principle, the procedure and results obtained with the inhibition assay of phenylalanine in blood.

METHOD

The inhibition assay for phenylalanine depends on the fact that *B. subtilis* spores will germinate and grow on agar only in the presence of phenylalanine. Beta-2-thienylalanine, which is an analog of phenylalanine, acts as an antimetabolite when it is added to the system. An amount of this antimetabolite is added which just prevents germination and growth of the *B. subtilis* spores, but which is not sufficient to inhibit the germination and growth of the spores of *B. subtilis* in the presence of phenylalanine. In practice, an agar plate is prepared which contains spores of *B. subtilis* suspended in special agar containing β-2-thienylalanine. Blood to be assayed is collected as spots on filter paper, and discs are cut from the blood spots with a paper punch. These discs are placed on the surface of the agar along with standard discs prepared from blood containing known amounts of L-phenylalanine. The plate, with the discs on the agar surface, is placed in an incubator for sixteen hours. During this time, phenylalanine diffuses from the blood spots into the agar. The phenylalanine antagonizes the inhibiting effect of β-2-thienylalanine, and, in this area of the plate, growth of the organism occurs. The diameter of the zone of growth is roughly proportional to the concentration of phenylalanine in the blood.

REAGENTS

1. *Modified Demain's Medium.* In a total of 890 ml of distilled water are dissolved 10.0 gm dextrose, 30.0 gm K_2HPO_4, 10.0 gm KH_2PO_4, 5.0 gm NH_4Cl, 1.0 gm NH_4NO_3, 1.0 gm Na_2SO_3, 1.0 gm glutamic acid, 1.0 gm asparagine, 0.5 gm L-alanine. Ten ml of salt solution (containing 1% $MgSO_4 \cdot 7H_2O$, 0.1% $MnCl_2 \cdot 4H_2O$, 0.1% $FeCl_3 \cdot 6H_2O$ and 0.05% $CaCl_2$) are added and mixed. This solution is dispensed into 90 ml aliquots and sterilized by autoclaving.

2. *10 Per Cent Dextrose.* 10.0 gm dextrose are dissolved in water and the volume is made to 100 ml. The solution is dispensed into 10 ml aliquots and sterilized by autoclaving.

3. *3 Per Cent Agar.* 30.0 gm agar are dissolved with heat in 1 liter of water. The solution is dispensed into 100 ml aliquots and sterilized by autoclaving.

4. *β-2-thienylalanine.* 17.0 mg are dissolved in water and made to a volume of 10 ml (0.01 M solution). The solution is dispensed in 0.3 ml quantities and dried.

5. *Bacillus subtilis ATCC 6051 Spores.* These may be prepared as a dry powder according to the method of Guthrie[5].

All material necessary for 325 tests is available commercially as PHENI-PLATE® from the Ames Company, Elkhart, Indiana. In the kits, agar, salts, dextrose and inhibitor are combined into one bottle of dry culture medium. The spores are supplied as a suspension in an ampule.

STANDARDS (CONTROL BLOOD SPOTS)

Blood from a normal healthy subject is assayed quantitatively for phenylalanine. Using stock solutions, of L-phenylalanine, small quantities of solution are added to aliquots of the blood to give total phenylalanine concentrations of 2, 4, 6, 8, 12 and 20 mg per 100 ml. The bloods are spotted on S & S #903 filter paper (to make spots at least $\frac{1}{4}$ in in diameter) and stored in a desiccator in the refrigerator. With PHENIPLATE, control blood spots are provided for each plate in a strip of eight spots with phenylalanine concentrations of 2, 4, 4, 6, 6, 8, 12 and 20 mg per 100 ml of blood.

SPECIAL APPARATUS

No highly specialized apparatus is required. In addition to a large clear flat dish for holding the agar, facilities for incubation of the agar plate for sixteen hours at 37 C are needed. Other common laboratory equipment such as a source of heat for dissolving the medium, a $\frac{1}{4}$ in paper punch for obtaining disks from blood spots and an autoclave for "fixing" blood spots on the filter paper are required.

PROCEDURE

1. Unknown blood spots, collected on S & S #903 paper and properly identified, are placed on wire racks and autoclaved for three minutes at 15 lbs pressure with the steam rapidly released from the autoclave. A series of control spots is autoclaved at the same time. (A box containing 25 printed instruction-record sheets with filter paper attached along with a package of 25 sterile lancets is available as Blood

Collection Kit from Ames Company.)

2. The contents of a bottle of culture medium from PHENIPLATE are mixed with 150 ml of distilled water and heated to boiling until just dissolved. The medium is cooled to a about 55 C — "comfortable to cheek" temperature — and an ampule of spore suspension is added and the mixture transferred to one of the plastic trays provided. (With the reagents prepared according to Guthrie and Susi, 90 ml modified Demain's medium, 10 ml dextrose, 100 ml warm (55 C) agar solution, 0.3 ml of 0.01 M β-2-thienylalanine and *B. subtilis* spores are mixed and poured into a flat clear plate such as a Pyrex baking dish.) Care is taken to be sure the agar plate is on a flat surface and the mixture is poured carefully to avoid air bubbles.

3. When the agar has hardened, disks are punched (with a ¼ in paper punch) from the control and unknown blood spots and are placed carefully on the surface of the agar with a forceps. Spots are placed about 1 in apart. A pattern sheet with horizontal and vertical lines drawn about 1 in apart and numbered at the intersections is placed under the agar plate to aid in positioning and identifying the spots.

4. The plate, with blood spots (unknowns and controls) on the surface of the agar, is covered with the lid provided and incubated upside down for sixteen hours at 37 C.

5. After incubation, the blood phenylalanine concentration is estimated by comparing the diameter of the zone of growth of *B. subtilis* around the unknown blood spots to the growth zones around the control spots.

DISCUSSION

There is an increasing amount of attention directed to the screening of newborn infants for phenylketonuria[2, 4]. The relative merits of blood studies[5, 6] or urine studies[1, 3, 7] for the recognition of phenylketonuria have been discussed by the proponents of each method. It appears that either approach is attractive and provides a means for finding the disease at a time when treatment can be effective.

The microbiological inhibition assay is well suited to mass usage, and the convenience of collecting a blood sample on a piece of paper and transporting it as a dry blood spot is unique. Blood specimens may be taken at several locations and the assays all carried out at a central laboratory. Ordinarily, in the infant with phenylketonuria, the blood phenylalanine increases above normal values within two or three days of food ingestion. This makes it practical to test most infants while still in the hospital if the microbiological inhibition method is employed for measuring blood phenylalanine. Testing the infant while still in the hospital insures good coverage of all babies, whereas testing urine following release from the hospital may not be as effective in providing tests to all babies. One drawback of the microbiological inhibition assay is that it is not readily adaptable to study of a small number of samples.

The phenylalanine inhibition assay appears to have a high degree of specificity. Although increased levels of blood phenylalanine may be encountered in certain infants who do not have phenylketonuria[6], the test has not been reported to give indication of elevated blood phenylalanine as a result of other substances causing a growth response of the *B. subtilis*.

Widespread screening for phenylketonuria has resulted in recognizing more cases of the disorder than had been initially predicted. The incidence of the genetic defect varies in different population groups. Certain groups who initially had been imagined to be free of the defect have been found to have a small number of affected members.

Source of Error

1. Improper collection of blood. The blood spots on the filter paper must be large enough to permit a ¼ in diameter disk to be punched out. With the Ames Blood Collecting Unit, the printed circles must be almost completely filled.

2. Failure to autoclave spots. It is necessary to "fix" the protein to the filter paper by autoclaving, or the hemoglobin will diffuse out of the paper and make interpretation of growth zone diameters difficult.

3. Improper incubation. Incubating for sixteen hours gives optimal results. Shorter times give less growth and longer times give fuzzy zone outlines. The plate must be incubated upside down so that the agar does not dry out.

4. Incubation temperature. The temperature of incubation should be carefully controlled. Growth will occur at temperatures above or below 37 C, but the sharpness of the growth zone boundaries will be decreased if recommended time-temperature relationships are not observed.

5. Exposure to excessive heat. Spores of *B. subtilis* are quite stable and can be exposed for short periods to relatively high temperatures. In preparing the medium by dissolving the solid constituents in boiling water to facilitate the solution of the agar, spores can be added to the hot solution. However, the medium must not be held at high temperatures after adding the spores but should be "poured" promptly.

Range of Values

Healthy full-term infants ordinarily have a blood phenylalanine level of 2 mg or less per 100 ml as indicated by the growth response of the organisms around the blood spot. A few infants may give a response indicating a level of 4 mg per 100 ml.

Blood spots from infants who have phenylketonuria will give a growth response comparable to 6 mg phenylalanine per 100 ml or greater. MacCready and Hussey[6] have reported that approximately one out of two thousand infants has a blood phenylalanine level of 6 mg per 100 ml or greater. These investigators stress the fact that an infant whose blood gives a response of 6 mg or more per 100 ml should be retested. In the MacCready series, approximately one case in five which gave elevated phenylalanine levels actually had phenylketonuria. The other cases were regarded as transient elevations which occur from time to time in normal babies and more frequently in premature babies.

RÉSUMÉ OF CLINICAL INTERPRETATION

Phenylketonuria is a genetic disorder characterized by an inadequate enzymatic mechanism for the conversion of phenylalanine to tyrosine. The result of this disorder is that phenylalanine contained in the diet will accumulate in the blood. A portion of the extra phenylalanine is excreted in the urine, during which process it is converted by deamination to phenylpyruvic acid. High levels of phenylalanine in the blood have a toxic influence on developing brain tissue with a resultant irreversible injury to the brain which is evident as severe mental retardation.

An increase of blood phenylalanine concentration will occur in the untreated phenylketonuric providing food is ingested. If there is not adequate food intake, there will not be an increase in blood phenylalanine in the phenylketonuric. Conversely, any condition involving excessive phenylalanine intake or inadequate conversion of phenylalanine to other compounds might increase the blood level of phenylalanine. An elevation of blood phenylalanine concentration in a newborn infant raises a definite question of the possibility of phenylketonuria but in no way establishes a diagnosis. Elevation of phenylalanine concentration of blood requires confirmation by one or more quantitative measurements of phenylalanine in the blood. These may be supplemented by additional tests carried out on urine and blood.

REFERENCES

1. Allen, R. J., and Wilson, J. L.: Urinary phenylpyruvic acid in phenylketonuria. JAMA, 188: 720-724, 1964.
2. Committee on Maternal and Child Care, Council on Medical Service, American Medical Association: Phenylketonuria and screening tests in the newborn and screening of newborn infants for metabolic diseases. J. Arkansas Med. Soc., 61:400-402, 1965.
3. Editorial: Urinary phenylpyruvic acid in phenylketonuria, JAMA, 188:748, 1964.
4. Fisch, R. O., and Davis, E.: Phenylketonuria in Minnesota. Programs for detection and treatment, Minnesota Med. 47:501-506, 1964.
5. Guthrie, R., and Susi, A.: A simple phenylalanine method for detecting phenylketonuria in large populations of newborn infants, Pediatrics, 32:338-343, 1963.
6. MacCready, R. A., and Hussey, M. G.: Newborn phenylketonuria detection program in Massachusetts, Amer. J. Public Health, 54: 2075-2081, 1964.
7. Martin, P. H.: County phenylketonuria screening program, J. Ind. Med. Ass., 57:856-858, 1964.

Identification of Reducing Substances in Urine by Paper Chromatography

HENRY A. TELOH, M.D.

Chromatography offers an easily performed and readily available technique for identification of various reducing substances in urine. In chromatographic separation of amino acids in urine, the number and complexity of compounds normally present necessitates a two-way chromatogram in order to identify the various amino acids. In the case of urinary sugars, the number of sugars present rarely exceeds two or, at the most, three, so that a simple one-way chromatogram is sufficient to effect adequate separation.

The demonstration of reducing substances in the urine is ordinarily equated with the presence of glucose, although this is by no means the only substance which may produce a positive result. Reducing action may be caused by: (a) carbohydrates (glucose, lactose, galactose, fructose, pentoses); (b) glucuronates (conjugates of glucuronic acid and various ingested drugs); (c) salicyluric acid (resulting from injestion of salicylates; (d) homogentisic acid; (e) ascorbic acid in large amounts; (f) uric acid in large amounts; and (g) creatinine in large amounts.

METHOD

In paper chromatography, there are two components: (a) a hydrophilic solid (cellulose); and (b) a solvent containing some proportion of water percolating through the solid. The stationary or solid phase consists of the solid (cellulose) with a quantity of imbibed water. The liquid phase consists of an appropriate organic solvent. The separation of different solutes (e.g., sugars) then depends upon specific differences in their differential distribution between the water-cellulose complex on the one hand and the water-containing organic solvent on the other hand. Many factors, such as size and shape of the molecule, as well as number, character and position of hydrophilic groups of the solute will determine the specific distribution of the solute between the two phases in a given system.

The ratio of the distance moved by a given substance from the origin to the distance of the liquid front from the origin is known as its R_f (relative front) value for that particular substance. Sugars generally separate in the same order in all non-phenolic solvents. However, there are minor differences due to content of water in the solvent system, type of organic solvent utilized, etc. The R_f value for any sugar is determined by the number as well as disposition of hydroxyl groups on the ring form (pyranose) of sugars, as well as the nature of the residue attached to either Carbon Atom 5 of the pyranose ring or Carbon Atom 4 of the furanose ring. A similar effect is observed with the residue attached to the reducing end of the sugar[5].

APPARATUS

Although many types of chromatographic apparatus have been designed and described[2], a simple apparatus satisfactory for identification of sugars can be constructed from equipment available in any clinical laboratory[3, 4].

1. *Test tubes*, approximately 25 x 200 mm. The Folin-Wu non-protein nitrogen digestion tube is satisfactory.

2. *Strips of filter paper* (Whatman No. 1, approximately 15 x 175 mm.

3. *Rubber stoppers*, No. 4. A slit approximately 1 cm deep is made in the bottom of the stopper so that the paper strip may be inserted and suspended in the test tube.

4. *Micropipettes* of 10 to 20 ul capacity. The Sahli hemoglobin pipette marked at 10 and 20 ul is satisfactory.

5. *Capillary glass tubes*, approximately 2 cm in length.

6. *Atomizer* for spraying the chromatographic strips.

7. *Drying oven* to operate at 100 to 105 C.

SOLVENT SYSTEMS

A number of solvent systems are utilized for ascending chromatography of sugars. In all of these solvents, the R^f values are generally low, and the solvent front should be permitted to travel the greatest possible distance in order to effect sufficient separation of individual compounds. In general, all solvent systems produce the same order of separation of sugars, namely pentoses, hexoses, disaccharides and trisaccharides in that order. In other words, separation and distance of migration occurs in order of chain length and molecular weight.

The R_f values for various solvents can be increased or decreased to meet specific needs by altering the composition of the solvent. In general, water and pyridine both cause an increase in migration, while ethyl acetate and butanol cause a decrease in migration.

The following solvent systems are commonly used and described for chromatography of sugars.

1. n-butanol, 60 ml; pyridine, 40 ml; water, 30 ml.

2. n-butanol, 80 ml; pyridine, 80 ml; water, 40 ml.

3. Isopropanol, 160 ml; water, 40 ml.

4. Ethyl acetate, 120 ml; pyridine, 50 ml; water, 40 ml.

5. Phenol. A stock solution containing 90 gm of phenol and 10 ml of water is prepared. This is liquid at room temperature. The mixture is shaken with an excess of water to obtain a water-saturated solution of phenol. The water layer is aspirated, and the phenol layer is used as the solvent.

6. Isopropanol, 120 ml; pyridine, 40 ml; water, 40 ml.

7. Isopropanol, 140 ml; ethyl acetate, 20 ml; water 40 ml.

8. Isopropanol, 140 ml; n-butanol, 20 ml; water, 40 ml.

9. n-butanol, 40 ml; glacial acetic acid, 10 ml; water, 50 ml. The mixture is shaken well. After separation, the aqueous layer is discarded.

10. Ethyl acetate, 140 ml; acetic acid, 30 ml; water, 30 ml.

STANDARD SOLUTIONS

Since R_f values for various sugars will vary depending on composition of solvent, type of chromatographic paper, ambient temperature and presence of extraneous interfering substances in the specimen to be analyzed, standard solutions of various sugars should be chromatographed simultaneously with the unknown material and under the same conditions. These standard solutions may be applied to separate strips to calculate R_f values under prevailing conditions or may be added to the unknown material for comparison.

Standard solutions may be made up either in aqueous solution or in organic solvents. A 1.0 per cent solution of a sugar in a saturated aqueous solution of benzoic acid is satisfactory. Standards may also be prepared as a 1.0 per cent solution in 10 per cent isopropanol.

LOCATION REAGENTS

The following color reagents will permit identification of most reducing substances in the urine.

1. *Dinitrosalicylic acid* (Eastman), 0.5 per cent solution in a 4 per cent aqueous solution of sodium hydroxide.

2. *Benzidine reagent*: 0.5 gm of benzidine base in glacial acetic acid, 20 ml, and absolute ethyl alcohol, 80 ml.

3. *Phloroglucinol reagent.* 0.2 gm phloroglucinol is dissolved in 80 ml of 90 per cent ethyl alcohol. The volume is made up to 100 ml with 25 per cent w/v trichloracetic acid.

4. *Ammoniacal silver nitrate.* The solution is freshly prepared by mixing equal parts of N/10 silver nitrate and 5 N ammonia solution. Any reagent not used is discarded, since dangerous explosive compounds may form on standing.

5. *Aniline hydrogen oxalate reagent.* .9 ml of redistilled aniline is shaken with 100 ml of N/10 oxalic acid solution.

6. *Aniline phthalate reagent.* 1.66 gm phthalic acid and 0.93 gm aniline are dissolved in water saturated with butyl alcohol. This reagent is similar to the aniline hydrogen oxalate reagent.

7. *m-phenylenediamine,* 2.16 gm per 100 ml of 76 per cent ethyl alcohol.

PROCEDURE

1. Using a pencil, a small dot is centrally placed approximately 20 mm from one end of a strip of filter paper. A second dot is similarly placed approximately 3 mm from the same end.

2. Using a micropipette or a Sahli 0.02 ml pipette, 0.01 to 0.02 ml of urine is placed at the point marked by the first dot, covering an area of approximately 5 mm. The spot is allowed to dry in air. To prevent spreading of the urine over too large an area, a small amount of urine is deposited on the paper. Then the paper is allowed to dry before the next application is made. In this manner, a relatively large volume of urine can be deposited and concentrated on a small area of the paper.

The volume of urine used varies with the amount of reducing substance present. If less than 0.2 per cent of reducing substance is present, 0.02 ml of urine is used; for 0.2 to 1 per cent of reducing substance, 0.01 ml is used; if more than 1 per cent of reducing substance is present, 0.005 ml of urine is used.

3. The opposite end of the paper strip is inserted into the slot in the rubber stopper. A segment of capillary glass tubing, approximately 20 mm long, is inserted through the paper at the second pencil dot, placed 3 mm from the end of the strip.

4. Approximately 15 ml of the solvent are placed in the test tube. The sides of the tube are allowed to drain. The amount of solvent should be sufficient so that the fluid level is approximately 5 mm above the end of the strip when the strip is inserted into position.

5. The chromatographic strip is carefully lowered into the tube. The strip must not touch the wall of the tube.

6. The solvent is permitted to migrate on the filter paper at room temperature for a period of two to two and one half hours and for a distance of approximately 130 mm. The actual time and distance of migration is not critical.

7. At the termination of the period of migration, the strip is carefully removed from the tube and detached from the cork. The capillary glass tube is removed from the opposite end of the strip. The upper limit attained by the migrating solvent is marked on the paper with pencil. Then the paper is dried in the oven at 100 to 105 C for ten minutes.

8. The paper is sprayed lightly, evenly and quickly with the color-developing solution. Care must be taken to avoid using too much solution.

9. Then the paper is heated in the oven at 100 to 105 C for ten minutes.

R_f VALUES

The R_f (relative front) value is defined as the ratio of the distance moved by a given substance to the distance of the solvent front from the origin when the solvent front is not allowed to run off the paper.

$$R_f = \frac{\text{distance substance has traveled from origin}}{\text{distance solvent front has traveled from origin}}$$

Although published R_f values are available for various solvent systems, these values will vary with the exact composition of the solvent system, ambient temperature, character of the carrier paper, presence of interfering substances in the unknown material to be analyzed, and other poorly defined factors. For this reason, known solutions of sugars should be chromatographed under identical conditions as the unknown and the R_f values determined. Since R_f values for most sugars are low, sharper separation of spots can be achieved by allowing the solvent front to run off the paper. Under these circumstances, reference markers are run in parallel with the solution to be examined. For example, glucose may be taken as a reference marker and an arbitrary R_g defined. Under these circumstances, the R_g for glucose will always be 100, and the values for all other sugars are determined from this reference point.

$$R_g = \frac{\text{distance substance travels from origin}}{\text{distance glucose travels from origin}} \times 100$$

A useful modification of the marker technique involves direct addition of known sugars to the unknown solution to be chromatographed. For example, in a case of suspected galactosemia, three chromatographic strips may be run: one with the unknown urine; one with the unknown urine plus added glucose; and one with the unknown urine plus added galactose. In the presence of galactose, Strips Number 1 and 3 will each have a single spot of identical location, while Strip Number 2 will have two spots due to presence of galactose and glucose.

Using the method described and the n-butanol-pyridine-water (60:40:30) solvent system, the following R_f values are usually obtained:

Lactose	0.22
Galactose	0.36
Glucose	0.41
Fructose	0.46
Pentose	0.52

DISCUSSION

Although the type of sugar involved in most mellituras may be identified by estimation of the R_f value of the sugar, additional information may be obtained by observation of the color reaction with various color reagents[1]. The first spraying with dinitrosalicylic acid or benzidine will indicate if a reducing sugar is present. Lactose, maltose, galactose, glucose and fructose form dark-brown spots on heating the strips within ten minutes. Pentoses give a chocolate-brown spot within five minutes of heating. Ascorbic acid gives a pale brown spot if more than ten μg is present. Large amounts of urates may produce a faint brown spot with dinitrosalicylic acid.

With phloroglucinol as color reagent, fructose gives an orange-brown spot. Sucrose produces a similar colored spot which should cause no confusion, since sucrose is a nonreducing substance. Galactose and ascorbic acid produce faint brown spots, while lactose, maltose, glucose, homogentisic acid and urates give no color reaction. Pentoses give a green-to-blue spot after prolonged heating or on standing at room temperature for a few hours.

Presence of a pentose can be confirmed by spraying with the aniline-oxalate or aniline-phthalate color reagents which give a bright red spot within five minutes. With these reagents, galactose and glucose give a brown spot, and ascorbic acid produces a faint yellow spot.

If no sugar is identified after spraying with dinitrosalicylic acid or benzidine base, the reducing action of the urine is due to a substance other than a sugar. Spraying with ammoniacal silver nitrate results in immediate production, at room temperature, of a black spot if ascorbic acid or homogentisic acid are present. Urine containing salicylates produces a brown spot on heating.

REFERENCES

1. Horrocks, R. H., and Manning, G. B.: Partition chromatography on paper: Identification of reducing substances in urine. Lancet, 1:1042-1045, 1949.
2. Sophian, L. H., and Connolly, V. J.: Chromatographic identification of reducing sugars in urine. Amer. J. Clin. Path., 22:41-45, 1952.
3. Sunderman, F. W., Copeland, B. E., Mac-Fate, R. P., Martens, V. E., Naumann, H. N., and Stevenson, G. F.: Manual of American Society of Clinical Pathologist Workshop on Glucose. Amer. J. Clin. Path., 26:1355-1372, 1956.

4. Teloh, H. A.: Identification of reducing substances in urine by paper chromatography. In Sunderman, F. W., and Sunderman, F. W., Jr. (eds.): Measurements of Exocrine and Endocrine Function of the Pancreas. Philadelphia, Lippincott, 1961, Chapter 20.

5. Isherwood, F. A.: Separation of carbohydrates and phosphoric esters on paper chromatograms. Brit. Med. Bull., 10:202-210, 1954.

Thin-Layer Chromatography of Urinary Sugars

MANFORD D. MORRIS, Ph.D., AND HOWARD QUITTNER, M.D.

INTRODUCTION

The appearance of one or more carbohydrates in the urine of the newborn may be of particular significance. Several hereditable disorders of carbohydrate metabolism are accompanied by severe clinical disease, and these diseases usually exhibit an associated melituria. Although galactosemia has received the most attention, reports have appeared with increasing frequency of clinical disease related to deficiency of intestinal disaccharidase(s) or abnormal fructose metabolism. These developments have expanded the need for a definitive methodology which can be used for the detection and identification of a number of simple sugars.

METHOD

Thin-layer chromatography is a technique for the separation of compounds of closely related molecular structure by means of a combination of adsorption and partition chromatography. The presence of either borate or acetate ions modifies the migration and enables the resolution of heretofore inseparable mixtures of biologically important simple sugars.

REAGENTS

1. *Silica gel G.*
2. *0.01 M boric acid.* 438 mg of boric acid USP are dissolved in 1000 ml of distilled water. The pH of the solution is not adjusted (approximate pH, 4.6).
3. *0.02 M sodium acetate.* 1.64 gm of sodium acetate AR are dissolved in 1000 ml of distilled water.
4. *Solvent.* Acetone AR and distilled water, 9:1 (v/v), is prepared just prior to use.
5. *Spray reagent*[1]. 100 mg of naphthoresorcinol (Calbiochem) are dissolved in a mixture of 50 ml of 95 per cent ethyl alcohol, reagent grade, and 1 ml concentrated sulfuric acid. The reagent is stable for three days at room temperature if kept in the dark.

STANDARD SOLUTIONS

1. *Stock Solutions.* Five mg per ml of the highest purity sugars (Mann Research Laboratories) are dissolved in 50 per cent ethanol. This strength of ethanol serves as an effective preservative at room temperature for prolonged periods.
2. *Working Solutions.* 1:5 dilutions of the single standards or mixtures of similar strength are prepared in 50 per

cent ethanol, so that the application of a 5μl volume to a standard plate does not deliver more than 5 μg of the known sugar.

SPECIAL APPARATUS

1. *Chromatography jars,* glass cylindrical form, 235 mm high, 60 mm diameter.*

2. *Caplug #250* as jar closure.*

3. *Flat glass plates,* smooth surfaced, 2-3 mm thickness, 200 × 50 mm.*

4. *Whatman #1 filter paper sheets* cut to 220 × 75 mm rectangles.

5. *Glass rod* 9-12 mm in diameter, 40 cm long; used as gel spreader.

6. *Masking tape* (Minnesota Mining and Manufacturing autoclave tape #1222); used as a gel form.

7. *Sprayer.* Device composed of a pressurized propellant can containing dichlorodifluoromethane attached to a reservoir bottle and atomizer nozzle. (Chromatosprayer)*

8. *Hot air oven* adjustable in the 80 to 120 C range.

9. *Micropipettes,* Sahli or other type, 20 μl and 5 μl.

10. *Optional equipment.* Desalter consisting of a power unit, electrodialysis unit and electrolyte delivery flask.*

PROCEDURE

A. *Preparation of Thin Layer Plates*[2]

1. Eight clean dry glass plates (precleaned by dipping in 95 per cent ethanol and rubbing dry) are lined up in a straight row on a smooth surface with their long edges closely apposed.

2. Single long strips of masking tape are placed along the opposite narrow

---

*Obtainable from Warner-Chilcott Laboratory Instrument Co.

ends so that 0.5 cm of the plate ends are covered by each of the tapes and the plates are secured to the smooth surface by the rest of the tapes.

3. Ten gm of silica gel G are slurried with 25 ml of either 0.01 M boric acid or 0.02 M sodium acetate in a 150 ml beaker. Thorough mixing is essential and can be easily achieved with a magnetic mixer.

4. The slurry is poured over the set of plates in a zig-zag pattern starting from one of the free edges of the set of plates.

5. The glass rod is grasped at its ends and is drawn over the plates in such a manner that the thumbs of the hands ride along the taped edges of the plates. The rod must not be allowed to roll on the surface of the tape. This procedure spreads the slurry evenly over the plates to a thickness determined by that of the masking tape.

6. The plates are allowed to air-dry until their surfaces glisten and are then placed in the oven at 110 C for thirty minutes. The plates must be stored in a dry-box or desiccator if not used within twenty-four hours but may be reactivated by another thirty-minute heating period.

7. The plates are shaped with a razor blade to produce an "hourglass" pattern (Fig. 1).

B. *Development of Chromatograms*

1. The specimens are spotted with a 20 μl pipette, 0.5 cm below the constriction, in a thin band extending across the width of the silica gel. Two plates are prepared for each specimen, one impregnated with acetate and one with borate. Care must be taken to deliver the liquid in small aliquots, drying under a fine jet of air between applica-

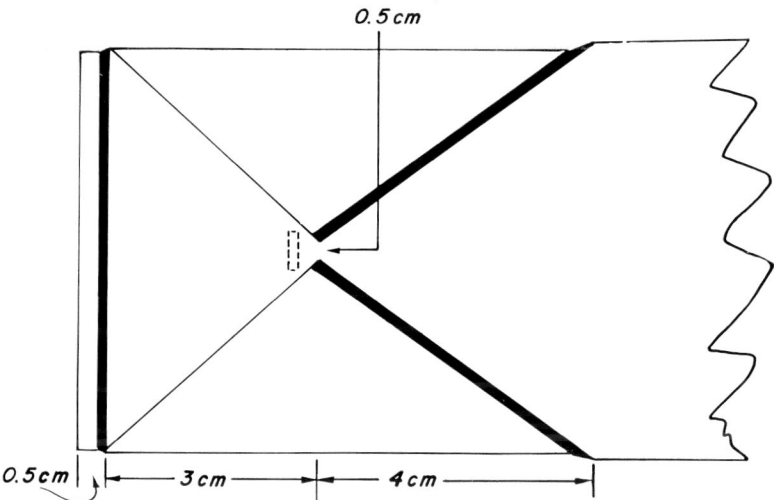

Fig. 1.   Shaping diagram of thin-layer plates.

tions. Suitable standards spotted with 5 μl pipettes are run with the specimens.

2. The jars are prepared by inserting the piece of filter paper along the wall to enhance saturation of the atmosphere in the jar. Thirty ml of the acetone-water mixture are placed in the jar, and it is capped. The jar is manipulated to saturate the paper, and one or two plates are then inserted in each jar in a manner that does not allow contact with the filter paper.

3. Solvent migration at room temperature is allowed to procede for a distance of at least 10 cm from the constriction (about 30 to 40 minutes).

4. The plates are removed from the chamber, the distance of solvent migration is scored in the gel, and the plates are air-dried.

5. The plates are placed at a steeply inclined angle in a well-vented hood and sprayed with the color reagent. They are then transferred to a hot-air oven at 85 C for fifteen minutes to develop the color.

6. R_f values and colors on both plates

are determined from the point of constriction. This should be done immediately, as the colors fade in a few minutes. A comparison of the colors and R_f values for the two silica gel systems allows a clear distinction of the six clinically important sugars: glucose; galactose; fructose; lactose; maltose; sucrose.

DISCUSSION

We have used one solvent and two buffers in an attempt to create a system which is simple, sensitive, rapid and easily interpreted. We have not been able to find a single solvent-buffer pair that would permit the complete resolution of the six clinically important sugars in a single mixture. This problem has been compounded since we have also repeatedly observed significant alterations in the migration distances of single sugars when they were incorporated into mixtures.

Although the colors produced with naphthoresorcinol fade quickly, the distinctiveness of the colors has made it the reagent of choice. Fructose and sucrose (which does not reduce copper reagents) produce a vivid purple-red color. While the remaining four sugars are blue, there are subtle differences in their hues. The colors allow ready recognition of maltose, which migrates in close proximity to sucrose. In contrast to other color reagents, the background with naphthoresorcinol remains essentially colorless.

The use of a shaped chromatoplate and the application of the specimen as a strip have produced relatively thin bands of each sugar spread out over the width of the plate as they ascend. This pattern minimizes overlapping of the sugars especially when they are present in large quantity.

The chromatographic identification of the sugars from among urinary reducing substances is not limited to the newborn period, nor is the method confined to urinalysis. Diagnostic information concerning the diseases of malabsorption, intestinal disaccharidase deficiency and "carbohydrate sensitivity" can be derived from the chromatography of aqueous extracts of stool[1].

SOURCES OF ERROR

No interfering substances have been encountered. The method is sensitive below the 5 μg range, (20 μl of urine containing 25 mg of sugar per 100 ml), which is less than the amount detectable by the screening test (100 mg per 100 ml). In fact, the optimal concentration to be applied is on the order of 2 μg. Desalting increases the clarity of the resolution but is not needed with the urines of newborns. Desalting is recommended for the urines of the older pediatric age group and for adults, but

is also not essential. It is possible that some medication may migrate in the solvent system used here and react with the color reagent, but none have as yet been encountered. The presence of such hypothetical substances should be very unlikely in the newborn period and also very readily identified by a careful history.

RANGE OF VALUES
(AVERAGE R_f)

Sugar	Acetate	Borate	Color
Dextrose	0.56	0.53	Green-blue
Sucrose	0.52	0.50	Purple-red
Maltose	0.49	0.47	Gray-blue
Galactose	0.47	0.39	Sky blue
Lactose	0.36	0.36	Pale blue
Fructose	0.47	0.15	Purple-red

RÉSUMÉ OF CLINICAL INTERPRETATIONS

The present methodology has disclosed the presence of one or more carbohydrates in the urine samples of every newborn under five days of age. The total reducing substance concentration in no case has been found to be as great as 100 mg per 100 ml. The significance of the presence of this minute "physiological" mellituria is unknown. Gross elevations are strong evidence for the presence of one of the hereditary metabolic diseases of carbohydrate metabolism.

Since our studies have indicated that the normal infant does not excrete as much as 100 mg per 100 ml of reducing substance in the urine, we have used a modified Benedict test to screen the urines of newborns at that level. The fact that a urine specimen reacts positively to a glucose oxidase test does not rule out the possibility that two or more sugars are present, only one being glucose. Accordingly, ten drops of urine and five drops of water are added to a Clinitest tablet[*] or to 2.5 ml of Benedict's solution. All urines showing a strong trace or a 1+ or greater reaction (approximately 100 mg per 100 ml of reducing substance) are chromatographed. This examination must be delayed until the infant has ingested and metabolized enough carbohydrate to allow for renal clearance of the various sugars. Therefore, the examina-

[*]Ames Co., Inc., Elkhart, Indiana.

tion should be deferred until the third day of life. If the mellituria is not glycosuria but is of significant degree, the offending carbohydrate can be removed easily from the diet until further diagnostic studies have been performed and potential damage to the infant thus averted.

REFERENCES

1. Masera, G., and Kaeser, H.: Una nuova technica per la separazione degli zuccheri: La chromatografia su strato sottile. Minerva Pediat., 16:14-16, 1964.
2. Lees, T. M., and DeMuria, P. J.: A simple method for the preparation of thin layer chromatography plates. J. Chromatogr., 8:108-109, 1962.

Chapter 15

Normal Values for Thyroid Function Tests in Infancy*

EVELYN B. MAN, Ph.D.

INTRODUCTION

The healthy full-term newborn during the first five days after birth has the highest values during the human life span for serum PBI (protein-bound iodine), or BEI (butanol extractable iodine, i.e., thyroxine-like iodine) [11, 25, 48, 53, 55, 58, 59, 60, 70, 72, 73, 89, 95]. Clinical advantages of the BEI over the PBI determination have been detailed [10, 12, 18, 47, 48, 54, 56].

In Figure 1 are plotted sixty-three measurements of BEI of forty-nine newborns during the first 120 hours of life [60]. Dots represent isolated values, and connected points portray serial determinations on the same healthy neonate during the first five days of life. At the bottom of the figure, solid lines define the minimum and maximum BEI values of normal adults, 3.2 through 5.6 μg per 100 ml for women, 3.3 through 6.7 for men [53]. The neonate is not just a little man in his circulating thyroxine-like iodine, since neonatal BEI concentrations of 7.2 through 15.2 μg per 100 ml are more than double the values of euthyroid adults.

*This investigation was supported in part by Public Health Service Grants HD-00415 and HD-01821 from the National Institute of Child Health and Human Development.

BEI VALUES BEFORE AND AFTER EXCHANGE TRANSFUSIONS

Why does the healthy newborn have the highest PBI or BEI observed during life [8, 9, 13, 24–26, 70–74, 92]? Are these high circulating thyroxine-like iodines the result of decreased removal from the bloodstream or an increased secretion rate of thyroxine-like iodine by the thyroid gland? Westphal obtained blood from full-term infants requiring exchange transfusions [95] (upper section, Fig. 2). Samples included pre-exchange, donor, immediately post-exchange and serial infants' bloods from one to ninety-six hours after an exchange transfusion. Infants with BEI concentrations over 9 μg per 100 ml, given donor serum with a BEI of approximately 4 μg per 100 ml, had a quick rebound to high BEI concentrations within one half to six hours after a single exchange or even after repeated transfusions. The rebound after two or three exchanges could not be calculated merely as transfer of thyroxine-like iodine from extravascular fluid, but suggested that the neonates' thyroids were secreting thyroxine-like iodine at an accelerated rate. Secondly, newborns over 2500 gm in birth weight,

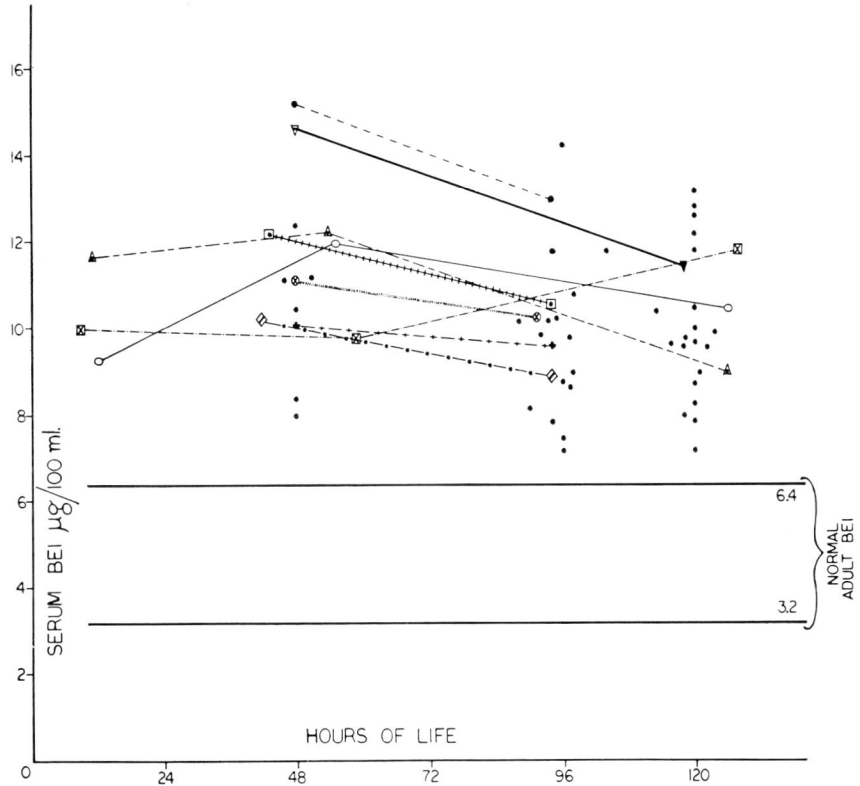

Fig. I.   Sixty-three measurements of BEI of forty-nine neonates plotted against hours after birth. All these neonates over 2500 gm in birth weight were considered healthy by routine standards, and at least one third of these children were subsequently contacted as control subjects who were found to be developing according to chronological ages (5 weeks to several years).[60] Connected points represent serial values on the same neonate. Reproduced by courtesy of Pediatrics, 35:753-758, 1965.

who required exchange transfusions, had as high BEI values and values compatible in thyroxine-like iodine with those of healthy neonates without exchange transfusions.

A wealth of neonatal blood of the first blood samples removed from newborns needing exchange transfusions was used for additional BEI determinations. Excluded were all infants who (or whose mothers) were known to have received therapy affecting BEI or thyroxine-binding protein values[27, 28, 33, 69, 83, 99, 100]. BEI concentrations during the first 126 hours of life are plotted

vertically *versus* birth weights (330 to 5046 gm) of 138 newborns in Figure 3.* Forty-one of the BEI values, 30 per cent, were from infants not needing exchange transfusions (see legend of Fig. 3). With our present technique, values on neonates not needing exchange transfusions are indistinguishable from values of infants requiring transfusions. Mean BEI values increased progressively (solid line through Δ) and were calculated by 500 gm incre-

*Additional values have been added to this figure since it was published[60].

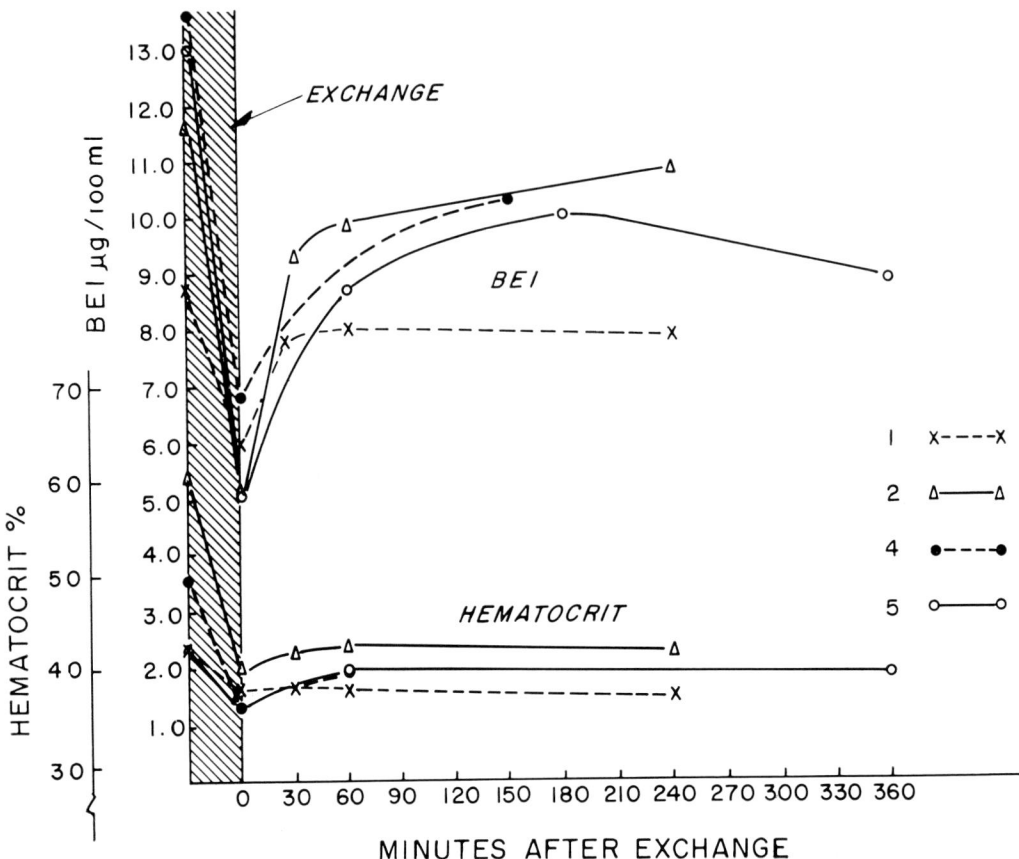

Fig. 2. Measurements of serum BEI and hematocrits of newborns from beginning to six hours after exchange transfusions. Shaded area represents exchange transfusion. Hematocrits determined for all four infants. Note overlapping of Infants I, 4 and 5. Reproduced by courtesy of J. Clin. Endocr., 22:452-456, 1962.

ments in birth weight from 2000 to 4000 gm.

BEI VALUES OF PREMATURES

Twenty-eight of the 138 newborns had "premature" birth weights of 330 through 2013 gm. Fourteen of the twenty-eight required exchange transfusions (crosses), and blood was obtained from fourteen prematures who did not need an exchange transfusion (dots or D for death, Fig. 3).

Twenty-five of the twenty-eight neonates of premature birth weight (89 per cent) had serum thyroxine-like iodines below the high normal range of full-term newborns. The three prematures having BEI values in the full-term range included one dehydrated newborn and two infants of thirty-eight and forty weeks gestation. One of the late gestational prematures was born to a women less than 5 ft. in height. BEI values of babies of less than 2014 gm in birth weight are obviously lower than BEI concentrations of full-term neonates (broken lines represent the BEI range of 7.2 through 15.2 μg per

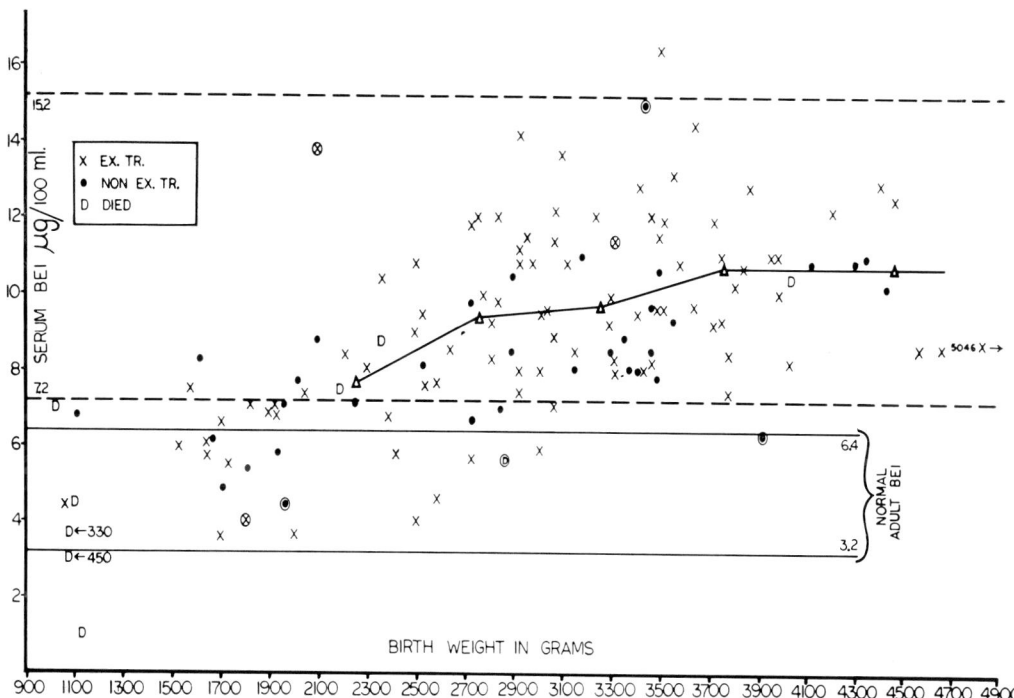

Fig. 3. Measurements of BEI of 138 neonates between 1½ and 126 hours old and ranging in weight from 330 to 5046 gm. Mean BEI's (△ connected by a heavy line) were calculated for the neonates as to birth weight by 500 gm increments beginning at 2000 gm. Seven encircled values were omitted from the means because neonates had recognized clinical abnormalities (high thyroxine-binding globulin [ ]; diabetic mother on insulin for years; neonatal death with autopsy findings of congenital anomalies and a transposed heart; two born to mothers with uncontrolled thyroid dysfunction during gestation; and two with definite clinical symptoms or bone x-ray confirmation of thyroid hypofunction).

Heavy broken lines at 7.2 and 15.2 μg/100 ml represent minimum and maximum BEI's of full-term normal neonates of Fig. 1.

Additional values have been added to this figure since it was published. Reproduced by courtesy of Pediatrics, 35:753-758, 1965.

100 ml for normal full-term infants). On the other hand, not only is gestational age a factor relative to BEI concentration, but, in certain instances, offspring of small parents have had lower birth weights and higher BEI's than anticipated until gestational age was considered.

Low PBI concentrations for prematures have been reported by Andreoli and Robbins, Starr and his associates and by Stevenson, Danowski and co-authors[1, 68, 81, 88].

SERUM TBG AND TBPA BINDING CAPACITIES DURING INFANCY

High BEI values of neonates were studied in relation to serum-binding capacities of TBG and TBPA (thyroxine-binding globulin and thyroxine-

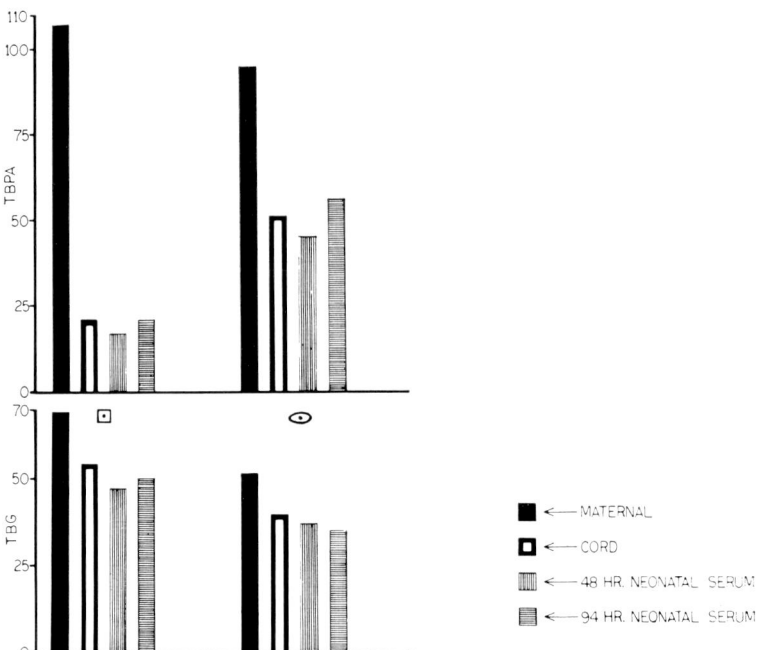

Fig. 4. Comparison of maternal, cord, forty-eight and ninety-four hour neonatal serum TBPA at top of graph, and in lower graph of TBG capacities to bind μg T_4/100 ml serum. These are examples that the neonate's TBPA is directly related to the cord TBPA concentration. Also, the height of the neonate's TBG is directly correlated with a high (left lower) or low (right lower) cord blood, serum TBG.

binding pre-albumin). TBG capacities are in the lower sections and TBPA in upper areas of Figures 4 through 6. Neonatal TBG binding capacities are high, almost double the values of non-pregnant adults, and TBPA capacities are low, less than half of maternal values. Binding capacities in sera of mothers at delivery, of cord blood and from healthy neonates at forty-eight and ninety-six hours of life were estimated by our slightly altered modification of Ingbar's tris buffer paper electrophoretic method[16, 43, 44, 85]. In Figure 4 are two representative examples. Serum TBG and TBPA of about 100 neonates at four or five days of age have been observed. The TBG of the mother at delivery usually exceeds the

serum TBG in cord blood; also, this cord TBG exceeds the neonate's values at two or four days of life (TBG binding capacity: 33 to 62 μg thyroxine per 100 ml serum).

Neonatal and cord TBPA capacities are significantly lower than in maternal sera (see open or shaded columns at right of solid black maternal column, Fig. 4). The neonatal binding capacities of TBPA at four days of age ranged from 14 to 56 μg T_4 per 100 ml and were usually less than half of maternal values.

Neonatal high TBG or low TBPA capacities have been reported by others[15, 39, 63, 78], but were confirmed by estimations on sera before and after exchange transfusions. At upper left of

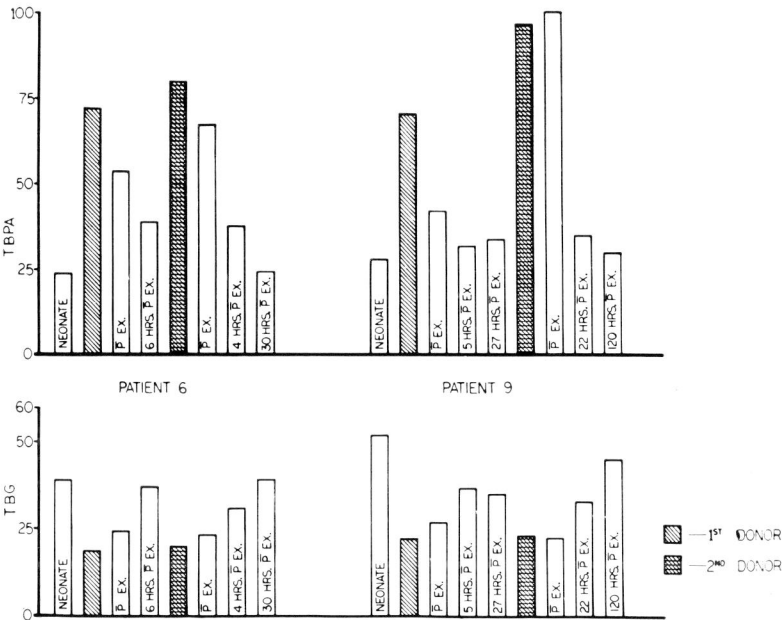

Fig. 5.   TBPA (upper graph) and TBG (lower graph) of two neonates before and after two exchange transfusions. This figure shows adult TBPA and TBG. Return of low TBPA and high TBG concentrations after two exchange transfusions illustrates the difference between neonatal and adult TBPA and TBG. Binding capacities in μg T_4/100 ml serum.

Figure 5, the low neonatal TBPA capacity is followed by the adult donor capacity in the barred column. Immediately after the exchange, the neonatal TBPA had risen but fell in six hours. A second exchange was needed and by thirty hours after the second exchange the neonate's TBPA was almost identical with the original pre-exchange value. In a second neonate requiring two exchanges, the same pattern is obvious: low TBPA capacity of the neonate, at left, higher value of donor; decreased neonatal TBPA capacities after each exchange to 35 and 30 μg T_4 per 100 ml. In the lower section of Figure 5, the increased TBG of both neonates fell after donor blood, but rose even after two exchanges to values within 8 μg T_4

per 100 ml of pre-exchange binding capacities.

In Figure 6, TBPA and TBG binding capacities of premature and full-term infants are compared at left of figure. The markedly lower BEI concentrations of prematures than of full-term newborns could not be correlated with any significant differences in TBG and TBPA binding capacities.

At the right of the figure are thyroxine-binding capacities of ten infants studied between six and eighteen weeks, and of seven infants observed at one year of age. TBG binding capacities fell to values between 24 and 35, and TBPA binding capacities rose to values between 50 and 92 μg T_4 per 100 ml.

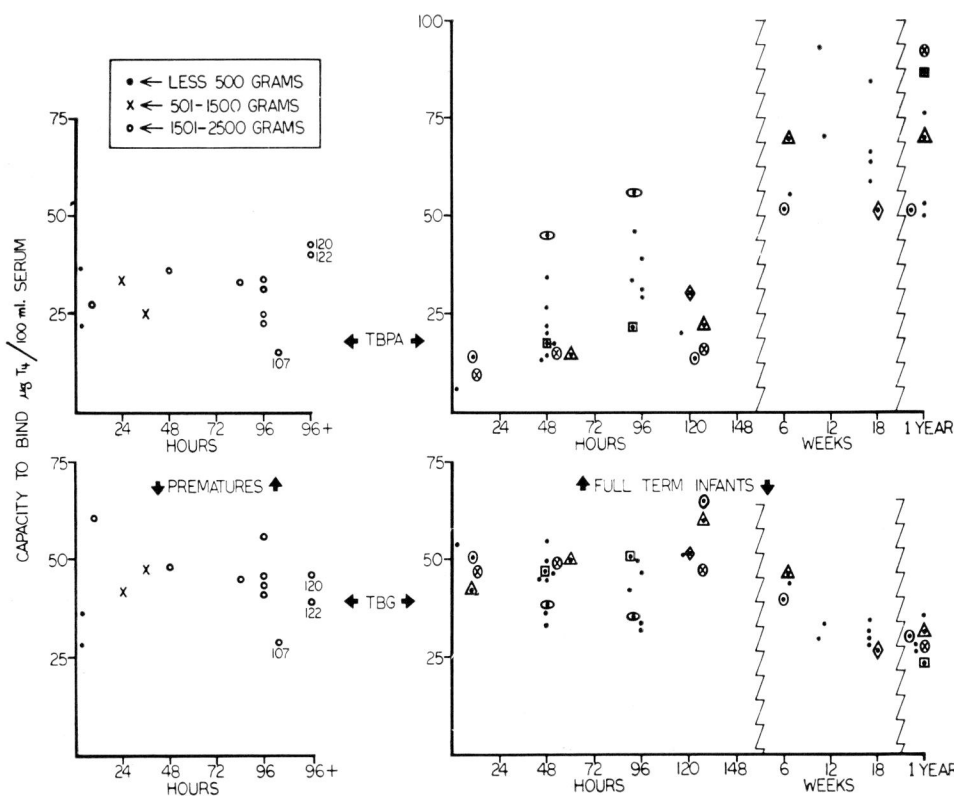

Fig. 6. TBG and TBPA of infants, binding capacity in μg T$_4$/100 ml serum. At the left are values on fourteen prematures through the first 122 hours after birth. The numbers between 107 and 122 refer to hours of age beyond the scale of 96 hours. Three different symbols are used for prematures with birth weights less than 500, between 500 and 1500, and between 1500 and 2500 gm.

At the right are values on forty-three sera of twenty-six infants who had been full term at birth. The symbols used in the right section are not related to the symbols for prematures. Sixteen were studied during the first 128 hours of life, and ten were studied between the ages of six weeks and one year. Vertical zigzags separate ages. Six full-term babies had determinations at more than one age. The symbols for these infants are listed below and may be compared at different ages.

TBPA IN TRANSPORT AND TURNOVER OF THYROXINE

Ingbar and Associates[43–45], Balfour and Tunnicliffe[2], Myant and Osorio[62], Robbins and Rall[77, 79] and Oppenheimer and associates[65–67, 90] have emphasized the role which TBPA probably plays in metabolism and utilization of thyroxine-like compounds. References to the excellent and large bibliographies of these investigators are pertinent. In addition, certain thyroidal enzyme dysfunctions and abnormalities in protein transport of thyroxine-like compounds are still challenging investigations[47, 51, 87]. Estimations of both TBG and TBPA capacities seemed significant in infancy when the TBPA is only a fraction of the adult capacity. Red cell or resin I^{131}-T_3 uptakes of neonates have not been measured in our laboratory. Enough serum was not available. Also I^{131}-T_3 tests reflect binding capacities of TBG and give no specific information about TBPA[52, 63, 77, 86].

Michener, Tauxe and Hayles[63] questioned whether thyroxine binding by proteins of the neonates differed from the binding by proteins in adult sera. Van Zyl has reported difficulties after transportation or delay in use of I^{131}-labelled 3, 5, 3′ triodo-L-thyronine from radiochemical breakdown or self-radiation[93, 94]. Pertinent references are given in the chapter on endocrine correlates in the newborn[22].

OTHER TESTS OF THYROID FUNCTION DURING INFANCY

Knee and foot x-rays of infants in relation to bone age are measures of thyroid function which should be evaluated by a pediatric radiologist.

I^{131}-uptake tests and references on this subject are given elsewhere in this book[22]. Thyroid antibodies in relation to autoimmunization have been reviewed by Blizzard, Doniach and Witebsky[4, 6, 40, 80, 98]. The unreliability of cholesterol values for thyroid underfunction of infants and children has been recognized[13, 4, 58].

DISCUSSION

LOW BEI CONCENTRATIONS OF PREMATURES

The low BEI values of prematures apparently occurred when birth weight was less than 2013 gm and the length of gestation less than thirty-six weeks (when gestational age could be estimated). Gestational age has been compared with maturation of thyroid function in fetal monkeys (*Macaca mulatta*) in experiments of Pickering and Fisher[71].

SERUM BEI OF CORD BLOOD

A correction should be made to a statement published in 1952. The statement was: "SPI and BEI of cord blood do not differ significantly from those of the mother's blood taken during delivery and therefore can not be used to measure the BEI of the infant during the first weeks of life"[58]. This has been found true for healthy full-term newborns born to euthyroid women. Twenty-eight mothers who delivered normal full-term infants at delivery had an average BEI of 7.2, an average cord blood BEI of 6.9, and sixteen of their infants at four or five days had an average BEI of 10.0 μg per 100 ml. This average BEI was significantly higher than the average for values of cord

BEI. Conversely, comparison of premature's cord blood BEI with the maternal BEI at delivery appears to give some indication of the premature's BEI, Table I. In seven premature births, the cord

TABLE I

Serum BEI's ($\mu g/100\ ml$)			Birth Weight (in gm)	Gesta- tion Weeks
Mother	Cord	Baby		
Av. for 28		for 16		
7.2	6.9	10.0	2500+	40
Prematures				
4.7*	2.3	—	365	22
3.8*	1.5	—	623	22
6.2	2.9	3.0	450	—
8.6	3.4	—	682	29
9.0	4.4	5.4	1814	33½
9.4	7.0	6.7	1616	37
7.9	4.7	—	1559	38

*From the same woman who was given Proloid during but not between 2 successful pregnancies.

BEI concentrations have been lower than the maternal BEI values near delivery, and significantly less in the five instances with gestation estimated as under thirty-four weeks.

In the three instances when blood was obtained on the newborn, the BEI of cord and neonates' blood correlated. Dr. Starr and his group have reported low PBI values in cord blood of prematures[68]. A contrasting situation should be emphasized. Cord and maternal BEI values have been low when a full-term newborn was delivered by a woman with hypothyroxinemia. If one is alert for this situation, comparison of maternal and cord blood serum BEI at premature birth may eliminate need for the premature's blood in the first days of life.

The father should not be ignored entirely. Paternal thyroid under-function has been mentioned, but usually in relation to sterility[20, 38, 61].

THYROXINE AND CNS MATURATION

Low BEI concentrations of prematures have been emphasized, and transient periods of replacement therapy have been tried[49, 88]. Thyroxine-like iodine compounds are essential for development of the central nervous system; in endemic goiter areas the incidence is high in deaf-mutism, mental retardation and neurologic deficits[3, 7, 14, 17, 19, 21, 23, 30–32, 34–37, 41, 42, 46, 49, 50, 61, 76, 82, 84, 91, 96, 97]. Beierwaltes and associates[3] reproduced a diagram which had also been used by Pickering and Fisher[29] to point out that at birth the weight of the brain is 20 to 30 per cent complete and by the end of the first year of life 65 per cent complete. A deficit of thyroxine *in utero* and in the early months after birth may be correlated with more severe mental retardation than occurs with thyroid under-function at an older age[30, 75, 84].

The question has recurred whether or not lower BEI concentrations of prematures were related to the environmental incubator temperature in contrast to lower nursery temperatures for full-term infants. Fisher and Oddie[25] studied and discussed PBI increases at forty-eight hours of life for full-term infants in usual nursery temperatures *versus* PBI increases for full-term infants transferred to an "isolette" heated sufficiently to prevent the usual neonatal fall in rectal temperatures. From the PBI values of the two groups of full-term newborns at forty-eight hours and from data recently available from Dr. Fisher[22], the lower BEI concentrations of premature neonates than of full-term newborns can not be attributed merely to incubator temperatures for prematures.

Thyroid Replacement Therapy for Infants

In Figure 7 are shown thyroid dosage and tapering of dosage by twelve months of age for two siblings born to a hyperthyroid woman treated with propylthiouracil and Lugol's during the pregnancies[57]. Each goitrous newborn had a BEI less than 2.0 μg per 100 ml and was given 45 mg of desiccated thyroid or Proloid per day. Since the time when desiccated thyroid was tapered at age one year, they have developed normally and are mentally equal to their siblings and are now at ages six and one half and seven and one half years respectively.

These two children were also reported by Burrow as the last infants, 4 and 5 in Table I, page 404[5]. The emphasis of his paper had been directed toward goiter in the offspring of women treated with propylthiouracil during pregnancy and not toward therapy for the babies. When therapy during the first year of life for Infants 4 and 5 was called to the attention of Dr. Burrow, records of other infants in Table I were re-examined. In addition to Newborns 4 and 5, Infants 1 and 3 (p. 404) were given thyroid replacement therapy. The child with the contaminated BEI received 45 mg of desiccated thyroid daily for the first month, and then this was increased to 100 mg a day and stopped in the sixth month. Also, the third child in Table I with the BEI of 1.9 μg per 100 ml serum was started on 45 mg of desiccated thyroid at the end of the first week and raised to 60 mg at seven weeks when the BEI was 3.8 μg per 100 ml and dosage was subsequently increased to 90 mg a day in the ninth week and 105 mg a day in

the eleventh week. This therapy was continued until the sixth month. These histories illustrate that infants given controlled amounts of desiccated thyroid during the first year of life may grow normally subsequently without recognizable impairment of endogenous thyroid function[101].

The administration of 45 mg desiccated thyroid per day for the two newborns in Figure 7 was less than 50 per cent of the dosage needed by hypothyroid infants during the first twelve months of life[57]. Most of the hypothyroid children treated early and given 90 to 120 mg of desiccated thyroid per day by twelve months of age have had good mental development in subsequent years to age eight[57]. Dosage was not increased after twelve months until age eight years. Pickering and Fisher[72] state: "In any infant in whom the suspected diagnosis cannot be satisfactorily ruled out, a therapeutic trial of optimal substitution therapy is indicated. . . In therapy, the serum hormonal iodine concentration should be maintained at 6 μg per 100 ml or above when Na-1-thyroxine is used and 5 μg per cent or above when thyroid (USP) is used."

High serum thyroxine-like iodines of full-term newborns, and high thyroidal replacement therapy during the first year of life accord with Van Middlesworth's[92] finding of a high turnover rate of I^{131} and agree with observations of Cottino et al.[8] and of Croughs et al.[9]. Cottino gave I^{131}-T_4 to newborns whose thyroid uptakes had been blocked by administration of iodine. Degradation rates of thyroxine iodine were over 4.0 μg per kg of body weight per day up to twelve months of age — over 2.0 up to about the third year and only 1.4

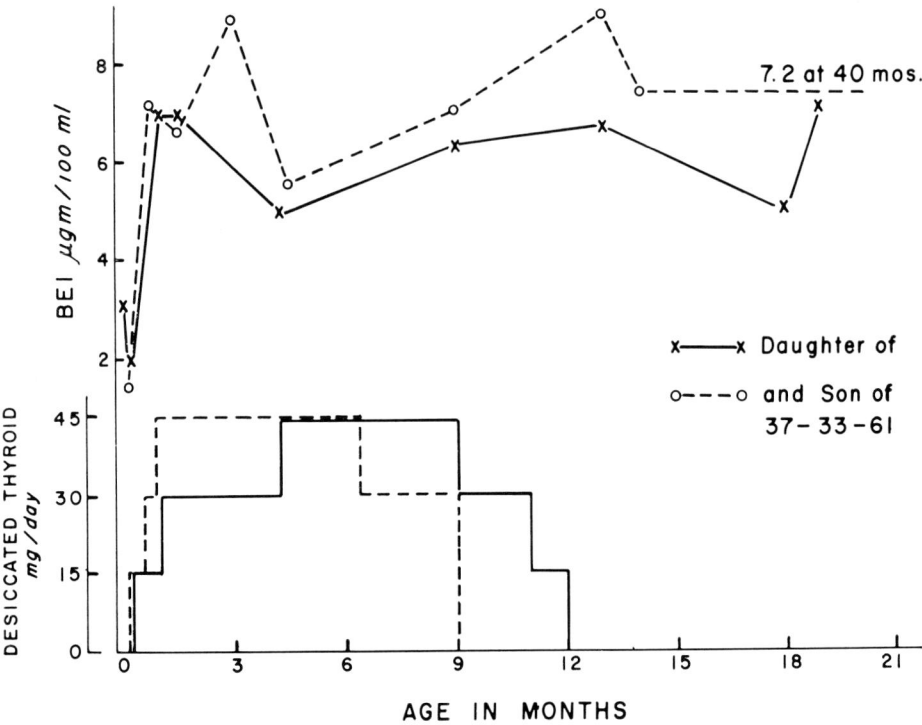

Fig. 7. Therapy with desiccated thyroid and serum BEI values of two goitrous infants born to a hyperthyroid woman who received medical treatment during these two successive pregnancies. For the female, height and weight percentiles were: fifth at five weeks; tenth at nine and nineteen weeks; twenty-fifth at ten months; thirty-fifth at one year, with growth and development normal when last evaluated at seven and one-half years. For the male, height and weight percentiles were: fifth at five weeks; third at nine weeks; fiftieth at six and eight months, with growth and development normal when last contacted for evaluation at six and one-half years. Reproduced by courtesy of J. Pediat., 63:926-941, 1963.

over three years. Croughs, Visser and Woldring[9] have reported thyroxin degradation rate per kg body weight and per sq m body surface for children as significantly higher than for adults. Their results "give further evidence for a higher metabolism of thyroxin in children compared with adults". Their values for adults are compatible with recent comparisons of iodine as thyroxine degraded per day by euthyroid volunteers[64].

SUMMARY

The range of normal values for butanol-extractable iodine in children, from age six months to ten years of age is 4.5 to 7.3 μg per 100 ml[18]. Normal ranges for BEI up to six months of age have not been established. In a small series of infants an average value for BEI at six weeks was 6.7, with only two values below 5.7 μg per 100 ml. Pickering and Fisher[73] reported transient low BEI values between twenty-one to thirty-five days of life, but with plateau values by thirty-five to forty days at a "level of 6.5 ± 1.0" μg per 100 ml. At four months of age, for a euthyroid infant in our series, the lowest value for BEI was 5.2 μg per 100 ml, a value obviously higher than the minimum for a euthyroid adult.

APPRECIATION

Dr. Milton Westphal is Co-investigator on data obtained on TBG and TBPA of blood serum from women in labor, from the cord and from the neonate. Dr. M. Gilda Marques' bibliography on thyroid function in pregnancy and infancy was invaluable in interpretation of data.

REFERENCES

1. Andreoli, M., and Robbins, J.: Serum proteins and thyroxine-protein interaction in early human fetuses. J. Clin. Invest., 41: 1070-1077, 1962.
2. Balfour, W. E., and Tunnicliffe, H. E.: Thyroxine binding by serum proteins. J. Physiol., 153:179-198, 1960.
3. Beierwaltes, W. H., Lowrey, G. H., Aster, R. A., Raman, G., and Carr, E. A.: Congenital hypothyroidism. A preventable cause of mental retardation. J. Mich. Med. Soc., 58:927-934, 1959.
4. Blizzard, R. M., and Chandler, R. W.: The history and present concepts of autoimmunization in thyroid disease. J. Pediat., 57:399-409, 1960.
5. Burrow, G. N.: Neonatal goiter after maternal propylthiouracil therapy. J. Clin. Endocr., 25:403-408, 1965.
6. Chandler, R. W., Blizzard, R. M., Hung, W., and Kyle, M.: Incidence of thyrocytotoxic factor and other antithyroid antibodies in the mothers of cretins. New Eng. J. Med., 267:376-380, 1962.
7. Christensen, J. F.: Prolonged icterus neonatorum and congenital myxedema. Acta Paediat., 45:367-371, 1956.
8. Cottino, F., Colombo, G., Ferrara, G. C., and Costa, A.: Investigations on the metabolism of the thyroid hormone in children by means of radiothyroxine. Panminerva Med., 3:471-474, 1961.
9. Croughs, W., Visser, H. K. A., and Woldring, M. G.: Studies of thyroxin secretion and degradation rate in children with different thyroidal functional states. Comparison of thyroid function in children and adults. J. Pediat., 67:343-352, 1965.
10. Danowski, T. S., Johnston, S. Y., and Greenman, J. H.: Alterations in serum iodine fractions induced by the administration of inorganic iodine in massive dosage. J. Clin. Endocr., 10:519-531, 1950.
11. Danowski, T. S., Johnston, S. Y., Price, W. C., McKelvy, M., Stevenson, S. S., and McCluskey, E. R.: Protein-bound iodine in infants from birth to one year of age. Pediatrics, 7:240-244, 1951.
12. Danowski, T. S., Mateer, F., Weigand, F. A., Peters, J. H., and Greenman, J. H.: Serum iodine fractions in subjects receiving potassium iodide in small dosage. J. Clin. Endocr., 10:532-539, 1950.
13. Deanesly, R.: Foetal endocrinology. Brit. Med. Bull., 17:91-95, 1961.
14. Dokumov, S. I.: The influence of endemic goiter on the course of pregnancy, labour and puerperium. Acta Endocr., 38:161-165, 1961.
15. Dowling, J. T., Freinkel, N., and Ingbar, S. H.: Thyroxine-binding by sera of pregnant women, newborn infants and women with spontaneous abortion. J. Clin. Invest., 35:1263-1276, 1956.
16. Dreyer, D. J., and Man, E. B.: Thyroxine-binding proteins and butanol-extractable iodine in sera of adolescent males. J. Clin. Endocr., 22:31-37, 1962.
17. Dumont, J. E., Ermans, A. M., and Bastenie, P. A.: Thyroidal function in a goiter endemic. IV. Hypothyroidism and endemic cretinism. J. Clin. Endocr., 23:325-335, 1963.
18. Durham, J. R., Cooke, R. E., Lancaster, J. W., and Man, E. B.: Serum butanol-extractable iodine values of children under ten years of age. Amer. J. Dis. Child., 87: 468-474, 1954.
19. Eayrs, J. T.: Effects of thyroid hormones on brain differentiation. In Cameron, M. P., and O'Connor, M. (eds.): Ciba Foundation Study Group on Brain-Thyroid Relationships. Boston, Little, Brown Co. pp. 60-74, 1964.
20. Faulkner, J. W.: Use of liothyronine to improve sperm counts after surgical correction of sterility. J. Urol., 88:262-265, 1962.
21. Federman, D., Robbins, J., and Rall, J. E.: Some observations on cretinism and its

treatment. New Eng. J. Med., **259**:610-615, 1958.

22. Fisher, D. A.: Endocrine adaptations of the newborn to the extra-uterine environment. In Sunderman, F. W., and Sunderman, F. W., Jr. (eds.): The Clinical Pathology of Infancy. Springfield, Thomas, 1966, Ch. 16.

23. Fisher, D. A., Hammond, G. D., and Pickering, D. E.: The hypothyroid infant and child. Therapy with sodium l-thyroxine. Amer. J. Dis. Child., **90**:6-21, 1955.

24. Fisher, D. A., and Oddie, T. H.: Thyroxine secretion rate during infancy: effect of estrogen. J. Clin. Endocr., **23**:811-819, 1963.

25. Fisher, D. A., and Oddie, T. H.: Neonatal thyroid hyperactivity. Response to cooling. Amer. J. Dis. Child., **107**:574-581, 1964.

26. Fisher, D. A., Oddie, T. H., and Burroughs, J. C.: Thyroidal radioiodine uptake rate. Measurement in infants. Amer. J. Dis. Child., **103**:42-53, 1962.

27. Fisher, D. A., Oddie, T. H., Epperson, D.: Interrelation of iodide clearance and adrenocortical activity. J. Clin. Endocr., **25**:1353-1360, 1965.

28. Fisher, D. A., and Panos, T. C.: "Due caution" and radioiodine in children. Amer. J. Dis. Child., **103**:729-737, 1962.

29. Fisher, D. A., and Pickering, D. E.: Infantile hypothyroidism. Pediat. Clin. N. Amer. Philadelphia, Saunders 1957, pp. 863-871.

30. French, F. S., and Van Wyk, J. J.: Fetal hypothyroidism. I. Effects of thyroxine on neural development. II. Fetal versus maternal contributions to fetal thyroxine requirements. III. Clinical implications. J. Pediat., **64**:589-600, 1964.

31. Gajdusek, D. C.: Congenital defects of the central nervous system associated with hyperendemic goiter in a neolithic highland society of Netherlands New Guinea. I. Epidemiology. Pediatrics, **29**:345-363, 1962.

32. Gardner, J. U., Hayles, A. B., Woolner, L. B., and Owen, C. A.: Iodine metabolism in goitrous cretins. J. Clin. Endocr., **19**:638-657, 1959.

33. Goldstein, D. J.: Uptake of iodine-131 by an 18-week human foetus. S. Afr. Med. J., **32**:239-241, 1958.

34. Gorbman, A., and Ishii, S.: Stimulation of neurosecretion in shark embryos by thyroid hormones. Proc. Soc. Exp. Biol. Med., **103**: 865-867, 1960.

35. Gordon, R. R.: Neonatal cold injury and hypothyroidism. Lancet, **1**:460-461, 1962.

36. Greenman, G. W., Gabrielson, M. O., Howard-Flanders, J., and Wessel, M. A.: Thyroid dysfunction in pregnancy (fetal loss and follow up evaluation of surviving infants). New Eng. J. Med., **267**:426-431, 1962.

37. Greenwald, I.: The relation of endemic goiter to deaf-mutism. Arch. Otolaryng. (Chicago), **70**:541-544, 1959.

38. Griboff, S. I.: Semen analysis in myxedema. Fertil. Steril., **13**:436-443, 1962.

39. Hirschfeld, J., and Soderberg, U.: The unsaturated capacity of the thyroxine-binding proteins in pregnant women and newborn infants. Acta Obstet. Gynec. Scand., **39**: 645-660, 1960.

40. Hjort, T., and Pedersen, G. T.: Thyroid antibodies and "thyroglobulin" in the serum. (In pregnant and parturient women and in newborn infants). Lancet, **2**:259-263, 1962.

41. Hoch, F. L.: Biochemical actions of thyroid hormones. Physiol. Rev., **42**:605-674, 1962.

42. Hodges, R. E., Hamilton, H. E., and Keettel, W. C.: Pregnancy in myxedema. Arch. Intern., Med., **90**:863-868, 1952.

43. Ingbar, S. H.: The interaction of the thyroid hormones with the proteins of human plasma. Ann. N. Y. Acad. Sci., **86**:440-453, 1960.

44. Ingbar, S. H.: Observations concerning the binding of thyroid hormones by human serum prealbumin. J. Clin. Invest., **42**:143-160, 1963.

45. Ingbar, S. H., Braverman, L. E., Dawber, N. A., and Lee, G. Y.: A new method for measuring the free thyroid hormone in human serum and an analysis of the factors that influence its concentration. J. Clin. Invest., **44**:1679-1689, 1965.

46. Johnsen, S.: Familial deafness and goitre in persons with a low serum level of protein-bound iodine: Preliminary report, Acta Oto-laryng. (Suppl.), **140**: 168-182, 1958.

47. Klevit, H. D., Eberlein, W. R., and Bongiovanni, A. M.: The iodoproteins in the iodotyrosyl coupling defect. J. Clin. Endocr., **25**:585-592, 1965.

48. Kontaxis, N. E., and Pickering, D. E.: A micro-method for the determination of butyl-alcohol extractable hormonal iodine in serum. J. Clin. Endocr., **18**:774-786, 1958.

49. Lees, M. H., and Ruthven, C. R. J.: The effect of triiodothyronine in neonatal hyperbilirubinaemia. Lancet, **2**:371-373, 1959.

50. Lowrey, G. H., Aster, R. H., Carr, E. A., Ramon, G., Beierwaltes, W. H., and Spafford, N. R.: Early diagnostic criteria of congenital hypothyroidism. Amer. J. Dis. Child., **96**:131-143, 1958.

51. McGirr, E. M., Hutchison, J. H., Clement,

W. E., Kennedy, J. S., and Currie, A. R.: Goitre and cretinism due to the production of an abnormal iodinated thyroid compound. Scot. Med. J., 5:189-203, 1960.

52. Malkasian, G. D., and Tauxe, W. N.: Uptake of 1-triiodothyronine-^{131}I by erythrocytes during pregnancy. J. Clin. Endocr., 25:923-926, 1965.

53. Man, E. B.: Differences in serum butanol-extractable iodines (BEIs) of children, men and women. Note on the preservation of serum BEIs with thiouracil. J. Lab. Clin. Med., 59:528-532, 1962.

54. Man, E. B.: Butanol-extractable iodine in serum. In Sunderman, F. W., and Sunderman, F. W., Jr. (eds.): Evaluation of Thyroid and Parathyroid Functions. Philadelphia, Lippincott, 1963, pp. 77-82.

55. Man, E. B., and Bondy, P. K.: Clinical significance of serum butanol-extractable iodine. J. Clin. Endocr., 17:1373-1382, 1957.

56. Man, E. B., Kydd, D. M., and Peters, J. P.: Butanol-extractable iodine of serum. J. Clin. Invest., 30:531-538, 1951.

57. Man, E. B., Mermann, A. C., and Cooke, R. E.: The development of children with congenital hypothyroidism. A note on early temporary replacement therapy for 2 goitrous infants. J. Pediat., 63:926-941, 1963.

58. Man, E. B., Pickering, D. E., Walker, J., and Cooke, R. E.: Butanol-extractable iodine in the serum of infants. Pediatrics, 9:32-37, 1952.

59. Man, E. B., Shaver, B. A., Jr., and Cooke, R. E.: Studies of children born to women with thyroid disease. Amer. J. Obstet. Gynec., 75:728-741, 1958.

60. Marks, A. N., and Man, E. B.: Serum butanol-extractable iodine concentrations in prematures. Pediatrics, 35:753-758, 1965.

61. Marques, M. G.: Interrelations of the thyroid gland in human pregnancy, infancy and childhood. In press from Med. Lit. Services, PRB, NINDB, NIH, Bethesda, Maryland.

62. Myant, N. B., and Osorio, C.: Paper electrophoresis of thyroxine in tris-malleate buffer. J. Physiol., 152:602-611, 1960.

63. Michener, W. M., Tauxe, W. N., and Hayles, A. B.: Capacity of thyroxine-binding globulin to bind triiodothyronine and thyroxine in maternal and cord blood. Pediatrics, 29:369-375, 1962.

64. Oddie, T. H., Fisher, D. A., and Epperson, D.: Effect of exogenous thyroxine on thyroid accumulation and secretion in euthyroid subjects. J. Clin. Endocr., 25:1196-1206, 1965.

65. Oppenheimer, J. H., Squef, R., Surks, M. I.,

and Hauer, H.: Binding of thyroxine by serum proteins evaluated by equilibrium dialysis and electrophoretic techniques. Alterations in non-thyroidal illness. J. Clin. Invest., 42:1769-1782, 1963.

66. Oppenheimer, J. H., Surks, M. I., Smith, J. C., and Squef, R.: Isolation and characterization of human thyroxine-binding prealbumin. J. Biol. Chem., 240:173-180, 1965.

67. Oppenheimer, J. H., and Tavernetti, R. R.: Displacement of thyroxine from human thyroxine-binding globulin by analogues of hydantoin. Steric aspects of the thyroxine-binding site. J. Clin. Invest., 41:2213-2220, 1962.

68. Perry, R. E., Hodgman, J. E., and Starr, P.: Maternal, cord, and serial venous blood: protein-bound iodine, thyroid-binding globulin, thyroid-binding albumin, and prealbumin values in premature infants. Pediatrics, 35:759-764, 1965.

69. Peters, J. P., German, W. J., Man, E. B., and Welt, L. G.: Functions of gonads, thyroid and adrenals in hypopituitarism. Metabolism, 3:118-137, 1954.

70. Pickering, D. E.: Clinical and laboratory aspects of thyroid function. Pediatrics, 29·692-702, 1962.

71. Pickering, D. E.: Maternal thyroid hormone in the developing fetus. Observations on monkeys (Macaca mulatta). Amer. J. Dis. Child., 107:567-573, 1964.

72. Pickering, D. E., and Fisher, D. A.: Therapeutic concepts relating to hypothyroidism in childhood. J. Chronic Dis., 7:242-263, 1958.

73. Pickering, D. E., Kontaxis, N. E., Benson, R. C., and Meechan, R. J.: Thyroid function in the perinatal period. Amer. J. Dis. Child., 95:616-621, 1958.

74. Pickering, D. E., Settergren, E. F., and Kontaxis, N. E.: Thyroid gland function in the infant macaque monkey (Macaca mulatta). Amer. J. Dis. Child., 105:77-80, 1963.

75. Pickering, D. E., Sheline, G. E., and Crane, J. T.: Sporadic familial goitrous hypothyroidism. Amer. J. Dis. Child., 93:510-518, 1957.

76. Raman, G., and Beierwaltes, W. H.: Correlation of goiter, deafmutism and mental retardation with serum thyroid hormone levels in noncretinous inhabitants of a severe endemic goiter area in India. J. Clin. Endocr., 19:221-233, 1959.

77. Robbins, J.: Measurement of thyroxine-binding proteins in serum with comments on the "T$_3$-RBC" test of thyroid function and method for measurement of thyroxine-bind-

ing proteins in serum. In Sunderman, F. W., and Sunderman, F. W., Jr. (eds.): Evaluation of Thyroid and Parathyroid Functions, Philadelphia, Lippincott, 1963, pp. 90-104.

78. Robbins, J., and Nelson, J. H.: Thyroxine binding by serum protein in pregnancy and in the newborn. J. Clin. Invest., **37**:153-159, 1958.

79. Robbins, J., and Rall, J. E.: Proteins associated with the thyroid hormones. Physiol. Rev., **40**:415-489, 1960.

80. Roitt, I. M., and Doniach, D.: Thyroid autoimmunity. Brit. Med. Bull., **16**:152-158, 1960.

81. Rose, H., Russell, K., and Starr, P.: The serum protein-bound iodine of mothers and new-borns at delivery in premature and term pregnancies. Amer. J. Obstet. Gynec., **86**:767-771, 1963.

82. Sanders, V.: Neurologic manifestations of myxedema. New Eng. J. Med., **266**:547-552, 599-603, 1962.

83. Shapiro, R., and Man, E. B.: Iophenoxic acid and serum-bound iodine values. JAMA, **173**: 1352, 1960.

84. Smith, D. W., Blizzard, R. M., and Wilkins, L.: The mental prognosis in hypothyroidism of infancy and childhood. Pediatrics, **19**: 1011-1022, 1957.

85. Socolow, E. L., Woeber, K. A., Purdy, R. H., Holloway, M. T., and Ingbar, S. H.: Preparation of I^{131}-labeled human serum prealbumin and its metabolism in normal and sick patients. J. Clin. Invest., **44**:1600-1609, 1965.

86. Spafford, N. R., Carr, E. A., Lowrey, G. H., and Beierwaltes, W. H.: I^{131} labeled triiodothyronine erythrocyte uptake of mothers and newborn infants. Amer. J. Dis. Child., **100**:844-849, 1960.

87. Stanbury, J. B.: Familial goiter. In Stanbury, J. B., Fredrickson, D. S., and Wyngaarden, J. B. (eds.): The Metabolic Basis of Inherited Disease. New York, McGraw, 1960, pp. 273-320.

88. Stevenson, S. S., Wirth, P., Bastiani, R., and Danowski, T. S.: Some effects of exogenous thyroid or thyroxin upon premature infants. Pediatrics, **12**:263-271, 1953.

89. Sunderman, F. W., Jr.: The measurement of serum protein-bound iodine. In Sunderman, F. W., and Sunderman, F. W., Jr. (eds.): Evaluation of Thyroid and Parathyroid Functions. Philadelphia, Lippincott, 1963, pp. 53-76.

90. Surks, M. I., and Oppenheimer, J. H.: Postoperative changes in the concentration of thyroxine-binding prealbumin and serum free thyroxine. J. Clin. Endocr., **24**:794-802, 1964.

91. Trotter, W. R.: The association of deafness with thyroid dysfunction. Brit. Med. Bull., **16**:92-98, 1960.

92. Van Middlesworth, L.: Radioactive iodide uptake of normal newborn infants. Amer. J. Dis. Child., **88**:439-442, 1954.

93. Van Zyl, A.: Self-radiation products formed from 3, 5, 3'-tri-iodo-l-thyronine labelled with ^{131}I. S. Afr. Med. J., **35**:631-632, 1961.

94. Van Zyl, A.: Radiochemical breakdown of ^{131}I-labelled 3, 5, 3', triiodo-L-thyronine. Clin. Chim. Acta, **7**:20-28, 1962.

95. Westphal, M., and Man, E. B.: Serum butanol-extractable iodine following exchange transfusion. J. Clin. Endocr., **22**:452-456, 1962.

96. Wettenhall, H. N. B.: Hypothyroidism in childhood. Med. J. Aust., **2**:653-655, 1961.

97. Wilkins, L.: The effects of thyroid deficiency upon the development of the brain. Ment. Retard., **39**:150-155, 1962.

98. Witebsky, E., and Rose, N. R.: Autoimmunity and its relationship to thyroid diseases. New York, J. Med., **63**:56-59, 1963.

99. Woeber, K. A., and Ingbar, S. H.: The effects of noncalorigenic congeners of salicylate on the peripheral metabolism of thyroxine. J. Clin. Invest., **43**:931-942, 1964.

100. Wolff, J., Stanbaert, M. E., and Rall, J. E.: Thyroxine displacement from serum proteins and depression of serum protein-bound iodine by certain drugs. J. Clin. Invest., **40**:1373-1379, 1961.

101. Beeson, P. B., Muschenheim, C., Castle, W. B., Harrison, T. R., Ingelfinger, F. J., and Bondy, P. K. (eds.): The Thyroid Gland. Year Book of Medicine, 1965-1966 Series. Chicago, Year Book, 1965, pp. 508-550, ed. note, pp. 529-530.

Chapter 16

Endocrine Correlates of Temperature Adaptation in the Newborn

DELBERT A. FISHER, M.D.

INTRODUCTION

In the intrauterine environment, fetal temperature regulation is a maternal function. At the time of birth, however, the precipitous exposure of the newborn infant to the extrauterine environment imposes the acute requirement for autonomous temperature control, since the usual ambient temperature of the delivery room and nursery (22 to 30 C) creates a profound acute cold stress. In such an environment, the rate of fall of deep body and skin temperatures of the newborn during the immediate neonatal period approximates 0.1 and 0.3 C per minute respectively[32]. The average fall in rectal temperature of newborn term infants during the first one to two hours of extrauterine life is 1.5 to 2.0 C and rectal temperatures of 34 to 35 C are not uncommon at two to four hours of age[49, 69].

Most term infants are capable of effective defense against this acute cold stress[49, 69]; rectal temperature usually increases to relatively normal levels by twelve to twenty-four hours of age[49, 69]. Enhanced peripheral vasoconstriction and increased muscular activity contribute significantly to this defense[2, 11, 12, 22, 50]. However, since the inherent physical characteristics of infants — the relatively large surface area to body mass ratio, smaller body shell and thinner layer of subcutaneous fat[11, 12, 22] — result in relatively high rates of heat loss in proportion to heat production, the predominant defense against hypothermia in the newborn is increased metabolic heat production or "nonshivering thermogenesis"[1, 2, 11, 12, 17, 30, 50, 53, 59, 62]. This enhancement of metabolic heat production is mediated largely by hormonal agents. Thus, the hormonal adaptations of the newborn to the extrauterine environment, now recognized to be largely oriented to temperature regulation[28], are of critical importance to extrauterine survival. This is especially true in the premature infant[10, 23, 36, 67].

ENDOCRINE RESPONSES

CATECHOLAMINES

Increased catecholamine, and especially noradrenaline, secretion has been demonstrated with acute cold exposure and during chronic cold acclimation in animals[43, 44, 66]. In the newborn infant, increased 3-methoxy-4-hydroxymandelic acid (VMA) and increased free catecholamine excretion have been observed in response to controlled environmental cold exposure[64, 75] and in association with acute increase in oxygen consumption[75]. These VMA and catecholamine data are summarized in Tables I and II. In addition, an increased sensitivity of the neonate to exogenous noradrenaline thermogenesis has been reported[37–39, 54]. This effect is similar to the enhanced thermogenic response to exogenous norepinephrine characteristic of cold acclimated animals[54, 66]. In the newborn, however, this increased sensitivity to noradrenaline is transient, disappearing after the first few weeks of life[37, 38].

In association with the increase in oxygen consumption in the newborn during the early neonatal period, serum glycerol and free fatty acid (FFA) levels have been observed to rise rapidly in the usual nursery environment[40, 56–58]. Maximum levels are reached by about twelve to twenty-four hours[57, 58]. Since this early postnatal rise in FFA occurs prior to feeding, the FFA is presumably derived from adipose tissue. It seems unlikely that decreased FFA utilization contributes to this effect since administration of glucose will suppress the rise and concomitant increase in serum ketone levels also occurs[58]. Moreover, the FFA content of adipose tissue in the newborn runs a course parallel to that of serum[58]. Dawkins and Hull[20, 21] have observed that adipose tissue, in addition to providing substrate for increased non-adipose tissue thermogenesis, appears to provide a highly

TABLE I   URINARY EXCRETION OF
3-METHOXY-4-HYDROXYMANDELIC ACID
(VMA) AT TWO INCUBATOR
TEMPERATURES IN NORMAL TERM
NEWBORNS*

Incubator Temperature†	Rectal Temperature	VMA Excretion (mg/24 hr)
85 F	98.7-99.8 F	0.344 ± 0.052
75 F	96.3-99.1 F	0.431 ± 0.059
Difference		0.087
P value		< 0.01

*Data from Sandler et al., Lancet, 1:485, 1961; mean ± SD

†24 hours at 85 F followed by 24 hours at 75 F; 16 infants.

TABLE II   EFFECT OF COLD ON URINARY CATECHOLAMINE EXCRETION
IN SIX NEWBORN TERM INFANTS*

	Noradrenaline (nanog/kg/min)	Adrenaline (nanog/kg/min)
Warm environmental range (32-34 C)	1.340 ± 0.16	0.103 ± 0.017
Cold environmental range (20-27 C)	2.719 ± 0.34	0.168 ± 0.037
Difference	1.379	0.065
P value	< 0.001	< 0.05

*From STERN, L., LEES, M. H., and LEDUC, J.: Pediatrics, 36:367, 1965.
Values recorded as mean ± SEM.

exothermic cycle of noradrenaline-stimulated hydrolysis and resynthesis of triglyceride within the adipose tissue cell. This process occurs in both white and brown adipose tissue, but is more active in "brown fat." This high metabolic activity of brown fat, its relative abundance in the newborn of several species including the human neonate and its localization to perivascular areas and areas of confluence of afferent vessels from the periphery have suggested a unique role for this tissue in neonatal thermogenesis[3, 20, 21, 72]. Silverman and colleagues[68] have reported that, during cold exposure of the newborn human infant, the nape of the neck, an area rich in brown fat, remains relatively warm in agreement with this hypothesis.

The infusion of noradrenaline into newborn animals and man produces changes similar to those observed spontaneously in the newborn in a cold environment. A prompt increase in oxygen consumption and CO_2 production and increased plasma glycerol and FFA levels are observed[20, 21, 37–39, 54, 55, 65]. The prompt increase in oxygen consumption and catecholamine excretion with cold exposure and the similarity of this cold-induced thermogenic and lipid response to the effects of noradrenaline infusion have led to the general belief that the utilization of fat and the sympathetic nervous system are of prime importance in the stimulation and maintenance of neonatal non-shivering thermogenesis[3, 56–58, 75].

Adamsons and colleagues[2] have shown that the increase in oxygen consumption in the neonate in response to cold exposure occurs within minutes and appears to be stimulated by thermal receptors in the skin. It seems likely, therefore, that the cold stimulus to catecholamine secretion is mediated by peripheral skin receptors. Brück[12] has suggested that the thermal receptors in the skin of the newborn may be more sensitive than those of the adult to changes in environmental temperature. He has observed that the increase in oxygen consumption in response to cold in the newborn occurs at higher ambient temperature and the rate of increase in oxygen consumption with decreasing ambient temperature is greater than in the cold-exposed adult.

THYROID HORMONES

During the first few days of extra-uterine life, serum hormonal iodine values have been observed to increase markedly[8, 19, 26, 27, 45, 61]. Thyroid hormone-binding protein concentrations remain essentially unchanged[60], with the result that increased saturation of binding proteins with thyroid hormones occurs. This is reflected in increased triiodothyronine I^{131} erythrocyte uptake[47, 73], triiodothyronine I^{131} resin uptake[27] and increased "free thyroxine" index[48] in the neonate. Thyroidal radio-iodine clearance is high, also, during this early neonatal period[26, 27].

The increase in the extra-thyroidal hormonal iodine pool, reflected by the increased serum hormonal iodine and increased saturation index values, during the first few days of life indicates that thyroid hormone secretion exceeds peripheral thyroid hormone utilization during this time. Feedback inhibition of thyrotropin (TSH) release and of thyroid hormone secretion by the increased thyroxine titers would normally be expected to limit promptly such

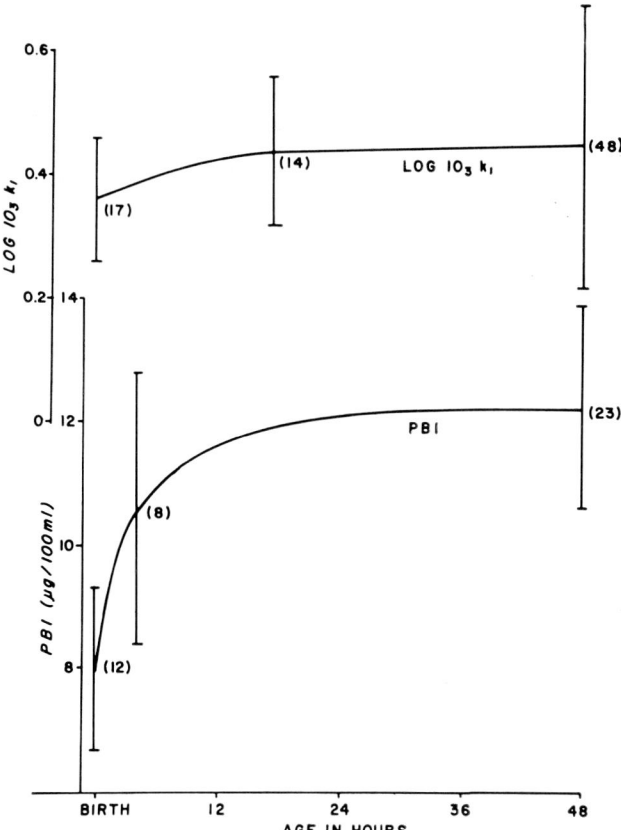

Fig. 1. Plot of thyroidal radioiodine clearance factor (log $10^3 k_1$) and PBI values at birth and during the first forty-eight hours of life in newborn infants kept at environmental temperatures of 22-29 C. Values recorded as mean ± SD. Numbers in parentheses indicate number of infants.

relatively excessive hormone secretion. That such is apparently not the case is indicated in Figure 1, where the logarithm of thyroidal radioiodine clearance factor (Log $10^3 k_1$)* and PBI values are plotted against age in hours in newborn infants kept at environmental temperatures of 22 to 29 C during the first forty-eight hours. It can be observed that thyroidal radioiodide clearance (and, presumably, TSH stimulation of thyronine release) remains high while PBI values are progressively increasing. This remains true during the first seventy-two to ninety-six hours of life. The feedback servomechanism therefore appears to be relatively ineffective or "short circuited" during this early neonatal period.

By four to five days of life, the feedback servomechanism appears to be-

---

*k_1 indicates fractional rate of removal per minute of radioiodine from the radioiodide space by the thyroid gland over the period 0-30 minutes after injection. Over this period the thyroid gland clears an average amount of 100 k_1% of the radioiodide pool each minute. Details of measurement and computation have been published[26].

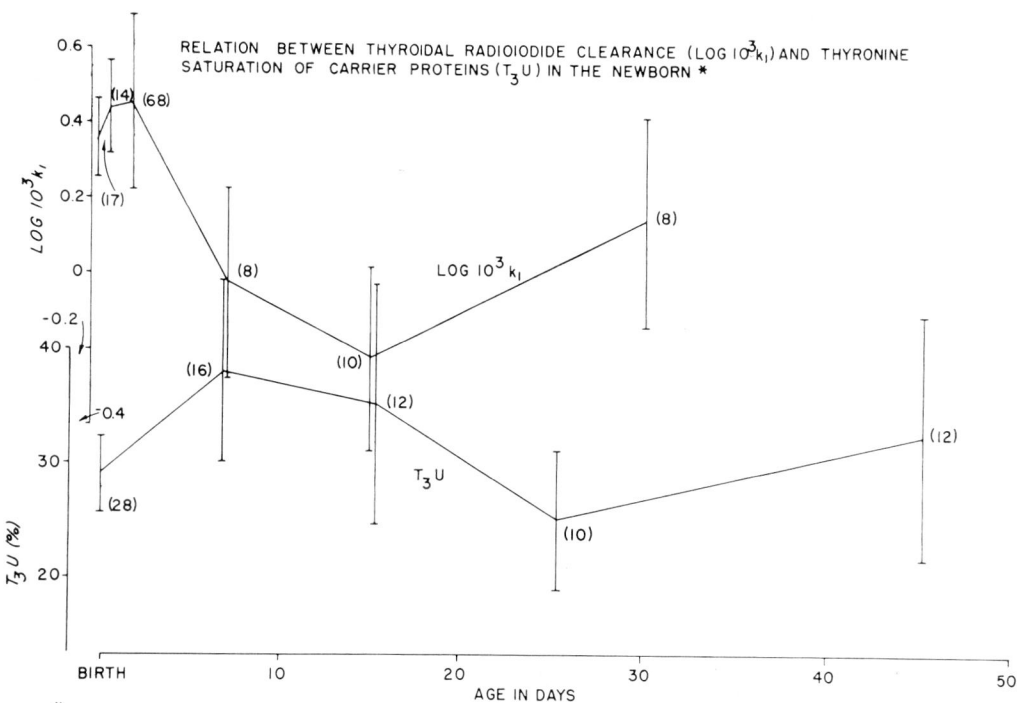

RELATION BETWEEN THYROIDAL RADIOIODIDE CLEARANCE (LOG $10^3 k_1$) AND THYRONINE
SATURATION OF CARRIER PROTEINS (T_3U) IN THE NEWBORN *

*MEAN ± SD – NUMBER IN PARENTHESES INDICATES NO. INFANTS

Fig. 2. Thyroidal radioiodine clearance (log $10^3 k_1$) and triiodothyronine I^{131} resin uptake values (T_3U) plotted against age in days during the first two months of life. Values recorded as mean ± SD. Numbers in parentheses indicate number of infants.

come operative. Figure 2 shows thyroidal radioiodide clearance (Log 10^3k_1) and triiodothyronine I^{131} resin uptake values (T_3U — which parallel PBI values) plotted against age in days during the first two months of life. It can be seen that, by five to six days, thyroidal radioiodide clearance progressively decreases in the presence of the high circulating T_3U (and PBI) values. Minimal clearance values are observed at two to three weeks and subsequently increase as T_3U and PBI values decrease further.

Investigations in newborn infants kept in a warm environment (31 to 39 C) in contrast to infants kept in a cool environment (22 to 29 C) have shown that the infants in the warm environment have significantly lesser increments in PBI levels during the first forty-eight hours (p value < 0.001)[27] and have significantly lower thyroidal radioiodine clearance values at forty-eight hours (p value 0.009)[29]. These data are graphically depicted in Figures 3 and 4. Thus, the neonatal "hyperthyroid state" appears to occur in response to neonatal cooling. The progressive increment in PBI values to

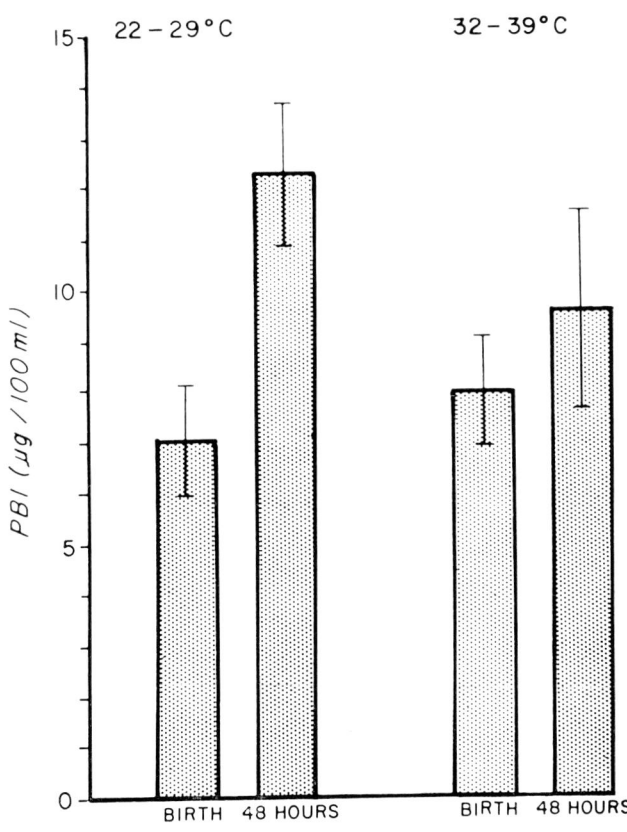

Fig. 3. PBI response of newborn term infants to environmental temperatures of 22-29 C (11 infants) and 31-39 C (10 infants) during the first forty-eight hours of life. Values recorded as mean ± SD.

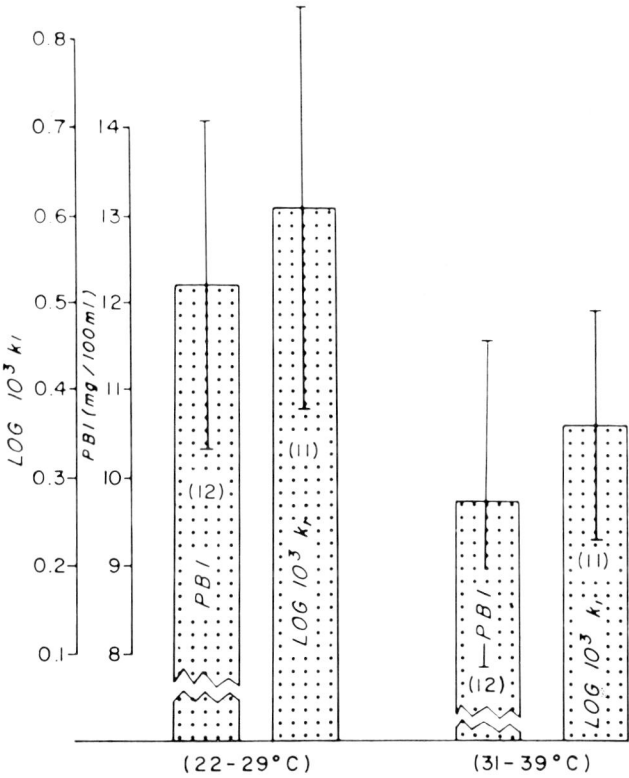

Fig. 4. Thyroidal radioiodine clearance factor (log $10^3 k_1$) and PBI values at forty-eight hours in newborn term infants kept at environmental temperatures of 22-29 C and 31-39 C. Values recorded as mean $\pm$ SD. Number in parenthesis indicates number of infants.

hyperthyroid levels in the cold infants in association with the significantly higher thyroidal radioiodide clearance would suggest a direct stimulation of thyrotropic hormone (TSH) secretion by the exposure to the cold environment.

In animals, stimulation of thyroid function in response to cold exposure is thought to occur reflexly via skin thermal receptors and the hypothalamic-pituitary system[4]. Interruption of this spinal-hypothalamic reflex pathway will prevent such stimulation[4, 18, 42]. Although the mechanism of the thyroid stimulation in the newborn is not known, analogy with animal data would suggest that, like the catecholamine response, the thyroidal hyperactivity is mediated by peripheral thermal receptors. Since infants with detectable thyroid stimulation are usually hypothermic, however, the possibility of central cold-receptor mediation cannot be excluded.

The role of thyroid hormones in cold exposure has not been completely defined. Thyroxine has been shown to potentiate the thermogenic effects of catecholamines[76, 77]. Oxygen consumption in response to adrenaline in thyroidectomized rats increases in proportion to the log dose of exogenous thyroxine[76]. The increased sensitivity of the neonate to noradrenaline thermogenesis during the first months of life[38, 39] correlates temporally with the period of increased serum hormonal iodine[27, 61] and presumably represents thyroid hormone potentiation of catecholamine thermogenesis. The progressive increase in oxygen consumption in response to acute cold exposure during the first days of life[11], during which time serum hormonal iodine values are progressively increasing (Fig. 1) might be explained similarly.

There is evidence to suggest that the capacity to increase catecholamine secretion is essential to maximal cold acclimation; adrenergic blockade inhibits or abolishes the increase in oxygen consumption and increases mortality with cold exposure in animals without altering the response to exogenous norepinephrine[44, 54]. The failure of propylthiouracil-treated rats to increase thermogenesis with acute cold exposure and the increased mortality with cold exposure of such animals also suggests an essential role of thyroid hormones[16].

ADRENAL CORTICOSTEROIDS

The hormonal response to cold exposure in animals may also include increased adrenal corticosteroid secretion[25]. This response shows species variation as well as a dependence upon the magnitude of the cold stress and the nutritional state of the animal[9, 71].

Ulstrom and colleagues[81], in studies of plasma 17-OH-CS levels in pooled venous samples of newborns at usual nursery temperatures, noted suggestively elevated values between three and twelve hours of life as contrasted with pooled cord blood or later twelve-hour plasma pools. Kenny and associates[41], however, noted essentially similar cortisol secretion rates in normal nursery infants during the first two weeks of life, and, more recently, Hillman and Giroud[34] have reported progressively decreasing plasma cortisol and cortisone levels in newborn term infants kept routinely in the nursery during the first twenty-four hours of life. Studies of forty-eight-hour urinary 17-OH-CS excretion in infants in a cool (22 to 29 C) environment contrasted with values in infants in a warm environment (32 to 39 C) are summarized in Table III. All infants were fed *ad*

TABLE III URINE 17-OH-CS EXCRETION IN NEWBORN INFANTS KEPT IN WARM AND COOL ENVIRONMENTS*

Environmental Temperature	No. Infants	48-hour 17-OH-CS Excretion (μg/kg)
23-29 C	11	141.9 ± 18.3
31-40 C	10	143.5 ± 30.0
Difference		1.6
P value		> 0.90

*Values recorded as mean ± SEM.

libitum at four-hour intervals beginning at four hours of age. No difference in forty-eight urinary 17-OH-CS excretion was noted in the two groups of infants[29]. Since many of the adrenal cortical secretory products characteristic of the neonate are not measured by the methylene chloride — Porter-Silber method — the present data are inadequate to characterize completely the adrenal response to neonatal cold stress.

WATER METABOLISM AND ANTIDIURETIC HORMONE (ADH)

Acute cold stress in animals and man results in a transient hemoconcentration secondary to a decrease in plasma volume[7]. Cold exposure has also been observed to provoke a water diuresis which occurs without associated change in glomerular filtration rate (GFR) or renal plasma flow and which can be prevented by pitressin administration[5]. This "cold diuresis" differs from the usual water diuresis in that a concomitant increase in sodium and chloride excretion may also be observed[5].

Similar marked increase in hematocrit and decrease in plasma volume have been reported in the neonate during the first few hours[15, 31, 74, 82]. That this hemoconcentration is temperature dependent is shown in Table IV, where it can be seen that infants in a cold environment (22 to 29 C) experience a marked increase in hematocrit during the first four hours, whereas those infants kept warm show only a small hematocrit increase[29]. This data is in agreement with observations of Celander[13] who, using plethysmographic methods, observed progressively increasing limb volume and an increased "capillary filtration coefficient" in newborns exposed to cold.

Significantly larger urine volumes have been observed in newborns exposed to a relatively cold environment[64]. More complete studies in newborn infants in a cool environment as contrasted with infants kept in a warm environment have shown that the colder infants on four hourly *ad libitum* feedings ingest more fluid and calories, excrete significantly more urine and tend to lose somewhat more body weight during the first two days of life than do the warm infants[29] (Table V). Although

TABLE IV EFFECT OF ENVIRONMENTAL TEMPERATURE ON HEMATOCRIT IN THE NEWBORN*

Environmental Temperature	No. Infants	Increase in Hematocrit Birth to 4 hours (%)
23-29 C	7	40.5 ± 8.6
31-40 C	7	9.4 ± 3.0
Difference		31.1
P value		< 0.01

*Values recorded as mean ± SEM.

TABLE V FLUID AND CALORIC INTAKE, URINE VOLUME AND WEIGHT CHANGE IN NEWBORN INFANTS KEPT IN WARM AND COOL ENVIRONMENTS*

Environmental Temperature	No. Infants	Fluid Intake (ml/kg/24 hr)	Calorie Intake (cal/kg/24 hr)	Urine Volume (ml/kg/24 hr)	Weight Change (gm/kg/24 hr)
23-29 C	16	97.1 ± 6.05	50.8 ± 4.52	48.9 ± 3.72	−14.1 ± 3.22†
32-40 C	15	72.6 ± 6.24	37.8 ± 2.94	20.6 ± 3.78	−6.7 ± 3.96‡
Difference		24.5	13.0	28.3	−7.4
P value		< 0.01	0.02	< 0.001	0.17

*Values recorded as mean ± SEM.
†n = 11.
‡n = 12.

the urine volume was greater in cold infants, GFR (determined as clearance of endogenous creatinine) and total osmolar excretion were similar in cold and warm infants (Tables VI and VII).

TABLE VI URINE VOLUME AND CREATININE CLEARANCE IN NEWBORN INFANTS KEPT IN WARM AND COOL ENVIRONMENTS*

Environmental Temperature	No. Infants	Urine Volume (ml/kg/24 hr)	Creatinine Clearance (ml/min)
23-29 C	7	58.9 ± 7.4	3.00 ± 0.42
31-40 C	7	18.0 ± 3.3	3.11 ± 0.45
Difference		40.9	0.11
P value		< 0.001	> 0.8

*Values recorded as mean ± SEM.

TABLE VII URINE VOLUME AND TOTAL OSMOLAR EXCRETION IN NEWBORN INFANTS KEPT IN WARM AND COOL ENVIRONMENTS*

Environmental Temperature	No. Infants	48-Hour Urine Volume (ml/kg)	48-Hour Osmolar Excretion (mOsm/kg)
23-29 C	11	98.2 ± 11.8	13.90 ± 1.51
31-40 C	10	44.4 ± 10.0	11.39 ± 1.64
Difference		53.8	2.51
P value		0.004	0.27

*Values recorded as mean ± SEM.

Urine osmolality was significantly less in the cooler infants[29].

The decrease in plasma volume with cold exposure can be prevented in animals by brainstem transection suggesting a CNS mediation[6]. It occurs, also, in spite of prevention of the water diuresis with pitressin[7], and in the new- born occurs prior to obvious water diuresis. This abrupt and marked de- crease in plasma volume[15, 31, 74, 82] pre- sumably is due to increased capillary hydrostatic pressure during the early minutes of life. Increased central venous pressure decreasing with time has been reported in the newborn during the first hours of life[35, 78] and seems to parallel the time course of decreasing plasma volume[15]. These data suggest that the hemoconcentration is related to early peripheral vasoconstriction and venoconstriction and that it may be due to the precipitate temperature- induced catecholamine secretion.

The significance of the water diuresis in the defense against cold is not clear. The newborn infant, similar to the adult, when acutely exposed to cold, experiences a water diuresis without change in GFR or total osmolar excre- tion. This water diuresis occurs in spite of a greater caloric and solute intake and tendency to greater weight loss (Table V). These data suggest that in cold infants there is an altered renal tubular water reabsorption which seems only partly accountable on the basis of increased water intake. It has been sug- gested that such "cold diuresis" may occur in response to cold-induced ADH inhibition, although this has not yet been demonstrated by direct analysis for antidiuretic activity of plasma or urine in cold-exposed subjects.

OTHER ENDOCRINE FACTORS

Other endocrine parameters in the newborn have been studied less com- pletely. Plasma growth hormone levels have been shown to be high in cord blood and in newborn plasma during the first few days of life as contrasted with values during later infancy[14]. The significance of these relatively elevated levels of growth hormone are not known. Whether growth hormone participates in the general cold response remains to be elucidated.

Plasma 17-ketosteroids have been shown to be elevated in the newborn as compared with concentrations in nonpregnant adults[33]. Plasma dehydro-epiandrosterone and androsterone levels are elevated in cord blood and decrease to undetectable levels during the first weeks of life[51, 52]. Relatively high levels of estrogens also exist in newborn plasma[24, 46, 63, 80]. These hormones appear to be largely of maternal or placental origin and are gradually excreted during the first week of life[70,79]. Again, there is no evidence, at present, to suggest that these maternally acquired estrogenic or androgenic hormones participate significantly in the acute neonatal adaptation of extrauterine life.

SUMMARY

The newborn infant precipitously transferred from the uterus to a relatively cold extrauterine environment experiences an abrupt hypothermia. Defense against this hypothermia occurs largely by way of increased non-shivering thermogenesis probably primarily stimulated by increased catecholamine secretion but progressively enhanced by increased thyroid hormone secretion. Adipose tissue stores appear to play a prime metabolic role in the enhanced thermogenesis by increasing local heat production as well as through the provision of free fatty acid substrate for non-adipose-tissue thermogenesis.

The increased catecholamine secretion probably secondarily produces an acute and transient shift in plasma volume by way of enhanced peripheral vasoconstriction and venoconstriction. An added cold-induced alteration in water metabolism observed in the newborn is a marked water diuresis occurring without change in creatinine or osmolar excretion and only partly accountable by increased water intake. It has been suggested that this water diuresis may be due to inhibition of antidiuretic hormone secretion by the cold exposure. The significance of this water diuresis to the defense against cold stress in the newborn has not been defined.

REFERENCES

1. Adams, F. H., Fujiwara, T., Spears, R., and Hodgman, J.: Temperature regulation in premature infants. Pediatrics, 33:487-495, 1964.
2. Adamsons, K., Jr., Gandy, G. M., and James, L. S.: The influence of thermal factors upon oxygen consumption of the newborn human infant. J. Pediat., 66:495-508, 1965.
3. Aherne, W., and Hull, D.: The site of heat production in the newborn infant. Proc. Roy. Soc. Med., 57:1172-1173, 1964.
4. Andersson, B., Ekman, L., Gale, C. C., and Sundsten, J. W.: Control of thyrotrophic hormone (TSH) secretion by the "heat loss center." Acta Physiol. Scand., 59:12-33, 1963.
5. Bader, R. A., Eliot, J. W., and Bass, D. E.: Hormonal and renal mechanisms of cold diuresis. J. Appl. Physiol., 4:649-658, 1952.
6. Barbour, H. G.: Localization of body vapor pressure reflexes to environmental temperature in the infundibular portion of the hypothalamus. Amer. J. Physiol., 109:4-5, 1934.
7. Bass, D. E., and Henschel, A.: Responses of body fluid compartments to heat and cold. Physiol. Rev., 36:128-144, 1956.
8. Benson, R. C., Pickering, D. E., Kontaxis, N. E., and Fisher, D. A.: Thyroid function in pregnancy. Obstet. Gynec., 14:11-19, 1959.
9. Boulouard, R.: Effects of cold and starvation on adrenocortical activity of rats. Fed. Proc., 22:750-753, 1963.
10. Buetow, K. C., and Klein, S. W.: Effect of maintenance of "normal" skin temperature on survival of infants of low birth weight. Pediatrics, 34:163-170, 1964.

11. Brück, K.: Temperature regulation in the newborn infant. Biol. Neonat., 3:65-119, 1961.

12. Brück, K.: General aspects of temperature regulation of small subjects. Maandschr. Kindergeneesk., 32:601-619, 1964.

13. Celander, O.: Discussion — Section IV — Temperature control of the newborn. In Jonxis, J. H. P., Visser, H. K. A., and Troelstra, J. A. (eds.): The Adaptation of the Newborn Infant to Extrauterine Life. Springfield, Thomas, 1964, pp. 292-296.

14. Cornblath, M., Parker, M. L., Reisner, S. H., Forbes, A. E., and Daughaday, W. H.: Secretion and metabolism of growth hormone in premature and full-term infants. J. Clin. Endocr., 25:209-218, 1965.

15. Cort, R. L., and Pribylova, H.: Placental transfusion and fluid metabolism on the first day of life. Arch. Dis. Child., 39:363-370, 1964.

16. Cottle, W. H.: Role of thyroid secretion in cold acclimation. Fed. Proc., 19 (Suppl. 5): 59-63, 1960.

17. Cross, K. W., Tizard, J. P. M., and Trythall, D. A. H.: The gaseous metabolism of the newborn infant. Acta Paediat., 46:265-285, 1957.

18. D'Angelo, S. A.: Adenohypophysial function in the guinea pig at low environmental temperature. Fed. Proc., 19 (Suppl. 5):51-58, 1960.

19. Danowski, T. S., Johnston, S. Y., Price, W. C., McKelvy, M., Stevenson, S, S., and McCluskey, E. R.: Protein-bound iodine in infants from birth to one year of age. Pediatrics, 7:240-244, 1951.

20. Dawkins, M. J. R., and Hull, D.: Brown adipose tissue and non-shivering thermogenesis in newborn animals. Maandschr. Kindergeneesk., 32:641-652, 1964.

21. Dawkins, M. J. R., and Hull, D.: The production of heat by fat. Sci. Amer., 213:62-67, 1965.

22. Day, R. L., Curtis, J., and Kelly, M.: Respiratory metabolism in infancy and in childhood. XXVII. Regulation of body temperature of premature infants. Amer. J. Dis. Child., 65:376-398, 1943.

23. Day, R. L., Caliguiri, L., Kamenski, C., and Ehrlich, F.: Body temperature and survival of premature infants. Pediatrics, 34:171-181, 1964.

24. Diczfalusy, E., and Magnusson, A.-M.: Estriol in blood. J, Clin Endocr., 20:1633-1634, 1960.

25. Egdahl, R. H., and Richards, J. B.: Effect of extreme cold exposure on adrenocortical function in the unanesthetized dog. Amer. J. Physiol., 185:239-242, 1956.

26. Fisher, D. A., Oddie, T. H., and Burroughs, J. C.: Thyroidal radioiodine uptake rate measurement in infants. Amer. J. Dis. Child., 103:738-749, 1962.

27. Fisher, D. A., and Oddie, T. H.: Neonatal thyroidal hyperactivity. Response to cooling. Amer. J. Dis. Child., 107:574-581, 1964.

28. Fisher, D. A., and Makoski, E. J.: Temperature adaptation of the newborn to the extrauterine environment. J. Lancet, 86:85-92, 1966.

29. Fisher, D. A., and Oddie, T. H.: The effect of environmental temperature on thyroid, adrenal and water metabolism in the newborn human infant. Pediatrics, 37:583-591, 1966.

30. Fujiwara, T.: Gaseous metabolism of premature infants in different environmental temperatures. Pediat. Jap., 3:68, 1960.

31. Gairdner, D., Marks, J., Roscoe, J. D., and Brettell, R. O.: The fluid shift from the vascular compartment immediately after birth. Arch. Dis. Child., 33:489-498, 1958.

32. Gandy, G. M., Adamsons, K., Jr., Cunningham, N., Silverman, W. A., and James, L. S.: Thermal environment and acid-base homeostasis in human infants during the first few hours of life. J. Clin. Invest., 43:751-758, 1964.

33. Gardner, L. I., and Walton, R. L.: Plasma 17-ketosteroids of full-term and premature infants. J. Clin. Invest., 33:1642-1645, 1954.

34. Hillman, D. A., and Giroud, C. J. P.: Plasma cortisone and cortisol levels at birth and during the neonatal period. J. Clin. Endocr., 25:243-248, 1965.

35. Jegier, W., Blankenship, W., and Lind, J.: Venous pressure in the first hour of life and its relationship to placental transfusion. Acta Paediat. (Upps.), 52:485-496, 1963.

36. Jolly, H., Molyneux, P., and Newell, D. J.: A controlled study of the effect of temperature on premature babies. J. Pediat., 60: 889-894, 1962.

37. Karlberg, P., Moore, R. E., and Oliver, T. K., Jr.: The thermogenic response of the newborn infant to noradrenaline. Acta Paediat. (Upps.), 51:284-292, 1962.

38. Karlberg, P., Moore, R. E., and Oliver, T. K., Jr.: The thermogenic response of the newborn infant to noradrenaline. Acta Paediat. (Upps.), Suppl. 140:53-54, 1963.

39. Karlberg, P., Moore, R. E., and Oliver, T. K., Jr.: Thermogenic and cardiovascular responses of the newborn baby to noradrenaline. Acta Paediat. Scand., **54**:225-238, 1965.

40. Kaye, R., and Kumagai, M.: Studies of unesterified fatty acid metabolism in infants. A.M.A. J. Dis. Child., **96**:527-528, 1958 (abstract).

41. Kenny, F. M., Malvaux, P., and Migeon, C. J.: Cortisol production rate in newborn babies, older infants and children. Pediatrics, 31:360-373, 1963.

42. Knigge, K. M.: Neuroendocrine mechanisms influencing ACTH and TSH secretion and their role in cold acclimation. Fed. Proc., **19** (Suppl. 5):45-51, 1960.

43. LeBlanc, J. A., and Nadeau, G.: Urinary excretion of adrenaline and noradrenaline in normal and cold-adapted animals. Canad. J. Biochem. Physiol., **39**:215-217, 1961.

44. Leduc, J.: Cathecholamine production and release in exposure and acclimation to cold. Acta Physiol. Scand., **53** (Suppl. 183):1-101, 1961.

45. Man, E. B., Pickering, D. E., Walker, J., and Cooke, R. E.: Butanol-estractable iodine in the serum of infants. Pediatrics, **9**:32-37, 1952.

46. Maner, F. D., Saffan, B. D., Wiggins, R. A., Thompson, J. D., and Preedy, J. R. K.: Interrelationship of estrogen concentrations in the maternal circulation, fetal circulation and maternal urine in late pregnancy. J. Clin. Endocr., **23**:445-458, 1963.

47. Marks, J., Wolfson, J., and Klein, R.: Neonatal thyroid function: erythrocyte T₃ uptake in early infancy. J. Pediat., **58**:32-38, 1961.

48. Marks, J. F.: "Free thyroxine" index in the newborn. J. Clin. Endocr., **25**:852, 1965.

49. McClure, J. H., and Caton, W. L.: Newborn temperature. I. Temperatures of term normal infants. J. Pediat., **47**:583-587, 1955.

50. Mestyan, G. Y., and Varga, F.: Chemical thermoregulation of full term and premature newborn infants. J. Pediat., **56**:623-629, 1960.

51. Migeon, C. J., Keller, A. R., and Holmstrom, E. G.: Dehydroepiandrosterone, androsterone and 17-hydroxycorticosteroid levels in maternal and cord plasma in cases of vaginal delivery. Bull. Hopkins Hosp., **97**:415-421, 1955.

52. Migeon, C. J.: The endocrine function of the newborn. Wolstenholme, G.E.W., and O'Connor, M. (eds.): In Somatic Stability in the Newly Born. Boston, Little, 1961, pp. 215-237.

53. Miller, H. C., Behrle, F. C., Nieman, J. L., Driver, R., and Dudding, B. A.: Oxygen consumption in newborn premature infants. Amer. J. Dis. Child., **103**:39-46, 1962.

54. Moore, R. E.: Control of heat production in newborn mammals: role of noradrenaline and mode of action. Fed. Proc., **22**:920-924, 1963.

55. Moore, R. E.: Chemical regulation of heat production in the neonate. Maandschr. Kindergeneesk., **32**:620-632, 1964.

56. Novák, M., Melichar, V., Hahn, P., and Koldovsky, O.: Levels of lipids in the blood of newborn infants and the effect of glucose administration. Physiol. Bohemoslov., **10**:488-492, 1961.

57. Novák, M., Melichar, V., and Hahn, P.: Postnatal changes in the blood serum content of glycerol and fatty acids in human infants. Biol. Neonat., **7**:179-184, 1964.

58. Novák, M., Melichar, V., Hahn, P., and Koldovsky, O.: Release of free fatty acids from adipose tissue obtained from newborn infants. J. Lipid Res., **6**:91-95, 1965.

59. Oliver, T. K., Jr., and Karlberg, P.: Gaseous metabolism in newly born human infants: the effects of environmental temperature and 15% oxygen in the inspired air. Amer. J. Dis. Child., **105**:427-435, 1963.

60. Perry, R. E., Hodgman, J. E., and Starr, P.: Maternal, cord and serial venous blood: protein-bound iodine, thyroid-binding globulin, thyroid-binding albumin and prealbumin values in premature infants. Pediatrics, **35**:759-764, 1965.

61. Pickering, D. E., Kontaxis, N. E., Benson, R. C., and Meechan, R. J.: Thyroid function in the perinatal period. A.M.A. J. Dis. Child., **95**:616-621, 1958.

62. Pribylova, H.: Environmental temperature: the effect on oxygen consumption, body and skin temperature and respiration in mature neonates. Ann. Paediat., **201**:399-409, 1963.

63. Roy, E. J.: The concentration of oestrogens in maternal and foetal blood obtained at caesarean section, and the effect of hospitalization on maternal blood estrogen levels. J. Obstet. Gynaec. Brit. Comm., **69**:196-202, 1962.

64. Sandler, M., Ruthven, C. R. J., Normand, I. C. S., and Moore, R. E.: Environmental temperature and urinary excretion of 3-methoxy-4-hydroxymandelic acid in the newborn. Lancet, 1:485-486, 1961.

65. Scopes, J. W., and Tizard, J. P. M.: The effect of intravenous noradrenaline on the

oxygen consumption of new-born mammals. J. Physiol. (London), **165**:305-326, 1963.

66. Sellers, E. A., and Schönbaum, E.: Catecholamines in acclimation to cold: historical survey. Fed. Proc., **22**:909-910, 1963.

67. Silverman, W. A., Fertig, J. W., and Berger, A. P.: The influence of the thermal environment upon the survival of newly born premature infants. Pediatrics, **22**:876-886, 1958.

68. Silverman, W. A., Zamelis, A., Sinclair, J. C., and Agate, F. J., Jr.: Warm nape of the newborn. Pediatrics, **33**:984-987, 1964.

69. Smith, C. A.: The Physiology of the Newborn Infant. Springfield, Thomas, 3rd ed., 1959, pp. 216-225.

70. Smith, C. A.: The sex hormones. In The Physiology of the Newborn Infant. Springfield, Thomas, 3rd ed., 1959, pp. 365-372.

71. Smith, R. E., and Hoijer, D. J.: Metabolism and cellular function in cold acclimation. Physiol. Rev., **42**:60-142, 1962.

72. Smith, R. E.: Symposium on temperature acclimation. Discussion of paper by L. E. Mount. Fed. Proc., **22**:822-823, 1963.

73. Spafford, N. R., Carr, E. A., Jr., Lowrey, G. H., and Beierwaltes, W. H.: I[131] labeled triiodothyronine erythrocyte uptake of mothers and newborn infants. Amer. J. Dis. Child., **100**:844-849, 1960.

74. Steele, M. W.: Plasma volume changes in the neonate. Amer. J. Dis. Child., **103**:10-18, 1962.

75. Stern, L., Lees, M. H., and Leduc, J.: Environmental temperature, oxygen consumption, and catecholamine excretion in newborn infants. Pediatrics, **36**:367-373, 1965.

76. Swanson, H. E.: Interrelations between thyroxin and adrenalin in the regulation of oxygen consumption in the albino rat. Endocrinology, **59**:217-225, 1956.

77. Swanson, H. E.: The effect of temperature on the potentiation of adrenalin by thyroxine in the albino rat. Endocrinology, **60**:205-213, 1957.

78. Taylor, P. M., Egan, T. J., Birchard, E. L., Bright, N. H., and Wolfson, J. H.: Venous hypertension in the newborn infant associated with delayed clamping of the umbilical cord. Acta Paediat. (Upps.), **50**:149-159, 1961.

79. Thorsen, T., Stoa, K. F., and Aarskog, D.: Identification of ring D α-ketolic oestrogens in the urine of newborn infants. Acta Endocr. (Kobenhavn), **45**:415-426, 1964.

80. Touchstone, J. C., and Greene, J. W., Jr.: Free estriol in blood plasma. J. Clin. Endocr., **20**:647-649, 1960.

81. Ulstrom, R. A., Colle, E., Reynolds, J. W., and Burley, J.: Adrenocortical steroid metabolism in newborn infants. IV. Plasma concentrations of cortisol in the early neonatal period. J. Clin. Endocr., **21**:414-425, 1961.

82. Usher, R., Shephard, M., and Lind, J.: The blood volume of the newborn infant and placental transfusion. Acta Paediat., **52**:497-512, 1963.

Chapter 17

Adrenocortical Dyscrasias in Infancy and Childhood: Discussion and Presentation of Cases and Tables of Hyperaldosteronism, Cushing's Syndrome and Adrenogenital Disease

MEYER M. MELICOW, M.D.

The versatility of the adrenal gland is astounding. The adult organ weighs only 5 to 6 gm, yet it plays a vital role in preserving life, maintaining electrolyte balance and hormonal homeostasis, responding to stress and strain, etc. If the volume of an endocrine gland varies with functional activity, then the fetal adrenal probably partakes significantly in prenatal development. Up to about the third month it is larger than the kidney. At term it is one third the weight of the kidney; whereas in the adult it is only one thirtieth in weight. At this time the adrenal weighs about 4 gm − 1 gm less than the adult organ. Thus, it is a veritable dynamo of activity during the early months of pregnancy. The cortex, particularly the dominant inner or "fetal" zone, undergoes resolution promptly after birth, and the gland loses about 50 per cent of its weight. Thence, during childhood and until puberty, i.e., during somatic growth, the gland remains stationary; but, soon after puberty, the adult weight of 5 to 6 gm is reached[21, 22, 32] (Fig. 1).

The adrenal cortex is composed of three merging zones of cells: glomerular; fascicular; and reticular. Zelander[35] concluded from his electron-microscope studies of the adrenals in the adult male mice that there are four zones (he divided the fascicular layer into an outer and inner zone). Some[2, 17, 36] have compared the interrelationship of the various layers to those of the epidermis, except that the direction is reversed. Sabatini *et al.*[29] and Greep and Deane[14], however, concluded from their studies that the layers are separate and that each has a specialized function. Messier and Leblond[23] used tritiated thymidine and observed that there "was not a significant degree of cell migration in the adrenal cortex of male rats." The func-

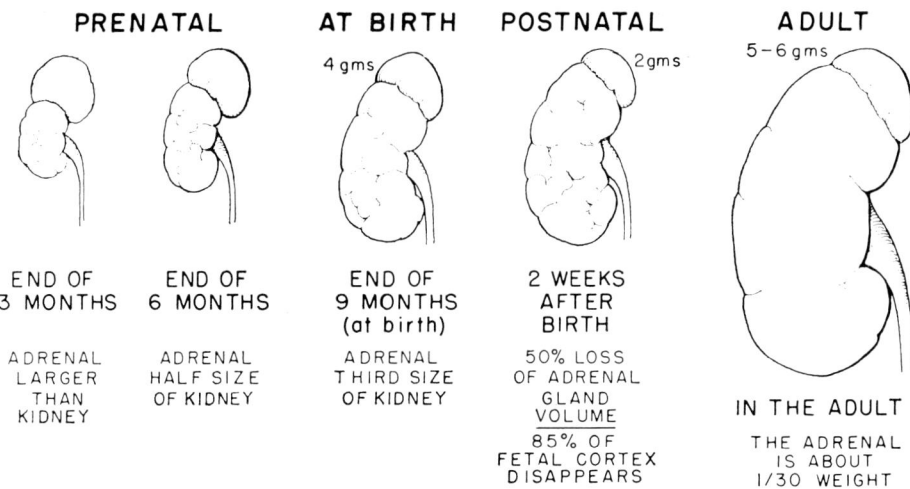

PRENATAL   **AT BIRTH** **POSTNATAL**   **ADULT**

4 gms   2gms   5-6 gms

END OF   END OF   END OF   2 WEEKS
3 MONTHS   6 MONTHS   9 MONTHS   AFTER
                                (at birth)   BIRTH

ADRENAL   ADRENAL   ADRENAL   50% LOSS
LARGER   HALF SIZE   THIRD SIZE   OF ADRENAL
THAN   OF KIDNEY   OF KIDNEY   GLAND
KIDNEY   VOLUME
                                                85% OF   IN THE ADULT
                                          FETAL CORTEX   THE ADRENAL
                                          DISAPPEARS   IS ABOUT
                                                                1/30 WEIGHT
                                                                OF KIDNEY

Fig. 1.   Comparison of weight of adrenal gland and kidney prenatally, at birth, post-
natally and during adult life (22).

tions of the zones of the adrenal cortex are outlined in Table I.

Accumulated case reports indicate that infants and children can suffer from adrenogenitalism, Cushing's syndrome and hyperaldosteronism. Gross and histologic changes in the adrenal cortex are not always consonant with these syndromes (Table II). Thus, any one of the disturbances can be associated with:

1. Hyperfunction or dysfunction *without* change in weight or size of the gland;

2. Bilateral hyperplasia; or

3. Neoplasia — adenoma, carcinoma.

Significant participation by the glomerular zone in primary hyperaldosteronism has not always been observed; in most instances, the component elements resemble the fascicular zone. On the other hand, in Cushing's syndrome,

TABLE I FUNCTION OF ZONES OF
ADRENAL CORTEX

1. Glomerulosa — mineralcorticoids (aldosterone)
2. Fasciculata — glucocorticoids
         mineralcorticoids (doca)
3. Reticularis — glucocorticoids
         ?androgens, estrogens

Gland contains high concentration ascorbid acid
Yellow color due to lipids (cholesterol, cholesterolesters, steroid hormones and their precursors).

TABLE II TYPE OF ADRENAL PATHOLOGY
SEEN IN CLINICAL ENTITIES INDUCED
BY CORTICAL DYSCRASIA

1. Hyperaldosteronism — none or bilateral hyperplasia, or adenoma, or carcinoma.
         site: glomerular zone, fascicular zone.

2. Congenital adrenogenital disease — none, or bilateral hyperplasia.
         site: fascicular ± reticular zone.

3. Postnatal adrenogenital disease — usually adenoma, or carcinoma.
         site: (?) reticular zone.

4. Cushing's syndrome — none, or bilateral hyperplasia, adenoma, carcinoma. Contralateral atrophy.
         site: fascicular zone.

as expected, the fascicular zone usually predominates. This association was observed and emphasized in 1948[21]. In neoplasms causing pure adrenogenital disease, granular cells in an array resembling the reticular zone were predominant in the majority of cases seen at the Squier Urological Clinic[5].

HYPERALDOSTERONISM

Aldosterone, the potent mineralocorticoid secreted by the glomerulosa is not dependent on ACTH but rather on the level of sodium in the circulation. A drop in the latter causes release of renin by the juxta-glomerular apparatus. Renin and blood globulin form angiotensin, which stimulates the glomerulosa to secrete larger amounts of aldosterone. The latter acts on the distal convoluted tubules, causing sodium retention and potassium excretion (Table III).

Excess aldosterone secretion due to hyperfunction of the glomerulosa or to hyperfunction associated with bilateral cortical hyperplasia or neoplasia causes hypokalemia, hypernatremia, hypochloremia, alkalosis and a rise in urine aldosterone level. The urine 17-ketogenic and 17-hydroxysteroids are normal.

TABLE III THE CHECK AND BALANCE OF ALDOSTERONE SECRETION AS RELATED TO SODIUM CONTENT IN CIRCULATION

```
              GLOMERULOSA
                secrets
              ALDOSTERONE
        (a salt retaining mineralcorticoid)

1) Secretion not depending on ACTH
2) Drop in Na    Release of RENIN by juxta-glomerular apparatus
   Renin & Blood Globulin ───► ANGIOTENSION
                                     │
                                     ▼
   vasopressor effect       ALDOSTERONE Secretion
                                     ▼
                                Rise in Na
```

Patients suffer from episodic weakness, headaches, tetany, hypertension, moderate retinopathy, cardiac hypertrophy, polyuria, polydypsia and nocturia.

Conn[7] reviewed 150 cases of aldosteronism in all age groups, and noted that single benign tumors occurred in 70 per cent, multiple adenomas in 15 per cent, bilateral hyperplasia in 9 per cent, and no significant change or nodular hyperplasia in 6 per cent. The fascicular zone predominated, occasionally the glomerular, and sometimes both zones were represented. Carcinoma was rare. He stated that hyperplasia occurred mostly in children or young adults. Kretchmer et al., in 1959[20], reported a nine-year-old boy suffering from primary aldosteronism. First one, then the opposite multinodular adrenal gland was removed. Both showed hyperplasia of the fascicular zone. The patient improved. Slater et al.[30] reported marked improvement following bilateral adrenalectomy in a five-year-old boy suffering from aldosteronism. The glands showed no significant change from the normal. Cavell et al., in 1964[6], reported primary aldosteronism in a three-year-old boy with a cortical adenoma weighing 15 gm. Sections revealed foci resembling all three zones of the cortex. It is of interest to note that the boy showed excessive hair, and his urine 17-ketosteroids were slightly elevated. A fascinating report of aldosteronism associated with precocious puberty, all due to an androblastoma of the ovary in a nine-year-old girl, was published by Ehrlich et al.[10]. There was hypertension (200/140), hypokalemia, increased excretion of aldosterone in the urine and irregular vaginal bleeding. It had been decided to do a bilateral

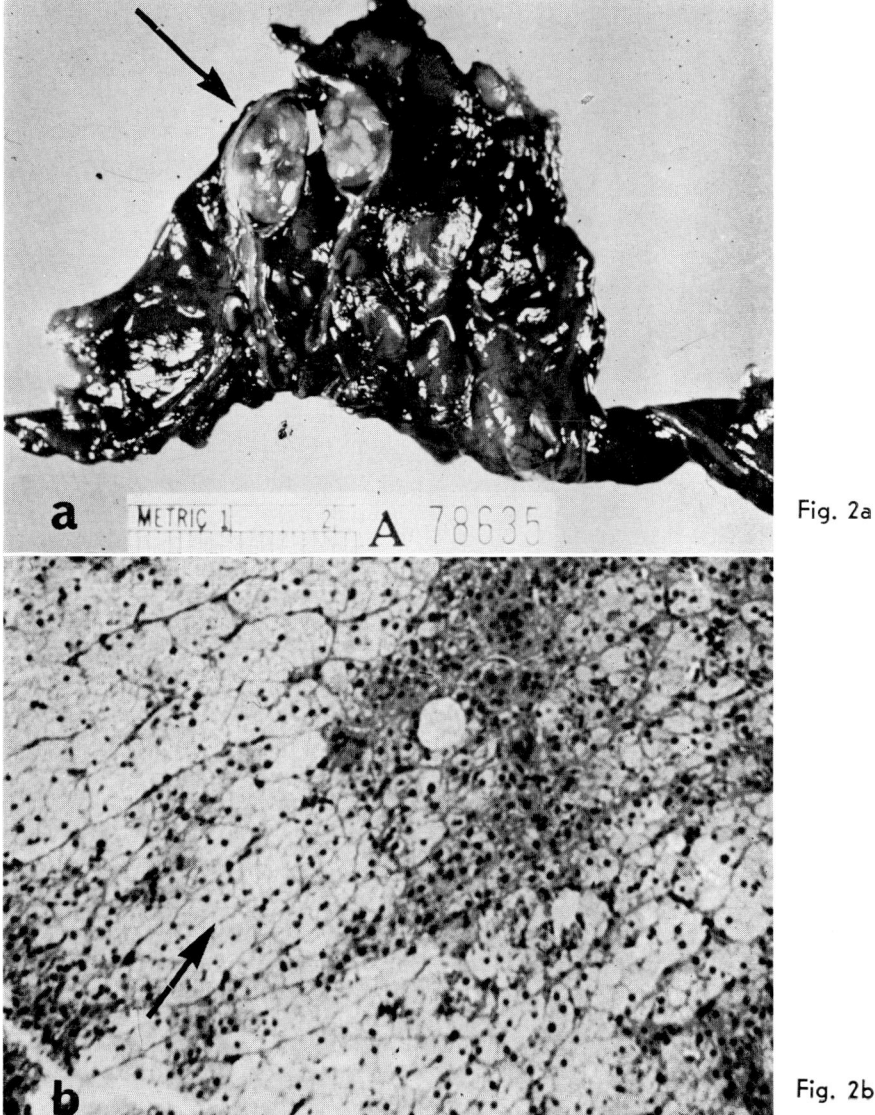

Fig. 2a

Fig. 2b

←————————

Fig. 2a and b.   L. J. (1411366) first complained of weakness, hypertension, polyuria, polydypsia, attacks of dyspnea and tachycardia, severe headaches and syncope when she was thirteen years of age. The symptoms persisted for three years and she was finally admitted to another hospital where, because radiographs revealed minor abnormality of the right kidney, a nephrectomy was performed. The right adrenal gland was said to be normal at that time. The patient's symptoms did not improve, and she was then referred to the Columbia Presbyterian Medical Center for further evaluation. The blood pressure ranged from 230 to 290 systolic and 120 to 180 diastolic. The results of laboratory examinations were as follows: serum sodium 146.8, potassium 2.5, chlorides 102.0 mEq/liter; the BUN 19 mg per 100 ml. The urine showed two plus protein, no glucose or acetone and occasional white blood cells. Because of the low potassium and relatively high sodium and an elevated aldosterone in the urine, a diagnosis of hyperaldosteronism was made, and the left adrenal was explored and removed. It weighed 5.15 gm and revealed no significant pathological change (A74873). The patient was discharged, but returned five months later with persistence of the original symptoms; and again a high sodium, low potassium and elevated urinary aldosterone were found. The right adrenal was enlarged and therefore excised. The gland (A78-635) weighed 15 gm and on section revealed a small adenoma whose component cells resembled those of the fascicular zone (b). Following this operation the patient's symptoms improved; the blood pressure ranged from around 120/70 mm Hg, and urine aldosterone was no longer elevated. Diagnosis: aldosteronoma of the right adrenal gland.

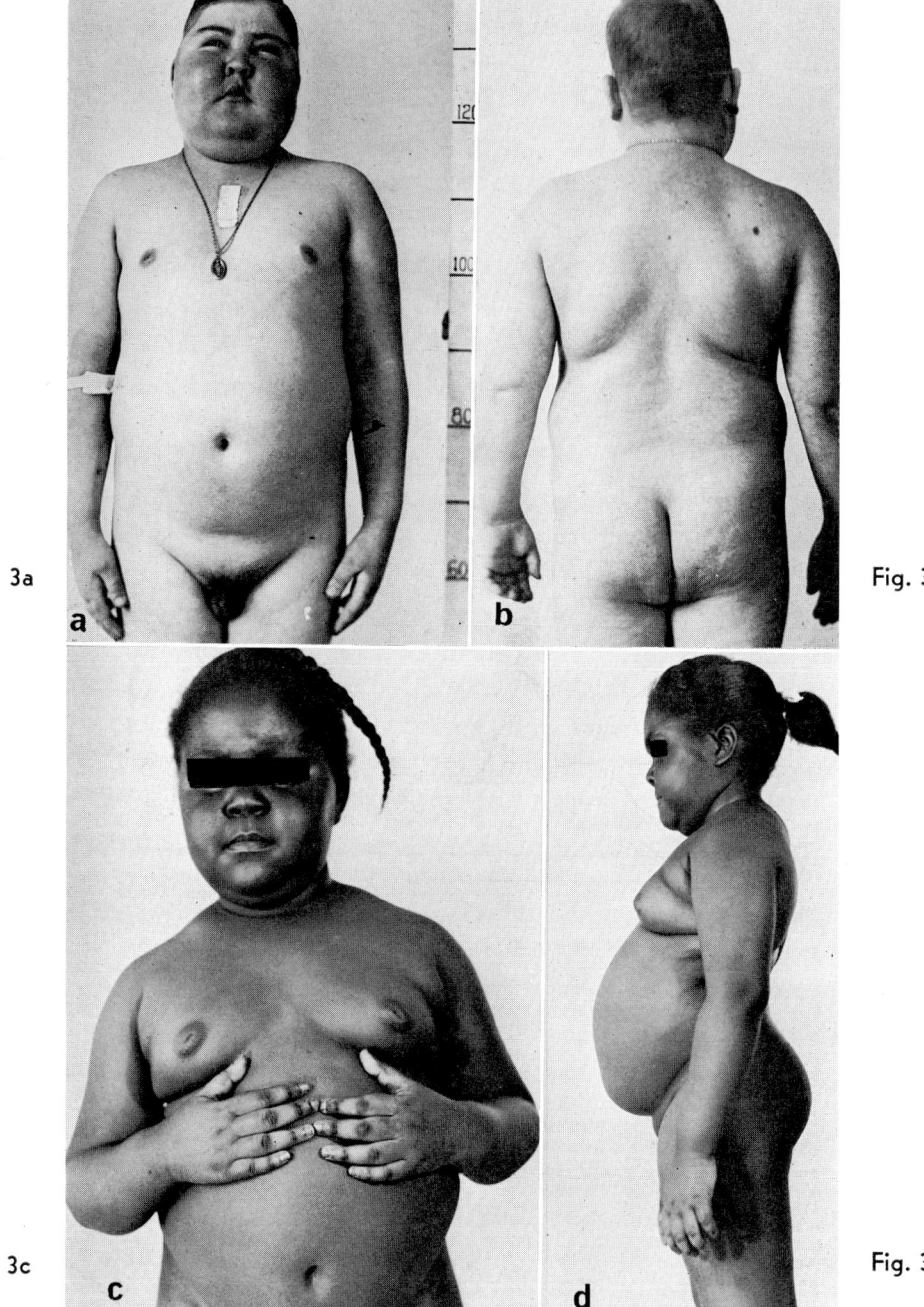

←———— ————

Fig. 3a and b.   A. G. (572037), age eleven years, was admitted to the Babies Hospital in 1939 because of excessive gain in weight and steady development of the clinical features of Cushing's syndrome (note moon face, obscurred ears, slit eyes, fish mouth and trunk obesity). Radiographs of the spine showed osteoporosis, and radiographs of the abdomen were suggestive of enlarged adrenal glands. At exploratory operation the glands were slightly enlarged and there was no evidence of tumor. The patient developed a severe postoperative hemolytic streptococcus infection and died of sepsis.

Diagnosis: Cushing's syndrome due to hyperfunction of the adrenal cortex.

Fig. 3c and d.   B. W. (938-601) was first seen when six years of age because of an excessive gain in weight, hirsutism and breast development; there were no menses. The blood pressure was 120/90 mm Hg. The clitoris was not enlarged. The result of laboratory tests were: sodium 144.4, potassium 4.8, chlorides 109 mEq/liter; and 25 mg of urine 17-ketosteroids per twenty-four hours. Fasting blood glucose was normal. There was an increase in circulating cortisone-like steroids following an injection of ACTH. Note the obesity and buffalo hump, suggestive of Cushing's syndrome (d). A bilateral adrenalectomy was performed. The glands were only slightly enlarged. Cortisone and sodium chloride were administered, and the patient improved, but within a year she returned with return of Cushing's syndrome. However, now she had an inoperable abdominal mass which was hard, irregular and apparently arose from the pancreas. The tumor was partially resected and a mass weighing 268 gm removed. The histologic studies showed (S-9383) an islet cell adenoma of the pancreas. The patient died on the eleventh postoperative day because of sepsis and aspiration of vomitus. At autopsy the pituitary gland was found to be smaller than normal (283 mg instead of 500 mg). Thus, it appears that this patient probably had a non-endocrine ACTH-producing tumor which clinically caused Cushing's syndrome, and at the same time inhibited the pituitary gland, causing partial atrophy.

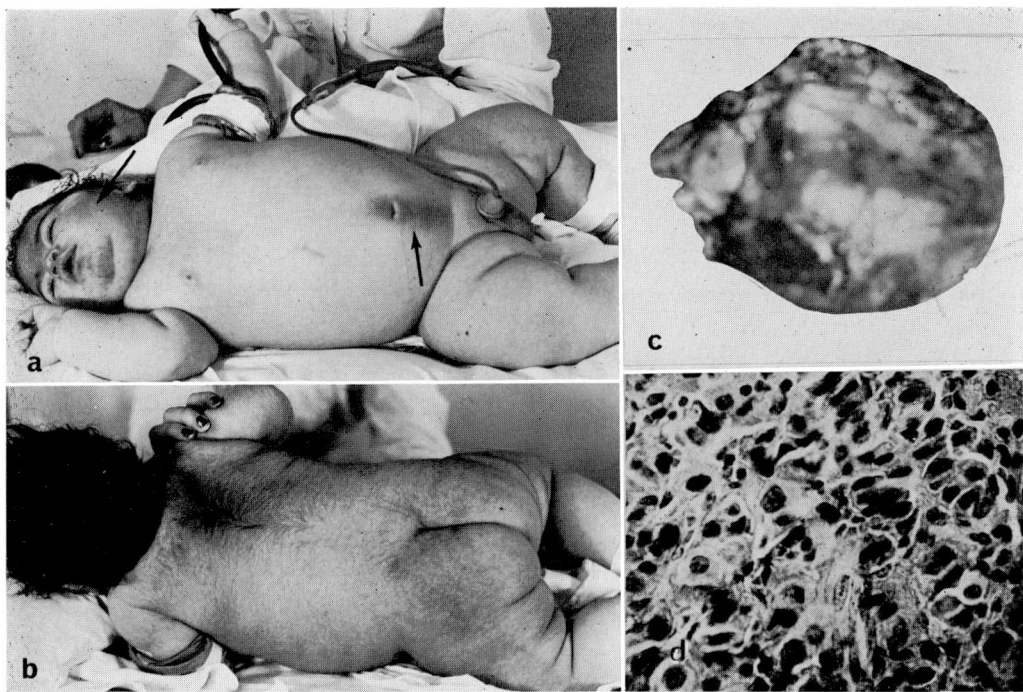

Fig. 4a, b, c and d. G. S. L. (226616) at the age of six months was admitted to the Babies Hospital because of pronounced gain in weight, hirsutism and acne. There was pronounced hyptertension (blood pressure: 280/230 mm Hg) osteoporosis, polycythemia and elevated urine 17-ketogenic steroids. Radiographs revealed a mass occupying the region of the right adrenal gland. A tumor weighing 110 gm was removed. Sections revealed a malignancy composed of pleomorphic, fairly large cells with irregular deep-staining nuclei. Areas of necrosis were present. The patient developed massive necrotizing cystitis, peritonitis and died within a week after the adrenalectomy. At autopsy a metastasis from the adrenal tumor to the frontal leptomeninges was found. The left adrenal showed cortical atrophy. Diagnosis: mixed Cushing and adrenogenital syndrome due to carcinoma of the adrenal cortex.

adrenalectomy, but, after removal of a normal right adrenal, suspicion was raised by the firm consistency of the right ovary. This led to further investigation and the discovery of the bright yellow tumor. All symptoms abated after oöphorectomy.

At the Squier Urological Clinic, one patient was seen whose symptoms of aldosteronism began when she was thirteen years of age (Fig. 2). However, the significance of these symptoms was not recognized until she reached sixteen years. Radiographs revealed no adrenal enlargement. The right adrenal area was explored, and a normal-appearing gland was removed, but symptoms persisted. The left gland was then excised, and, on section, a small adenoma (Fig. 2) was found. The histologic picture showed predominance of the fascicular zone.

CUSHING'S SYNDROME

The glucocorticoids, secreted by the cells of the fascicular zone, affect vascular homeostasis, gluconeogenesis, protein and salt water metabolism, gastro-

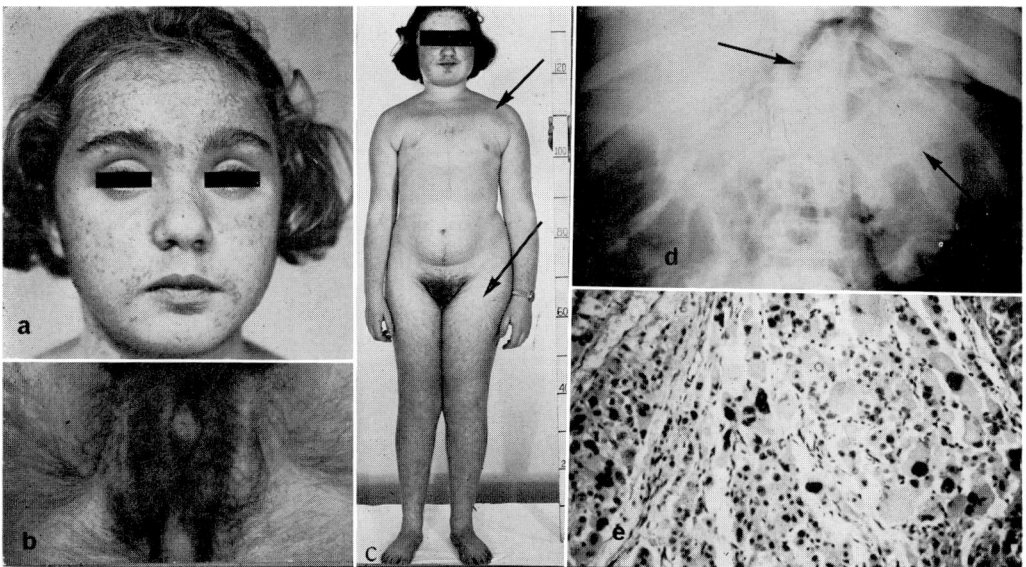

Fig. 5a and b.   C. A. (754001), a seven-year old girl, was admitted to the Babies Hospital of the Squier Urological Clinic, with a five months' history of acne, hirsutism and enlargement of the clitoris.   The blood pressure was 140/85 mm Hg.   The urinary 17-ketosteroids were 76.8 mg per twenty-four hours.   A large, partly calcified, non-resectable mass was found in the right suprarenal region.   Sections revealed an anaplastic cortical carcinoma.

Fig. 5c, d and e.   A. P. (072857), an eleven-year-old girl, was admitted to the Babies Hospital because of hirsutism, deepening of voice and weight gain of one year's duration. Note the moon face, hirsutism and acne (c). There was a peculiar hemi-hypertrophy of the left half of the body. A soft tissue mass anterior to and superior to the left kidney was noted by airogram (d). The 17-ketosteroids were elevated (39.4, 30.2 mg in 24 hours), and there was no drop following four days of cortisone therapy. The glucose tolerance curve was of the diabetic type. The benzodioxane test was negative. The impression was carcinoma of the left adrenal cortex secreting hormones which induced virilism and Cushing's. The blood pressure was 190/155 mm Hg. The patient underwent left adrenalectomy. Sections showed an anaplastic tumor; hyperchromatism was frequent, and some areas resembled the fascicular zone (e). The blood pressure fell from 180/120 to 100/60, and shock continued in spite of the administration of cortisone, ACTH, norepinephrine, etc. She expired on the first postoperative day, after voiding approximately 50 cc of bloody fluid. It was surmised that death was caused by irreversible shock and that the contralateral adrenal was either absent or completely atrophied.

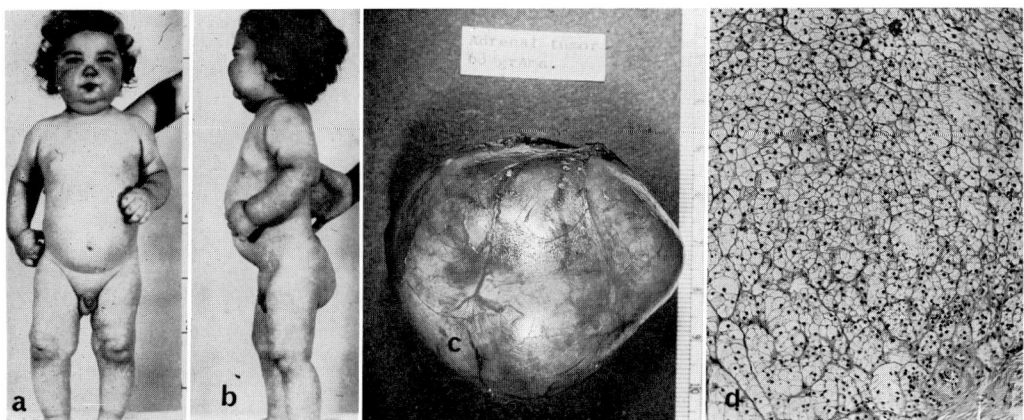

Fig. 6a, b, c and d.   J. S. (138-25-31), a nineteen-month-old boy, was admitted to the Babies Hospital with a picture characteristic of Cushing's syndrome. The latter condition was first noted about seven months earlier and had steadily grown worse. A mass involving the right adrenal gland was removed. It weighed 63 gm. The component cells resembled the fascicular zone. The patient made an uneventful recovery, lost the plethoric look, and his blood pressure, which, prior to operation, ranged from 140 to 180 systolic and from 100 to 130 diastolic, now averaged 96/65 mm Hg.

intestinal absorption, immunologic and inflammatory response and resistance to stress. An increased production of glucocorticoids produces Cushing's syndrome, with obesity, hyperglycemia, polycythemia, demineralization of bone, salt and water retention, and hypertension, as the predominant symptoms. Cushing's syndrome can also be induced iatrogenically, but the spontaneous types result from disturbances in the following areas.

1. In the adrenal cortex, or in ectopic cortical tissue by: (a) hyperplasia, usually bilateral and secondary to excess ACTH from any source, usually the pituitary; or (b) neoplasia — adenoma or carcinoma.

2. In the pituitary by an ACTH-secreting tumor.

3. In a non-endocrine tumor, secreting ACTH (carcinoma of the lung,

tumors of the pancreas[13], thymus, etc.).

There are numerous case reports of Cushing's syndrome in infants and children[8, 16, 18, 28, 31, 33]. In the majority of the cases seen at the Squier Urological Clinic, adrenocortical malignancies were found, and in many instances there was evidence, clinical and chemical, of a mixture of ketogenic steroids (glucocorticoids) and androgenic hormones. These patients showed a somatic metamorphosis toward a florid moon face and trunk ballooning, and often there was hirsutism, acne and, in some of the females, moderate clitoral enlargement. In Figures 3, 4 and 5 are presented some of the cases seen at the Squier Urological Clinic and Babies Hospital of the Columbia Presbyterian Center in New York[15].

Since Cushing's syndrome can develop as the result of a disturbance in three different sites, and can be due to hyperplasia or neoplasia, it is necessary to obtain and employ differential diagnostic procedures. These are itemized and correlated in Table IV.

DISCUSSION OF TABLE IV

The common finding in all types of Cushing's syndrome was an elevation of urinary 17-hydroxycorticosteroids. In all, the diurnal variation was lost. However, rhythm in adrenocortical secretion can also be upset by emotional or physical stress[26]. In obese children with slightly elevated urine 17-ketogenic steroids, the question of Cushing's syndrome may arise. They retain diurnal variation and respond promptly with marked suppression of the urinary corticoids with even a small dose (0.5 mg) of dexamethasone[25] (Table IV).

Cortical hyperplasia, being dependent on pituitary activity, produced a prompt rise in urinary 17-ketogenic steroids following infusion of ACTH, whereas tumors, adenoma or carcinoma, being autonomous, showed no response. Dexamethasone, a synthetic corticoid which blocks ACTH, caused suppression in patients with the hyperplasia[25]. However, in normal subjects, Pavlatos et al.[26] found the suppressibility of morning plasma 17-hydroxycorticosteroid levels by 1 mg dexamethasone given by mouth at 11 PM the preceding night to be greater than that in patients with Cushing's syndrome. Dexamethasone had no affect on patients with adrenal carcinoma. Methapyrapone (Metopirone®) caused an elevation of ketogenic steroids in hyperplasia but had no effect on adrenal tumors. The measurable peripheral plasma ACTH was only slightly elevated in early stages, but rose to high levels in later stages (in 12% of the latter, pituitary tumors were present)[25]. An enlarged sella turcica was usually observed in the radiographs of patients with Cushing's syndrome caused by an ACTH-producing pituitary growth; whereas the pituitary bed in cases with adrenal adenoma or carcinoma was usually small. Suspicion as to the presence of a non-endocrine tumor secreting ACTH should arise when positive evidence for adrenal participation is lacking, particularly if the response to the chemicals enumerated above is unremarkable, and certainly if there is radiographic evidence or a positive history of a primary carcinoma of the lung, etc. or of an abdominal mass, etc.

ADRENOGENITALISM

The syndrome complexes of congenital adrenogenitalism are well known. The significance of enzyme blocks in genesis of the congenital type has been established[4]. In Table V, modified after Eberlein[9], are tabulated the progressive stages in the metabolism of intra-adrenal cholesterol which, by means of a series of enzymes in progressive steps, finally yields corticosterol, aldosterone and cortisol (Compound F). Enzyme Block no. 1, fortunately, is rare, because it is incompatible with survival. The condition is a form of congenital lipoid adrenal hyperplasia, and males afflicted with this condition show pseudohermaphrodism[3]. An enzyme block of Δ 5-pregnenolone (Block no. 2) allows accumulation of pregnenolone and development of the type of adrenogenital disease which is accompanied by a

TABLE IV CUSHINGS'S SYNDROME:
TESTS USEFUL IN DIFFERENTIAL DIAGNOSIS AS TO CAUSE

| Pathological Condition | Base Line in 24 hrs | Diurnal Variation | Level of Urine 17-Hydroxycorticosteroids | | | Response to Metapyrapone (Metopirone) S U 4885 750mg/q 4hrs x6 | Measurable Peripheral Plasma ACTH |
| | | | Response to Infusion of ACTH | Response to Dexamethasone | | | |
				Low Dosage 0.5mg/q 6 hrs x4	High Dosage 2.0mg/q 6h x4		
Cortical hyperplasia	elevated	usually lost	marked rise	slight or no suppression	distinct suppression	marked rise	elevated, very high in adrenalectomized patients with pituitary tumors
Cortical adenoma	elevated	usually lost	usually none, rise in some	slight or no suppression	slight or no suppression	none	not elevated
Cortical carcinoma	elevated	usually lost	none	slight or no suppression	slight or no suppression	none	not elevated
Anterior pituitary tumor secreting ACTH	elevated	usually lost	rise in some (due to resultant cortical hyperplasia)	slight or no suppression	distinct suppression	rise	elevated
Non-endocrine tumor secreting ACTH	elevated	usually lost	slight rise in some	slight or no suppression	slight or no suppression	usually none	elevated
Obesity with hypertension	slightly elevated	retained	moderate rise	distinct suppression	distinct suppression	normal rise	not elevated

TABLE V TYPES OF CONGENITAL ADRENOGENITAL SYNDROMES RESULTING
FROM INBORN ERRORS OF CORTISOL SYNTHESIS

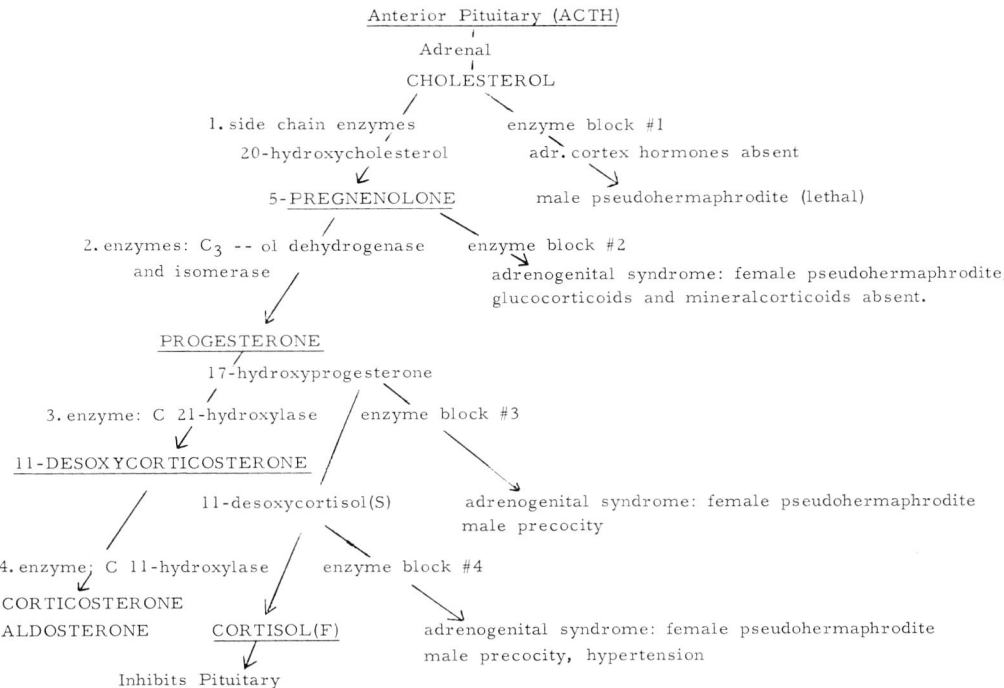

salt-losing component. Enzyme Block no. 3, of C 21-hydroxylase, allows accumulation of 17-hydroxyprogesterone and is the cause of the *most common* form of congenital adrenogenital hyperplasia. Enzyme Block no. 4 (or C 11-hydroxylase) allows accumulation of 11-desoxycortisol, resulting in an adrenogenital syndrome which is accompanied by *hypertension.*

The problem in the management of a patient with congenital adrenogenital disease is threefold.

1. Assignment of sex in neonatal genotypical females with ambiguous genitalia and, later, surgical procedures when feasible or advisable, particularly if an error in sex assignment has been made.

2. Prompt correction and manage-

ment of the salt-losing component, when present.

3. Steroid maintenance therapy.

FEMINIZING ADRENOCORTICAL TUMORS IN MALE INFANTS

The congenital and postnatal adrenogenital syndrome usually causes virilization in females and precocity in males. A feminizing adrenogenital syndrome in male infants is rare. The outstanding symptom is gynecomastia. Some show precocious somatic growths and axillary hair.

Gabrilove *et al.*[12], in a review of feminizing adrenal cortical tumors in males, tabulated four patients. Two were five years old[34, 11]; one was seven years old[24]; and one was fourteen years old[27]. In two, adenomas were present, and the condition improved after operation. One patient with an inoperable carcinoma died, and another boy with a tumor diagnosed as a carcinoma was developing normally ten years after adrenalectomy. Bacon and Lowry[1] report the case of a boy who developed fatal metastases seven years after the removal of a feminizing malignant tumor. (The boy was six years old at the time of the first operation.)

PROCEDURES REQUIRED IN THE ASSIGNMENT OF SEX IN NEWBORN WITH AMBIGUOUS GENITALIA

Since male and female pseudohermaphrodites and true hermaphrodites often have similar appearing genital ambiguities, it is necessary to have a plan of procedure leading to the diagnosis of the true sex or the assignment of that sex in which the genital material at hand can best function. This plan is presented in Table VI.

DISCUSSION OF TABLE VI

It is presupposed that a thorough history and physical examination of the patient has been performed. It is important to document whether hormones were administered to the mother during pregnancy. The status of siblings and other significant familial factors should be recorded. Radiographs of the urinary tracts should be obtained, because, in 10 to 15 per cent of the patients with sexual ambiguities, anomalies in the upper urinary tracts have been found. Having checked the foregoing, the following steps should be taken.

1. Demonstrate the sex chromatin pattern of cells obtained by buccal smear. Karyotype studies may be required in some cases to rule out mosaicism.

2. Recheck genitalia and palpate for "nodules" in the cleft-like scrotum, labioscrotal folds or inguinal regions. These may turn out to be hernial sacs or gonads.

3. Check levels of the twenty-four-hour output of 17-ketosteroids in the urine. (Rise becomes perceptible by the third or fourth postnatal week.)

INFANTS WITH SEX CHROMATIN POSITIVE PATTERN

The external genitalia are incongruous because of: a phallus too large for a clitoris, yet too small for a penis; a urethral meatus which is either of the female type or is incompletely male, i.e. hypospadic; a clitoral urethra *versus* a true penile urethra (this is rare); a small vagina or persistent urogenital sinus; or large or fused labia *versus* cleft or true scrotum. The internal genitalia may show representative elements in varying degree of Mullerian and/or Wolffian elements.

(a) If there is a surprise finding of palpable "nodules" in the labioscrotal or inguinal areas (which may turn out to be hernias or gonads), then the evaluation of the level of the urine 17-ketosteroids will be helpful in determining the type of sexual anomaly.

If the 17-ketosteroids are normal, then the possibility of Klinefelter syndrome, or a true hermaphrodite should be considered. Karyotype evalution is advis-

TABLE VI STEPS IN THE DIAGNOSIS OF TYPE OF ANOMALY IN INFANTS WITH AMBIGUOUS GENITALIA

Sex Chromatin Pattern	Positive				Negative			
"Gonads" in inguino-genital area	Clinically Palpable		Clinically Not Palpable		Clinically Palpable		Clinically Not Palpable	
Level Urine 17-ketosteroids	Normal	Elevated	Normal	Elevated	Normal	Elevated	Normal	Elevated
	(A)	(B)	(C)	(D)	(E)	(F)	(G)	(H)
Types of clinical syndromes	Klinefelter's syndrome true hermaphrodite	congenital adrenogenital ♀ pseudohermaphrodite with inguinal or labial hernias	non-adrenal ♀ pseudohermaphrodite true hermaphrodite	congenital adrenogenital ♀ pseudohermaphrodite "iatrogenic" ♀ pseudohermaphrodite (hormones administered to mother)	♂ pseudohermaphrodite feminizing testis true hermaphrodite	rare type of congenital lipoid adrenal hyperplasia in ♂ pseudohermaphrodites	♂ pseudohermaphrodite with undescended testes Turner's syndrome feminizing testis true hermaphrodite anorchism	like (F)

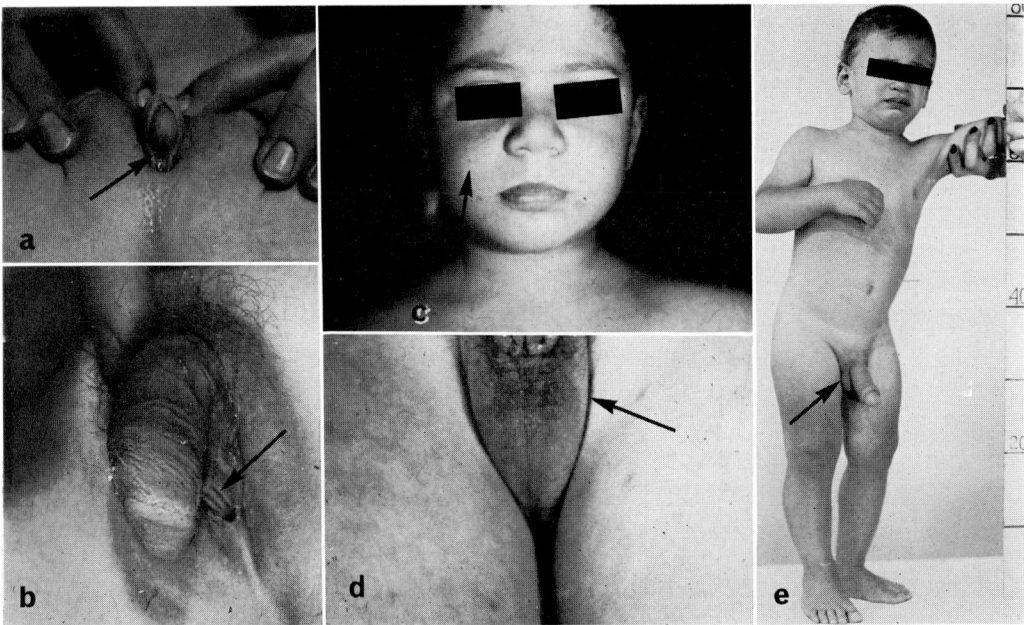

Fig. 7a.   J. L. (591160), in whom clitoral enlargement was first noted at the age of three years, was brought to the Pediatric Clinic of the Babies Hospital when she was 4.5 years old (a). The bone age was that of a seven-year-old girl. Airograms revealed bilaterally enlarged adrenal glands. Portions of the latter were excised and the hypertrophied clitoris subtotally amputated. However, the clitoral enlargement recurred. At this stage cortisone was administered, and for the first time a drop in the urinary 17-ketosteroids was obtained from 14.8 to 2.2 mg per twenty-four hours. A second partial clitorectomy was performed, and treatment with cortisone was continued. Though the patient, now twelve years of age, still shows precocious somatic development and acne, evidence of feminization is noted by the enlarged breasts and the onset of menses.

Fig. 7b.   S. W. (1339565) was brought to the Babies Hospital when two and one-half weeks of age because of bizarre genitalia and doubt as to the assigned sex. Because of the extremely large phallus it was thought she was a male with undescended testes and hypospadias. Note the urogenital sinus. The urine 17-ketosteroids were 3.2 mg per twenty-four hours. The sex chromatin pattern was positive. The pelvis was explored and found to contain a normal uterus and ovaries. The patient was given cortisone and a clitorectomy was performed. Diagnosis: female pseudohermaphrodite due to congenital adrenogenital hyperplasia.

Fig. 7c and d. R. A. L. (1372233) was admitted at the age of three years with a diagnosis of congenital adrenogenital syndrome. The patient had been reared as a boy because of a penile urethra and fused labia which looked like a scrotum. The boy had been completely oriented toward masculinity, and the parents insisted that the child be reared as a boy, in spite of the positive sex chromatin and of the laboratory findings which indicated the presence of the adrenogenital syndrome. A hysterectomy and bilateral oophorectomy were performed as was circumcision. The 17-ketosteroids, which had been as high as 13.7 mg per twenty-four hours before the administration of cortisone, dropped to 0.2 mg per twenty-four hours. Testicular plasticies are to be inserted at a future date. Diagnosis: female pseudohermaphrodite due to adreno-genital syndrome, reared as a male.

Fig. 7e. D. Z. (169930) was first seen at seven weeks of age because of fever, vomit-ing, diarrhea, dehydration and weight loss of one month's duration. The penis was enlarged. Laboratory examinations revealed serum sodium 128, chlorides 119 and potassium 6.5 mEq/liter. The NPN was 85 mg per 100 ml. The urine 17-ketosteroids were 8.9 mg per twenty-four hours. A diagnosis of congenital adrenogenital syndrome with salt-losing component was made. Doca and salt were administered, and later cortisone, as well as antibiotics. The patient, however, went downhill and expired within a week after admission. At autopsy, the combined weight of both adrenals was 15 gm.

able, because mosaicism and/or other aberrations may be present. Biopsy of the "nodules" may show testicular or ovotesticular tissue. If the nodules prove to be hernias, gonads may still be pres-ent, and laparotomy is required to rule out abdominal testes or ovotestes. Mul-lerian remnants in varying degree may also be found.

If the urine 17-ketosteroids are ele-vated, then a congenital adrenogenital female pseudohermaphrodite with in-guinal hernias should be considered. The latter may, in rare instances, con-tain herniated gonads (ovaries).

(b) If the ambiguous external genitalia and groins are *devoid* of palpable nodules, then again it is helpful to eval-uate the level of urine 17-ketosteroids.

If the urine 17-ketosteroids are nor-mal, then a true hermaphrodite or a female pseudohermaphrodite on a non-adrenal basis would seem likely. Lap-arotomy, in addition to the biopsy of the gonads, may be required to estab-lish the diagnosis.

If the urine 17-ketosteroids are ele-vated, then the patient probably has the *most common* type of *female pseu-dohermaphrodism*, i.e., the *congenital adrenogenital syndrome*. It is important to remember that gonadal differentia-tion is completed by the eighth week and ductal differentiation by the fifth month; hence, the earlier in the stage of ductal differentiation during which the disturbance occurs, the less the inhibition of the Wolffian system and the greater the heterosexual dominance (Fig. 7). The history of hormone intake by the mother will aid in the diagnosis

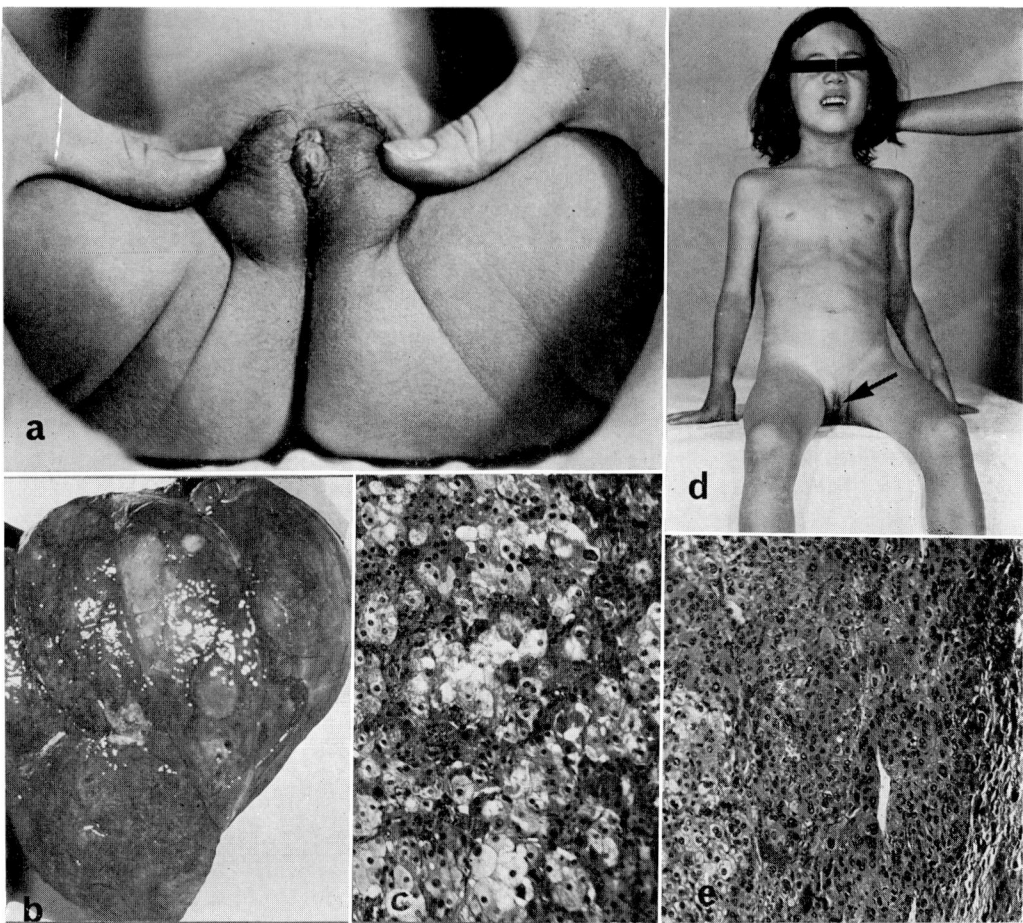

Fig. 8a, b and c.   A. F. (097760) was first seen at the age of four and one-half years because of abnormal pubic hair growth. The child has been raised as a girl, and symptoms of hirsutism and enlargement of the clitoris had been observed for the last few months. The urine 17-ketosteroids measured 23.6 mg per twenty-four hours, and the bone development was that of a girl eight to nine years of age. The airogram suggested the presence of a mass in the right adrenal gland. A right adrenalectomy was performed, and a tumor weighing 15.5 gm was removed. Diagnosis: adenoma of the adrenal cortex. The patient made a uneventful recovery and developed as a phenotypical female.

Fig. 8d and e.   A. F., a four and one-half year old girl whose family physician noted some pubic hair and an enlarged clitoris during a general physical examination which was required prior to her entering school. The parents had observed the change over a period of two months. The blood pressure was 93/63 mm Hg, and the urine 17-ketosteroids were 23.6 mg per twenty-four hours. The bone age was that of a girl of nine years of age. Radiographs revealed an enlarged right adrenal. which was removed. It weighed 15.5 gm, and sections revealed the pattern of a cortical adenoma.

of the iatrogenic type of genital ambiguity.

INFANTS WITH SEX CHROMATIN NEGATIVE PATTERN

The external genitalia are deficient or completely ambiguous and not in harmony with the genotype and may resemble the ambiguities described above.

(a) If the tiny nodules are palpable in the labioscrotal or diminutive scrotum, then evaluation of the urine 17-keto-steroids is helpful in establishing the type of sexual anomaly.

If the urine 17-ketosteroids are normal, then there are three possibilities.

1. Male pseudohermaphrodite with inguinal or scrotal testes which are defective (tiny penis with persistence of the urogenital sinus, vagina, etc.). This is the *commonest type of male pseudohermaphrodism*. Biopsy of the nodules is essential, and decision as to sex assignment will be dependent on the estimation of the probable future competency of masculine apparatus at hand. If the penis is tiny, devoid of a urethra, and the gonads are completely deficient testes, one might consider orchiectomy and plastic surgery on the genitalia, and rearing the infant as a female. If, however, it is surgically feasible to improve the masculine apparatus, then a series of procedures should be planned involving herniotomy, orchiopexy (if needed), correction of hypospadias, excision of vagina and other Mullerian elements. This may cover a period of years. The possibility of a neoplastic change in the dysgenetic gonad should be kept in mind.

2. The syndrome of feminizing testis. The infants are completely phenotypical females and are possessed of external female genitalia, but their gonads show tubules lined by Sertoli cells only. It is advisable to raise these infants as females.

3. A true hermaphordite. Gonadal biopsy is indicated.

If the urine 17-ketosteroids are elevated, a type of congenital lipoid adrenal hyperplasia inducing male pseudohermaphrodism should be considered.

(b) If the ambiguous genitalia are devoid of nodules in the genital or groin areas, then, again, evaluation of the urinary 17-ketosteroids will be helpful in differential diagnosis.

If the urine 17-ketosteroids are normal, then there are five possibilities:

1. A male pseudohermaphrodite with abdominal testes (deficient testes);

2. Turner's syndrome, the presence of a webbed neck or of lymphedema (Bonnevie Ullrich syndrome) are pathognomonic; mosaicism should be ruled out;

3. Feminizing testes (gonads are in abdomen and tubules are lined by Sertoli cells only);

4. True hermaphrodite; or

5. Anorchism (laparotomy with examination of pelvic contents and biopsy of gonadal tissue or remnants are usually performed).

If the urine 17-ketosteroids are elevated, then the infant may be a male pseudohermaphrodite of the congenital lipoid adrenal hyperplasia type with abdominal gonads.

SUMMARY

Three types of syndromes can be caused by adrenal hyperfunction or dysfunction. These are hyperaldosteronism, Cushing's syndrome and adrenogenital disease.

There may be no gross change in the size of the adrenal gland, or there may be bilateral enlargement due to hyperplasia (zonal or nodular) or to neoplasia (adenoma, carcinoma). Zonal correlation with type of syndrome was not always observed. In hyperaldosteronism, the fascicular zone was more frequently involved than the glomerular. In Cushing's syndrome involving the adrenal cortex, it was the fascicular zone which most frequently showed hyperactivity. The histologic picture in the congenital adrenogenital hyperplasia showed fascicular and/or reticular zone participation, while, in the postnatal type with adenoma, the component cells resembled the reticular zone.

The characteristic symptoms, signs and findings in hyperaldosteronism were presented, and some of the cases reported in the medical literature were mentioned.

Cushing's Syndrome can be caused by: (a) cortical hyperfunction and/or hyperplasia, usually bilateral, secondary to excess ACTH from any source (usually the pituitary); (b) an ACTH-producing tumor of the pituitary; or (c) a non-endocrine tumor secreting ACTH (carcinoma of the lung, tumors of the pancreas, thymus, etc.).

A table presenting tests which can aid in the differential diagnosis of the types of Cushing's syndrome was presented. An iatrogenic source of corticoids should be ruled out.

The three important types of congenital adrenogenital syndrome and their causes were presented. The postnatal adrenogenital syndrome was discussed, and feminizing tumors of the adrenal cortex in boys were reviewed.

A table showing three steps in the differential diagnosis of the various sexual anomalies has been presented. The steps are: (a) determination of sex chromatin pattern; (b) determining whether palpable nodules (gonads) are present in inguino-genital areas; and (c) evaluation of the excretion of 17-ketosteroids in the urine.

REFERENCES

1. Bacon, G. E., and Lowry, G. H.: Feminizing adrenal tumor in a six-year old boy. J. Clin. Endocr., **25**:1403-1406, 1965.
2. Bennett, H. S.: The life history and secretion of the cells of the adrenal cortex of the cat. Amer. J. Anat., **67**:151-227, 1940.
3. Black, M. M., and Wagner, B. W.: Dynamic Pathology. St. Louis, Mosby, 1964, Chapter III, p. 71.
4. Bongiovanni, A. M., and Root, A. W.: The adrenogenital syndrome. New Eng. J. Med., **268**:1283-1289, 1342-1351, 1391-1399, 1963.
5. Cahill, G. F., and Melicow, M. M.: Tumors of the adrenal gland. J. Urol., **64**:1-25, 1950.
6. Cavell, B., Sandegard, E., and Hokfelt, B.: Primary aldosteronism due to an adrenal adenoma in a three-year old child. Acta Paediat. (Stockholm), **53**:205-212, 1964.
7. Conn, J. W.: Evolution of primary aldosteronism as a highly specific clinical entity. JAMA, **172**:162-165, 1960.
8. Davies, D. M.: Cushing's syndrome in a child of 2½ years. Proc. Roy. Soc. Med., **46**:307-308, 1953.
9. Eberlein, W. R.: Congenital adrenal hyperplasia. Proceedings of the Post-Graduate Course in Endocrinology. Given at the 17th Postgraduate Assembly of the Endocrine Society, Miami Beach, Florida, Oct. 29, 1965, pp. 53-55.
10. Ehrlich, E. N., Dominguez, O. V., Samuels, L. T., Lynch, D., Oberhelman, H. Jr., and Warner, N. E.: Aldosteronism and precocious puberty due to an ovarian androblastoma

(sertoli cell tumor). J. Clin. Endocr., **23**: 358-367, 1963.

11. Fontaine, R., Sacrez, R., Klein, M., Frank, P., Lausecker, Ch., Stoll, G., and Kahn, R.: Puberté précoce avec developpment des seins chez un garcon porteur d'une tumeur de la surrènale. Arch. Franc. Pediat., 11:417-420, 1954.

12. Gabrilove, J. L., Sharma, D. C., Wotiz, H. H. and Dorfman R. I.: Feminizing adrenocortical tumors in the male. Medicine (Balt.), **44**:37-39, 1965.

13. Geokas, M. C., Chun, J. Y., Dinan, J. J., and Beck, I. T.: Islet-cell carcinoma with hypercorticism. Canad. Med. Ass. J., **93**:137-143, 1965.

14. Greep, R. O., and Deane, H. W.: Cytology and cytochemistry of adrenal cortex. Ann. N.Y. Acad. Sci., **50**:596-615, 1949.

15. Grumbach, M. M.: Some considerations of the pathogenesis and classification of anomalies of sex in Man. Clin. Endocrinology. New York, Grune, Chapter VI, pp. 407-436, 1960.

16. Guin, G. H., and Gilbert, E. F.: Cushing's syndrome in children associated with adrenocortical carcinoma. A case report and review of the literature. J. Dis. Child., **42**:297-307, 1956.

17. Hoerr, N.: The cells of the suprarenal cortex in the guinea pig, their reaction to injury and their replacement. Amer. J. Anat., **48**:139-197, 1931.

18. Jackson, W. P. U., Zilberg, B., Lewis, B., and McKenzie, D.: Cushing's syndrome in childhood: Report of case of adrenocortical carcinoma with excessive aldosterone production. Brit. Med. J., **2**:130-133, 1958.

19. Kepler, E. J., Dockerty, M. B., and Priestley, J. T.: Adrenal-like ovarian tumor associated with Cushing's syndrome (so-called masculinovoblastoma, luteoma, hypernephroma, adrenal cortical carcinoma of the ovary). Amer. J. Obstet. Gynec., **47**:43-62, 1944.

20. Kretchmer, N., Dickinson, A., McNamara, H., and Karl, R.: Primary aldosteronism in a 9-year-old child. Pediatrics, **23**:1115-1124, 1959.

21. Melicow, M. M.: Hyperfunction, hyperplasia and neoplasia of the adrenal gland: A clinicopathologic analysis. Med. Ann. D.C., **17**: 429-436, 1948.

22. Melicow, M. M.: Tumors and hyperplasias of the adrenal gland. In Ariel, I. M., and Pack, G, T.: Cancer and Allied Diseases of Infancy and Childhood. Boston, Little, 1960, Chapter 14, pp. 275-339.

23. Messier, B., and Leblond, C. P.: Cell proliferation and migration as revealed by radioautography by after injection of THYMIDINE-H³ into male rats and mice. Amer. J. Anat., **106**:247-285, 1960.

24. Moiser, H. D., and Goodwin, W. E.: Feminizing adrenal adenoma in a 7-year-old boy. Pediatrics, **27**:1016-1021, 1961.

25. Nelson, D. H.: Methods of evaluating adrenal cortical function. Proceedings of the Postgraduate Course in Endocrinology. Given at the 17th Postgraduate Assembly of the Endocrine Society, Miami Beach, Florida, Oct. 29, 1965, pp. 48-52.

26. Pavlatos, C. F., Smilo, R. P., and Forsham, P. H.: A rapid screening test for Cushing's syndrome. JAMA, **193**:720-723, 1965.

27. Picard, R., Horeau, J., Kerneis, J., Hardy, M., Guenot, U., and Ranger, J.: Tumeur corticosurrenale chez un garcon de 14 ans avec hyperfolliculism. Bull. Soc. Med. Hop. Paris, **68**:72-75, 1952.

28. Silver, H. K., and Ginsburg, M. M.: Cushing's syndrome in an eight-year old girl. Amer. J. Dis. Child., **100**:405-411, 1960.

29. Sabatini, D. D., De Robertis, E. P., and Bleichmar, H. D.: Submicroscopic study of the pituitary action on the adrenocortex of the rat. Endocrinology, **70**:390-406, 1962.

30. Slater, R. J., Geiger, D. W., Leeson, J., and Gornall, A. G.: Aldosteronism and hypertension: The influence of complete adrenalectomy upon essential hypertension in a child. Pediatrics, **23**:1125-1135, 1959.

31. Sobel, E. H., Lee, C. M., Jr., Esselborn, V. M., and Clark, L. C. Jr.: Functioning adrenal tumors in childhood. Amer. J. Dis. Child., **86**: 733-751, 1953.

32. Swinyard, C. A.: Growth of the suprarenal glands. Anat. Rec., **141**:87-97, 1943.

33. Thursby-Pelham, D. C., and Crowe, G. G.: Cushing's syndrome in childhood due to adrenal hyperplasia. Brit. Med. J., **5266**: 1536-1539, 1961.

34. Wilkins, L.: Feminizing adrenal tumor causing gynecomastia in a boy of five contrasted with a virilizing tumor in a 5-year-old girl. J. Clin. Endocr., **8**:111-132, 1948.

35. Zelander, T.: The ultrastructure of mouse adrenocortex: An electron microscopical study in intact and hydrocortisone treated male adults. J. Ultrastruct. Res., May, 1959, pp. 1-11.

36. Zwemer, R. L., Wotton, R. M., and Norkus, M. G.: A study of corticoadrenal cells. Anat. Rec., **72**:249-263, 1938.

Biochemical Diagnosis of Disorders of the Adrenal Medulla and Chromaffin Tissues in Infancy

F. WILLIAM SUNDERMAN, JR., M.D. AND
CAROLYN R. SUNDERMAN, M.D.

Biochemical measurements of catecholamine metabolites in infancy are primarily directed to the diagnosis of three disorders: (a) pheochromocytoma; (b) neuroblastoma and related tumors; and (c) familial dysautonomia (the "Riley-Day syndrome"). Inasmuch as each of these disorders is characterized by specific alterations in the urinary excretions of vanilmandelic and homovanillic acids, principal attention will be focused upon the clinical interpretations of measurements of these catabolites during infancy.

For purposes of orientation, the major pathways of norepinephrine metabolism are summarized in Figure 1, based upon the results of recent investigations[3, 4, 6, 9, 25, 76, 78, 115, 117, 124, 226]. Only 3 to 6 per cent of norepinephrine is excreted in the urine without metabolic alteration, and the remainder is distributed among five or more urinary metabolites[79]. By action of catechol O-methyltransferase, norepinephrine undergoes O-methylation to form normetanephrine[6, 9]. A portion of the normetanephrine is excreted in the urine in unconjugated form and as sulfate and glucuronide conjugates. A second portion of normetanephrine is deaminated by action of monoamine oxidase to yield 3-methoxy-4-hydroxymandelic aldehyde. A fraction of this intermediate is reduced to 3-methoxy-4-hydroxyphenylglycol[8], which is excreted in the urine, but the major fraction is oxidized to vanilmandelic acid. As an alternative pathway, norepinephrine may be deaminated to yield 3,4-dihydroxymandelic aldehyde[124]. This intermediate may be reduced to 3,4-dihydroxyphenylglycol[116], or oxidized to 3,4-dihydroxymandelic acid. A portion of 3,4-dihydroxymandelic acid appears in the urine, and a small fraction is oxidized to protocatechuic aldehyde and protocatechuic acid[199]. The major portion of 3,4-dihydroxymandelic acid undergoes O-methylation to yield vanilmandelic acid (VMA). VMA is the principal urinary metabolite of norepinephrine. VMA is largely excreted in the urine without metabolic alteration, but a small proportion is oxidized to vanillin[214] and vanillic acid[37, 155, 156, 204]. The metabolic pathways of epinephrine are

METABOLISM of NOREPINEPHRINE

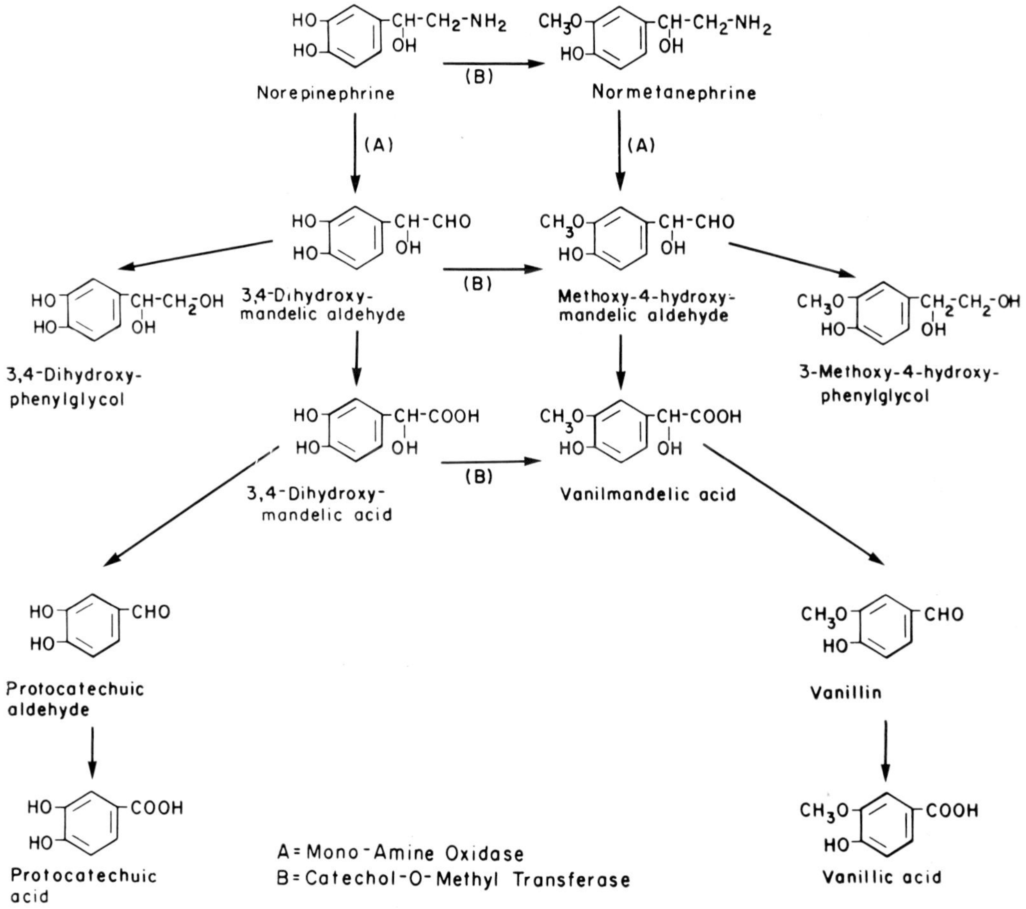

Fig. I

analogous to those of norepinephrine, and lead to the urinary excretion of metanephrine and the deaminated metabolites which are illustrated in Figure 1[6, 25]. In addition, N-methyl-epinephrine and N-methylmetanephrine have been identified as minor metabolites of epinephrine[7, 64, 96, 151].

In patients with pheochromocytoma, increases are observed in the urinary excretion of the catecholamines and all of their metabolites[31, 69, 82, 83, 91, 99, 107,] [108, 120, 152, 161, 192, 206, 207, 209, 239]. Methods have been developed for the quantitative determination of catecholamines[5, 26,] [39, 42, 43, 46, 54, 75, 84, 90, 98, 101, 129, 130, 131, 175,] [176, 187, 224], metanephrines[12, 20, 34, 119, 144,] [160, 183, 211, 233, 235, 236], phenylglycols[160, 233], dihydroxymandelic acid[36, 132, 133, 223, 231], vanillic acid[204] and vanilmandelic acid[2,] [30, 34, 35, 40, 49, 55, 56, 58, 59, 61, 71, 72, 89, 109, 129,] [133, 134, 143, 145, 150, 153, 154, 162, 163, 164, 167, 169,] [171, 195, 200, 202, 205, 208, 210, 225, 227, 232, 237]. In the hands of various investigators, each of these biochemical methods has proven to be satisfactory as a screening procedure for pheochromocytoma. In our own laboratory, quantitative measurements of catecholamines, metanephrines and VMA have been undertaken, as well as qualitative chromatographic separations of the urinary phenolic amines, aldehydes and acids. In our estimation, the measurement of VMA is the most logical selection as a screening procedure for pheochromocytoma, inasmuch as VMA is the predominant urinary metabolite of the catecholamines in patients with pheochromocytoma[31] as well as in normal subjects[78, 79, 122, 148].

The results of several studies have suggested that the primary metabolic disorder in neuroblastoma and related neural tumors is an increase in the synthesis of dihydroxy-phenylalanine (DOPA) and dopamine[14, 16, 24, 121, 140, 177, 186, 196]. Pertinent pathways of the metabolism of dihydroxyphenylalanine are outlined in Figure 2, based upon the results of recent investigations[44, 62–68, 121, 196, 197, 203]. A major portion of dihydroxyphenylalanine undergoes decarboxylation to dopamine; dopamine is then hydroxylated at the β carbon to form norepinephrine. Patients with neuroblastomas usually have increased urinary excretion of dihydroxyphenylalanine, dopamine, norepinephrine, epinephrine and all of the metabolic products of the catecholamines which have previously been discussed[23, 94, 97, 140, 186, 189, 196, 217–221]. These patients also excrete increased amounts of several additional metabolites of dihydroxyphenylalanine and dopamine, which are illustrated in Figure 2, including especially vanillactic[65, 184,] vanilpyruvic[67, 68]

and homovanillic acids. To aid in the diagnosis of neuroblastomas, several analytical procedures have been developed for the quantitative determination of homovanillic acid[41, 139, 158, 166, 168, 173, 198, 229].

The pattern of urinary excretion of catechol metabolites in neuroblastomas is more variable than in pheochromocytomas[6, 47, 138, 202, 217–221]. Numerous investigations have demonstrated that the metabolic abnormalities which are most consistently observed in neuroblastomas and related neural tumors are increased excretion of vanilmandelic and homovanillic acids[13, 102, 103, 104, 112, 113, 114, 138, 177, 203, 228, 230]. The excretion of homovanillic acid is usually normal in pheochromocytomas. Therefore, measurements of homovanillic acid in conjunction with measurements of vanilmandelic acid provide a biochemical means for the differentiation of neuroblastoma and pheochromocytoma.

Familial dysautonomia (the "Riley-Day Syndrome") is a genetically determined alteration in the metabolism of the catecholamines which leads to incapacitating alterations in the functions of the autonomic nervous system[50, 53]. Consideration will be given subsequently to the clinical manifestations and diagnostic findings in this disorder. Although the precise biochemical defects in familial dysautonomia have not been elucidated, the most consistent biochemical findings which have been observed in patients with this syndrome have been increased urinary excretion of homovanillic acid and diminished urinary excretion of vanilmandelic acid[60, 182].

Thus, to recapitulate, in pheochromocytoma there is usually normal excretion of homovanillic acid and increased excretion of vanilmandelic acid. In neuroblastoma and related neural tu- mors there is usually increased excretion of both homovanillic and vanilmandelic acids, and in familial dysautonomia

METABOLISM OF DIHYDROXYPHENYLALANINE

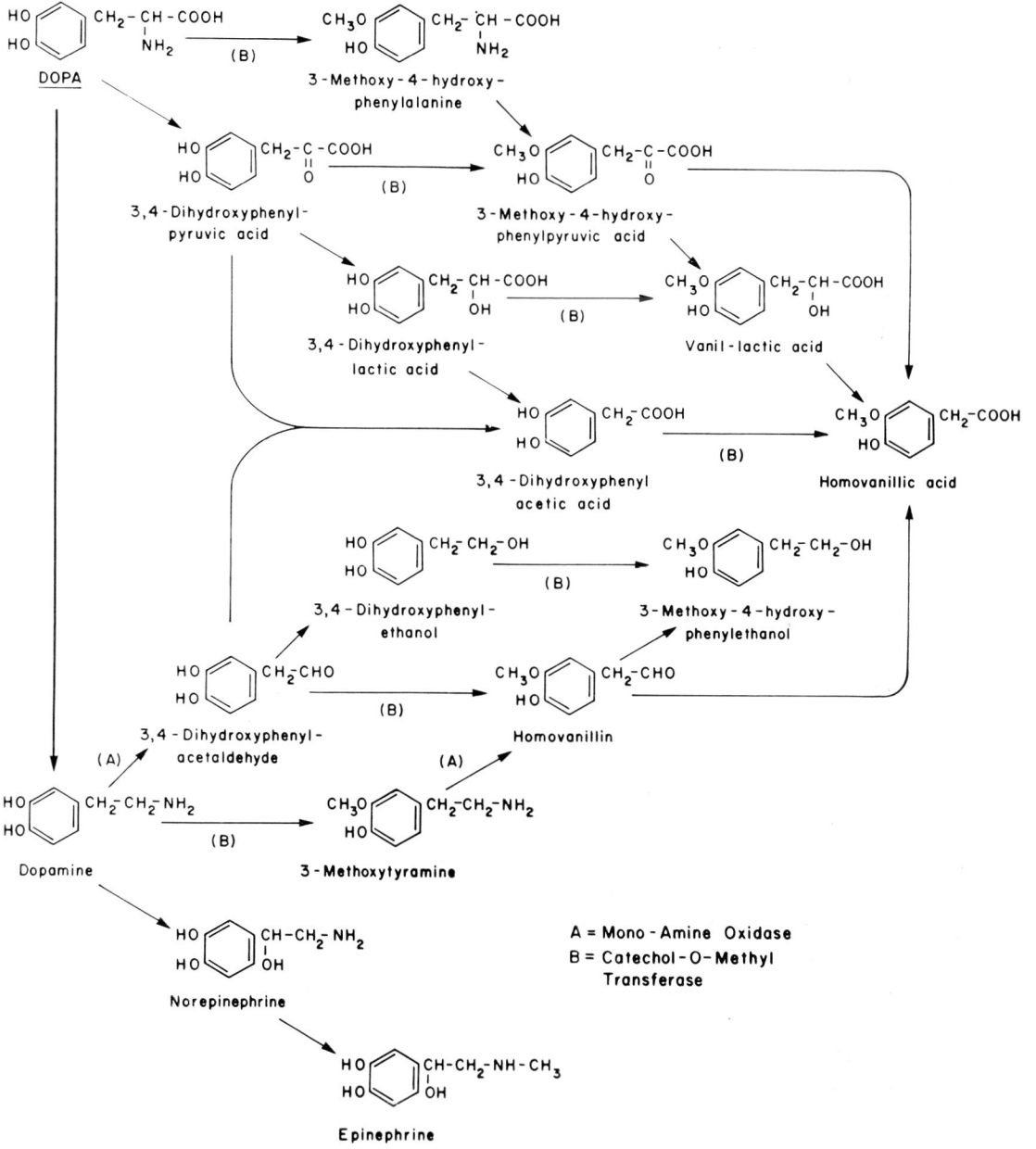

Fig. 2

there is usually increased excretion of homovanillic acid and diminished excretion of vanilmandelic acid.

A specific colorimetric procedure for the determination of vanilmandelic acid was developed in our laboratory in 1960[208]. As shown in Figure 3, potassium the other procedures, the method is entirely specific for vanilmandelic acid. Moreover, the procedure is relatively simple and employs instrumentation which is commonly available in clinical laboratories.

In Table I, the normal values for

DETERMINATION OF VANILMANDELIC ACID

FERRICYANIDE OXIDATION:

Fig. 3

ferricyanide is employed for oxidation of vanilmandelic acid to vanillin. To accelerate the oxidation, one of the reaction products, potassium ferrocyanide, is precipitated as insoluble potassium zinc ferrocyanide. Vanillin subsequently reacts with indole and sulfuric acid, in the presence of concentrated phosphoric acid, to yield a salmon-colored carbonium salt which may be measured colorimetrically. The coefficient of variation of replicate analyses by this procedure is 3.4 per cent, a degree of precision which has not been equalled by any of the other published techniques for VMA. Unlike most of urinary excretion of VMA by our procedure are contrasted with published values obtained by a variety of analytical procedure. There is general agreement between the normal values achieved by paper chromatography, paper electrophoresis, spectrophotometric methods and isotope dilution, although it may be noted that the normal values reported by Woiwod and Knight[232] are higher than those observed by others. By our procedure, the mean excretion of VMA in urine from sixty-eight normal adults was 4.0 mg per twenty-four hours (SD $\pm$ 1.5), with a range from 0.7 to 6.8. The mean

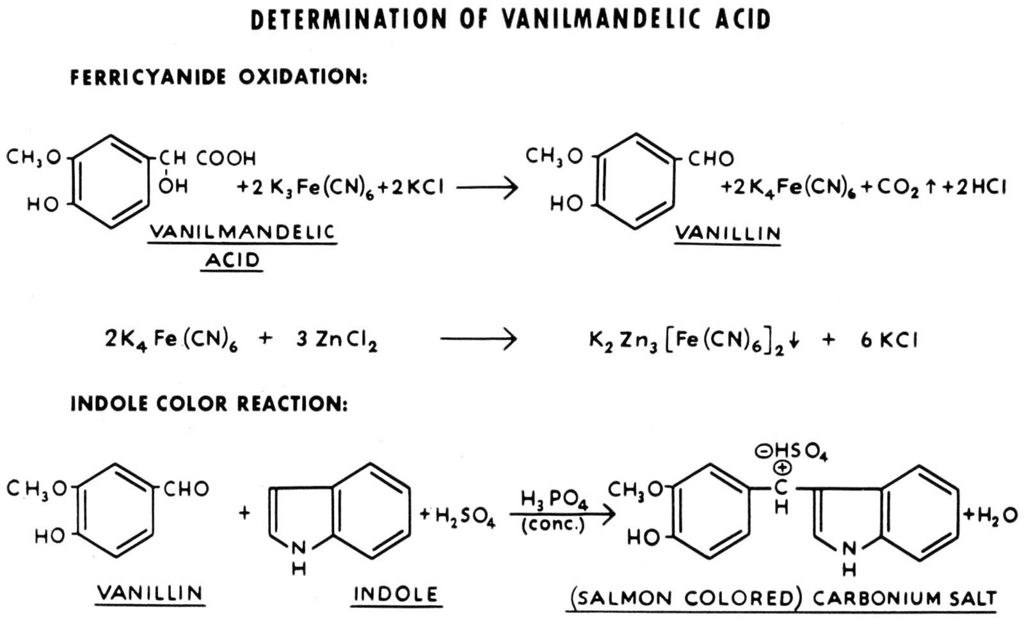

TABLE I NORMAL VALUES FOR URINARY EXCRETION OF VANILMANDELIC ACID

Authors	Year	No. of Subjects	Method	Mean (mg/24 hr)	Range (mg/24 hr)
Armstrong and McMillan[3]	1957		chromatography		2.0- 4.0
Robinson et al.[150]	1959	30	chromatography		1.4- 3.6
Ziegler[239]	1960		chromatography		2.0- 6.0
von Studnitz[195]	1960	62	electrophoresis	4.8	3.2- 6.4
Moolenaar and Graeff[134]	1960		electrophoresis		3.5- 7.5
Sato[167]	1960	22	electrophoresis	3.1	2.0- 4.0
Klein and Chernaik[109]	1961	12	electrophoresis	3.2	1.7- 4.9
Sunderman et al.[208]	1960	68	spectrophotometry	4.0	0.7- 6.8
Sandler and Ruthven[164]	1961	15	spectrophotometry	3.9	2.1- 5.2
Woiwod and Knight	1961	9	spectrophotometry		9.0-17.9
Mahler and Humoller[129]	1962	14	spectrophotometry	5.4	1.8-10.8
Miyake et al.[133]	1962	20	spectrophotometry	3.7	2.1- 5.3
Fellman et al.[49]	1962		spectrophotometry	3.3	0.5- 7.0
Connelian and Godfrey[30]	1964	52	spectrophotometry	4.1	1.7- 7.4
Weise et al.[227]	1961	10♂	isotope dilution	3.7	2.6- 4.6
Weise et al.[227]	1961	14♀	isotope dilution	2.9	1.7- 3.7

excretion of VMA in 1489 hypertensive patients, excluding cases of pheochromocytoma, was 3.9 mg per twenty-four hours (SD ± 2.2), with a range from 0.2 to 10.3[206].

Normal values for the excretion of vanilmandelic acid in urine of infants and children are summarized in Table II, expressed as mg per day, mg per kg per day, and μg per mg of creatinine. Von Studnitz[195] and Zeisel[238] observed relatively increased excretion of VMA during the first week of life, presumably attributable to the stress of parturition and adaptation to the extrauterine environment. Thereafter, there is a pro-

TABLE II VANILMANDELIC ACID IN URINE OF INFANTS AND CHILDREN

Authors		No. of Subjects	Age	mg/day	mg/kg/day	μg/mg of creatinine
Infants						
von Studnitz[195]	1960	6	1st day	—	—	6.3 (5.0-8.3)
Zeisel[238]	1961	8	1st wk	0.27	80	—
Zeisel[238]	1961	7	1st mo	0.19	54	—
Zeisel[238]	1961	8	2-5 mo	0.30	60	—
Gitlow et al.[60]	1965	—	<12 mo			7.0 (1.5-15)
Children						
von Studnitz[195]	1960	10	4-10 yr	2.3 (1.2-3.4)	—	5.9 (3.0-8.0)
Zeisel[238]	1961	10	2-5 yr	0.60	46	—
Zeisel[238]	1961	8	5-10 yr	0.98	40	—
Zeisel[238]	1961	10	10-15 yr	1.30	32	—
Gitlow et al.[60]	1965	—	2-5 yr	—	—	4.3 (1.5-7.5)
Gitlow et al.[60]	1965	—	5-10 yr	—	—	2.3 (0.5-5.5)
Gitlow et al.[60]	1965	—	10-15 yr	—	—	1.9 (0.3-3.3)

TABLE III   NORMAL VALUES FOR HOMOVANILLIC ACID IN URINE

Authors		No. of Subjects	Method	Mean	Range
Adults					*mg/24 hr*
Sankoff and Sourkes[166]	1963	18	thin-layer chromatography	8.2	4.5-15.6
Ruthven and Sandler[159]	1964	18	colorimetry	5.1	3.4- 7.3
Sato[168]	1965	5	fluorometry	5.4	3.7- 7.5
Children, (1 mo to 15 yr)					*μg/mg creatinine*
von Studnitz[198]	1962	12	electrophoresis	16.8	4.0-30.0
Sankoff and Sourkes[166]	1963	6	thin-layer chromatography	14.6	7.3-24.5
Williams and Greer[230]	1963	24	gas chromatography	6.5	1.2-10.0
Gitlow et al.[60]	1965	106	paper chromatography		
(3-5 yr)				7.3	4-12
(5-10 yr)				4.9	0.5- 8.5
(10-15 yr)				2.1	0.5-12
(>15 yr)				1.0	0.5- 2.0

gressive decrease in the urinary excretion of VMA, whether the output is expressed on the basis of body weight or on the basis of creatinine excretion[22, 195, 238].

Normal values for the urinary excretion of homovanillic acid in urine are listed in Table III. The most reliable methods for determinations of homovanillic acid are probably the colorimetric procedure of Ruthven and Sandler[159] or the fluorometric procedure of Sato[168]. By these techniques, the mean adult excretions of HVA are 5.1 and 5.4 mg per twenty-four hours, respectively, with ranges of values from 3.4 and 3.7 to 7.3 and 7.5. Most of the reported measurements of excretion of homovanillic acid in children have been expressed as μg of HVA per mg of creatinine. The data of Gitlow and associates[60] indicate that, during childhood, there is a progressive diminution in the urinary excretion of HVA relative to creatinine.

During the past six years, measurements of vanilmandelic acid have been performed in our laboratory upon urine

collections from twenty patients with pheochromocytomas[206]. Four of these twenty pheochromocytomas occurred in childhood[27, 28, 29, 188]. The preoperative excretions of VMA in urine from these four children are listed in Table IV.

The clinical findings in Patient no. 1 conformed to the classical description of a benign pheochromocytoma of the adrenal gland. Surgical resection of the tumor was complicated by protracted postoperative hypotension, requiring Levophed® infusions for more than forty-eight hours. Such hypotension is generally attributable to the sudden expansion in blood volume which occurs following removal of the pheochromocytoma[19, 85, 100].

Patient 2 suffered from multiple pheochromocytomas involving ten para-aortic ganglia and both adrenal glands. Continued elevation of urinary VMA following the initial surgical procedure indicated the persistence of pheochromocytomas, and repeated operations were necessary to excise all the tumors[52]. Localization of the tumors was facilitated by measurements of plasma cate-

TABLE IV PHEOCHROMOCYTOMAS IN CHILDREN

Patient	Location	Preoperative VMA (mg/24 hr)	Remarks
1. J. M. ♀ 8	adrenal (benign)	12	protracted postoperative hypotension
2. C. T. ♂ 10	para-aortic ganglia° (benign)	21	multiple pheochromocytomas involving 10 para-aortic ganglia and both adrenal glands
3. C. R. ♂ 11	cervical sympathetic ganglion (benign)	11	familial pheochromocytoma
4. C. N. ♀ 11	organ of Zuckerkandl (malignant, with retro-peritoneal metastases)	17	familial pheochromocytoma

°Localized by measurements of plasma catecholamines upon specimens obtained by vena cava catheterization.

cholamines upon samples obtained from multiple locations by venous catheterizations[33, 48, 88, 127, 128, 135, 212].

Several investigators have reported the familial occurrence of pheochromocytoma[28, 181, 215], such as was noted in the family of Patients 3 and 4. This familial predisposition to pheochromocytoma is so noteworthy that, in our estimation, it is advisable to measure VMA excretion in the urine of relatives of patients with pheochromocytoma, in an endeavor to detect latent tumors. Moreover, such a screening program seems to be indicated in patients with von Recklinghausen's neurofibromatosis. Approximately 5 per cent of patients with neurofibromatosis have been reported to harbor a pheochromocytoma[86].

Patient 4 developed a malignant recurrence of a pheochromocytoma which had originally been classified histologically as a benign tumor[29]. Similar malignant recurrences of pheochromocytomas have occurred in five of the twenty patients in our series[17, 206], as well as in other series[57, 73, 95, 137]. In

one patient who is currently being studied in our hospital, local malignant recurrence of an adrenal pheochromocytoma developed sixteen years following resection of the original tumor. Therefore, it is our opinion that patients who have had a pheochromocytoma resected should be followed throughout life by periodic measurements of VMA excretion.

As shown in Table V, the excretion of vanilmandelic acid ranged from 22 to 58 mg per twenty-four hours in urine from three children with neuroblastomas and one child with ganglio-neuroblastoma. In Patients 1 and 2, serial measurements of urinary vanilmandelic acid provided close correlation with the temporary clinical responses which followed surgery, chemotherapy and x-ray therapy. Patient 3 was an infant, three months of age, who died one month after the diagnosis of a neuroblastoma. In the final child in the series, a ganglio-neuroblastoma of the left adrenal gland was resected at the age of one year. The patient received chemo-

TABLE V   TUMORS OF NEURAL CREST ORIGIN

Patient	Tumor	Location	Preoperative VMA (mg/24 hr)	Remarks
1. J. M. ♂ 4	neuroblastoma	right adrenal gland; metastases to peri-aortic nodes and left orbit	58	temporary response to x-ray and chemotherapy
2. L. W. ♂ 6	neuroblastoma	left adrenal gland; metastases to vertebrae	35	died after 5 months despite x-ray and chemotherapy
3. P. G. ♀ 3	neuroblastoma	right adrenal gland; metastases to vertebrae, spinal cord and mediastinum	22	death within 1 month
4. C. P. ♀ 1	ganglio-neuro-blastoma	left adrenal gland	25	presenting symptom: diarrhea; 2-year survival

therapy postoperatively and has survived for two years without evidence of recurrence of the tumor. Although several investigators[80, 81, 157, 190, 191] have emphasized the occurrence of diarrhea in tumors of neural crest origin, Patient 4 was the only one of the children in this series in whom diarrhea was a presenting symptom. No data are given for the excretion of homovanillic acid, since these patients were studied before measurements of urinary homovanillic acid became available in our laboratory.

The clinical and biochemical findings in patients with familial dysautonomia are summarized in Table VI. The clinical findings[50, 53] include alacrimia (lack of tears), sialozemia (profuse drooling), blotchy erythema of the skin, increased sweating, hyporeflexia and disturbance of speech. There is lability of the blood pressure and temperature, and relative indifference to pain. The patients are usually of Jewish lineage. There is equal distribution between the sexes.

Diagnostic reactions in patients with familial dysautonomia include: (a) the lack of an axon flare following intradermal injection of histamine[178]; (b) marked pupillary constriction following

TABLE VI   FAMILIAL DYSAUTONOMIA (RILEY-DAY SYNDROME)

Clinical Findings

Alacrimia   Sialozemia   Skin Blotching
Hyperhidrosis   Hyporeflexia   Dysarthria
Labile blood pressure and temperature
Indifference to pain
Familial inheritance (Jewish lineage)

Diagnostic Reactions

No axon flare following intradermal histamine
Miotic response of pupils to mecholyl
Exaggerated hypertensive response to norepinephrine
Diminished taste perception for sucrose
Decreased sensitivity of respiratory center to CO_2

Biochemical Findings

Increased urinary homovanillic acid (HVA)
Diminished urinary vanilmandelic acid (VMA)
Normal urinary metanephrines (MN + NMN)

Pathological Findings

Vacuolar cytoplasmic changes in peripheral autonomic ganglia and plexuses instillation of 1 per cent Mecholyl®[50, 53]; (c) exaggerated hypertensive response to the intravenous infusion of low concentrations of norepinephrine[180]; (d) diminished taste perception for sucrose solutions[179]; and (e) decreased sensitivity of the respiratory center to CO_2[51].

As previously mentioned, the urinary excretion of homovanillic acid is increased, and the excretion of vanilmandelic acid is decreased in patients with familial dysautonomia[60, 182]. The excretion of urinary metanephrines is within the normal range[60]. Solitaire and Cohen[185] have reported the presence of vacuolar cytoplasmic changes in the peripheral autonomic system ganglia and plexuses in a patient with familial dysautonomia. These authors suggest the use of rectal biopsies for investigating these pathologic changes in patients suspected of suffering from the disorder[185].

The pathologic and physiologic conditions which have been reported to be associated with alterations in the urinary excretion of vanilmandelic acid are listed in Table VII. In addition to the tumors which have already been considered, increased excretion of vanilmandelic acid has been observed in association with retinoblastoma[113], carotid body tumors[38, 70], malignant carcinoid tumors[92, 194], and acrodynia[149]. Increased excretion of vanilmandelic acid has also been reported following parturition[18], surgery[151], burns[40, 151, 195], trauma[151], shock[142], and gravitational[11, 77, 226], thermal[165], and hypobaric stresses[11, 151]. The excretion of VMA is increased following athletics, such as bicycle racing, in amateurs, but not in seasoned athletes[110]. Increased excretion of VMA has been observed following psychological stress in jet pilots[111] and automobile chauffeurs[172]. Passengers on long automobile trips may also develop increased excretion of VMA[172].

In addition to familial dysautonomia, diminished excretion of vanilmandelic acid has been observed in the paraplegia which follows transection of the cervical spinal cord[93, 151], and in malnutrition[87]. In thyrotoxicosis, the excretion of vanilmandelic acid has been reported to be in the lower normal range[125]. Cession reported the excretion of vanilmandelic acid by ten patients during the third trimester of pregnancy to be within the normal range for nonpregnant subjects[21].

Dietary and pharmacologic factors which influence the urinary excretion of vanilmandelic acid are summarized in Table VIII. Several investigators have reported an increase in the excretion of catecholamines following the ingestion of bananas, owing to their content of norepinephrine[10, 31, 222]. Shaw and Trevarthen[174] observed an increase in vanilmandelic acid in urine from an apparently normal person following the consumption of four bananas. The excre-

TABLE VII PATHOLOGIC AND PHYSIOLOGIC ALTERATIONS IN URINARY EXCRETION OF VANILMANDELIC ACID

Increased Excretion

Pheochromocytoma	Retinoblastoma
Neuroblastoma	Carotid body tumor
Ganglio-neuroblastoma	Malignant carcinoid
Ganglioneuroma	Acrodynia

Parturition, surgery, burns, trauma and shock, gravitational, thermal, hypobaric, athletic and psychological stress

Decreased Excretion

Familial dysautonomia
Transection of cervical spinal cord
Malnutrition

TABLE VIII DIETARY AND PHARMACOLOGIC ALTERATIONS IN
URINARY EXCRETION OF VANILMANDELIC ACID

Increased Excretion	Decreased Excretion	No Influence
Bananas	pentobarbital	coffee
Epinephrine	morphine	citrus fruits
Norepinephrine	p-hydroxy-amphetamine	amphetamine
Histamine	Iproniazid	guanethidine
Insulin Shock	phenelzine	α-methyl-DOPA
Reserpine (acute)	reserpine (chronic)	meprobamate
	chlorpromazine	isopropylarterenol
	imipramine	ephedrine
	segontin	angiotensin

tion of vanilmandelic acid did not, however, exceed the normal range.

Numerous studies have demonstrated increased vanilmandelic acid in urine following the parenteral administration of epinephrine and norepinephrine[78, 79, 122, 174], and Resnick[147] has reported increased excretion of vanilmandelic acid following oral administration of epinephrine. Theil and Garcia[213] observed a slight increase in urinary excretion of VMA following intravenous infusion of histamine in normal subjects.

In view of the increase in excretion of catecholamines which follows the injection of insulin[45, 74, 123, 141], it might be anticipated that insulin would likewise cause increased excretion of vanilmandelic acid[136]. Von Studnitz and Hanson[202] observed increased excretion of vanilmandelic acid during insulin shock therapy, but Kaser and associates[105] failed to demonstrate consistent increases of vanilmandelic acid following the injection of insulin in moderate dosages.

McDonald and Weise reported increased excretion of vanilmandelic acid by normal persons immediately after a single intramuscular injection of reserpine[126]. Allegranza and co-workers[1]

observed diminished excretion of VMA following chronic administration of reserpine to schizophrenic patients.

A profound diminution in the excretion of vanilmandelic acid follows the administration of monoamine oxidase inhibitors, such as iproniazid and phenelzine[155, 170, 193, 239]. McDonald and Weise[126] observed moderate diminution in excretion of vanilmandelic acid following the oral administration of chlorpromazine. Borderline diminutions in urinary VMA follow injections of morphine[102] pentobarbital sodium[102] and p-hydroxyamphetamine[201]. Raven and Albert reported diminished excretion of VMA following administration of segontin[146]. Schildkraut and associates[170] found similar depression in the excretion of VMA in patients receiving imipramine.

Guanethidine[234], meprobamate[126], amphetamine[126], angiotensin[216] and sympathomimetic amines, including isopropylarterenol and ephedrine, seem to have little effect upon the excretion of vanilmandelic acid.

In the investigations of Booth and co-workers[15], vanilmandelic acid was not present among the metabolites of caffeic acid, which were demonstrated to include vanillic acid, vanilloylglycine and several related phenolic compounds with 3-methoxy-4-hydroxy substituents. Metabolites of caffeic acid and hesperidin cause interference in the rapid screening procedures for vanilmandelic acid[61], but have not been found to influence analyses for vanilmandelic acid by specific procedures[169, 174].

SUMMARY

A resume has been presented of the biochemical diagnosis of disorders of the adrenal medulla and chromaffin tissues in infancy. Particular attention has been focused upon measurements of homovanillic and vanilmandelic acids in the diagnosis of pheochromocytoma, neuroblastoma and familial dysautonomia.

REFERENCES

1. Allengranza, A., Bozzi, R., and Bruno, A.: Urinary excretion of 5-hydroxyindoleacetic, homovanillic and vanilmandelic acids in schizophrenics taking reserpine and chlorpromazine. J. Nerv. Ment. Dis., 140:207-214, 1965.
2. Anino, J. S., Lipson, M., and Williams, L. A.: Determination of 3-methoxy-4-hydroxymandelic acid (VMA) in urine by thin-layer chromatography. Clin. Chem., 11:905-913, 1965.
3. Armstrong, M. D., and McMillan, A.: Identification of a major urinary metabolite of norepinephrine. Fed. Proc., 16:146, 1957.
4. Armstrong, M. D., McMillan, A., and Shaw, K. N.: 3-Methoxy-4-hydroxy-D-mandelic acid, urinary metabolite of norepinephrine. Biochim. Biophys. Acta, 25:422-423, 1957.
5. Atkinson, R., and Wynne, N. A.: A method for the estimation of adrenaline and noradrenaline in urine. J. Pharm. Pharmacol., 14:794-797, 1962.
6. Axelrod, J.: Metabolism of epinephrine and other sympathomimetic amines. Physiol. Rev., 39:751-776, 1959.
7. Axelrod, J.: N-Methyladrenaline, a new catecholamine in the adrenal gland. Biochim. Biophys. Acta, 45:614-615, 1960.
8. Axelrod, J., Kopin, I. J., and Mann, J. D.: 3-Methoxy-4-hydroxyphenylglycol sulfate, a new metabolite of epinephrine and norepinephrine. Biochim. Biophys. Acta, 36: 576-577, 1959.
9. Axelrod, J., Whitby, L. G., Hertting, G., and Kopin, I. L.: Studies on the metabolism of catecholamines. Circ. Res., 9:715-720, 1961.
10. Barbeau, A., and Wilkoff, L. J.: Fruits, serotonin, and catecholamines. Canad. Med. Ass. J., 80:717-719, 1959.
11. Berman, M. L., and Pettitt, J. A.: Urinary excretion of 3-methoxy-4-hydroxymandelic acid after several stress situations. J. Lab. Clin. Med., 57:126-135, 1961.
12. Bertler, A., Carlsson, A., and Rosengren, E.: Fluorimetric method for differential estimation of the 3-0-methylated derivatives of adrenaline and noradrenaline (metanephrine and normetanephrine). Clin. Chim. Acta, 4:456-457, 1959.
13. Bettex, M., and Kaser, H.: Diagnostic and prognostic value of the determination of urinary output of vanillyl-mandelic acid in tumours of sympathetic nervous system. Arch. Dis. Child., 37:138-141, 1962.
14. Bohuon, C.: Biochemical findings in neuroblastomas. Ann. Biol. Clin. (Paris), 23:779-789, 1965.
15. Booth, A. N., Emerson, O. H., Jones, F. T., and DeEds, F.: Urinary metabolites of caffeic and chlorogenic acids. J. Biol. Chem., 229:51-59, 1957.
16. Brett, E. M., Oppé, T. E., Ruthven, C. R. J., and Sandler, M.: Congenital dopamine-secreting neuroblastoma with clinical and biochemical remission. Arch. Dis. Child., 39: 403-405, 1964.
17. Brown, R. B., and Borowsky, M.: Further observations on intestinal lesions associated with pheochromocytomas. A case of malignant pheochromocytoma in pregnancy. Ann. Surg., 151:683-692, 1960.
18. Brundin, J., and Engstrom, L.: Urinary excretion of free catecholamines during spontaneous and oxytocin-induced labor. Obstet. Gynec., 17:99-102, 1961.
19. Brunjes, S., Johns, V. J., Jr., and Crane, M. G.: Pheochromocytoma: Postoperative shock and blood volume. New Eng. J. Med., 262: 393-396, 1960.
20. Brunjes, S., Wybenga, D., and Johns, V. L., Jr.: Fluorimetric determination of urinary metanephrine and normetanephrine. Clin. Chem., 10:1-12, 1964.
21. Cession, G.: Urinary elimination of 4-hy-

droxy-3-methoxy-mandelic acid in the normal pregnant woman. C. R. Soc. Biol. (Paris), 157:1326-1328, 1963.

22. Cession-Fossion, A., Libotte, G., and Chantraine, J. M.: Urinary elimination of catecholamines and their metabolite, vanllylmandelic acid in normal children. Acta Paediat. Belg., 18:104-107, 1964.

23. Chaptal, J., Jean, R., Crastes de Pauleta, A., and Bonnet, H.: Hyperexcretion of catecholamines and vanillin-mandelic acid in 2 cases of sympathoblastoma. Pediatrie, 18:417-425, 1963.

24. Clarkson, P. M.: Neuroblastoma and catecholamine metabolism. Clin. Pediat. (Phila.), 4:397-403, 1965.

25. Cohen, R. A., Bridgers, W. F., Axelrod, J., Weil-Malherbe, H., LaBrosse, E. H., Bunney, W. E., Jr., Cardon, P. V., Jr., and Kety, S. S.: Clinical Staff Conference of the National Institutes of Health: The metabolism of the catecholamines. Ann. Intern. Med., 56:960-988, 1962.

26. Comens, P., Perry, H. M., Jr., and Schroeder, H. A.: Evaluation of bioassay for urinary catecholamines with strips of rabbit aorta. J. Lab. Clin. Med., 55:748-756, 1960.

27. Cone, T. E., Jr.: Recurrent pheochromocytoma. Report of a case in a previously treated child. Pediatrics, 21:994-999, 1958.

28. Cone, T. E., Jr., Allen, M. S., and Pearson, H. A.: Pheochromocytoma in children. Report of three familial cases in two related families. Pediatrics, 19:44-56, 1957.

29. Cone, T. E., Jr., and Pearson, H. A.: Malignant pheochromocytoma. Report of a case in a 12-year-old girl. Pediatrics, 32:531-539, 1963.

30. Connelian, T. P., and Godfrey, J. M.: The routine determination of urinary 4-hydroxy-3-methoxy-mandelic acid. Clin. Chim. Acta, 9:410-412, 1964.

31. Crout, J. R., Pisano, J. J., and Sjoerdsma, A.: Urinary excretion of catecholamines and their metabolites in pheochromocytoma. Amer. Heart J., 61:375-381, 1961.

32. Crout, J. R., and Sjoerdsma, A.: The clinical and laboratory significance of serotonin and catecholamines in bananas. New Eng. J. Med., 261:23-26, 1959.

33. Crout, J. R., and Sjoerdsma, A.: Catecholamines in the localization of pheochromocytoma. Circulation, 22:516-525, 1960.

34. Dauchy, F., and Giudicelli, J. F.: New methods for measurement of vanilmandelic acid, metadrenaline and normetadrenaline

in urine. Ann. Biol. Clin. (Paris), 23:769-778, 1965.

35. Dauchy, F., and Schwartz, J. C.: Colorimetric measurement of vanilmandelic acid in urine. Path. Biol. (Paris), 10:527-530, 1962.

36. Dequattro, V.: Determination of urinary 3,4-dihydroxymandelic acid. J. Lab. Clin. Med., 63:864-878, 1964.

37. Dirscherl, W., Thomas, H., and Schriefers, H.: Vanillic acid as the end product of the catabolism of adrenaline and noradrenaline. Acta Endocr., 39:385-394, 1962.

38. Duke, W. M., Phillips, M. W., Donald, J. M., Jr., and Boshell, B. R.: A nor-epinephrine secreting glomic tissue tumor (chemodectoma). JAMA, 193:108-110, 1965.

39. Eade, N. R.: Biologic assay of tissue catecholamines. Meth. Med. Res., 9:159-168, 1961.

40. Eichhorn, F., and Rutenberg, A.: A simple low-voltage paper electrophoretic method for the determination of urinary vanillylmandelic acid (VMA). Clin. Chem., 9:615-619, 1963.

41. Eichhorn, F., and Rutenberg, A.: A simple and rapid method for estimating 3,4-dihydroxyphenylethylamine (Dopamine), 3,4-di-hydroxyphenylalamine (Dopa) and homovanillic acid (HVA) with "two-solutions" paper electrophoresis. Clin. Chem., 11:563-569, 1965.

42. Ettman, S. L., and Gordon, H. S.: A shortened screening test for catecholamines. Clin. Chem., 10:959-961, 1964.

43. Euler, U. S. von, and Floding, I.: A fluorimetric micromethod for differential estimation of adrenaline and noradrenaline. Acta Physiol. Scand., 33 (Suppl. 118):45-56, 1955.

44. Euler, U. S. von, Floding, I., and Lishajko, F.: The presence of free and conjugated 3,4-dihydroxyphenylacetic acid (Dopac) in urine and blood plasma. Acta Soc. Med. Upsal., 64:217, 1959.

45. Euler, U. S. von, Ikkos, D., and Luft, R.: Adrenaline excretion during resting conditions and after insulin in adrenolectomized human subjects. Acta Endocr., 38:441-448, 1961.

46. Euler, U. S. von, and Lishajko, F.: Improved technique for the fluorimetric estimation of catecholamines. Acta Physiol. Scand., 51:348-355, 1961.

47. Evans, A. R.: Congenital neuroblastoma. J. Clin. Path., 18:54-62, 1965.

48. Faivre, G., Sommelet, J., Gilgenkrantz, J.

M., Cherrier, F., and Masse, G.: Topographical diagnosis of a pheochromoyctoma by determination of catecholamines at various levels of the venacaval system. Bull. Soc. Med. Hop. Paris, 113:129-137, 1962.

49. Fellman, J. H., Severson, L. J., Robinson, E. H., and Fujita, T. S.: A chemical method for the quantitative determination of 3-methoxy-4-hydroxymandelic acid (VMA) in urine. Fed. Proc., 21:114, 1962.

50. Fellner, M. J.: Manifestations of familial autonomic dysautonomia. Report of a case with analyses of 125 cases in the literature. Arch. Derm. (Chicago), 89:190-195, 1964.

51. Filler, J., Smith, A. A., Stone, S., and Davies, J.: Respiratory control in familial dysautonomia. J. Pediat., 66:509-516, 1965.

52. Fleisher, D. S., Voci, G., Cresson, S. L., and Karafin, L.: Preoperative localization of pheochromocytoma. J. Pediat., 64:711-715, 1964.

53. Geltzer, A. I., Gluck, L., Talner, N. S., and Polesky, H. F.: Familial dysautonomia. Studies in a newborn infant. New Eng. J. Med., 271:436-440, 1964.

54. Georges, P., and Savel, J.: The biochemical diagnosis of pheochromocytoma by determination of urinary catecholamines. Critical study of the fluorometric method. Path. Biol. (Paris), 11:472-479, 1963.

55. Georges, R. J.: A colorimetric modification of the Pisano method for the estimation of 3-methoxy-4-hydroxymandelic acid in urine. Clin. Chim. Acta, 10:583-585, 1964.

56. Georges, R. J., and Small, N. A.: The determination of 3-methoxy-4-hydroxymandelic acid in urine. J. Clin. Path., 15:388-389, 1962.

57. Gifford, R. W., Jr., Kvale, W. F., Maher, F. T., Roth, G. M., and Priestley, J. T.: Clinical features, diagnosis and treatment of pheochromocytoma: A review of 76 cases. Mayo Clin. Proc., 39:281-301, 1964.

58. Gitlow, S. E., Mendlowitz, M., Khassis, S., Cohen, G., and Sha, J.: The diagnosis of pheochromocytoma by determination of urinary 3-methoxy-4-hydroxymandelic acid. J. Clin. Invest., 39:221-226, 1960.

59. Gitlow, S. E., Mendlowitz, M., Kruk, E., and Khassis, S.: Diagnosis of pheochromocytoma by assay of catecholamine metabolites. Circ. Res., 9:746-754, 1961.

60. Gitlow, S., Mandlowitz, M., Wilk, E. K., Wolf, R., and Glick, J.: Excretion of catecholamine metabolites by normal children and those with familial dysautonomia. J. Clin. Invest., 44:1049-1050, 1965.

61. Gitlow, S. E., Ornstein, L., Mendlowitz, M., Khassis, S., and Kruk, E.: A simple colorimetric urine test for pheochromocytoma. Amer. J. Med., 28:921-926, 1960.

62. Gjessing, L.: Quantitative chemical diagnosis of pheochromocytoma, neuroblastoma, carcinoid syndrome and Folling's syndrome. T. Norsk. Laegeforen., 81:1209-1210, 1961.

63. Gjessing, L. R.: Biochemical study of urine in tumors of the sympathetic nervous system. T. Norsk. Laegeforen., 82:1145-1147, 1962.

64. Gjessing, L. R.: Studies of functional neural tumors. I. Urinary 3-methoxy-4-hydroxyphenyl metabolites. Scand. J. Clin. Lab. Invest., 15:463-473, 1963.

65. Gjessing, L. R.: Studies of functional neural tumors. V. Urinary excretion of 3-methoxy-4-hydroxyphenyl-lactic acid. Scand. J. Clin. Lab. Invest., 15:649-653, 1963.

66. Gjessing, L. R.: Studies of functional neural tumors. VII. Biochemical diagnosis. Scand. J. Clin. Lab. Invest., 16:661-669, 1964.

67. Gjessing, L. R., and Borud, O.: Studies of functional neural tumors. VII. Urinary excretion of phenolic pyruvic acids. Scand. J. Clin. Lab. Invest., 17:80-84, 1964.

68. Gjessing, L. R., and Borud, O.: Urinary vanilpyruvic acid neuroblastoma. Lancet, 2:818, 1964.

69. Gjessing, L. R., and Hjermann, I.: Difficulties in chemical diagnosis of pheochromocytoma. Lancet, 2:1014-1015, 1964.

70. Glenner, G. G., Crout, J. R., and Roberts, W. C.: A functional carotid body-like tumor. Arch. Path. (Chicago), 73:230-240, 1962.

71. Godicke, W.: The determination of 3-methoxy-4-hydroxymandelic acid in the urine. Deutsch. Gesundh., 19:1643-1648, 1964.

72. Godicke, W., and Brosowski, K. H.: Isolation of 3-methoxy-4-hydroxymandelic acid from urine by means of the wedge-strip method. J. Chromatogr., 15:88-89, 1964.

73. Goldberg, W. M., and Johnson, A. C.: Malignant pheochromocytoma: report of two cases. Canad. Med. Ass. J., 89:410-413, 1963.

74. Goldfien, A., Moore, R., Zileli, S., Havens, L. L., Boling, L., and Thorn, G. W.: Plasma epinephrine and norepinephrine levels during insulin-induced hypoglycemia in man. J. Clin. Endocr., 21:296-304, 1961.

75. Goldfien, A., Zileli, S., Goodman, D., and Thorn, G. W.: The estimation of epinephrine and norepinephrine in human plasma. J. Clin. Endocr., 21:281-295, 1961.

76. Goodall, M., Alton, H., and Rosen, L.: Normetadrenaline metabolism in man. Biochem. Pharmacol., 13:703-711, 1964.

77. Goodall, M., and Berman, M. L.: Urinary output of adrenaline, noradrenaline, and 3-methoxy-4-hydroxymandelic acid following certrifugation and anticipation of centrifugation. J. Clin. Invest., 39:1533-1538, 1960.

78. Goodall, M., Kirshner, N., and Rosen, L.: Metabolism of noradrenaline in the human. J. Clin. Invest., 38:707-714, 1959.

79. Goodall, M., and Rosen, L.: Urinary excretion of noradrenaline and its metabolites at 10-minute intervals after intravenous injection of DL-noradrenaline-2-C. J. Clin. Invest., 42:1578-1588, 1963.

80. Green, M., Cooke, R. E., and Lattanzi, W.: Occurrence of chronic diarrhea in 3 patients with ganglioneuromas. Pediatrics, 23:951-955, 1950.

81. Greenberg, R. E., and Gardner, L. I.: New diagnostic test for neural tumors in infancy; increased urinary excretion of 3-methoxy-4-hydroxymandelic acid and norepinephrine in ganglioneuroma with chronic diarrhea. Pediatrics, 24:683-684, 1959.

82. Greenberg, R. E., and Gardner, L. I.: Catecholamine metabolism in a functional neural tumor. J. Clin. Invest., 39:1729-1736, 1960.

83. Greer, M., and Williams, C. M.: The sympathetic neurohormones in pheochromocytoma, neuroblastoma and dysautonomia. Trans. Amer. Neurol. Ass., 82:223-224, 1963.

84. Haggendal, J.: Fluorimetric determination of 3-0-methylated derivatives of adrenaline and noradrenaline in tissues and body fluids. Acta Physiol. Scand., 56:258-266, 1962.

85. Hardy, J. D., McPhail, J. L., and Gallagher, W. B., Jr.: Pheochromocytoma: Shock following resection. Notes on mechanism with catecholamine measurements in case during pregnancy. JAMA, 179:107-111, 1962.

86. Healey, F. H., Jr., and Mekelatos, C. J.: Pheochromocytoma and neurofibromatosis. Report of a case. New Eng. J. Med., 258:540-543, 1958.

87. Henrotte, J. G., Libotte, G., and Dresse, A.: The urinary excretion of vanillylmandelic acid in different human populations. Arch. Int. Pharmacodyn., 142:282-285, 1963.

88. Herbeuval, R., Cuny, G., and Masse, G.: The topographic diagnosis of paragangliomas by the plasma catecholamine determination in the vena cava system. Presse Med., 73:77-79, 1965.

89. Hermann, G. A.: The determination of urinary 3-methoxy-4-hydroxymandelic (vanilmandelic) acid by means of electrophoresis with cellulose acetate membrane. Amer. J. Clin. Path., 41:373-376, 1964.

90. Hermann, H., Berger, M., Peyrin, L., Mornex, R., and Vial, J.: Critical study of the determination of urinary catecholamines. Comparison of fluorimetric and biological methods. Path. Biol. (Paris), 9:2229-2241, 1961.

91. Hruska, V., and Duchon, J.: 3-Methoxy-4-hydroxymandelic acid in the diagnosis of pheochromocytoma. Cas. Lek. Cesk., 102:962-967, 1963.

92. Huebner, G. D., and Reed, P. A.: Secreting tumors of chromaffin tissue. Ann. Surg., 158:216-221, 1963.

93. Imhof, P., Hediger, F., and Kaser, H.: The regulation and excretion of 3-methoxy-4-hydroxy-mandelic acid in urine after traumatic transverse lesion of the spinal cord. Helv. Med. Acta, 29:183-210, 1962.

94. Isaacs, H., Medalie, M., and Politzer, W. M.: Noradrenaline-secreting neuroblastoma. Brit. Med. J., 1:401-404, 1959.

95. Isaacson, C., Rosenzweig, D., and Seftel, H. C.: Malignant pheochromocytoma of the organs of Zuckerkandl. Arch. Path. (Chicago), 70:725-729, 1960.

96. Itoh, C., Yoshinaga, K., Sato, T., Ishida, N., and Wada, Y.: Presence of N-methyl-metadrenaline in human urine and tumour tissue of phaeochromocytoma. Nature (London), 193:477-478, 1962.

97. Jacob, N. H., Jr.: Relation of phenolic acid excretion to tumors of neural crest origin. Texas J. Med., 58:893-896, 1962.

98. Jacobs, S. L., Sobel, C., and Henry, R. J.: Specificity of the trihydroxyindole method for determination of urinary catecholamines. J. Clin. Endocr., 21:305-314, 1961.

99. Jacobs, S. L., Sobel, C., and Henry, R. J.: Excretion of 3-methoxy-4-hydroxymandelic acid and catecholamines in patients with pheochromocytoma. J. Clin. Endocr., 21:315-320, 1961.

100. Johns, V. J., Jr., and Brunjes, S.: Pheochromocytoma. Amer. J. Cardiol., 9:120-125, 1962.

101. Kahane, Z., and Vestergaard, P.: An improved method for measurement of free epinephrine and nor-epinephrine with a phosphate-metaphosphate buffer in the trihydroxyindole procedure. J. Lab. Clin. Med., 65:848-858, 1965.

102. Kaser, H.: The value of 3-methoxy-4-hy-

droxymandelic acid for the differential diagnosis of neural tumors in childhood. Schweiz. Med. Wschr., 91:586-589, 1961.

103. Kaser, H.: The excretion of catecholamine metabolites in the urine in cases of sympathetic nerve tumors. Bull. Schweiz. Akad. Med. Wiss., 17:322-328, 1962.

104. Kaser, H., Better, M., and Studnitz, W. von: Further observations on the determination of catecholamine metabolites in tumors of sympathetic nervous system. Arch. Dis. Child., 39:168-171, 1964.

105. Kaser, H., Eberhardt, M., Sellei, K., and Cornu, F.: On the content of 3-methoxy-4-hydroxymandelic acid in the urine under diagnostic insulin loading. Helv. Paediat. Acta, 18:17-31, 1963.

106. Kaser, H., and Studnitz, W. von: Urine of children with sympathetic tumors. The excretion of 3-methoxy-4-hydroxymandelic acid. Amer. J. Dis. Child., 102:199-204, 1961.

107. Kelleher, J., Walters, G., Robinson, R., and Smith, P.: Chemical tests for pheochromocytoma. J. Clin. Path., 17:399-404, 1964.

108. Kirkendall, W. M., Liechty, R. D., and Culp, D. A.: Diagnosis and treatment of patients with pheochromocytoma. Experiences at university hospitals from 1941-1964. Arch. Intern. Med., 115:529-536, 1965.

109. Klein, D., and Chernaik, J. M.: Determination of urinary 3-methoxy-4-hydroxymandelic acid (vanillylmandelic acid") by paper electrophoresis. Clin. Chem., 7:257-264, 1961.

110. Klepping, J., Truchot, R., Didier, J. P., Escousse, A., and Eygonnet, J. P.: Study of the urinary excretion of vanillylmandelic acid (VMA) during exertion as a criterion of capacity of adaptation to muscular exercise. C. R. Soc. Biol. (Paris), 158:2007-2009, 1964.

111. Klepping, J.: Truchot, R., Mounie, J., and Eygonnet, J. P.: Evaluation of the urinary elimination of 3-methoxy-4-hydroxymandelic acid (VMA) in jet pilots during training flights of different types. C. R. Soc. Biol. (Paris), 158:1815-1817, 1964.

112. Kontras, S. B.: Urinary excretion of 3-methyl-4-hydroxymandelic acid in children with neuroblastoma. Cancer Chemother. Rep., 16:443-453, 1962.

113. Kontras, S. B.: Urinary excretion of 3-methoxy-4-hydroxymandelic acid in children with neuroblastoma. Cancer, 15:978-986, 1962.

114. Koop, C. E., and Hernandez, J. R.: Neuro-

115. Kopin, I. J.: Storage and metabolism of catecholamines: the role of monoamine oxidase. Pharmacol. Rev., 16:179-191, 1964.

116. Kopin, I. J., and Axelrod, J.: 3,4-Dihydroxyphenylglycol, a metabolite of epinephrine. Arch. Biochem., 89:148, 1960.

117. Kopin, I. J., Axelrod, J., and Gordon, E.: The metabolic fate of H^3-epinephrine and C^{14} metanephrine in the rat. J. Biol. Chem., 236:2109-2113, 1961.

118. Kough, R. H., Brown, H. E., and Manwiller, C. E., Jr.: Pheochromocytoma: report of 2 cases and a brief review of the literature. Bull. Geisinger Med. Cent., 13:157-162, 1961.

119. Kraupp, O., Bernheimer, H., and Papistas, D.: Isolation and quantitative determination of 3-0-methyladrenaline and 3-0-methylnoradrenaline in urine. Clin. Chim. Acta, 6:851-860, 1961.

120. Kraupp, O., Stormann, H., Bernheimer, H., and Obenaus, H.: Presence and diagnostic significance of phenolic acids in urine in pheochromocytoma. Klin. Wschr., 37:76-80, 1959.

121. Labrosse, E. H., and Karon, M.: Catechol-0-methyltransferase activity in neuroblastoma tumour. Nature (London), 196:1222-1223, 1962.

122. Labrosse, E. H., Mann, J. D., and Kety, S. S.: The physiological and psychological effects of intravenously administered epinephrine, and its metabolism in normal and schizophrenic men. III. Metabolism of 7-H3-epinephrine as determined in studies on blood and urine. J. Psychiat. Res., 1:68-75, 1961.

123. Leak, D., Brunjes, S., Johns, V. J., Jr., and Starr, P.: Adrenal medullary response to insulin hypoglycemia in hypothyroid patients. J. Lab. Clin. Med., 60:811-817, 1962.

124. Leeper, L. C., Weissbach, H., and Udenfriend, S.: Studies on the metabolism of norepinephrine, epinephrine and their O-methyl analogs by partially purified enzyme preparations. Arch. Biochem., 77:417-427, 1958.

125. Levine, R. J., Oates, J. A., Vendsalu, A., and Sjoerdsma, A.: Studies on the metabolism of aromatic amines in relation to altered thyroid function in man. J. Clin. Endocr., 22:1242-1250, 1962.

126. McDonald, R. K., and Weise, V. K.: The effect of certain psychotropic drugs on the urinary excretion of 3-methoxy-4-hydroxy-

blastoma: experience with 100 cases in children. Surgery, 56:726-733, 1964.

mandelic acid in man. J. Pharmacol. Exp. Ther., **136**:25-30, 1962.

127. McGuire, L. B., and Fox, L. M.: Recurrent pheochromocytoma with recognition of site of metastasis by means of venous catheterization. Ann. Intern. Med., **60**:125-130, 1964.

128. Mahaux, J. E., Schaeporyver, A. F. de., Verniory, A., Enderle, J., Smets, W., Reinhold, H., Rood, M. de., and Meunier, A.: Pheochromocytoma with pseudohyperthyroid symptoms. Localization of the tumor by retropneumoperitoneum and by graded determination of catecholamines in the interior vena cava. Ann. Endocr. (Paris), **24**:93-101, 1963.

129. Mahler, D. J., and Humoller, F. L.: A comparison of methods for determining catecholamines and 3-methoxy-4-hydroxymandelic acid in urine. Clin. Chem., **8**:47-55, 1962.

130. Merrills, R. J.: An autoanalytical method for the estimation of adrenaline and noradrenaline. Nature (London), **193**:988, 1962.

131. Merrills, R. J.: A semiautomatic method for determination of catecholamines. Anal. Biochem., **6**:272-282, 1963.

132. Miyake, H., Miyazaki, M., and Imaizumi, R.: Determination of urinary 3,4-dihydroxymandelic acid (DOMA). Jap. J. Pharmacol., **12**:162-165, 1965.

133. Miyake, H., Yoshida, H., and Imaizumi, R.: Determination methods for urinary 3-methoxy-4-hydroxymandelic acid and 3,4-dihydroxymandelic acid. Jap. J. Pharmacol., **12**:79-92, 1962.

134. Moolenaar, A. J., and Graeff, J. de: Experiences with Studnitz's and Hanson's method for determination of 3-methoxy-4-hydroxymandelic acid in urine and its value for the diagnosis of pheochromocytoma. Nederl. T. Geneesk., **104**:1723-1726, 1960.

135. Neimann, N., Pierson, M., Lesure, J., Vert, P., and Gilgenkranz, G.: Pheochromocytoma in a 10-year-old girl. Topographic diagnosis by determination of blood catecholamines at different levels. Arch. Franc. Pediat., **16**:1372-1377, 1959.

136. Otsuka, A.: Studies on the relation of carbohydrate metabolism to urinary catecholamines. 2. Studies on urinary catecholamines and urinary excretion of vanillylmandelic acid under various conditions of carbohydrate metabolism. Folia Endocr. Jap., **37**:977-991, 1961.

137. Palmieri, G., Ikkos, D., and Luft, R.: Malig-

nant pheochromocytoma. Acta Endocr., **36**:549-560, 1961.

138. Petrasek, J., and Dubovsky, J.: Isolation of 3-methoxy-4-hydroxymandelic acid (vanillinmandelic acid) and 3-methoxy-4-hydroxyphenylacetic acid (homovanillic acid) in tumors of the sympathoadrenal system. Cas. Lek. Cesk., **101**:1457-1460, 1962.

139. Petrasek, J., and Dubovsky, J.: Excretion of 3-methoxy-4-hydroxyphenylacetic acid (homovanillic acid). II. Clinical applications. Sborn. Lek., **65**:107-113, 1963.

140. Petrasek, J., Dubovsky, J., and Vich, Z.: Excretion of some catecholamine metabolites in sympathoblastomas. Cas. Lek. Cesk., **100**:1335-1336, 1961.

141. Peyrin, L., Mornex, R., and Pellet, M.: Adrenalinuria induced in the course of insulin hypoglycemia. Method of exploration of the adrenal medulla. Rev. Franc. Etud. Clin. Biol., **8**:271-275, 1963.

142. Piliego, N., and Rossini, P.: Increase of catecholamines and vanillmandelic acid in traumatic shock. Boll. Soc. Ital. Biol. Sper., **39**:603-606, 1963.

143. Pisano, J. J., Crout, J. R., and Abraham, D.: Determination of 3-methoxy-4-hydroxymandelic acid in urine. Clin. Chim. Acta, **7**:285-291, 1962.

144. Randrup, A.: On the differential fluorimetric determination of metadrenaline and normetadrenaline. Clin. Chim. Acta, **6**:584-586, 1961.

145. Randrup, A.: Determination of urinary 3-methoxy-4-hydroxymandelic (vanilmandelic) acid by electrophoresis at low pH. Scand. J. Clin. Lab. Invest., **14**:262-266, 1962.

146. Raven, H. M., and Albert, I.: The excretion of 3-methoxy-4-hydroxymandelic acid in man after segontin administration. Klin. Wschr., **42**:443-445, 1964.

147. Resnick, O.: The metabolism of orally ingested epinephrine in man. Life Sci., **9**:629-636, 1963.

148. Resnick, O., and Freeman, H.: Epinephrine metabolism in normal and psychotic man. Arch. Gen. Psychiat. (Chicago), **6**:388-394, 1962.

149. Ritzel, G., Berger, H., and Roulet, D. L.: Increased catecholamine excretion in a case of acrodynia (Pink disease). Ann. Paediat. (Basel), **198**:81-88, 1962.

150. Robinson, R., Ratcliffe, J., and Smith, P.: A screening test for phaeochromocytoma. J. Clin. Path., **12**:541-543, 1959.

151. Robinson, R., and Smith, P.: Urinary

phenols in stress. Nature (London), **186**: 240, 1960.

152. Robinson, R., and Smith, P.: Urinary amines in phaeochromocytoma. Clin. Chim. Acta, **7**:29-33, 1962.

153. Rosano, C. L.: Enzymatic method for determination of vanillyl mandelic acid. Clin. Chem., **10**:673-677, 1964.

154. Rosano, C. L., and Fiore, J. M.: An enzymatic method for determining vanillyl-mandelic acid. Clin. Chem., **8**:452, 1962.

155. Rosen, L., and Goodall, M.: Effect of iproniazid on metabolism of noradrenaline in man. Amer. J. Physiol., **202**:883-887, 1962.

156. Rosen, L., and Goodall, M.: Identification of vanillic acid as a catabolite of noradrenaline metabolism in the human. Proc. Soc. Exp. Biol. Med., **110**:767-769, 1962.

157. Rosenstein, B. J., and Engelman, K.: Diarrhea in a child with a catecholamine secreting ganglioneuroma. Case report and review of the literature. J. Pediat., **63**:217-226, 1963.

158. Ruthven, C. R. J., and Sandler, M.: The estimation of homovanillic acid in urine. Biochem. J., **83**:30 p., 1962.

159. Ruthven, C. R. J., and Sandler, M.: Estimation of homovanillic acid in urine. Anal. Biochem., **8**:282-292, 1964.

160. Ruthven, C. R. J., and Sandler, M.: The estimation of 4-hydroxy-3-methoxyphenylglycol and total metadrenalines in human urine. Clin. Chim. Acta, **12**:318-324, 1965.

161. Sandler, M.: The laboratory investigation of catecholamine secreting tumors. J. Med. Lab. Techn., **21**:306-309, 1964.

162. Sandler, M., and Ruthven, C. R.: Quantitative colorimetric method for estimating 3-methoxy-4-hydroxymandelic acid in urine; value in diagnosis of phaeochromocytoma. Lancet, **2**:114-115, 1959.

163. Sandler, M., and Ruthven, C. R.: Colorimetric estimation of 3-methoxy-4-hydroxy-mandelic acid in urine. Lancet, **2**:1043, 1959.

164. Sandler, M., and Ruthven, C. R.: The estimation of 4-hydroxy-3-methoxymandelic acid in urine. Biochem. J., **80**:78-82, 1961.

165. Sandler, M., Ruthven, C. R., Normand, I. C., and Moore, R. E.: Environmental temperature and urinary excretion of 3-methoxy-4-hydroxymandelic acid in the newborn. Lancet, **1**:485-486, 1961.

166. Sankoff, I., and Sourkes, T. L.: Determination by thin layer chromatography of urinary homovanillic acid in normal and disease states. Canad. J. Biochem. Physiol., **41**: 1381-1388, 1963.

167. Sato, T.: Determination of urinary 3-methoxy-4-hydroxy-mandelic acid by high voltage electrophoresis. Nisshin Igaku., **47**: 827-833, 1960.

168. Sato, T.: The quantitative determination of 3-methoxy-4-hydroxy-phenylacetic acid (homovanillic acid) in urine. J. Lab. Clin. Med., **66**:517-525, 1965.

169. Sato, T., Wada, Y., and Moebashi, M.: Simultaneous determination of urinary vanillylmandelic acid and 5-hydroxyindole acetic acid. Tohaku J. Exp. Med., **80**:1, 1963.

170. Schildkraut, J. J., Klerman, G. L., Hammond, R., and Friend, D. G.: Excretion of 3-methoxy-4-hydroxymandelic acid in depressed patients treated with anti-depressant drugs. J. Psychiat. Res., **2**:257-266, 1964.

171. Schmid, E., and Henning, N.: On the demonstration of 3-methoxy-4-hydroxy-mandelic acid in the urine. Klin. Wschr., **41**:566-567, 1963.

172. Schmid, E., and Meythaler, C.: Measurement of sympatho-adrenal response of automobile driving with estimations of vanilmandelic acid in urine. Klin. Wschr., **42**: 139-140, 1964.

173. Sharman, D. F.: A fluorimetric method for the estimation of 4-hydroxy-3-methoxy-phenylacetic acid (homovanillic acid) and its identification in brain tissue. Brit. J. Pharmacol., **20**:204-213, 1963.

174. Shaw, K. N. F., and Trevarthen, J.: Exogenous sources of urinary phenol and indole acids. Nature (London), **182**:797-798, 1958.

175. Sheppard, H., and Zimmerman, J.: Increased sensitivity of ethylene diamine analyses for norepinephrine. Nature (London), **194**:578, 1962.

176. Small, N. A.: The fluorimetric determination of total catecholamines in urine. Clin. Chim. Acta, **8**:803-806, 1963 .

177. Smellie, J. M., and Sandler, M.: Secreting intrathoracic ganglio-neuroma. Proc. Roy. Soc. Med., **54**:327-329, 1961.

178. Smith, A. A.: Response to intradermal histamine in familial dysautonomia — a diagnostic test. J. Pediat., **63**:889-894, 1963.

179. Smith, A. A., and Davies, J.: Taste discrimination in familial dysautonomia. Pediatrics, **33**:441-443, 1964.

180. Smith, A. A., and Davies, J.: Exaggerated response to infused norepinephrine in familial dysautonomia. New Eng. J. Med., **270**:704-707, 1964.

181. Smith, A. A., and Davies, J.: Familial pheochromocytoma presenting as familial dysautonomia: A case report. J. Pediat., 65:463-465, 1964.

182. Smith, A. A., Taylor, T., and Wortis, S. B.: Abnormal catecholamine metabolism in familial dysautonomia. New Eng. J. Med., 268:705-707, 1963.

183. Smith, E. R., and Weil-Malherbe, H.: Metanephrine and normetanephrine in human urine: method and results. J. Lab. Clin. Med., 60:212-223, 1962.

184. Smith, P.: Pathological excretion of 4-hydroxy-3-methoxy-phenyllactic acid. Nature (London), 205:1236, 1965.

185. Solitaire, G. B., and Cohen, G. S.: Peripheral autonomia nervous system lesions in congenital or familial dysautonomia (Riley-Day Syndrome). Neurology (Minneap.), 15:321-327, 1965.

186. Sourkes, T. L., Denton, R. L., Murphy, G. F., Chavez, B., and Saint Cyr, S.: The excretion of dihydroxyphenylalanine, dopamine, and dihydroxyphenylacetic acid in neuroblastoma. Pediatrics, 31:660-668, 1963.

187. Sourkes, T. L., and Murphy, G. F.: Determination of catecholamines and catecholamino acids by differential spectrophotofluorimetry. Meth. Med. Res., 9:147-152, 1961.

188. Stackpole, R. H., Melicow, M. M., and Uson, A. C.: Pheochromocytoma in children. Report of 9 cases and review of the first 100 published cases with follow-up studies. J. Pediat., 63:314-330, 1963.

189. Stickler, G. B., and Flock, E. V.: Neuroblastoma and ganglio-neuroblastoma: associated increased urinary excretion of catecholamines. Cancer Chemother. Rep., 16:439-442, 1962.

190. Stickler, G. B., Hallenbeck, G. A., and Flock, E. V.: Ganglio-neuroblastoma associated with chronic diarrhea and increased excretion of catecholamines: preliminary report. Mayo Clin. Proc., 34:548-549, 1959.

191. Stickler, G. B., Hallenbeck, G. A., Flock, E. V., and Rosevear, J. W.: Catecholamines and diarrhea in ganglioneuroblastoma. Amer. J. Dis. Child., 104:598-604, 1962.

192. Straus, R., and Wurm, M.: Catecholamines and the diagnosis of pheochromocytoma. A review and evaluation. Amer. J. Clin. Path., 34:403-425, 1960.

193. Studnitz, W. von: Effect of marsilid on excretion of 3-methoxy-4-hydroxymandelic acid in man. Scand. J. Clin. Lab. Invest., 11:224-225, 1959.

194. Studnitz, W. von: On the excretion of 3-methoxy-4-hydroxymandelic acid in patients with serotonin producing tumours. Scand. J. Clin. Lab. Invest., 11:309-310, 1959.

195. Studnitz, W. von: Methodical and clinical studies of the excretion of 3-methoxy-4-hydroxymandelic acid in urine. Scand. J. Clin. Lab. Invest., 12 (Suppl. 48):3-73, 1960.

196. Studnitz, W. von: Neuroblastoma and catecholamine excretion. Lancet, 2:215, 1961.

197. Studnitz, W. von: Occurrence, isolation and identification of 3-methoxy-4-hydroxy-phenylalanine. Clin. Chim. Acta, 6:526-530, 1961.

198. Studnitz, W. von: On the excretion of 3-methoxy-4-hydroxyphenylacetic acid (homovanillic acid) in neuroblastoma and other neural tumors. Klin. Wschr., 40:163-167, 1962.

199. Studnitz, W. von: On the occurrence of protocatechuic aldehyde in urine. Clin. Chim. Acta, 10:565, 1964.

200. Studnitz, W. von: Comparative studies of 3-hydroxy-4-methoxymandelic acid and 3-methoxy-4-hydroxymandelic acid. Clin. Chim. Acta, 12:330-334, 1965.

201. Studnitz, W. von: Effect of p-hydroxy-amphetamine on catecholamine excretion in man. Acta Pharmacol., 22:172-176, 1965.

202. Studnitz, W. von, and Hanson, A.: Determination of 3-methoxy-4-hydroxymandelic acid in urine by high-voltage paper electrophoresis. Scand. J. Clin. Lab. Invest., 11:101-105, 1959.

203. Studnitz, W. von, Kaser, H., and Sjoerdsma, A.: Spectrum of catecholamine biochemistry in patients with neuroblastoma. New Eng. J. Med., 269:232-235, 1963.

204. Sturm, A., Jr.: Determination and significance of increased urinary excretion of vanillic acid in pheochromocytoma. Deutsch. Med. Wschr., 88:1000-1005, 1963.

205. Sunderman, C. R., Sunderman, F. W., Jr., and Ballinger, W. F. II.: Measurements of serum vanilmandelic acid in a patient with pheochromocytoma. Amer. J. Clin. Path., 43:122-129, 1965.

206. Sunderman, F. W., Jr.: Measurements of vanilmandelic acid for the diagnosis of pheochromocytoma and neuroblastoma. Amer. J. Clin. Path., 42:481-497, 1964.

207. Sunderman, F. W., Jr., and Sunderman, F. W.: Urinary excretion of catecholamines and mandelic acid derivatives. Trans. Coll. Physicians Phila., 27:222, 1960.

208. Sunderman, F. W., Jr., Cleveland, P. D., Law, N. C., and Sunderman, F. W.: A method for the determination of 3-methoxy-4-hydroxymandelic acid (vanilmandelic acid) for the diagnosis of pheochromocytoma. Amer. J. Clin. Path., 34:293-312, 1960.

209. Sunderman, F. W., Jr., Cleveland, P. D., and Sunderman, F. W.: Estimations of urinary mandelic acid derivatives and catecholamines in the diagnosis of pheochromocytoma. Fed. Proc., 19:155, 1960.

210. Sweeley, C. C., and Williams, C. M.: Microanalytical determinations of urinary aromatic acids by gas chromatography. Anal. Biochem., 2:83-86, 1961.

211. Taniguchi, K., Kakimoto, Y., and Armstrong, M. D.: Quantitative determination of metanephrine and nor-metanephrine in urine. J. Lab. Clin. Med., 64:469-484, 1964.

212. Tcherdakoff, P., Idatte, J. M., Alexandre, J. M., Samarcq, P., and Milliez, P.: Pheochromocytomas: Problems concerning clinical and biological aspects, localization and classification. Ann. Biol. Clin. (Paris), 23:791-831, 1965.

213. Theil, G. B., and Garcia, V. C.: The effect of intravenous histamine on the urinary excretion of epinephrine, nor-epinephrine and 3-methoxy-4-hydroxymandelic acid in essential hypertension. Amer. J. Med. Sci., 249:654-662, 1965.

214. Thomas, H., and Dirscherl, W.: 3-Methoxy-4-hydroxy benzaldehyde (vanillin) as a metabolite of adrenaline and noradrenaline. Acta Endocr., 47:69-75, 1964.

215. Tisherman, S. E., Gregg, F. J., and Danowski, T. S.: Familial pheochromocytoma. JAMA, 182:152-156, 1962.

216. Vincent, W. A., Kashemsant, V., Cuddy, R. P., Fried, A. H., Smulyan, H., and Eich, R. H.: Vanillylmandelic acid excretion in labile hypertensive subjects: its variation and response to norepinephrine and angiotensin infusion. Amer. J. Med. Sci., 249:79-85, 1965.

217. Voorhess, M. L., and Gardner, L. I.: Urinary excretion of norepinephrine, epinephrine, and 3-methoxy-4-hydroxymandelic acid by children with neuroblastoma. J. Clin. Endocr., 21:321-335, 1961.

218. Voorhess, M. L., and Gardner, L. I.: The value of serial catecholamine determinations in children with neuroblastoma. Pediatrics, 30:241-246, 1962.

219. Voorhess, M. L., and Gardner, L. I.: Studies of catecholamine excretion by children with neural tumors. J. Clin. Endocr., 22:126-133, 1962.

220. Voorhess, M. L., Pickett, L. K., and Gardner, L. I.: Functioning tumors of neural crest origin in childhood. Follow-up report. Amer. J. Surg., 106:33-35, 1963.

221. Voorhess, M. L., and Whalen, J. P.: Role of catecholamine excretion in diagnosis and treatment of neuroblastoma. Radiology, 83:92-97, 1964.

222. Waalkes, P. T., Sjoerdsma, A., Creveling, C. R., Weissbach, H., and Udenfriend, S.: Serotonin, norepinephrine, and related compounds in bananas. Science 127:648-650, 1958.

223. Wada, Y.: Quantitative determination of 3,4-dihydroxymandelic acid in human urine. Tohoku J. Exp. Med., 79:389, 1963.

224. Weil-Malherbe, H.: The fluorimetric estimation of catecholamines. Meth. Med. Res., 9:130-146, 1961.

225. Weil-Malherbe, H.: Studies on the estimation of 3-methoxy-4-hydroxy-mandelic acid (VMA) in human urine. Anal. Biochem., 7:485-494, 1964.

226. Weil-Malherbe, H., and Smith, E. R.: Metabolites of catecholamines in urine and tissues. J. Neuropsychiat., 4:113-118, 1962.

227. Weise, V. K., McDonald, R. K., and Labrosse, E. H.: Determination of urinary 3-methoxy-4-hydroxymandelic acid in man. Clin. Chim. Acta, 6:79-86, 1961.

228. Williams, C. M.: Biochemical diagnosis of neuroblastoma. Postgrad. Med., 36:A95-A98, 1964.

229. Williams, C. M., and Greer, M.: Diagnosis of neuroblastoma by quantitative gas chromatographic analysis of urinary homovanillic and vanilmandelic acid. Clin. Chim. Acta, 7:880-883, 1962.

230. Williams, C. M., and Greer, M.: Honovanillic acid and vanilmandelic acid in diagnosis of neuroblastoma. JAMA, 183:836-840, 1963.

231. Williams, C. M., and Leonard, R. H.: Microanalytical determination of dihydroxy-aromatic acids by gas chromatography. Anal. Biochem., 5:362-366, 1963.

232. Woiwod, A. J., and Knight, R.: The determination of 3-methoxy-4-hydroxymandelic acid in urine. J. Clin. Path., 14:502-504, 1961.

233. Wolf, R. L., Mendlowitz, M., Roboz, J., and Gitlow, S. E.: New rapid test for pheochromocytoma: urinary assay of normetanephrine, metanephrine and 3-methoxy-4-hydroxy-phenylglycol. JAMA, 188:859-861, 1964.

234. Woods, J. W., and Ajzen, H.: Effect of reserpine and guanethidine on excretion of 3-methoxy-4-hydroxymandelic acid in man. Proc. Soc. Exp. Biol. Med., **114**:107-109, 1963.

235. Yoshinaga, K., Itoh, C., Ishida, N., Sato, T., and Wada, Y.: Quantitative determination of metadrenaline and normetadrenaline in human urine. Tohoku J. Exp. Med., **74**:105-112, 1961.

236. Yoshinaga, K., Itoh, C., Ishida, N., Sato, T., and Wada, Y.: Quantitative determination of metadrenaline and normetadrenaline in normal human urine. Nature (London), **191**:599-600, 1961.

237. Young, R. B., Steiker, D. D., Bongiovanni, A. M., Koop, C. E., and Eberlein, W. R.: Urinary vanilmandelic acid (VMA) excretion in children: Use of a simple semiquantitative test. J. Pediat., **62**:844-854, 1963.

238. Zeisel, H.: Degradation products of catecholamines in urine of children. Z. Kinderheilk., **86**:89-101, 1961.

239. Ziegler, W.: The significance of 3-methoxy-4-hydroxymandelic acid (VMS) for the diagnosis of pheochromocytoma and for a study of catecholamine metabolism. Helv. Med. Acta, **27**:647-651, 1960.

Determination of Vanilmandelic Acid in Urine

F. WILLIAM SUNDERMAN, JR., M.D.

INTRODUCTION

In 1957, Armstrong, McMillan and Shaw[1, 2] reported that vanilmandelic acid (3 - methoxy - 4 - hydroxymandelic acid) is a major urinary metabolite of the catecholamines and noted that the urinary excretion of vanilmandelic acid is increased in cases of pheochromocytoma. Numerous investigators have confirmed these observations and have employed measurements of urinary vanilmandelic acid for the diagnosis of pheochromocytoma, neuroblastoma and related tumors. The metabolic pathways leading to the formation of vanilmandelic acid, as well as the methodology and clinical interpretation of measurements of vanilmandelic acid, have been reviewed in the previous section and in previous publications[3-7].

PRINCIPLE

Pigments are removed from acidified urine by adsorption upon activated magnesium silicate. Vanilmandelic acid is extracted from the urine filtrate with ethyl acetate and is re-extracted from the ethyl acetate with potassium carbonate. Vanilmandelic acid is oxidized to vanillin by potassium ferricyanide at acid pH in the presence of zinc. Under these conditions, the ferrocyanide produced by the oxidation reaction is precipitated as potassium zinc ferrocyanide. Vanillin is extracted from the oxidation mixture with toluene and is recovered from the toluene by re-extraction with potassium carbonate. The carbonate extract is acidified with sulfuric acid. Indole and phosphoric acid are added to develop a salmon-colored complex with vanillin. Photometric measurements are made at 495 mμ. The absorbance of the sample, minus that of a "urine blank" which has not been subjected to oxidation, yields the absorbance attributable to vanilmandelic acid.

REAGENTS

1. *Vanilmandelic acid stock standard.* Fifty mg of vanilmandelic acid (3-methoxy-4-hydroxymandelic acid)[*] are transferred into a 50 ml volumetric flask and dissolved in 0.01 N HCl. The contents are diluted to the mark with 0.01 N HCl and transferred to a glass-stoppered brown bottle. The solution is stored in the refrigerator and discarded after three months.

2. *Vanilmandelic acid working stand-*

---

[*]California Corporation for Biochemical Research, Los Angeles 63, California.

ard. Five ml of the vanilmandelic acid stock standard are transferred to a 100 ml volumetric flask and diluted to the mark with distilled water. The solution is stored in the refrigerator and discarded after one week. One ml of this working standard contains 50 μg of vanilmandelic acid.

3. *Potassium carbonate,* 0.4 M. Exactly 55.3 gm of K_2CO_3 (anhydrous, reagent grade) are transferred into a 1 liter volumetric flask. The contents are dissolved in distilled water and diluted to the mark. The solution is stored at room temperature and discarded after one month.

4. *Potassium ferricyanide* (0.6 per cent w/v). Exactly 0.60 gm of $K_3Fe(CN)_6$ are transferred into a 100 ml volumetric flask. The contents are dissolved in distilled water and diluted to the mark. The solution is stored in the refrigerator in a glass-stoppered, brown bottle and discarded after three days.

5. *Zinc sulfate* (1.2 per cent w/v). 1.2 gm of $ZnSO_4 \cdot 7H_2O$ are transferred into a 100 ml volumetric flask. The contents are dissolved in distilled water and diluted to the mark. The solution is stored at room temperature and discarded after three months.

6. *Ethanolic indole reagent.* Exactly 0.50 mg of indole (reagent grade) are transferred into a 100 ml volumetric flask. The contents are dissolved in absolute ethanol and diluted to the mark with absolute ethanol. The solution is stored in the refrigerator and discarded after one month.

7. *Phosphoric acid,* 85 per cent, reagent grade. The phosphoric acid is stored in the refrigerator so that it is cold at the time of analysis. Occasional batches of phosphoric acid contain aldehydes which produce an orange color in the reagent blank. If the reagent blank is not water-clear, contamination of the phosphoric acid should be suspected.

8. *Mixed indole-phosphoric acid reagent.* One ml of indole reagent is transferred into a 50 ml glass-stoppered mixing cylinder and diluted to 40 ml with cold 85 per cent phosphoric acid. This mixed reagent is prepared immediately before use and kept immersed in an ice bath.

9. *Hydrochloric acid,* concentrated, reagent grade.

10. *Sulfuric acid,* concentrated, reagent grade.

11. *Ethyl acetate,* reagent grade.

12. *Toluene,* reagent grade.

13. *Activated magnesium silicate* (Florisil, 60/100 mesh).*

SPECIAL APPARATUS

1. *Centrifuge tubes,* 50 ml, with ground glass stoppers.**

2. *Aspiration assembly.* A glass Pasteur pipette with a fine bore, 6 in in length, is connected to gentle suction by thin-walled rubber tubing. The rate of aspiration is regulated by digital pressure on the tubing.

NOTE: Steel needles are *not* satisfactory for aspiration because of reaction with ferricyanide.

3. *Water bath,* 37 C, fitted with metal cover.

---

*Florsil may be obtained from the Fisher Scientific Company.

**Centrifuge tubes No. 45168, Kimble Glass Co., Toledo, Ohio. These tubes fit centrifuge cups No. 367 with rubber cushions No. 575, metal shields No. 572, and trunnion rings No. 366, International Equipment Co., Boston, Massachusetts.

4. *Cuvettes,* glass-stoppered, 19 x 150 mm, optically matched.†

OBTAINING AND STORING SPECIMENS

The patient is instructed to abstain from medications and from coffee, tea, chocolate and bananas for two days prior to collection of urine. The twenty-four-hour specimen of urine is collected in a brown glass bottle which contains 30 ml of 6 N HCl. The bottle is stored in the refrigerator during the collection period. The urine may be stored in the refrigerator at 4 C for a least one week before analysis. If the urine is frozen and stored in a deep freeze at -30 C, the concentration of vanilmandelic acid remains stable for at least one year.

PROCEDURE

1. Fifty ml of urine are transferred to a 125 ml Erlenmeyer flask which contains 5 ml of concentrated HCl.

2. Five gm of Florisil are added.

3. The contents of the flask are agitated for ten minutes, using either a rotating shaking apparatus, a wrist-action shaker or a magnetic stirring apparatus.

4. The contents of the flask are filtered through Whatman No. 1 filter paper.

5. Ten ml aliquots of the urinary filtrate are transferred to each of two 50 ml centrifuge tubes labelled "UR" (urine reaction) and "UB" (urine blank).

6. To prepare the standard sample, 1 ml of vanilmandelic acid working standard and 1 ml of concentrated hy-

drochloric acid are transferred to another centrifuge tube and diluted with distilled water to 10 ml.

7. To prepare the reagent blank, 1 ml of concentrated hydrochloric acid is transferred to another centrifuge tube and diluted with distilled water to 10 ml.

8. Approximately 45 ml of ethyl acetate are added to each tube.

9. The contents of the tubes are mixed vigorously for two minutes, either shaking by hand, or with a "Vortex" mixer or wrist-action shaker.

10. The tubes are centrifuged at 2000 rpm for five minutes.

11. The aqueous infranatants are aspirated and discarded.

12. The tubes are recentrifuged for one minute and the drop of aqueous phase which usually collects at the tip of each tube is aspirated.

13. Five ml of potassium carbonate are added to each tube.

14. The contents of the tube are mixed vigorously for two minutes.

15. Without delay, the tubes are centrifuged at 2000 rpm for five minutes.

16. The supernatant organic phases are aspirated and discarded, using gentle suction to ensure a quantitative separation.

17. Two and one half ml of concentrated HCl are added to each carbonate extract.

18. The tubes are shaken vigorously and allowed to stand unstoppered for at least five minutes to ensure complete evolution of CO_2. The carbonate extraction procedure must be performed as rapidly as possible, since vanilmandelic acid is relatively unstable in an alkaline medium.

†Test tubes, glass-stoppered, 19 x 150 mm, No. 45100, Kimble Glass Co., Toledo, Ohio. Optically matched tubes are selected in the laboratory.

19. The laboratory is darkened, extinguishing fluorescent lights and closing window blinds. The specimens should be protected from intense light throughout the ferricyanide oxidation procedure. A small incandescent bulb provides sufficient light for the pipetting.

20. One ml of potassium ferricyanide solution is added to the standard, the reagent blank and to one of the urine extracts (UR). Ferricyanide is *not* added to the duplicate urine extract (UB) which serves as the "urine blank."

21. One ml of zinc sulfate solution is added to all the centrifuge tubes.

22. The contents of the tubes are mixed and those which contain ferricyanide are placed in the 37 C water bath in the dark for two hours. Tube UB is placed in the refrigerator.

23. Approximately 45 ml of toluene are added to each centrifuge tube.

24. The contents of the tubes are mixed vigorously for two minutes.

25. The tubes are centrifuged at 2000 rpm for five minutes.

26. Each aqueous infranatant is aspirated and discarded.

27. The tubes are recentrifuged for two minutes to pack the precipitated potassium zinc ferrocyanide in the tips of the tubes.

28. The drop of aqueous phase which usually collects at the tip of each tube is aspirated and discarded.

29. Each toluene extract is decanted into another 50 ml centrifuge tube with care not to dislodge the precipitate.

30. Using a graduated Mohr pipette, 3.4 ml of potassium carbonate reagent are added to each tube.

31. The contents of the tubes are mixed vigorously for two minutes.

32. Without delay, the tubes are centrifuged at 2000 rpm for five minutes.

33. A 3 ml volumetric pipette is inserted through the toluene layer into each infranatant carbonate extract. The analyst blows gently through the pipette to express the drop of toluene which enters the pipette during its insertion.

34. Three ml of each carbonate extract are transferred to a 19 x 150 mm glass stoppered colorimeter cuvette which contains 0.5 ml of concentrated sulfuric acid. It is convenient to add the sulfuric acid to the cuvettes during step 32. The rack containing the cuvettes is placed in an ice bath. Agitation of each cuvette in the ice bath during addition of the carbonate extract ensures complete evolution of carbon dioxide without excessive foaming or heating.

35. Using a 5 ml Mohr pipette, 4 ml of cold indole-phosphoric acid reagent are added to each cuvette.

36. The cuvettes are stoppered immediately and the contents are mixed by gentle inversion. The cuvettes are not replaced in the ice bath.

37. The absorbances of the cuvettes at 495 mμ are determined precisely five minutes after addition of the indole-phosphoric acid reagent. If eight cuvettes are to be measured in a group of analyses (e.g., standard, blank and three sets of urine samples), it is convenient to add the indole-phosphoric acid reagent at thirty-second intervals. Measurements of absorbance are then also made at thirty-second intervals after a delay of five minutes. If measurements of absorbance exceed 0.8, the analysis is repeated, using 5 ml of the urine filtrate instead of 10 ml. The absorbance of

the standard (50 μg of VMA) should be approximately 0.55.

CALCULATIONS

The concentration of vanilmandelic acid is calculated from the following equation which incorporates the factors for urine dilution and the concentration of the standard:

$$Vanilmandelic\ acid\ (mg/100\ ml\ ) =$$
$$\frac{A\ of\ urine\ sample\ (UR) - A\ of\ urine\ blank\ (UB)}{A\ of\ standard - A\ of\ reagent\ blank} \times 0.55$$
$$Vanilmandelic\ acid\ (mg/24\ hr) =$$
$$\frac{Vanilmandelic\ acid\ (mg/100\ ml) \times urine\ volume\ (ml)}{100}$$

CALIBRATION CHART

A calibration chart is prepared by treating standard samples containing 0, 10, 20, 30 . . . 80 μg of vanilmandelic acid according to the procedure as outlined. The calibration chart should be linear in the range of absorbance less than 0.8.

DISCUSSION

The experimental studies which were undertaken in the development of this procedure are described in the original publication[5]. The recovery of vanilmandelic acid added to urine averages 94 per cent (SD ± 7.6), and the coefficient of variation of replicate determinations is 3.4 per cent. The specificity of the method has been verified by: (a) comparisons of spectral absorption curves of urine extracts with those of purified compounds; (b) screening of related aromatic aldehydes, acids and amines for interference; and (c) chromatographic separations of compounds which participate in the indole color reaction[5].

The urinary excretion of vanilmandelic acid in sixty-eight normal adults ranged from 0.7 to 6.8 mg per twenty-four hours (mean 4.0, SD ± 1.5). In 1,489 hypertensive patients, excluding cases of pheochromocytoma, the excretion of vanilmandelic acid ranged from 0.2 to 10.3 mg per twenty-four hours (mean 3.9, SD ± 2.2)[6].

The colorimetric method for the determination of vanilmandelic acid has been adapted for the measurements of vanilmandelic acid in the serum of a patient with pheochromocytoma[7]. By means of intravascular catheterization, specimens of blood were obtained simultaneously from several locations in the vasculature. The highest concentration of serum vanilmandelic acid (47 μg per 100 ml) was present in the sample from the inferior vena cava at the level of the hepatic veins. The lowest concentration of serum vanilmandelic acid (18 μg per 100 ml) was found in the sample from the inferior vena cava at the level of the adrenal veins. Intermediate concentrations were found in samples from the superior vena cava and from the femoral artery, averaging 42 and 35 μg per 100 ml, respectively. These observations support the hypothesis that the liver is a major site for the catabolism of catecholamines to vanilmandelic acid. The limit of detection of vanilmandelic acid in serum is approximately 5 μg per 100 ml. Serums from normal persons do not contain detectable concentrations of vanilmandelic acid.

REFERENCES

1. Armstrong, M. D., and McMillan, A.: Identification of a major urinary metabolite of norepinephrine. Fed. Proc., **16**:146, 1957.

2. Armstrong, M. D., McMillan, A., and Shaw, K. N.: 3-Methoxy-4-hydroxy-D-mandelic acid, an urinary metabolite of norepinephrine. Biochim. Biophys. Acta, **25**:422-423, 1957.

3. Sunderman, F. W., Jr., and Sunderman, F. W.: Urinary excretion of catecholamines and mandelic acid derivatives. Trans. Coll. Physicians Phila., **27**:222, 1960.

4. Sunderman, F. W., Jr., Cleveland, P. D., and Sunderman, F. W.: Estimations of urinary mandelic acid derivatives and catecholamines in the diagnosis of pheochromocytoma. Fed. Proc., **19**:115, 1960.

5. Sunderman, F. W., Jr., Cleveland, P. D., Law, N. C., and Sunderman, F. W.: A method for the determination of 3-methoxy-4-hydroxy-mandelic acid (vanilmandelic acid) for the diagnosis of pheochromocytoma. Amer. J. Clin. Path., **34**:293-311, 1960.

6. Sunderman, F. W., Jr.: Measurements of vanilmandelic acid for the diagnosis of pheochromocytoma and neuroblastoma. Amer J. Clin. Path., **42**:481-497, 1964.

7. Sunderman, C. R., Sunderman, F. W., Jr., and Ballinger, W. F., II.: Measurements of serum vanilmandelic acid in a patient with pheochromocytoma. Amer. J. Clin. Path., **43**:121-129, 1965.

Chapter 19

Classification of Sexual Abnormalities in Infancy and Childhood:

Based on a Periodic Table of Sexual Development

MEYER M. MELICOW, M.D.

Sex chromosomal aberrations, gonadal alterations and deficiencies, genital ambiguities, geno-phenotypical incongruities and gender role deviations in varying degree are not uncommon[59, 18, 24, 30]. In the young, early recognition and judicious management of the abnormalities are vital to prevent subsequent physical, psychic and emotional inadequacies, malfunctions and maladjustments[33, 47]. This may be difficult, particularly in the newborn, because many intersexes resemble one another superficially, regardless of cause (Fig. 1). Careful investigation, however, will often reveal certain features in the anomalous structures which, when viewed in the light of the genotype and phenotype, aid in differential diagnosis and management. The severity and character of the somato-sexual abnormality varies primarily with the stage, or period of fetal and/or postnatal development, during which the damage

occurs, and subsequently with the age period when correction is sought. Awareness of such a cause and effect in time relationship, i.e., a *periodic table*, should guide one in selecting those tests essential for correct diagnosis and institution of adequate therapy.

What are these periods? Before answering this question, it should be emphasized that somato-sexual development is normally a variable continuum. There are, however, critical loci in time when a calamitous event can modify significantly and characteristically, the appearance of the end product. These are the stages, or periods, as presented in chronological order in Table I.

DISCUSSION OF TABLE I

Sex chromosomes carry the master plan or blueprint for sexual development[46]. They play a determinant role during the process of meiosis, later, during syngamy, and subsequently,

267

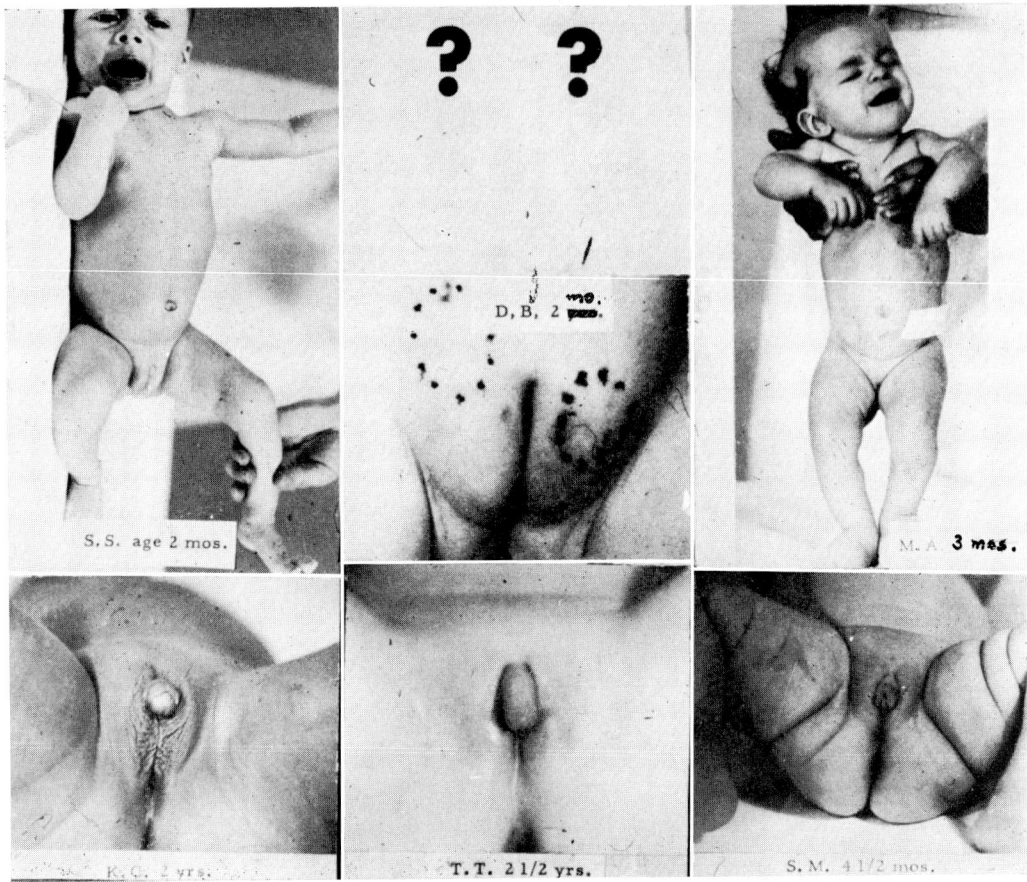

Fig. I. Diagnosis please? These infants presented with ambiguous genitalia, and sex was in doubt. See end of chapter for the result of the examination and tests which led to the decision as to the assigned sex.

when the blastomeres multiply. This is the *chromosomal period* of sexual development, and any error during this stage will result in sexual anomalies which are included in the first group of Table II. At syngamy, the future differentiation of the bipotential gonad is determined which, in normal course, means induction of the medulla in xy, and of the cortex in xx embryos. Differentiation of the selected zone then follows with inhibition of the opposing zone. The totipotent germ cells migrate to the genital ridge and, in the gonad, become the primitive sex cells, i.e., the

future spermatogones, if within the medulla; or ovocytes, if in the cortex. This is the *gonadal period* of sexual development, and any abnormalities during this stage can cause sexual anomalies which comprise the second group of Table II. It is, of course, possible that an abnormal gene in the sex chromosome can cause gonadal anomalies, but it is the gonadal defect which is responsible for the ductal and genital abnormalities.

Following induction of the bipotential gonad and its organization and development into a normal testis (or

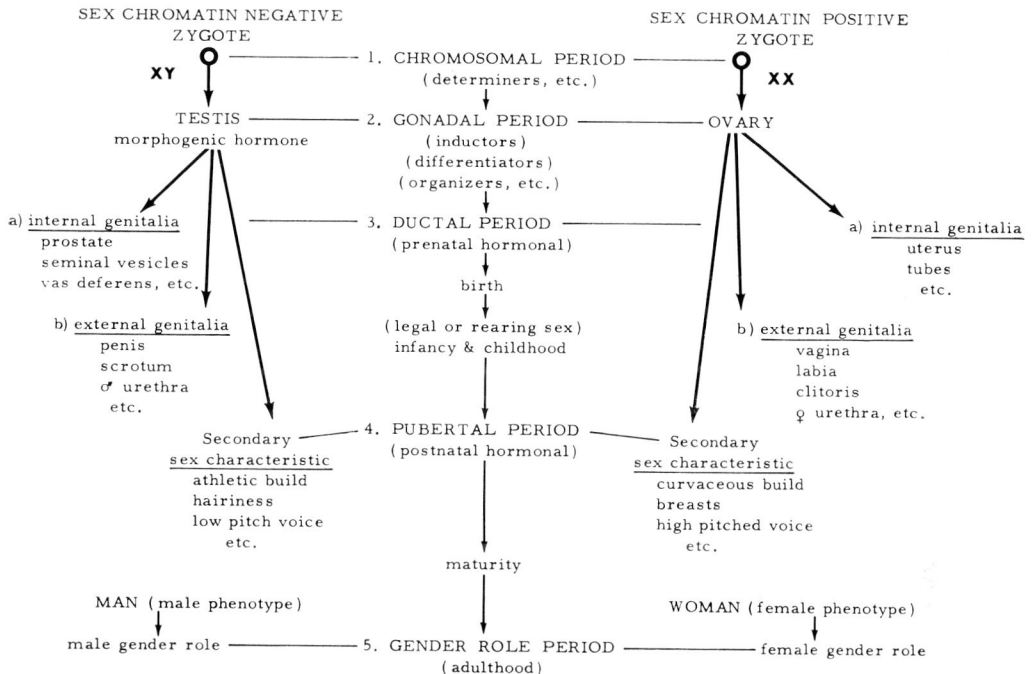

TABLE I NORMAL SEXUAL DEVELOPMENT

ovary), the differentiation of the bisexual ducts and external genitalia is determined[61]. In the normal course, this means induction and differentiation of the Wolffian ducts and male external genitalia in the presence of a testis, for which the latter elaborates a morphogenic hormone, and of the Mullerian ducts and female external genitalia in the presence of an ovary. This is the *ductal period* (or prenatal hormonal), and any disturbance during this stage induces alterations which are included in the third group of Table II. The morphogenic hormone of the testis probably aids in its descent.

At birth, the configuration of the external genitalia usually influences the decision as to the assigned, legal or nursery sex. From birth through infancy and childhood there is normally an interlude in sexual differentiation, and somatic growth is predominant. Thus, this is a relatively negative period as far as sexual development is concerned; however, sexual precocity due to gonadal hyperfunction, dysfunction or neoplasia may occur. Disturbances in other endocrine organs, some types of neoplasms and lesions in the cerebrum or cerebellum can also affect sexual maturation.

The next stage is the *puberal* or *postnatal hormonal period,* and now secretions of the pituitary, thyroid, adrenal, etc., as well as those from the gonads, further sexual development, culminating in maturity. A variety of endocrine dyscrasias during this stage can cause sexual abnormalities, some of which are listed under the fourth group in Table II.

TABLE II PERIODIC TABLE OF ABNORMAL SEXUAL DEVELOPMENT

I. Chromosomal Period

Abnormality in number, morphology, etc. of sex chromosomes.
Effect is direct on gonads, indirect on ducts, ultimately on phenotype.

    A. Turner's syndrome: 44 autosomes + xo sex chromosomes, total 45

    B. Klinefelter's syndrome: 44 autosomes + triple chromosomes, total 47

    C. Mosaicism and variations of A and B

    D. Klinefelter's plus mongolism: trisomy at 21 autosome, + XXY, etc.

II. Gonadal Period

Abnormality is due to zonal or total, unilateral or bilateral inhibition, deficiency or ablation. Affects not only function of gonads, but also development of ducts and external genitalia. *Is the commonest cause of male pseudohermaphroditism.*

    A. True hermaphrodites: ovotestes, etc.

    B. Male pseudohermaphrodites(deficient "males")

        1. Testes: mild to severe deficiency or morphogenic hormone

            a. Cryptorchism

            b. Ambigous internal and external genitalia

            c. "Feminizing" testes

            d. Anorchism, etc.

    C. Deficient females: mild to severe ovarian damage

            a. Cystic ovaries

            b. Dysgenetic ovaries, etc.

III. Ductal Period (prenatal hormonal)

Abnormality is due to hormonal dyscrasia with inhibition of isosexual and stimulation of heterosexual ducts. Affects not only sex ducts but also external genitalia. *Is the commonest cause of female pseudohermaphroditism.*

    A. Female pseudohermaphrodites:

        1. Congenital adrenal hyperplasia

            a. Virilism and salt-losing component

            b. Virilism only

            c. Virilism and hypertension

        2. Congenital (maternal) arrhenoblastoma

        3. Iatrogenic masculinizing hormones administered during pregnancy, etc.

    B. Male pseudohermaphrodites: rare type of congenital adrenal hyperplasia with feminization

IV. Pubertal Period (postnatal hormonal)

Abnormality is due to postnatal altered, or excessive androgen or estrogen production. Effects varies with age of onset and involves mainly external genitalia and secondary sex characteristic.

    A. During infancy and childhood

        1. In girls

            a. Isosexual precocity

                Constitutional, familial or racial

                Granulosa cell tumor of ovary,

                Tumors of central nervous system, etc.

      b. Heterosexual change

          Postnatal adrenal hyperplasia, adenoma or carcinoma

          Arrhenoblastoma

          Cystic disease of ovaries (Stein-Leventhal syndrome) etc.

      c. Isosexual retardation

          Constitutional, etc.

          Bilateral oophoritis, mumps, etc.

          Bilateral oophorectomy

          Deficiency of pituitary, thyroid etc.

          Obesity, etc.

  2. In boys

      a. Isosexual precocity

          Constitutional, familial or racial

          Postnatal adrenal hyperplasia, adenoma or carcinoma

          Interstitial cell tumors of testis

          Tumor of pineal, or C.N.S., or liver, etc.

      b. Eunuchoid

          Constitutional, etc.

          Bilateral orchitis, mumps, etc.

          Bilateral orchitis, orchiectomy

          (?) Sertoli cell tumor

          Deficiency: pituitary (Froehlich Syndrome), thyroid, etc.

          Obesity, etc.

B. During puberty and onset of adulthood

  1. Women: same as in A1

  2. Men: same as A2

      Adrenal cortical tumor may be feminizing

      Interstitial cell tumor may be feminizing

      Gynandroblastoma, etc.

V. Gender Role Period

Abnormality is in sex gender role behavior and may be contrary to phenotypic sex. Causes are deep seated and frequently in psycho-emotional sphere.

A. In men

  1. Impotentia (rule out diabetes, etc.)

  2. Homosexuality

  3. Abnormal sexual gratification

  4. Satyriasis

  5. Transvestism, transsexualism, etc.

B. In women

  1. Frigidity

  2. Homosexuality

  3. Abnormal sexual gratification

  4. Nymphomania

  5. Transvestism, transsexualism, etc.

At maturity, the phenotypical man and phenotypical woman finally emerge (phenotypic sex). The *gender role period* now becomes manifest and normally is heterosexual. Gender role is the summation and crystallization of hormonal factors plus the influence of environment, training, sex customs, mores, psycho-emotional experiences, etc. Some of the aberrations and deviations during this stage of sexual function are mentioned in the fifth group of Table II. It is important to emphasize that the periods in normal sexual development are not self-contained, but overlap.

DISCUSSION OF TABLE II

It is not our purpose to review in detail or itemize *all* of the varieties and multitudinous errors in sexual development. The field of cytogenetics, for example, has become quite complex, with an ever-growing, at times baffling terminology, particularly for chromosomal aberrations[18]. Our object is to call attention to the more common ambiguities which one may be called upon to diagnose and correct, and, wherever possible, to establish the period during which the calamitous viral, radiant, chemical, vascular, anoxic, apoplectic, etc. event occurred which disturbed, damaged or destroyed the determiners, inductors, organizers, differentiators, etc. It is felt that this concept will aid in carrying out measures which would lead to early diagnosis and to the institution of logical, adequate corrective procedures. Classification is by no means complete; there is no sharp line of demarcation between adjacent periods; and, in regard to some of the syndromes, opinions and postulates vary as to the

time during fetal development when the trouble occurred. Nevertheless, a plan, however wanting, is needed in order to find one's way through this hazy maze of sexual anomalies. Such a plan has been presented in Table II. For some of the tests and procedures in differential diagnosis and for corrective measures, see Table III.

Sexual abnormalities resulting from errors occurring during the chromosomal period are due to defects in the sex chromosomes and, at times, the autosomes. Thus, the effect is profound and widespread. It is direct on the gonads, indirect on the ducts, external genitalia and eventually the phenotype, and can result in "asexuality," or sex "reversal," etc.

Turner's Syndrome (Fig. 2)

The phenotype is at variance with the nuclear sex chromatin. The patients appear feminine, yet their nuclear sex shows a negative or male (xy) pattern. This is suggestive of sex reversal; however, the karyotype often reveals forty-four autosomes and only one sex chromosome. Thus, these patients are really xo and possess only forty-five chromosomes. Lacking an additional x or a y, they are probably neither male nor female (asexual). In some, mosaicism (xo/xx, xo/xxx, etc.) has been found. In extreme degree types, gonadal and ductal tissues do not develop (agenesis). In many cases, however, a remnant of gonadal tissue (a "knob" or "streak") of indeterminate character (gonadal dysgenesis or dysplasia) is present; while, in a few, other hypoplastic Mullerian elements (infantile uterus and/or adnexa) may be found. Germinal cell aplasia[10, 38] is the common denominator.

TABLE III STEPS IN THE DIAGNOSIS OF TYPE OF SEXUAL ANOMALY
IN INFANTS OR CHILDREN WITH AMBIGOUS GENITALIA

1. Sex Chromatin Pattern	2. Gonad (s)			
	Clinically palpable		Clinically not palpable	
	3. Urine 17-Ketosteroids, etc.			
	Normal	Elevated	Normal	Elevated
Positive	Klinefelter's syndrome true hermaphrodite	?	true hermaphrodite female pseudohermaphrodite (non-adrenal)	congenital adrenogenital syndrome (female pseudohermaphrodite) iatrogenic
Negative	male pseudohermaphrodite (deficient testes) true hermaphrodite feminizing testes (inguinal or labial)	Male pseudohermaphrodite (rare type of congenital adrenal hyperplasia)	male pseudohermaphrodite. true hermaphrodite. Turner's syndrome. feminizing testes (abdominal)	male pseudohermaphrodite (rare type of congenital adrenogenital hyperplasia)

In some, the stroma in the gonadal tissue may resemble immature ovarian parenchyma containing some clear cells (hilus cells), but no ovocytes.

In 1930, Ullrich[58] described a syndrome, now often referred to as the Bonnevie-Ullrich syndrome[4, 13] which is comprised of a webbed neck, shield-shaped thorax, neonatal retardation, lymphangiectatic edema of hands and feet (cutis laxa) and small stature. Later, many patients with this complex were found to have sex chromosomal abnormalities and gonadal dysgenesis. In 1938, Turner[57] described a triad consisting of sexual infantilism, webbed neck and cubitis valgus. It has since been observed that these patients were female phenotypes with negative nuclear sex chromatin. Many had associated cardiac defects, coarctation of the aorta, hypertension, low intelligence, etc. In 1947, Dell Castilo[10, 11] described phenotypical females with senile facies, short stature and skeletal deformities. Many of these patients also showed a negative nuclear sex chromatin pattern. Thus, what is now termed Turner's syndrome is a heterologous group of patients composed of female phenotypes with antithetical nuclear sex chromatin and xo karyotypes and, at times, mosaicism. These patients have associated somatic abnormalities of varying severity.

At birth, the assigned sex is usually feminine, and no suspicion of any abnormality arises unless there are somatic defects. At puberty, medical advice may be solicited because of athelia and failure of onset of pubarche or menarche. The

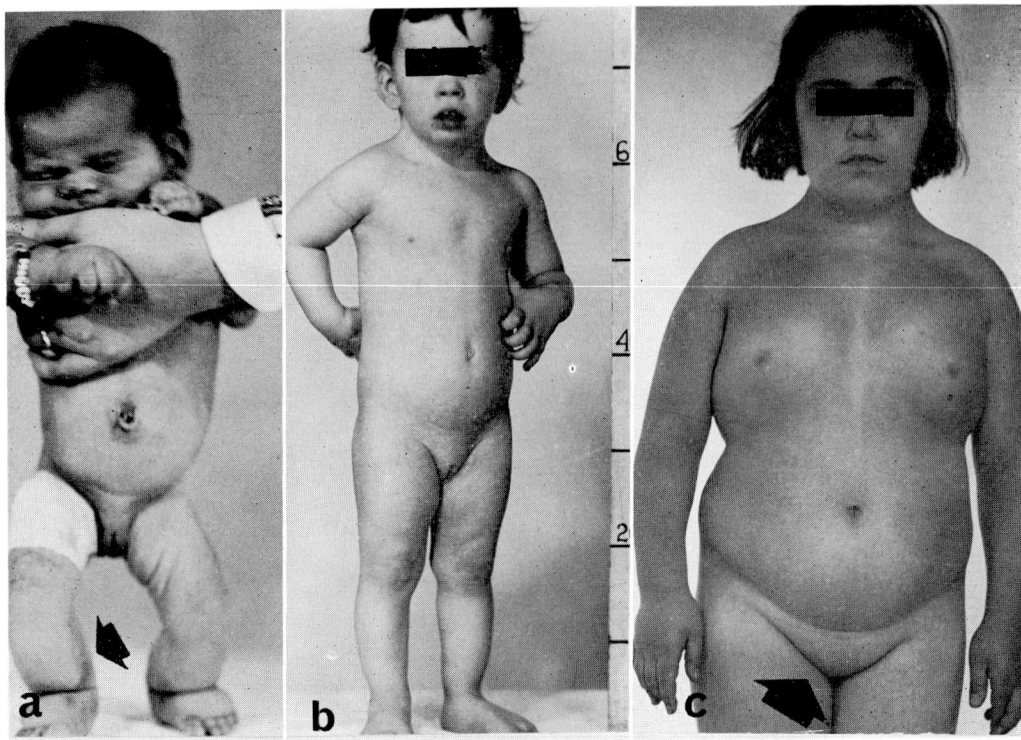

Fig. 2a, b and c.   Sexual abnormality resulting from errors during chromosomal period (Turner's syndrome). (a) E. O., three days of age, phenotypical female with negative sex chromatin pattern and lymphedema of legs and feet (Bonnevie-Ullrich type). (b) same patient at six years. Front view reveals webbed neck. (c) I. K., eleven-year-old phenotypical female, mentally retarded. Note webbed neck. Patient also had hypertension, coarctation of the aorta, abnormalities of hands and feet and was sex chromatin negative.

vulva is infantile, the clitoris, tiny; and the vagina, narrow and shallow. Later, there is a rise in gonadotrophin output; hypertensive episodes and hot flushes may occur. Administration of female hormones may induce enlargement of breasts and vaginal bleeding in those patients who possess a uterine anlage. Marriage is possible, but the patients are sterile.

Klinefelter's Syndrome[53] (Fig. 3)

The phenotype is at variance with the nuclear sex chromatin; i.e., the patients are masculine, but their nuclear sex reveals a positive or female (xx) pattern[5]. This is suggestive of sex reversal. However, the karyotype often shows, in addition to forty-four autosomes, three or more sex chromosomes, one of which is a y — a total of forty-seven chromosomes. Mosaicism is frequently present (xx/xxy or xxy/xxxxy, etc.). The condition has occurred in siblings and in twins[19]. The association of Klinefelter's syndrome with mongolism (trisomy at 21, with 45 autonomes and 3 sex chromosomes, making a total of 48 chromosomes), has been reported[23]. At birth, the assigned sex is masculine, and no suspicion of any sexual abnormality arises until puberty or adulthood. Many of the patients show mental retardation. At puberty, gynecomastia develops, and may on occasion be unilateral. The patients are tall, with large hands and feet, but with poor musculature. The buttocks are round and full. The penis and testes are small, and the sparse public hair shows a female escutcheon. The usual chief complaints are gynecomastia and sterility.

The prepuberal testis is hypoplastic,

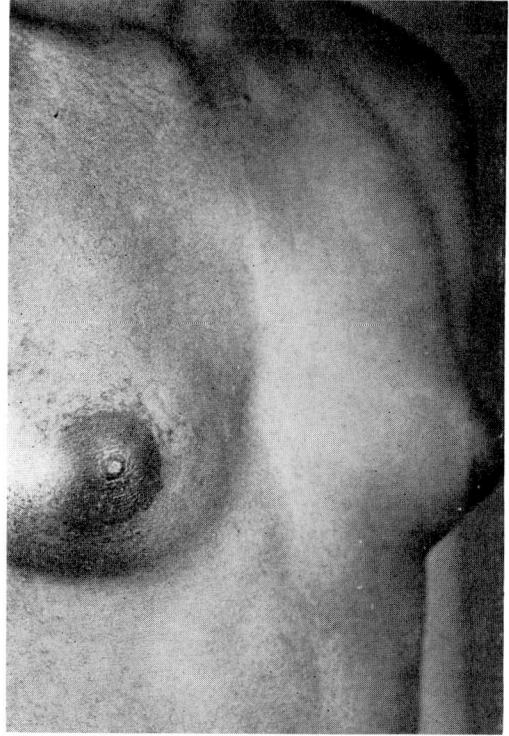

Fig. 3. Sexual abnormality resulting from error during chromosomal period (Klinefelter's syndrome). S. O., age fifteen years, phenotypical male (large build, poor musculature) with gynecomastia. The penis was normal in size, the scrotum well developed and contained immature testes. The sex chromatin pattern was positive.

its tubules are small, irregular and lined by indeterminate sex cells. Characteristic germ cells are absent or greatly reduced. Intratubular concentric concentrations or bodies, sometimes simulating ovocytes, are occasionally encountered. Interstitial cells are not prominent. It is after puberty that progressive tubular degeneration occurs. Germ cells are absent or greatly reduced, and only very rarely does complete spermatogenesis occur. Sertoli cells, many showing degenerative changes, line the tubules. The walls show progressive fibrosis and hyalinization. The Leydig cells are numerous, yet the urine 17-ketosteroids are normal and androgens low. An increase in gonadotropin excretion is noted at puberty.

SEXUAL ABNORMALITIES RESULTING FROM ERRORS OCCURRING DURING THE GONADAL PERIOD

It is presupposed that the chromosomal period was normal and that the disturbances involved mainly the gonads. There is partial or complete, unilateral or bilateral, zonal (i.e. cortical or medullary) damage. The gonadal defects affect the development of the sexual ducts, external genitalia and even the phenotype, particularly in cases with bilateral damage[34, 35].

True Hermaphrodite (Fig. 4)

Partial failure of the isosexual gonadal zone, i.e., the zone which is consonant with the chromatin sex, and concomitant only partial inhibition of the heterosexual zone, ends in persistence of the bipotential gonad and the devel-

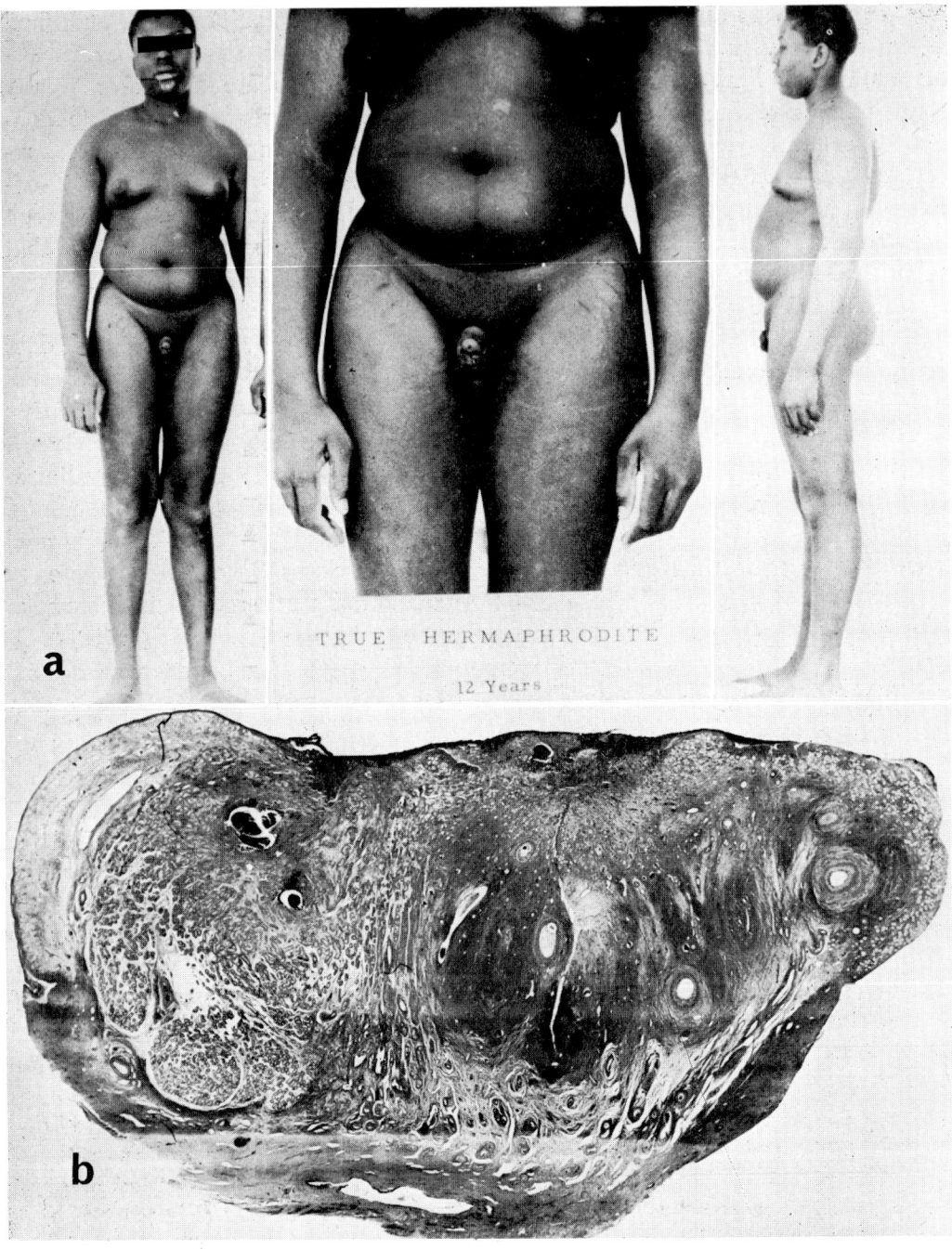

Fig. 4a, b and c. Zonal damage to the bipotential gonad occurring during the gonadal period can lead to failure by the chromosomally induced "dominant" zone (i.e., the cortex in xx, the medulla in xy) to inhibit the heterosexual zone. The error may be partial, total, unilateral or bilateral and result in the devolpment of an ovotestis, etc. (the true hermaphrodite). (a and b) K. C., a two-year-old child, was raised as a female, but sex was in doubt due to anomalous external genitalia. The clitoris was

in social orientation on the part of the patient and family and a horrendous psycho-emotional complex for all. A series of operations to correct the chordee, the hypospadias and post-operative fistulae, and to bring down the undescended testes had to be performed and at times repeated because of faulty healing. The end result, in some cases, was a psychophysical misfit with inadequate and distorted genitalia. It has been our experience that plastic construction of an anatomically adequate and sexually functioning penis from a micropenis, particularly if devoid of a urethra, is a most difficult task. The decision as to reassignment of sex requires a careful evaluation of all the material at hand, and it may be wiser in many instances to remove the dysgenetic testes (they tend to undergo neoplasia), and let the "error" in sex assignment remain.

The "Feminizing Testis" (Fig. 6)

The babies are sex chromatin negative phenotypical females with tiny testes in or near the labia[15, 25, 36, 37]. The vagina is small. The testes contain tubules lined mainly by Sertoli cells. Apparently, the dysgenetic testes not only lack the androgenic hormone, but instead manufacture estrogens. The children are raised as girls, but, in some cases, medical advice may be sought early because of swellings in the labia interpreted as hernias, but which turn out to be testes at operation. During puberty the breasts develop, but failure to menstruate may lead to medical investigation and discovery of the anomaly. Later, when these individuals reach maturity, their phenotype is strikingly feminine, but they are sterile. It is then that some seek an explanation of their difficulty. The clitoris is usually small, the vagina shallow; there is no cervix, and, at laparotomy, there is, as a rule, no uterus or tubes; dysgenetic undescended testes are usually found near the internal inguinal ring. Removal of the latter may be followed by the symptoms of menopause, i.e., hot flashes, dizzy spells, etc. The testes may contain Sertoli cell adenomas[8, 9, 20]. In a few cases, persistent hilar cells become hyperplastic and cause virilism.

In females, varying degrees of cortical (ovarian) deficiency can occur, but this does not result in a female pseudohermaphrodite (see *ductal period*), but rather in the hypogonadal or "deficient female" whose status may not be detectable until puberty (Fig. 7). The individuals fail to mature sexually. They

laparotomy no Mullerian elements were found. Operation disclosed small undescended testes near inguinal rings. (c) R. I., age two and one-half years, with ambiguous genitalia, male sex chromatin, fairly well developed phallus with hypospadias and persistent urogenital sinus. Laparotomy revealed a uterus, tubes and gonads (near internal ring) which on biopsy proved to be testes. Hysterectomy was performed and hypospadias repaired. (d) E. D., age six years, sex chromatin negative, cleft scrotum, small penis. Testes high in inguinal regions. Orchiopexy. (e) A. D., a nine-year-old sex chromatin individual, brought up as a male, but doubt persisted as to "true sex." Note fairly well developed "penis," moderate hypospadias, cleft scrotum and remnants of vagina (f and g). Following several operations for orchiopexy (testes were in inguinal ring) and plastic operations on penis and urethra, function now is fairly adequate (h)

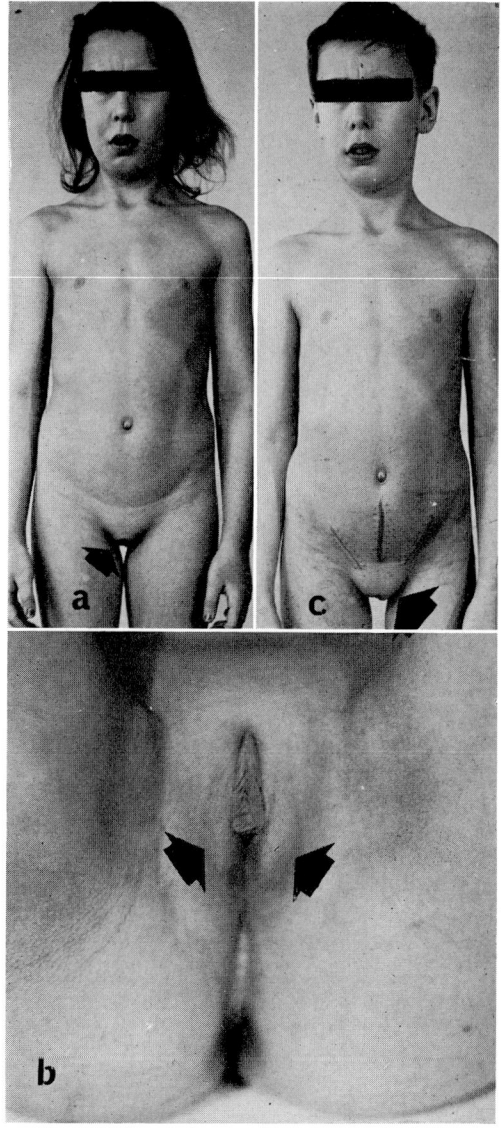

Fig. 6a, b and c.   Sexual anomalies resulting from disturbances occurring during the gonadal period of sexual development in genotypical males may be associated with the "feminizing testis." The latter is indeed a fascinating pathological entity, particularly in view of the clinical appearance of the patients. They are sex chromatin negative phenotypical "females" with small testes which are usually located in the inguinal or "labial" areas. There is a miniature penis and bifid or empty scrotum. A uterus or tubes, however, are not present as a rule. The outstanding features are: seminiferous tubules lined by Sertoli cells plus, in many cases, gross or microscopic tubular adenomas. The picture suggests that the totipotent germ cells failed to reach the developing medulla or were destroyed when they arrived. The medulla had inhibited the cortex, but the predominating estrogen-producing Sertoli cells fortified the maternal hormones which molded the fetus into a feminine phenotype.

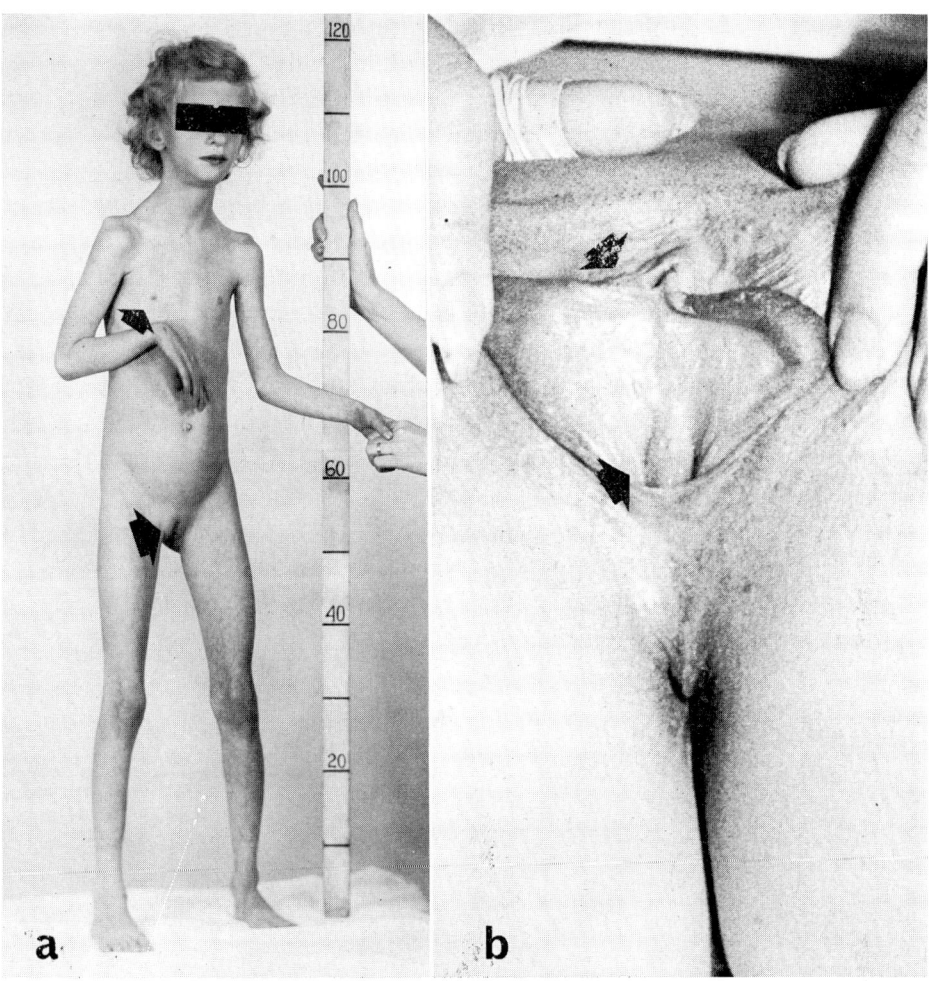

Fig. 7a and b. Anomalous sexual development due to errors during gonadal period. Deficient ovaries. (a) J. K., age eighteen years, sex chromatin positive, was short, had underdeveloped breasts and primary amenorrhea. She was a hypogonadal female. (b) J. N., twenty-three years old, sex chromatin positive, had amenorrhea, short vagina, immature ovarian tissue.

have little breast tissue; the pubic and axillary hair is sparse. The vagina is small, and there may be synechiae; the uterus and/or adnexae may be absent or, if present, are infantile. The ovaries are small and undeveloped, and thus,

(a, b, c) S. S., a ten-year-old child, raised as a girl, was brought to the hospital because of bilateral swelling in labia (c) which were thought to be inguinal hernias. At operation, however, the swellings proved to be gonads which, on biopsy, revealed seminiferous tubules lined mainly by Sertoli cells. Microtubular adenomas were present. At laparotomy, no uterus or tubes were found. It was, therefore, decided to change the patient's sex. Note appearance of "boy" following futile attempts to construct a scrotum, etc.

there is amenorrhea and sterility. In ovarian dysplasia, heterosexual changes can occur. Thus, virilization (female pseudohermaphroditism) is seen in the Stein-Leventhal syndrome[51] and in arrhenoblastoma (of fetal or maternal origin) etc.

Tumors in Intersexes (Fig. 8)

The majority of the gonads in intersexes are immature and dysgenetic. Normal differentiation is often arrested, and for that reason it is not possible to identify in some cases, whether one is dealing with testicular or ovarian elements. The histologic features in these defective gonads are as follows: (a) There are clusters of clear cells containing prominent round, deep stain-ing nuclei. These have been labeled "neuter" cells[50]. (b) There are also concretions which at times appear laminated. In some dysgenetic gonads, cells resembling spermatogones or ovocytes are also present, as well as scattered foci of Sertoli or granulosa cells and/or interstitial or theca cells. The natural history of the gonads varies. They usually show progressive degeneration and calcification, but sometimes undergo a neoplastic change[1, 14, 28, 29, 31, 39, 43, 48, 49, 52, 54, 55]. Such tumors characteristically are composed of "neuter" cells interspersed with calific concretions (Figs. 8, 9) and have been termed gonadoblastomas or dysgenetic gonadomas[28, 48]. These neoplasms are slow

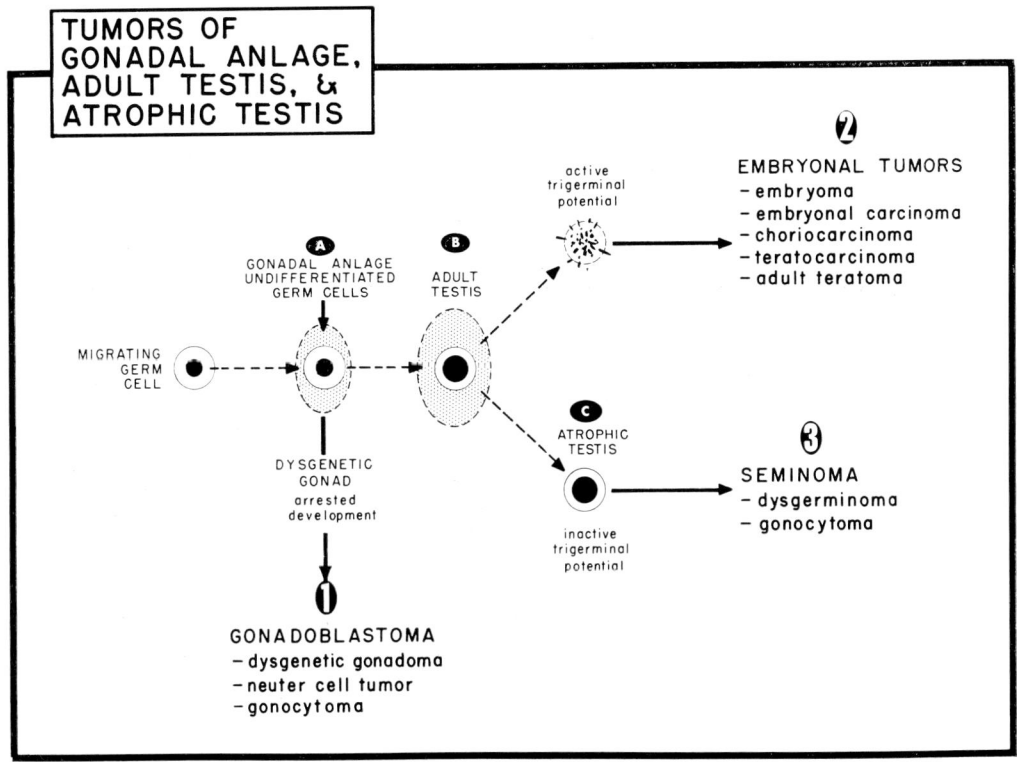

Fig. 8. Diagram indicates place of gonadoblastoma, the tumor arising from undifferentiated "neuter" cells of the dysgenetic gonad, in testicular oncology.

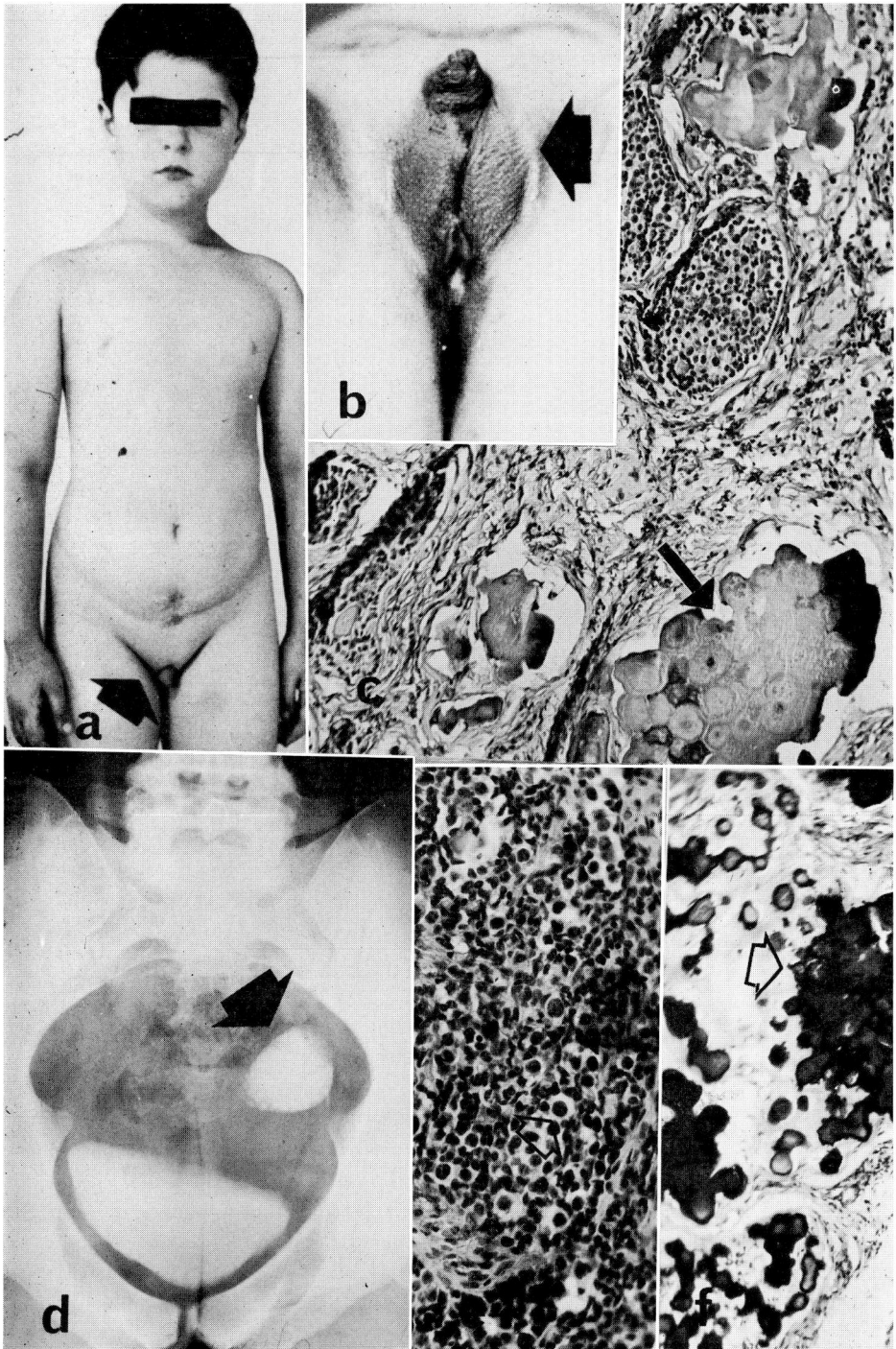

Fig. 9a, b, c and d. Gonadoblastoma in intersexes (a, b and c) G. K., a nine-year-old boy presented with urogenital sinus and vaginal canal at birth, and, because of this, sex was in doubt. Bifid scrotum was empty, but oval masses were palpated in inguinal

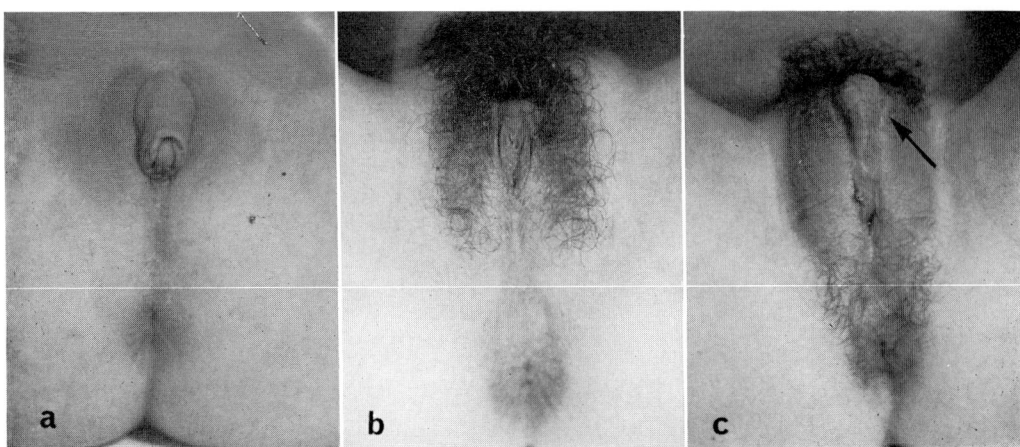

Fig. 10a, b and c.   Sexual anomalies resulting from disturbances occurring during ductal period (prenatal hormonal) of sexual development. It is presumed that normal differentiation had occurred during chromosomal and gonadal periods, but that further development was altered by hormonal factors which in most instances emanate from enzymal disturbances arising within adrenal cortex. This is usually associated with androgen excess, but at times also with salt-losing syndrome and/or hypertension. Adrenogenital syndrome is the commonest cause of female pseudohermaphroditism. In male patients, isosexual precocity occurs. Rarely, estrogen-producing hormone emanating from adrenal gland has been reported in male patients. (a) T. T., a twenty-one-month-old girl with an enlarged clitoris and high level urine 17-ketosteroids (5.3 mg per twenty-four hours). (b) J. B., a three-year-old girl with enlarged clitoris since birth. The urine 17-ketosteroids ranged from 7.6 to 23 mg per twenty-four hours. (c) J. L., a similar history in a three-year-old girl.

growing and rarely metastasize. However, in some, the associated germ cells when present develop into malignancies such as seminomas (dysgerminomas), or embryonal carcinomas, teratocarcinomas or choriocarcinomas. The non-germinal cells may show hyperplasia or neoplasia (Sertoli or granulosa cell tumors, or interstitial or theca cell tumors[26, 27, 31]). A new concept regarding

canals. Many operations were performed to correct chordee and hypospadias and to bring down both inguinal masses (biopsies showed immature testicular tissue) into small, newly built scrotum. Mullerian elements (uterus, tubes) were removed. Sex chromatin pattern was negative. Bilateral dysgenetic gonadomas were excised eight years later and prostheses inserted. (d, e and f) J. M., a twenty-two-year-old intersex, was brought up as a male. His ambiguous genitalia plagued him since childhood. The phallus was well developed (patient had had coitus with women). There was hypospadias, a urogenital sinus and a vagina. Note colpogram (d) and the shadow of a calcified mass above and to the left of the bladder shadow. At laparotomy a uterus and tubes were present and removed. Biopsy of the right gonad showed testicular tissue. The left gonad was removed and found to be a gonadoblastoma.

the place of gonadoblastoma in the oncology of all types of gonadal tumors has been presented by the author[31].

SEXUAL ABNORMALITIES RESULTING FROM ERRORS OCCURRING DURING THE DUCTAL PERIOD (PRENATAL HORMONAL)
(Fig. 10)

It is presupposed that the chromosomal and gonadal periods have been normal and that the disturbances, hormonal ones, occurred during the differentiation of the sex ducts and external genitalia. The enzyme systems of the adrenal gland are usually at fault, causing the abnormality[3]. Congenital adrenogenital hyperplasia is accompanied by an excess of androgen and is the *commonest cause of female pseudohermaphroditism*[30, 59]. The clitoris

ongenital adreno-
ow macrogenito-
ecocious puberty.
 pseudohermaph-
sed by congenital
ssociated with an
 lack of mineral-

olved in some of
turbed organizers[61]
 vascular supply.
isorganization, dis-
iency of elements
em or of the Wolf-

IES RESULTING FROM
 DURING INFANCY
 AND PUBERTY
 PERIOD)

d that the chromo-
ductal periods were
normal, consonant with another, and that normal birth and delivery had occurred. Though somatic development and growth during infancy and childhood supersede sexual maturation, cer-

result from an arrhenoblastoma or the ovary, or from ovarian dysfunction accompanying the Stein-Leventhal syndrome, etc.

Boys with congenital adrenogenital hyperplasia show macrogenitosomia and pseudo-precocious puberty. A rare type of male pseudohermaphroditism can be caused by adrenal hyperplasia or tumor associated with an estrogen effect and lack of mineralcorticoids.

An estrogen excess in females promotes isosexual precocity and results in precocious puberty or pseudo-puberty. Causes may be constitutional, familial or polyostotic fibrous dysplasia[41], granulosa cell tumors of the ovary, retroperitoneal masses[6], tumors of the hypothalamus, etc. (Fig. 12). Estrogen deficiency may be constitutional, familial or the result of bilateral oophoritis or following oophorectomy, diseases of the pituitary, thyroid, etc., or obesity.

Phenotypical sex chromatin negative boys, with hitherto normal external and internal genitalia, can develop an adro-

pigmentation around nipples and the fine pubic hair. The labia were hypertrophied. On abdominal exploration the uterus was found to be enlarged and the ovaries normal except for cysts in the right. The long bones showed some cystic changes. The findings were suggestive of periostotic fibrous dysplasia. (Reprinted by courtesy of Dr. M. G. Peterman, J. Pediat., 49, p. 722, Figs. 5-7, 1956.)

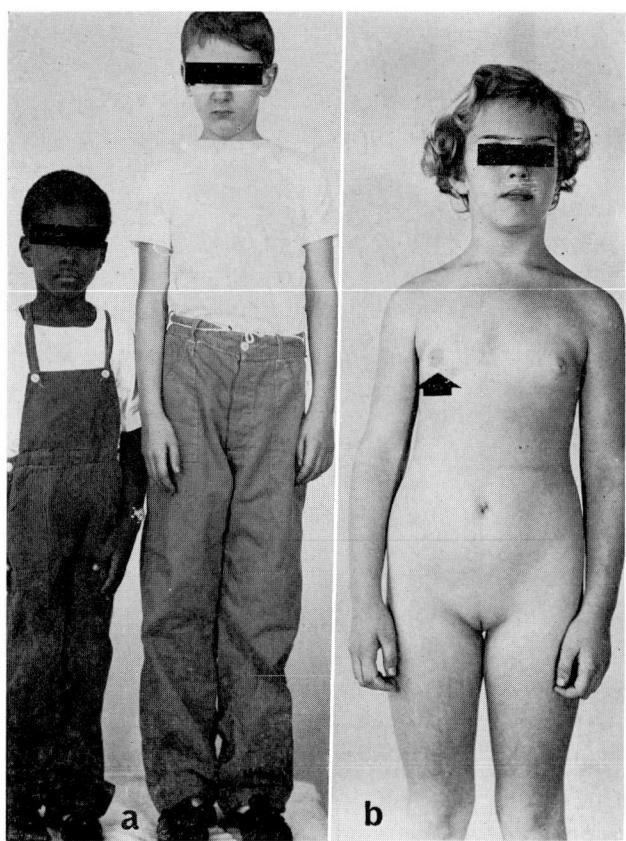

Fig. 13a and b.   Isosexual precocity in childhood, probably on a constitutional basis.
(a) J. E. and E. B. are the same age (six years). J. E. shows normal development for
his age; E. B. is much taller. (b) F. M. at seven and one-half years is large for her age,
shows breast enlargement and has a history of vaginal bleeding.

gen deficiency or estrogen excess causing feminization. The cause may be
constitutional, familial or bilateral orchi-
tis with atrophy, bilateral orchiectomy,
pituitary deficiency, hypothyroidism,
obesity, sertolioma, gynandroblastoma,
etc. An androgen excess induces isosexual precocity resulting in precocious
puberty or pseudo-puberty. The cause
may be "constitutional" (Fig. 13) or a
tumor of the adrenal cortex (postnatal
adrenogenital syndrome[30], interstitioma,
tumors of the nervous system, adrenal
rests in the testis[16], pineal; hepatoma[44]
and presacral teratoma[45], etc.).

SEXUAL ABNORMALITIES DEVELOPING
DURING THE GENDER ROLE PERIOD

A discussion of the sexual aberration
and abnormalities in adults is not within
the scope of this article[2, 30]. The type
of disturbances are listed in Table II.

SOME OF THE MEASURES
EMPLOYED IN THE DIAGNOSIS
OF INTERSEXUALITY IN
INFANCY AND CHILDHOOD

There are three zones in the genital
area which require a careful check in
the newborn with doubtful sexual

status: (a) phallus — note size, site of meatal opening and whether urogenital sinus is present; (b) labia-scrotal area — determine if area resembles fused labia or cleft scrotum, or is an unduly small scrotum; (c) gonads — check whether there are palpable nodules in the inguinal, labial or scrotal areas, and if hernias are present.

Measures employed in establishing the diagnosis as to the cause of the sexual ambiguity are present in Table III. It is important to emphasize that, in addition to determining the sex chromatin pattern and evaluation of urinary 17-ketosteroids, it is often necessary to perform a gonadal biopsy in the clinically palpable gonads. Depending on age and other anatomical indications, vaginograms, cystoscopy, intravenous pyelography and laparotomy with inspection of internal genitalia and biopsy of gonads (if present) are carried out. In all cases, a careful family history should be obtained regarding any sexual abnormalities, the status of siblings and inquiry as to whether the mother has received hormones, etc. during pregnancy.

SUMMARY

1. A classification, based on the concept that sexual anomalies result from errors occurring during five critical period of sexual development, has been presented. The critical periods are: (a) chromosomal; (b) gonadal; (c) ductal (prenatal hormonal); (d) postnatal hormonal (puberal); (e) gender role. Clinical examples of sexual abnormalities characteristic of the first four periods, involving infants and children, have been presented.

2. The sex chromosomes carry the master plan or blueprint of sexual development. Therefore, any sex chromosomal error can result in a variety of profound sexual anomalies affecting gonads, ducts, external genitalia and sex characteristics, resulting in asexuality or in phenotypical sex reversal as seen in Turner's and Klinefelter's syndrome. Somatic abnormalities, due to associated autosomal errors, are often concomitant, particularly in Turner's syndrome. Mental retardation is frequent.

3. Since it is necessary to have a normal functioning testis in order to obtain adequate differentiation of the Wolffian system, errors affecting the medulla in the bipotential gonads (testicular dysgenesis, hypofunction, dysfunction) become manifest in sex chromatin negative individuals and are the *commonest cause of male pseudohermaphroditism*. The latter group, neonatally, may resemble the female congenital adrenogenital pseudohermaphrodite. The negative sex chromatin pattern and normal urinary 17-ketosteroids characterize the male anomaly. Cortical or ovarian deficiency (ovarian dysgenesis) results only in poorly developed phenotypical females with deficient internal and external genitalia. The phenomenon of the feminizing testis and of the various combinations of ovariotestis (true hermaphrodite) are discussed, and postulates as to cause are presented.

4. Gonadal differentiation may be relatively adequate, but the differentiation of the bisexual ducts can later be markedly affected by prenatal hormonal excess or alterations such as occur in congenital adrenal hyperplasia or androgen formation from other sources (maternal arrhenoblastoma, iatrogenic,

etc.). Since androgen excess is more frequent than that of estrogens, the former is the *commonest cause of female pseudohermaphroditism*. The positive sex chromatin pattern and elevated urinary 17-ketosteroids characterize this female anomaly.

5. Normal differentation and maturation of the secondary sex characteristics are accompanied during the postnatal hormonal period by a check and balance of secretions from the entire endocrine chain. Retardation or acceleration can be induced by a variety of disturbances: on the one hand, constitutional factors and functioning hyperplasia or neoplasia of endocrine organs; on the other hand, functional deficiencies or deprivations of the same systems. A variety of syndromes in these categories is mentioned.

6. During normal sexual development, the bipotential gonad gives way to the unipotential testis or ovary, consonant with the sex chromatin pattern; thereafter, the bisexual ducts, in a similar way, give up their heterosexual components; finally, the ambisexual external genitalia likewise blossom into an isosexual predominance. Is there also a duality in the sex gender role behavior? Phenotypism, the maturation of external genitalia, secondary sex characteristics, physical and psycho-emotional factors in the environment, together with parental example, training, dress, habits, and society's mores, taboos, etc. all tend to stimulate that role which coincides with the genital and hormonal sex.

7. This concept and classification is proposed as a guide in diagnosis and management. The physician is apt to be consulted at certain periods: (a)

in the newborn, because of ambigous genitalia, necessitating careful investigation in order to arrive at a decision regarding the assigned sex; (b) *in infancy or childhood*, because sexual development is apparently contrary to the sex which had been assigned; (c) *during the same period*, because of a heterosexual change in a hitherto normally developed child, or because of isosexual precocity in either sex; (d) *during or after puberty*, in phenotypical girls who do not menstruate or whose breasts do not develop, or in phenotypical boys who have become obese or have developed gynecomastia or eunuchoidism; (e) *during the same period*, in girls, because of virilism and hirsutism and clitoral enlargement.

8. An outline of procedures helpful in establishing the diagnosis in hermaphrodism and other genital and gonadal abnormalities has been presented.

Answers to Problem Cases in Figure 1

1. S. S., age two months: (a) sex chromatin negative (xy); (b) tiny penis with normal urethra and meatus, bifid scrotum with palpable nodules which on biopsy showed defective testicular tissue; (c) urine 17-ketosteroids normal. Diagnosis: male pseudohermaphrodite due to testicular deficiency which probably occurred during gonadal period.

2. D. B., age two months: (a) sex chromatin negative (xy); (b) small clitoris, female urethra; dots indicate area where nodules were palpated; biopsy showed testis with seminiferous tubules lined by Sertoli cells only; (c) urine 17-ketosteroids normal. Diagnosis: male pseudohermaphrodite due to "feminizing testis."

3. M. A., age three months: (a) sex chromatin pattern negative (karyotype

xo); (b) external genitalia feminine; no palpable nodules; (c) urine 17-ketosteroids normal; webbed neck. Diagnosis: Turner's syndrome (laparotomy to be performed).

4. K. C., age two years: (a) sex chromatin pattern positive; (b) large phallus looks like penis with hypospadias; small vagina; no plapable masses; (c) urine 17-ketosteroids normal; laparotomy indicated; at operation, uterus, tubes and gonads were found; biopsy of latter showed ovariotestes. Diagnosis: true hermaphrodite with positive sex chromatin pattern.

5. T. T., age two and one half years: (a) sex chromatin positive; (b) progressively enlarging phallus since birth, female urethra, large labia; no palpable nodules; (c) urine 17-ketosteroids elevated. Diagnosis: congenital adrenogenital syndrome in girl.

6. S. M., age four and one half months: (a) sex chromatin positive; (b) moderately enlarged clitoris since birth, female urethra, labia and vagina; no palpable nodules; (c) urine 17-ketosteroids slightly elevated (mother had received hormone injections during pregnancy). Diagnosis: iatrogenic adrenogenital syndrome.

REFERENCES

1. Abbata, G., Perlow, V., Crampton, R. S.: Malignant neoplasms in non descended testes. New York J. Med., 64:3012-3014, 1964.
2. Armstrong, C. N.: Transvestism. In Robertson Smith, D., and Davidson, W. M.: Symposium on Nuclear Sex. London, Heineman, New York, Interscience, 1958, Chapter 12, pp. 84-92.
3. Bongiovanni, A. M., and Eberlein, W. R.: Clinical and metabolic variations in the androgenital syndrome. Pediatrics, 16:628-635, 1955.
4. Bonnevie, K.: Embryological analysis of gene manifestation in Little and Bagg abnormal mouse tribes. J. Exp. Zool., 67:443-520, 1934.
5. Bunge, R. G., and Bradbury, J. T.: Three atypical chromatin positive male patients. Trans. Amer. Ass. Genitourin. Surg., 53:167-174, 1961.
6. Cabrera, A., and De la Para, S.: Isosexual precocious pseudopuberty associated with retroperitoneal carcinoma. New York, J. Med., 63:1360-1367, 1963.
7. Clayton, G. W., Smith, J. D., and Rosenberg, H. S.: Familial true hermaphrodism in pre- and post-pubertal genetic females: Hormonal and morphologic studies. J. Clin. Endocr., 18:1349-1358, 1958.
8. Culp, D. A., Frazier, R. G., and Butler, J. J.: Sertoli cell tumors in an infant. J. Urol., 76:162-167, 1956.
9. Daino, J. A., Tchertkoff, V., Akhavan, T. H., and Ober, W. B.: Leydig cell tumor of testis. Pseudohermaphrodite with testicular feminization. New York J. Med., 63:2258-2262, 1963.
10. Del Castillo, E. B., Trabucco, A., and De la Balze, F. A.: Syndrome produced by absence of the germinal epithelium without impairment of the Sertoli or Leydig cells. J. Clin. Endocr., 7:493-502, 1947.
11. Del Castillo, E. B., Argonz, J., Trabucco, A., and Trabucco, A.: Anomalies renalis en el sindrome de la gonada rudimentaria. Rev. Argent. Endocr., 3:21-35, 1957.
12. Dempsey, H., and Richardson, Hill, S., Jr.: Feminizing adrenocortical tumors. J. Clin. Endocr., 23:173-180, 1963.
13. Engle, E. T., Yeaw, R. C., and Lattimer, J. K.: True hermaphroditism. Supplementary report of a case. J. Urol., 56:731-736, 1946.
14. Frazer, A.: Gonadoblastoma in monozygous twins with gonadal dysgeneses. J. Pediat., 64:740-745, 1964.
15. Flor, F. S., Schadt, D. S., and Benz, E. J.: Gonadal dysgenesis with male chromatin pattern: testicular feminization syndrome. JAMA, 181:103-107, 1962.
16. Glenn, J. F., and Boyce, Wm. H.: Adrenogenitalism with testicular adrenal rests simulating adrenal tumor. Trans. Amer. Ass. Genitourin. Surg., 54:59-66, 1962.
17. Grumbach, M. M., Ducharme, J. R., and Moloshek, R. E.: On the fetal masculinizing action of certain oral progestins. J. Clin. Endocr., XIX:1369-1380, 1959.
18. Grumbach, M. M.: Some considerations of

Acknowledgment: For the use of material, the author is indebted to Drs. J. K. Lattimer, Director of Urology of the Squier Urological Clinic; and M. M. Grumbach, formerly of the Babies Hospital, Columbia-Presbyterian Medical Center.

the pathogenesis and classification of anomalies of Sex in man. In "The Reproductive System," Clinical Endocrinology, New York, Grune, 1960, Chapter VI, pp. 407-436.

19. Holub, D. A., Grumbach, M. M., and Jailer, J. W.: Seminiferous tubule dysgenesis (Klinefelter's syndrome) in identical twins. J. Clin. Endocr., 18:1359-1368, 1958.

20. Huggins, C., and Moulder, P. V.: Estrogen production by Sertoli cell tumors of the testis. Cancer Res., 5:510-514, 1945.

21. Jost, A.: Reserches sur l a différentiation de l'embryon de lapin. 3. Rôle des gonades foetales dans la différentiation sexuelle somatique. Arch. Anat. Micr. Morph. Exp., 36: 271-315, 1947.

22. Klinefelter, H. F. Jr., Reifenstein, E. C., Jr., and Albright, F.: Syndrome characterized by gynecomastia, aspermatogenesis without a — Leydigism, and increased excretion of follicule-stimulating hormone. J. Clin. Endocr., 2:615-627, 1942.

23. Lanman, J. T., Sklarin, B. S., Cooper, H. L., and Hirschhorn, K.: Klinefelter's syndrome in a ten month-old mongolian idiot. New Eng. J. Med., 263:887-890, 1960.

24. Lisser, H., and Escamilla, R. F.: Atlas of Clinical Endocrinology. St. Louis, Mosby, 2nd ed., 1962.

25. Lubs, H. A. Jr., Vilar, O., and Bergenstal, D. M.: Familial male pseudohermaphroditism and labial testes and partial feminization. Endocrine studies and genetic aspects. J. Clin. Endocr., XIX:1110-1120, 1959.

26. Melicow, M. M.: Embryoma of testis. Report of case and a classification of neoplasms of testis. J. Urol., 44:333-344, 1940.

27. Melicow, M. M.: Classification of tumor of the testis. A clinical and pathological study based on 105 primary and 13 secondary cases in adults and 3 primary and 4 secondary cases in children. J. Urol., 73:547-574, 1955.

28. Melicow, M. M., and Uson, A. C.: Dysgenetic gonadomas and othe gonadal neoplasms in intersexes: Report of 5 cases and review of literature. Cancer, 12:552-572, 1959.

29. Melicow, M. M., and Uson, A. C.: Classification of tumors of testis. New York J. Med., 64:2191-2200, 1964.

30. Melicow, M. M., and Uson, A. C.: A periodic table of sexual anomalies. J. Urol., 91:402-425, 1964.

31. Melicow, M. M.: Tumors of dysgenetic gonads in intersexes; Case report and discussion regarding their place in gonadal oncology. Bull. N. Y. Acad. Med., 42:3-20, 1966.

32. Milner, W. A.: Hermaphrodite siblings. J. Urol., 79:1003-1009, 1958.

33. Money, J.: Problems in sexual development. Endocrinologic and psychologic aspects. New York J. Med., 63:2348-2354, 1963.

34. Moore, C. R.: Gonad hormones and sex differentiation. Amer. Natur., 78:97-130, 1944.

35. Moore, C. R.: Embryonic Sex Hormones and Sexual Differentiation. Springfield, Thomas, 1947.

36. Morris, J. D.: The syndrome of testicular feminization in male pseudohermaphrodites. Amer. J. Obstet. Gynec., 65:1192-1211, 1953.

37. Neubecker, R. D., and Theiss, E. A.: Sertoli cell adenoma in patients with testicular feminization. Amer. J. Clin. Path., 38:52-59, 1962.

38. Nowakowski, H.: Der Hypogonadismus im Knaben und Mannesalter. Ergebn. Inn. Med. Kinderheilk., NF 12:219-230, 1959.

39. Ober, W. B.: Embryonal carcinoma of testicular type arising in the gonad of a true hermaphrodite. Jew. Mem. Hosp. Bull. (N.Y.), 6:94-97, 1962.

40. Oettlé, A. G., Rabinowitz, M. B., and Seftel, H. C.: The Laurence-Moon syndrome with germinal aplasia of the testis: Report of a case and review. J. Clin. Endocr., 20:683-699, 1960.

41. Peterman, M. G.: Polyostotic fibrous dysplasia (with precocious puberty and pigmentation). J. Pediat., 49:719-727, 1956.

42. Prader, A., and Siebenmann, R. E.: Nebenniereninsuffizienz bei kongenitaler Lipoidhyperplasie der Nebenneieren. Helv. Paediat. Acta, 12:569-595, 1957.

43. Reddy, D. J., Ramani, C., Sarojini, J. S., and Sivaramakrishna, G.: Seminoma in a male pseudohermaphrodite. Indian J. Surg., XXXII: 167-172, 1960.

44. Reeves, R. L., Tesluk, H., and Harrison, C. E.: Precocious puberty associated with hepatoma. J. Clin. Endocr., 19:1651-1660, 1959.

45. Rhoden, A. E.: Precocious sexual and somatic development in a male infant with a presacral teratoma containing androgen-producing tissue. J. Clin. Endocr., 4:185-193, 1944.

46. Robertson Smith, D., and Davidson, W.: Symposium on Nuclear Sex. London, Heineman, New York, Interscience, 1958.

47. Schutt, A. J., and Hayles, A. B.: Intersex. Mayo Clin. Proc., 39:363-379, 1964.

48. Scully, R, E., Gonadoblastoma: A gonadal tumor related to dysgerminoma (seminoma) and capable of sex hormone production. Cancer, 6:455-463, 1953.

49. Sohval, A. R.: Testicular dysgenesis in relation to neoplasms of the testicle. J. Urol., 75:285-291, 1956.

50. Spielman, F., and Motyloff, L.: Hermaphroditism and dysgerminoma (neuter cell tumor). New York, J. Med., **55**:2168-2178, 1955.

51. Stein, I. F., and Leventhal, M. L.: Amenorrhea associated with bilateral polycystic ovaries. Amer. J. Obstet. Gynec., **29**:181-191, 1935.

52. Taub, J.: Malignant testis tumor, cryptorchidism, and polyorchidism in a pseudohermaphrodite. J. Urol., **71**:475-482, 1954.

53. Takai, Sh., Morita, T., Shimamura, S., Tonomura, A., and Matsunaga, E.: Clinical and chromosomal features in two cases of Klinefelter's syndrome. J. Urol., **88**:533-538, 1962.

54. Teter, J.: An unusual gonadal tumor (gonadoblastoma) in a female patient with testicular dysgenesis. J. Obstet. Gynaec. Brit. Comm., **67**:238-242, 1960.

55. Teter, J.: Mixed form of feminizing germ cell tumor (gonocytoma II). Amer. J. Obstet. Gynec., **84**:722-739, 1962.

56. Teter, J., Janozewski, Z., Wigura, A., and Melicow, M. M.: Congenital anorchism with anomalous external genitalia: A report of two cases. J. Urol., **87**:964-971, 1962.

57. Turner, H. H.: Syndrome of infantilism, congenital webbed neck, and cubitus valgus. Endocrinology, **23**:566-574, 1938.

58. Ullrich, O.: Über typische Combinations Multipler Abartungen. Z. Kinderheilk., **49**: 271-276, 1930.

59. Wilkins, L.: The Diagnosis and Treatment of Endocrine Disorders in Childhood and Adolescence. Springfield, 1957. Thomas, 2nd ed., 1957.

60. Witschi, E.: Genes and inductors of sex differentiation in amphibians. Biol. Rev., **9**: 460-488, 1934.

61. Witschi, E.: Modification of the development of sex in lower vertebrates and in mammals. In Sex and Internal Secretions. Baltimore, Williams & Wilkins, 1939.

62. Witschi, E.: Migration of the germ cells of human embryos from the yolk sac to the primitive gonadal folds. Contr. Embryology, Carnegie Inst., Washington, **32**:67-80, 1948.

The Detection and Diagnosis of Cystic Fibrosis

EARL B. WERT, M.D.

Early reports, including that of Lansteiner in 1905, described many features of cystic fibrosis. In 1936, Fanconi[1] associated fibrosis of the pancreas with bronchiectasis in the young. However, it remained for Anderson[2] to describe this distinct disease entity in 1938. Rarely diagnosed except at the autopsy table until the development of the sweat test in 1953, the disease may now be categorized as follows.

HEREDITY

Transmitted as a Mendelian recessive trait, cystic fibrosis is seen almost exclusively in the homozygous form. Heterozygotes may show partial patterns, such as increased sweat electrolytes, chronic respiratory infections, etc., suggesting a break through of the heterozygotic recessive trait. However, clinical observation and the sweat test separate the homozygotic and heterozygotic forms in approximately 99 per cent of cases.

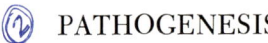 PATHOGENESIS

The structural changes are seen chiefly in tissues containing mucus-secreting glands, and can be traced to abnormal mucus, which is low in sodium chloride, in contrast to the high concentration of salt in the sweat, and to the ease with which this mucus is denatured and rendered insoluble. This viscous material produces mechanical obstruction with retention, and subsequent infection, fibrosis and destruction of the gland and adjacent tissues. Although the secretion of mucous and non-mucous-producing glands are abnormal, pathologic changes are limited to the former. Thus, obstruction of the mucous glands of the pancreas and liver, lungs and sinuses, result in chronic infection and fibrosis. The offending organism is usually the hemolytic staphylococcus.

DIAGNOSIS

In about 98 per cent of cases the homozygotic form of the disease produces elevations in the sodium and chloride in sweat from three to six times normal concentrations, the concentration of each ion being raised from approximately 20 mEq per liter to about 100 mEq per liter. With the possible exception of untreated adrenocortical insufficiency, no other disease is known to produce such elevations. It may be noted that sweat electrolyte concentrations increase with age, and that the normal adult ranges extend into the lowest infant levels consistent with cystic fibrosis. The age of the patient, however, and the ancillary clinical data usually suffice to distinguish the heterozygotic and homozygotic forms. At present, the pilocarpine iontophoresis of sweat, with elution and analysis for sodium and chloride stands as the most reliable index of cystic fibrosis, and is the cornerstone for the diagnosis or exclusion of this disease.

THE SWEAT TEST

Although sweat may be obtained by heat applied generally or locally, the iontophoresis of pilocarpine is so simple, safe and effective that it is generally regarded as a procedure of choice. A flat fleshy surface is selected, such as the forearm or leg, although abdomen or back may be used in small infants, and the electrodes applied. Since burns may be produced by any equipment now available, the following safeguards are recommended.

First, the possibility of burns and the importance of the test should be explained to the parents, and signed permission should be obtained. Second, only experienced personnel should perform the test, keeping the pads of the electrodes soaked with solution and pressure evenly distributed, avoiding wrinkling of the pads and undue pressure over bony prominences. The positive (red) electrode is saturated with freshly prepared 0.5 per cent pilocarpine nitrate and placed on the inner aspect of the limb. The negative (black) electrode is saturated with 1.0 per cent sodium nitrate and applied to the outer surface of the limb.

Burns occur exclusively at the negative electrode. The current is maintained at 1.5 to 2.0 ma for five minutes. The skin is allowed to sweat for ten minutes while dried salt is purged from the ducts. The salt is cleansed from the skin with distilled water, and a previously weighed pad is applied at the site of the pilocarpine using forceps to avoid finger contamination. Covered by Parafilm and bound securely, the pad collects the sweat for one hour. The pad is then returned to a tared bottle to avoid evaporation, weighed, and appropriate diluent is added. The salt is squeezed from the sponge; sodium is determined by flame photometry, chloride by any reliable method.

The iontophoresis of two sites, either simultaneously using two power supplies, or consecutively using the same power unit, has proved helpful. At one site, sweat may be collected in a small plastic cup for analysis of total ions by conductivity methods, and, at the second site, a sponge may be used for elution techniques; or, a sponge may be used at each site.

In the presence of clinical evidence of cystic fibrosis, a sweat sodium of 70 mEq per liter, and a chloride of 60 mEq per liter or greater are compatible with the homozygous form of the disease. Both sodium and chloride should be determined as a control measure. If differences greater than 10 mEq per liter are found, the test should be repeated. A small number of values will fall in an intermediate zone, of 50 to 70 mEq per liter. These patients should be advised that the diagnosis is still in doubt. The sweat test should be repeated at intervals and further observations made. In no case should the diagnosis be made categorically on the basis of a single test, regardless of the clinical or sweat test pattern. It would seem better, usually, to allow events to prove the diagnosis, provided treatment is instituted promptly to avoid irreversible changes, and provided the parents understand the nature of the problem.

No relationship exists between the severity of the disease and the volume of the sweat or the concentration of electrolytes. Rarely, one may fail to obtain sweat in adequate amounts, owing to acute illness or dehydration, to decomposed pilocarpine or to inadequate electrical stimulation. Two (2) milliamperes of current should not be exceeded in the interest of avoiding burns.

Other tests for cystic fibrosis include the use of silver nitrate and potassium chromate on agar or filter paper to estimate the concentrations of chloride in sweat. These tests require some skill in reading, but if carefully done and repeated, may serve to rule out the disease. For physicians with access to a modern clinical laboratory, the techniques are not recommended. The analysis of finger nails for sodium and potassium has been found to be of some value. Owing to technical problems incident to cleaning and dissolving nails, the procedure is not recommended for routine hospital analysis. Siblings of cystic fibrosis patients, but not parents, can be separated into two groups, those having high and low sodium and potassium values respectively.

Recently, conductivity methods have served to simplify the analysis of sweat. Electrodes designed to measure sodium or chloride directly on the skin (hydrogen ion, or combination silver-silver chloride types) have been reported as promising, and may soon be marketed for general use. Their expense, maintenance and calibration may limit their use.

Trypsin studies on duodenal contents or stools need be done only in special cases, and are rarely the deciding factor.

CLINICAL ASPECTS

Early diagnosis and vigorous treatment are of extreme importance, with treatment directed especially to relieving bronchial obstruction and surpressing staphylococcal infection in the lung. Efforts directed at the early liquification of bronchial mucus and the control of the infection have been accompanied by remarkable clinical improvement, so that the disease, while serious, is no longer uniformly fatal at an early age. Frequently, all respiratory symptoms are absent early in the disease, appearing only months or years after birth, and may be accompanied by paranasal sinus disease, frequently with polyposis. Meconium ileus is seen in less than 10 per cent of the cases, but the 60 per cent mortality rate at operation, and the 80 per cent mortality rate during the first year in these patients, document the seriousness of this manifestation. Malnutrition, as a result of pancreatic enzyme deficiency occurs in over 80 per cent of patients. Pancreatic deficiency may be accompanied by abdominal distention, bulky, foul stools, abdominal pain, inspissated fecal masses and prolapsed rectum.

Intolerance to hot weather, or to febrile episodes, with circulatory collapse and occasional death, is attributable to the excessive loss of electrolytes through the sweat. Indeed, one mother of a mildly affected infant found, while kissing her infant, that the sweat was saltier than her other children, providing the clue to a somewhat belated diagnosis in this case.

A high degree of clinical awareness and of the varying clinical appearance of the illness is essential. Often, a robust child with excellent development, but with a history of recurring respiratory infections, or intolerance to heat or to fatty foods may be shown to have the homozygotic form of the disease, and over the ensuing months or years may develop the typical course. Although these cases may be mild, most are severe, and all require careful management. Any or all of the triad of respiratory symptoms, failure to thrive and gastrointestinal symptoms suggest the diagnosis. Thus, pertussis, bronchopneumonia, bronchitis, sinusitis, asthma, bronchiectasis, tuberculosis, agammaglobulinemia, as well as celiac disease, should be indications for undertaking the sweat test.

REFERENCES

1. Fanconi, G., Uehlinger, E., and Knauer, C.: Das Coeliakiesyndrom bei angerborener zystischer Pankreasfibromatose und Bronchiektasien. Wien Med. Wschr., 86:753-756, 1936.
2. Andersen, D. H.: Cystic fibrosis of the pancreas and its relation to celiac disease. A clinical and pathological study. Amer. J. Dis. Child., 56:344-399, 1938.
3. di Sant'Agnese, P. A.: Cystic fibrosis of the pancreas, edited transcription of a combined clinical staff conference at the Clinical Center, Bethesda, Maryland, by the National Institutes of Health Service, Department of Health, Education and Welfare. Ann. Intern. Med., 54:482, 1961.
4. Shwachman, H., and Gohm, N.: Studies in cystic fibrosis of the pancreas: A simple test for the detection of excessive chloride on the skin. New Eng. J. Med., 255:999, 1956.
5. Gibson, L. E., and Cooke, R. E.: A test for concentration of electrolytes in sweat in cystic fibrosis of the pancreas utilizing pilocarpine by iontophoresis. Pediatrics, 23:545, 1959.
6. Hsai, D. Y.: The laboratory detection of heterozygotes. Amer. J. Hum. Genet., 9:98-116, June, 1957.
7. Bulletin: The National Cystic Fibrosis Research Foundation, 521 5th Ave., N.Y. 17, N.Y. Cystic Fibrosis News Bulletin.
8. Kulezycki, L. L., MacLeod, K. I. E., and Shwachman, H.: A survey of school children for cystic fibrosis. Amer. J. Dis. Child., 100:174, 1960.
9. Andersen, D. H.: Cystic fibrosis of the pancreas. J. Chronic Dis., 7:58-90, 1958.
10. di Sant'Agnese, P. A., and Vidaurreta, A. M.: Cystic fibrosis of the pancreas. JAMA, 172:2065, 1960.
11. Shwachman, H., Laubner, H., and Catzel, P.: Mucoviscidosis. In Levine, S. Z. (ed.): Advances in Pediatrics. Chicago, Year Book, 7:249-323, 1955.
12. Shlaes, W. H., et al: Sweat test for mucovicidosis. Amer. J. Gastroent., 40:247-254, 1963.
13. Troutman, E. G.: A new method of iontophoresis and analysis of sweat electrolytes. Amer. J. Resp. Dis., Nov., 736-741, 1964.
14. Mendelsohn, R. S., and Cohen, B. M.: Otorhinolaryngologic aspects of cystic fibrosis. Arch. Otolarygn. (Chicago), 79:312-317, 1964.
15. Shwashman, H., Dunham, B. S., and Phillips, W. R.: Electrical conductivity of sweat, a simple diagnostic test in children. Pediatrics, 32:85-88, Vol. 1, 85-88, 1963.
16. Meskin, L. H., Bernard, B., and Warwick, W.: Biopsy of labial mucous salivary glands in cystic fibrosis. JAMA, 188, 1:202-203.
17. Goldbloom, R. B., and Sekelj, Paul: Cystic fibrosis of the pancreas diagnosis by application of a sodium electrode to the skin. New Eng. J. Med., 269:1349-1352, 1963.
18. Kopito, L., et. al.: Studies in cystic fibrosis: Analysis of nail clippings for sodium and potassium. New Eng. J. Med., 272:10 pp. 504-509, 1965.
19. Andersen, Dorothy H., et. al. Problems in cystic fibrosis. Ann. N.Y. Acad. Sci., 93:Art. 12, pp. 485-624 (Aug. 15), 1962.
20. Warwick, W., et. al.: A quantitative sweat chloride test for routine use in the newborn nursery. Cystic Fibrosis Club Abstracts, 6th Annual Meeting. May 3, 1965, pp. 15.

Iontophoresis of Sweat and Determination of Sweat Electrolytes

EARL B. WERT, M.D.

INTRODUCTION

The concentration of sodium and chloride in sweat is a reliable diagnostic feature of cystic fibrosis and is the cornerstone for the diagnosis or exclusion of this disease. The pilocarpine iontophoresis of sweat, its collection on gauze with subsequent elution and analysis for sodium and chloride is the recommended procedure. Conductivity methods for the analysis of sweat, both directly on the skin using a specially designed electrode, or on sweat collected in capillary tubes, have also received endorsement.

PRINCIPLE

Sweat glands, in a localized area on the arm or leg, are stimulated by pilocarpine introduced by iontophoresis. The positive electrode contains pilocarpine nitrate, the negative electrode at another position on the skin contains another electrolyte. A difference of potential is applied, the positively charged pilocarpine radicals move into the skin toward the negative electrode, with the stimulation of the sweat glands. Special care must be exercised with the negative electrodes to avoid electrical burns, which may be severe. After removal of the electrodes, the sweat secreted is collected on weighed gauze, using scrupulous technique to prevent contamination by salt, or loss of water. The sweat collected averages 0.2 to 0.4 gm, although, in dehydrated or malnourished infants, the yield may be somewhat less. After suitable elution and dilution of the sweat in the sponge, the sodium content is determined by flame photometry; the chloride content, by one of several methods.

REAGENTS AND STANDARD SOLUTIONS

1. *Pilocarpine nitrate solution,* 0.5 per cent. Approximately 1.25 gm of pilocarpine nitrate is dissolved in 250 ml of distilled water and kept refrigerated.

2. *Sodium nitrate solution,* 1.0 per cent. One gm of sodium nitrate is dissolved in 100 ml of distilled water.

3. *Distilled water.*

4. *Sodium chloride standard,* 50 mEq per liter. Exactly 0.2925 gm of dry sodium chloride is diluted to 1 liter with distilled water.

SPECIAL APPARATUS

1. *Iontophoresis power unit.*[*]
2. *Two electrodes* and *filter paper disks.*
3. *Perforated rubber strap* to secure electrodes.
4. *Parafilm* (paraffin film).
5. *Scissors, forceps, adhesive tape* (Micropore).
6. Unopened packages of 4 x 4 in and 2 x 2 in *gauze sponges.*
7. *"Plastainer"* snap-cap plastic vials with caps, 9 dram size. (Owens — Illinois #P-9 or similar air tight vial.)
8. *Analytical balance.*
9. *Interval clock timer.*

---

[*]Although the power supply for iontophoresis may be constructed from readily available elements, complete instruments may be purchased at reasonable prices. Two companies manufacturing standard models are: Farrall Instruments, P.O. 658, Grand Island, Nebraska; and Alloyd Laboratories, P.O. 225, Huntsville, Alabama. Both provide battery- and line-operated units that have given good service. The Alloyd instrument supplies newly patented electrodes which are hollow to receive the pilocarpine and electrolyte.

The Heat Technology Laboratory, Inc. (4308 Governors Drive, Huntsville, Alabama) instrument combines circuitry for power supply and conductivity measurements. The glass capillary tubes require some skill in filling, but this is easily acquired. The tubes must be carefully cleaned, (alcohol is essential). The capacity of the capillary tube is 0.001 to 0.002 ml. Thus, the patch is placed on the arm without gauze, the tiny beads of sweat are taken up by capillarity, and the readings made from a calibration curve and confirmed by standard solutions of electrolyte.

The Solu-meter (Industrial Instruments, Inc., 89 Commerce Road, Cedar Grove, New Jersey) is a standard conductivity meter used in industry. Using a micropipette-type conductivity cell of 0.02 ml capacity, Dr. Harry Shwachman, Children's Hospital, Boston, Massachusetts, has reported good results, although some difficulty may be anticipated in filling the pipette, due to small amounts of sweat secreted. Marginal values (conductivity values between 80 and 100 scale units) should be confirmed by elution techniques.

PROCEDURE

NOTE: Care must be exercised in handling of materials used for the collection of sweat, since contamination with perspiration from the fingers must be avoided.

A. *Preparation*

1. Parafilm squares. Parafilm can be purchased in rolls of 8 or 24 in widths and is free of sodium chloride. The Parafilm is cut into 3 in by 3 in squares without removing the paper backing thus preventing contamination of the covered surface.

2. Sweat collection sponges. A new package of 2 in x 2 in gauze sponges is opened. One sponge is placed in each of four clean "Plastainer" vials, using forceps. Two such vials are prepared for each patient ("test" and "blank"), and two are used for controls. The caps are replaced; each "test" sponge-vial is weighed on an analytical balance to the third decimal place.

B. *Iontophoresis*

1. The power supply is plugged into an electrical outlet of 110 v and the leads into the color-coded jacks on the front of the power supply. (Red = positive terminal; black = negative terminal.)

2. The positive electrode is filled with 0.5 per cent pilocarpine nitrate solution. One filter paper disk is placed over the bottom of this electrode, making certain that the metal portion of the electrode is covered.

3. The negative electrode is filled with 1.0 per cent sodium nitrate solution, and the bottom is covered by a filter paper disk.

4. A relatively hair-free area of the flexor surface of the forearm is selected in older children and adults; the calf area is used in infants and young children. The pilocarpine nitrate-filled positive electrode is placed on this surface. The sodium nitrate-filled negative electrode is placed on the opposite side of the arm and positioned so that both electrodes can be secured by the rubber strap. The electrodes are held firmly but without decreasing the circulation in the extremity. It should be ascertained that the position of the filter paper disk on each electrode does not allow the metal portion of the electrode to touch the patient's skin.

5. The lead connected to the red jack on the power supply is plugged into the red-coded pilocarpine-filled electrode on the flexor surface of the arm. The lead connected to the black jack on the power supply is plugged into the negative electrode stem on the opposite side of the arm.

6. The current is turned on by rotating the knob on the power supply in a clockwise direction. The current slowly is increased until the meter reads 1.5 ma. This step should take one to two minutes.

NOTE: The patient should feel no pain or shock. However, a mild tingling or prickling may be noticed. This is harmless, and does not require reducing current.

7. The current is turned off after five minutes of iontophoresis at 1.5 ma.

8. The electrodes and strap are removed. Five minutes are allowed for the sweat glands to flush out accumulated salt secretions. This is a convenient time to rinse the electrodes with distilled water, as is required after each use.

9. After the five-minute waiting period, the flexor surface of the arm, or leg is cleaned with distilled water and blotted dry with a clean 4 x 4 in gauze sponge.

10. Using forceps, the pre-weighed "test" sponge is removed from the vial and placed directly over the skin area of the pilocarpine-filled postive electrode. The paper backing from one of the 3 x 3 in Parafilm squares is removed, and the clean, salt-free surface is placed over the sponge.

11. All four sides of the Parafilm are taped down, using two strips of tape on each side. Then the exposed center portion of the Parafilm is covered with tape as well, to prevent tearing. The patch must be airtight.

12. The patient, nurse or parent is informed that the airtight patch must be worn for 60 to 120 minutes while the sweat collects on the gauze sponge. During this time the patient may be ambulatory and may drink liquids freely.

13. After one to two hours, one corner of the patch is lifted and, using forceps, the sweat-containing sponge is removed immediately and placed into the "test" vial. The vial is capped.

14. The adhesive tape and Parafilm are discarded.

15. Immediately, the sponge-vial and cap are weighed accurately to the third decimal place.

16. The sweat collected is calculated by subtracting the weight of the sponge-vial and cap before collection of sweat from the weight after collection of sweat.

17. 0.2 ml of the 50 mEq per liter

Example:

Weight of vial, cap, sponge and sweat	9.297 gm
Weight of vial, cap and sponge	9.086 gm
Therefore, sweat collected	= 0.211 gm

NaCl standard (control no. 1) is added to the pre-weighed control "test" vial. This is treated exactly as the sample of sweat. It is re-weighed, and the weight of "control" is determined.

18. The previously prepared "blank" sponge-vials are used to determine the sodium and chloride content of the sponge. This value is subtracted from the "test" value. The "blank" is treated in the same manner as the "test" when performing the sodium and chloride determinations.

C. Removal of Sweat from Sponges for Sodium and Chloride Determinations

1. The sweat may be eluted from the sponges by using any diluent which is compatible with the methods of choice for the determinations of sodium and chloride.

2. The sweat can be centrifuged out of the sponges rather than eluted. This method yields a higher number of unsatisfactory tests when small volumes of sweat are secreted. A golf tee or other support in the tip of a centrifuge tube will hold the sponge above the level of fluid as it is centrifuged.

DISCUSSION

Generally held to be an inborn error of metabolism genetically transmitted as a Mendelian dominant, cystic fibrosis occurs in about 0.1 to 0.5 per cent of live births, or about 4,000 cases per year in the United States. About 25,000 cases are under treatment. Estimates hold 2 to 5 per cent of population to be carriers of the C/F gene.

SOURCES OF ERROR

Errors may arise from evaporation of water from sweat during collection. Parafilm should be carefully placed and sealed at its edges on the skin by two overlapping strips of tape along each edge; the gauze should be quickly placed in a tared bottle, using forceps, when Parafilm is removed. False high values may also result from failure to allow sweat to wash out salt accumulations in skin and from failure to wash the site thoroughly with distilled water before beginning the collection. Sponge must be used as a "blank," as some gauze contains appreciable amounts of salt.

Values are subject to variation by salt intake, fluid intake and rate of sweating, but these effects have not seemed to produce misleading results. Marginal values, of course, must be repeated and carefully correlated with clinical data. Schlaes has reported that desoxycorticosterone reduces sweat sodium to normal in the heterozygote with increased levels. Untreated adrenal insufficiency may lead to increased concentration of electrolytes in sweat. In general, however, steroids seem not to effect the level of sweat electrolytes.

Failure to obtain adequate amounts of sweat will occur in about 5 per cent of cases, chiefly in dehydrated or malnourished infants, and may be somewhat more common in hot, humid weather. Forcing fluids for several hours and repeating the test usually produces adequate amounts.

RANGE OF VALUES

Values are somewhat higher in the newborn and in adults, but these usually do not extend into diagnostic levels.

Normal: 20 to 30 mEq per liter sodium or chloride
Compatible with cystic fibrosis: above 60 mEq per liter of chloride
above 70 mEq per liter of sodium
Marginal values (should be repeated): 50 to 60 mEq per liter of sodium or chloride
Cystic fibrosis, average values: 120 mEq per liter of sodium or chloride
Highest values reported in cystic fibrosis: 150 mEq per liter of sodium or chloride

RESUME OF CLINICAL INTERPRETATIONS

Although the marked elevation of sweat electrolyte levels in cystic fibrosis is not found in any other disease with which it can be confused, and the test is said to be about 98 per cent accurate, care must be exercised in the interpretation of the results. The pathologist should confer with the patient's physician, and each should understand the limitations of a single test before deciding the child has cystic fibrosis, with its serious implications. When normal values are found in a child showing chronic infections, or failure to thrive or gastrointestinal complaints, etc., one test, satisfactorily performed, may suffice to rule out cystic fibrosis. Marginal values, of 50 to 70 mEq per liter of sodium or chloride, or even higher in a child with an incomplete clinical pattern of cystic fibrosis, present difficulty. The problem as to whether this represents a "mild case" of true cystic fibrosis, a "variant," a symptomatic heterozygote bearing the gene for cystic fibrosis, etc., cannot be stated with certainty. These patients may require lifelong therapy, but have a more benign prognosis.

Cystic fibrosis is not invariably fatal at an early age. In general, however, there is little or no correlation between the electrolyte concentration and the severity of the disease. Thus, values in excess of 100 mEq per liter of sodium or chloride, in the absence of a clear clinical pattern of cystic fibrosis, may not be associated with an early demise. As an example: A physician told the parents of a robust child (chronic cough, wheezing, sinusitis) that life expectancy was limited on the basis of three sweat tests (Na = 94, 188, 71 mEq per liter). The child subsequently has developed a partial pattern of cystic fibrosis, requires postural drainage, liquifying agents, and antibotics, but at age seventeen years maintains robust appearance and excellent development.

Although the parents of children with cystic fibrosis do show statistically significant elevations of sweat electrolytes over normal controls, considerable overlapping is present. There is no premarital method for identification of heterozygotes at present; that is, the electrolyte level in heterozygotes is of theoretical interest but is not dependably used in genetic counseling.[*]

---

[*]Physicians should apply to National Cystic Fibrosis Research Foundation, 521 Fifth Avenue, New York 17, New York for available literature.

REFERENCES

1. Fanconi, G., Uehlinger, E., and Knauer, C.: Das Coeliakiesyndrom bei angerborener zystischer Pankreasfibromatose und Bronchiektasien. Wien Med. Wschr., **86**:753-756, 1936.

2. Andersen, D. H.: Cystic fibrosis of the pancreas and its relation to celiac disease. A clinical and pathological study. Amer. J. Dis. Child, **56**:344-399, 1938.

3. di Sant'Agnese, P. A.: Cystic fibrosis of the pancreas, edited transcription of a combined clinical staff conference at the Clinical Center, Bethesda, Maryland, by the National Institutes of Health Service, Department of Health, Education, and Welfare. Ann. Intern. Med., **54**:482, 1961.

4. Shwachman, H., and Gohm, N.: Studies in cystic fibrosis of the pancreas: A simple test for the detection of excessive chloride on the skin. New Eng. J. Med., **255**:999, 1956.

5. Gibson, L. E., and Cooke, R. E.: A test for concentration of electrolytes in sweat in cystic fibrosis of the pancreas utilizing pilocarpine by iontophoresis. Pediatrics, **23**:545, 1959.

6. Hsai, D. Y.: The laboratory detection of heterozygotes. Amer. J. Hum. Genet., **9**:98-116, June, 1957.

7. Bulletin: The National Cystic Fibrosis Research Foundation, 521 Fifth Avenue, New York 17, New York. Cystic Fibrosis News Bulletin.

8. Kulczycki, L. L., MacLeod, K. I. E., and Shwachman, H.: A survey of school children for cystic fibrosis. Amer. J. Dis. Child, **100**:174, 1960.

9. Andersen, D. H.: Cystic fibrosis of the pancreas. J. Chronic. Dis., **7**:58-90, 1958. .

10. di Sant'Agnese, P. A., and Vidaurreta, A. M.: Cystic fibrosis of the pancreas. JAMA, **172**:2065, 1960.

11. Shwachman, H., Laubner, H., and Catzel, P.: Mucoviscidosis. In Levine, S. Z. (ed.): Advances in Pediatrics. Chicago, Year Book, 7:249-323, 1955.

12. Shlaes, W. H., et. al.: Sweat test for mucovicidosis. Amer. J. Gastroent., **40**:247-254, 1963.

13. Troutman, E. G.: A new method of iontophoresis and analysis of sweat electrolytes. Amer. J. Resp. Dis., Nov., 736-741, 1964.

14. Mendelsohn, R. S., and Cohen, B. M.: Otorhinolaryngologic aspects of cystic fibrosis. Arch. Otolarygn. (Chicago), **79**:312-317, 1964.

15. Shwachman, H., Dunham, B. S., and Phillips, W. R.: Electrical conductivity of sweat, a simple diagnostic test in children. Pediatrics, **32**:85-88, Vol. 1, 1963.

16. Meskin, L. H., Bernard, B., and Warwich, W.: Biopsy of labial mucous salivary glands in cystic fibrosis. JAMA, **188**, 1:202-203.

17. Goldbloom, R. B., and Sekelj, P.: Cystic fibrosis of the pancreas, diagnosis by application of a sodium electrode to the skin. New Eng. J. Med., **269**:1349-1352, 1963.

18. Kopito, L., et. al.: Studies in cystic fibrosis: Analysis of nail clippings for sodium and potassium. New Eng. J. Med., **272**:10 pp., 504-509, 1965.

19. Andersen, D. H., et. al.: Problems in cystic fibrosis. Ann. N.Y. Acad. Sci., **93**:Art. 12, pp. 485-624 (Aug. 15), 1962.

Chapter 21

Disorders of Bilirubin Metabolism

IRWIN M. ARIAS, M.D.

Advances in understanding of the mechanism and regulation of bilirubin metabolism have resulted in recognition of new disease syndromes. Study of these disorders has increased knowledge regarding normal bilirubin metabolism[1-5]. This chapter will review briefly the hepatic metabolism of bilirubin and present a pathophysiologic classification of jaundice.

The serum bilirubin concentration in man normally does not exceed 1 mg per 100 ml. All the bilirubin found in normal serum is unconjugated and is mainly derived from the systematic degradation of mature, circulating erythrocytes. These cells have an average life span of 120 days and are destroyed in the reticuloendothelial system. The initial bile pigment formed is biliverdin, which is enzymatically reduced to bilirubin in the reticuloendothelial system. Approximately 15 per cent of the bilirubin formed each day is derived from sources other than the destruction of mature, circulating erythrocytes. Bilirubin is transported in plasma bound to albumin. At present there are no known pathways for the catabolism of bilirubin *in vivo*.

Bilirubin in plasma is primarily transported to the liver. The hepatic metabolism of bilirubin may be conveniently divided into three general processes:

(a) uptake; (b) conjugation; and (c) excretion. Virtually nothing is known about the mechanisms responsible for the transfer of unconjugated bilirubin from plasma into the liver cell (i.e., uptake) except that the transfer is too rapid to be linked to albumin. Presumably, an exchange occurs in the lateral cell membrane facing the hepatic sinusoid; unconjugated bilirubin enters the cytoplasm of the parenchymal liver cell and is bound by unidentified receptor molecules. Bilirubin is then conjugated with glucuronic acid in the endoplasmic reticulum. Conjugation converts bilirubin from a lipid-soluble aglycone to a water-soluble conjugate. In man, the major (and possibly only) conjugate formed is an ester glucuronide. In the rat, a small amount of ethereal sulfate conjugate of bilirubin is found in bile. The rate-limiting step in the biosynthesis of bilirubin glucuronide involves the enzymatic transfer of glucuronic acid from uridine diphosphate glucuronic acid (UDPGA) to bilirubin. This reaction is catalyzed by glucuronyl transferase, an enzyme found in the microsomal fraction of liver homogenates. Glucuronic acid used in glucuronide biosynthesis is derived from glucose and not from exogenous glucuronic acid. Conjugated bilirubin is subsequently transferred from the cytoplasm of the liver cell into the bile (i.e., excretion). This intracellular excretory process limits the overall transfer of bilirubin from blood to bile.

Virtually all of the bilirubin present in freshly obtained mammalian bile is conjugated. The bilirubin conjugates are subsequently hydrolyzed in the intestine. Bilirubin is partially reabsorbed in an enterohepatic circulation but primarily undergoes a series of reductions resulting in the formation of colorless compounds called *urobilinogens*. Urobilinogens are largely re-absorbed by an enterohepatic circulation and subsequently excreted in the bile. A small fraction is excreted in the urine. Normal fecal excretion of urobilinogen ranges from 80 to 250 mg per day. Normal urinary excretion ranges from 1 to 4 mg per day.

Jaundice is observed clinically when the serum bilirubin concentration exceeds approximately 2 mg per 100 ml. The reasons for the selective distribution of bilirubin in certain tissues (e.g., sclerae, elastic tissue and fat) are poorly understood. Chemical quantitation of conjugated and unconjugated bilirubin in serum is technically difficult; however, the concentrations of these pigments in serum are approximated by the direct and indirect van den Bergh's reactions, respectively.

Hyperbilirubinemia may be generally classified into two forms, depending upon whether the serum concentration of unconjugated or conjugated bilirubin is primarily increased. Table I is a pathophysiologic classification of jaundice.

Unconjugated hyperbilirubinemia can

TABLE I PATHOPHYSIOLOGIC CLASSIFICATION OF HYPERBILIRUBINEMIA

Unconjugated Hyperbilirubinemia

1. Hemolysis: increased bile pigment production
2. Physiologic jaundice of the newborn: normal delayed development of the glucuronide conjugating system
3. Transient familial neonatal hyperbilirubinemia: *ibid.*, and ? role of inhibitory effect of sera on bilirubin conjugation by rat liver slices
4. Neonatal jaundice associated with breast feeding: *ibid.*, and maternal excretion of pregnane 3(α),20(β)-diol in milk
5. Crigler-Najjar syndrome: glucuronyl transferase deficiency
6. Homozygous Gunn rat: glucuronyl transferase deficiency
7. Gilbert syndrome: etiologic heterogeneity

Conjugated Hyperbilirubinemia

1. Extrahepatic biliary obstruction
2. "Intrahepatic obstructive" jaundice
   a. Acquired defects in hepatic excretory function
      (i) Drugs
      (ii) Viral hepatitis
      (iii) Cirrhosis
   b. Inherited defects in hepatic cell excretory function
      (i) Rotor syndrome
      (ii) Dubin-Johnson syndrome
      (iii) Black liver disease in Corriedale sheep

theoretically result from increased bilirubin production, impaired hepatic uptake of unconjugated bilirubin or defective conjugation of bilirubin. There is no reliable method for estimating the hepatic uptake of bilirubin and, therefore, the role of this process in the pathogenesis of jaundice remains obscure.

Increased destruction of circulating erythrocytes in adults is only rarely associated with marked unconjugated hyperbilirubinemia. This presumably reflects the large functional reserve of the normal liver regarding the metabolism of bilirubin. The superimposition of erythrocyte hemolysis on structural or functional liver damage results in severe hyperbilirubinemia. The bilirubin in serum, however, is usually divided between conjugated and unconjugated.

Transient unconjugated hyperbilirubinemia is observed in virtually every full-term newborn infant. The serum bilirubin concentration rarely exceeds 5 to 6 mg per 100 ml and disappears by the third to fifth day of life. This "physiologic jaundice" of the newborn is believed to result from normally occurring delayed development of glucuronyl transferase activity[6, 7]. This disorder is of little clinical consequence, but, when additional factors are superimposed, kernicterus, which is a serious clinical disorder, can result[4]. Kernicterus results from unconjugated bilirubin toxicity to the central nervous system and may occur in full-term infants when the serum unconjugated bilirubin concentration exceeds approximately 20 mg per 100 ml during the first five days of life. The various factors known to facilitate the development of kernicterus are hemolysis (ABO and Rh incompatibility), infections of various types, metabolic disorders, prematurity and several familial disorders.

Transient familial neonatal hyperbilirubinemia is a rare syndrome in which all of a mother's infants develop transient but severe unconjugated hyperbilirubinemia and, frequently, kernicterus[8]. Beginning in the second trimester of normal pregnancy, serum from pregnant women inhibits glucuronyl transferase activity *in vitro*. The titer of inhibition increases until term and then disappears from postpartum and neonatal serum within seven to ten days[9]. Various progestins have been isolated from pregnancy serum and are responsible for the observed inhibition[10] which is competitive on kinetic analysis[11]. As shown in Figure 1, sera obtained from mothers of infants who develop transient familial neonatal hyperbilirubinemia have significantly increased inhibitory activity *in vitro*. The inhibitor has not been identified in this disorder, but its association with pregnancy suggests that it may be a progestational steroid. Its presence is believed to be of importance in the pathogenesis of this syndrome.

Some mothers excrete pregnane-3(α), 20(β)-diol in their breast milk[12]. Their breast-fed infants develop severe and prolonged unconjugated hyperbilirubinemia, probably due to inhibition of hepatic glucuronyl transferase activity by the steroid in milk[13]. Abrupt cessation of breast feeding results in prompt amelioration of jaundice.

An inherited deficiency of glucuronyl transferase activity is responsible for the rare, lifelong non-hemolytic unconjugated hyperbilirubinemia observed in the Crigler-Najjar syndrome[14] and in the

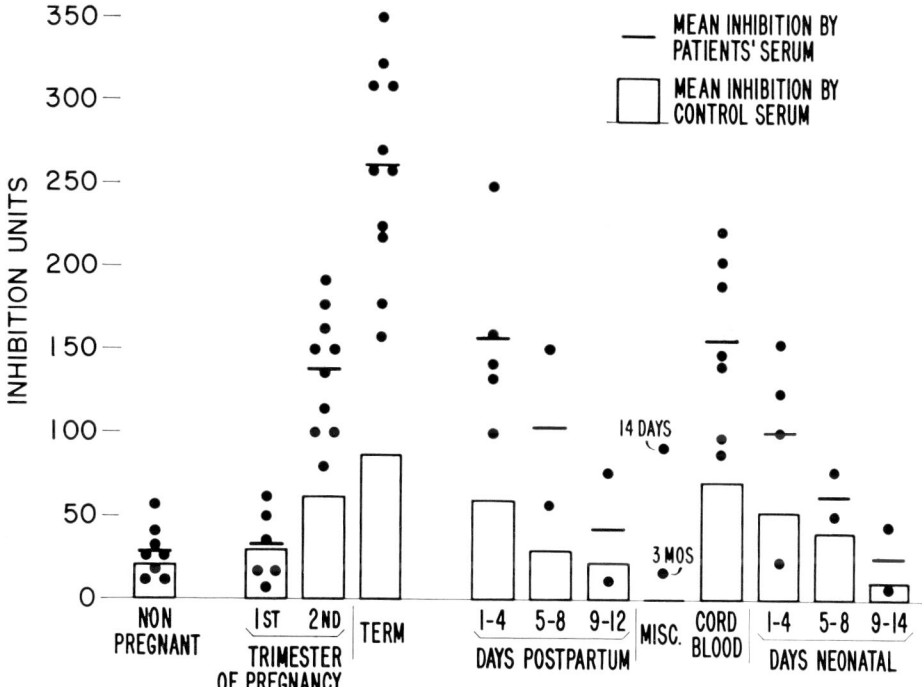

INHIBITION OF O-AMINOPHENOL GLUCURONIDE FORMATION BY RAT LIVER
HOMOGENATES BY SERUM FROM INFANTS WITH TRANSIENT FAMILIAL
NEONATAL HYPERBILIRUBINEMIA AND THEIR PREGNANT MOTHERS.

Figure I.

mutant Gunn rat[15]. These disorders are inherited with the characteristics of autosomal recessive genes. Bilirubin must be conjugated to be excreted by the liver or kidney; there is no compensatory increase in the formation of non-glucuronide conjugates, and due to the inherited deficiency in glucuronyl transferase, unconjugated bilirubin accumulates in plasma and tissues.

Mild to severe unconjugated hyperbilirubinemia unassociated with overt hemolysis is frequently observed in adolescents and adults and is usually termed Gilbert's disease or constitutional hepatic dysfunction. This syndrome results from etiologic heterogeneity[16]. An inherited deficiency of glucuronyl transferase activity has been demonstrated in a group of patients with this syndrome. Other mechanisms are compensated hemolytic states, postviral hepatitis, and increased production of bile pigment from sources other than mature, circulating erythrocytes[17]. In many patients, no etiologic mechanism can be demonstrated, and a defect in the transfer of bilirubin from plasma into the liver has been proposed.

Mechanical obstruction of the biliary tree and so called "intrahepatic obstructive" jaundice produced by virus, drugs and inherited disorders are characterized primarily by conjugated hyperbilirubinemia. Conjugated bilirubin is excreted by the kidney, whereas unconjugated bilirubin is not; therefore, as regards bile pigment metabolism, obstructive jaundice is characterized by conjugated hyperbilirubinemia and bilirubinuria.

There is no single biochemical or morphologic test or examination whereby "intrahepatic obstructive" jaundice can be differentiated from extrahepatic biliary obstruction. Studies of plasma bile pigments have not clarified this differential diagnosis.

Two inherited disorders involving the transfer of conjugated bilirubin from the liver into the bile have been described. The Rotor syndrome is characterized by chronic conjugated hyperbilirubinemia, bilirubinuria and bromsulfophthalein (BSP) retention[18]. The abnormality is transmitted with the characteristics of an autosomal dominant gene. The Dubin-Johnon syndrome is characterized by mild, intermittent conjugated hyperbilirubinemia, bilirubinuria, BSP retention and impaired radiologic visualization of the gall bladder following ingestion of cholecystographic agents[19]. In addition, the liver cells contain a black pigment which has physical and chemical characteristics of a melanin. The pigment probably results from accumulation, oxidation and polymerization of metabolites which are normally excreted in the bile. The mode of inheritance of the Dubin-Johnson syndrome is unknown. Similar functional and morphologic features have been described in mutant Corriedale sheep[20, 21].

"Intrahepatic obstructive" jaundice associated with hepatitis, various drugs and cirrhosis probably represents a functional disorder within the liver cell involving the poorly understood mechanisms whereby bilirubin conjugates are transferred from the liver cell into the bile. Previous attempts to explain the pathogenesis of these disorders by morphologic intrahepatic obstructive phenomena have not met with general acceptance. It is anticipated that further understanding of the precise mechanisms of hepatic cellular excretory function will clarify the pathogenesis and diagnosis of "intrahepatic obstructive" jaundice.

Whereas recent knowledge of bilirubin metabolism has clarified the pathogenesis of many inherited types of jaundice, this knowledge has not proven useful in understanding the mechanisms responsible for jaundice in acquired diseases, such as hepatitis and cirrhosis. The heterogeneity of the pathologic processes probably affects every aspect of the hepatic metabolism of bilirubin and accounts for the variable results in studies of the pathogenesis of jaundice in acquired diseases.

BIBLIOGRAPHY

1. Klatskin, G.: Bile pigment metabolism. Ann. Rev. Med., 12:211, 1961.
2. Billing, B. H.: The metabolism of bilirubin. In Advances Clin. Chem., 2:268, 1959.
3. Schmid, R.: Hyperbilirubinemia. In Stanbury, J. B., Wyngaarden, J. B., and Fredrickson, D. S. (eds.): Metabolic Basis of Inherited Disease. New York, McGraw, 1960.
4. Arias, I. M.: The chemical basis of kernicterus. Advances Clin. Chem., 3:35, 1960.
5. Arias, I. M.: The transport of bilirubin in the liver. In Popper, H., and Schaffner, F. (eds.): Progress in Liver Disease. New York, Grune, 1961, p. 363.
6. Brown, A. K., and Zuelzer, W. W.: Studies on the neonatal development of the glucuronide conjugating system. J. Clin. Invest., 37: 332, 1958.
7. Gartner, L., and Arias, I. M.: Developmental pattern of glucuronide formation in rat and guinea pig liver. Amer. J. Physiol., 205:663, 1963.
8. Arias, I. M., Wolfson, S., Lucey, J. F., and and McKay, R., Jr.: Transient familial neo-

natal hyperbilirubinemia. J. Clin. Invest., **44**: 1442, 1965.

9. Lathe, G. H., and Walker, M.: Inhibition of bilirubin conjugation in rat liver slices by human pregnancy and neonatal serum and steroids. Quart. J. Exp. Physiol., **43**:257, 1958.

10. Hsia, D. Y. Y., Dowben, R. M., Shaw, R., and Grossman, A.: Inhibition of glucuronyl transferase by progestational agents from serum of pregnant women. Nature (London), **187**:693, 1960.

11. Hsia, D. Y. Y., Riabov, S., Dowben, R. M.: Inhibition of glucuronosyl transferase by steroid hormones. Arch. Biochem., **103**:181, 1963.

12. Arias, I. M., Gartner, L. M., Seifter, S., and Furman, M.: Prolonged neonatal unconjugated hyperbilirubinemia associated with breast feeding and a steroid pregnane-3(alpha), 20 (beta)-diol, in maternal milk that inhibits glucuronide formation in vitro. J. Clin. Invest., **43**:2037, 1964.

13. Arias, I. M., and Gartner, L. M.: Production of unconjugated hyperbilirubinemia in full term newborn infants following administration of pregnane-3(alpha), 20(beta)-diol. Nature (London), **203**:1292, 1964.

14. Crigler, J. F., and Najjar, V. A.: Congenital familial nonhemolytic jaundice with kernic-

terus. Pediatrics, **23**:903, 1959.

15. Schmid, R., Axelrod, J., Hammaker, L., and Swarm, R. L.: Congenital jaundice in rats due to defect in glucuronide formation. J. Clin. Invest., **37**:1123, 1958.

16. Arias, I. M.: Chronic unconjugated hyperbilirubinemia without overt signs of hemolysis in adolescents and adults. J. Clin. Invest., **41**:2233, 1962.

17. Israels, L. G., Sunderman, H. J., and Ritzman, S. E.: Hyperbilirubinemia due to an alternate path of bilirubin production. Ann. J. Med., **27**:693, 1959.

18. Rotor, A. B., Manahan, L., and Florentin, A.: Familial nonhemolytic jaundice with direct van den Bergh reaction. Acta Med. Philipp., **5** (2):37, 1948.

19. Dubin, N., and Johnson, F. B.: Chronic idiopathic jaundice with unidentified pigment in liver cells. Medicine, **33**:155, 1954.

20. Arias, I. M., Bernstein, L. H., Toffler, R., Cornelius, C. E., Novikoff, A. B., and Essner, E.: Black liver disease in Corriedale sheep: A new mutation affecting hepatic excretory function. J. Clin. Invest., **43**:1249, 1964.

21. Cornelius, C. E., Arias, I. M., and Osburn, B. I.: Hepatic pigmentation with photosensitivity: A syndrome in Corriedale sheep resembling Dubin-Johnson syndrome in man. J. Amer. Vet. Med. Ass., **146**:709, 1965.

Microanalysis of Serum Bilirubin by a Diazotization Procedure

J. DE LA HUERGA, M.D., Ph.D., GEORGE W. SMETTERS, M.D. AND JOSEPH C. SHERRICK, M.D.

INTRODUCTION

Bilirubin is a yellow tetrapyrrol pigment derived from hemoglobin breakdown. It is conjugated with glucuronic acid by the liver, and the product is excreted into the intestine. Normally, a small amount is present in the circulating blood, bound to albumin. Under certain conditions, intercellular binding forces may be strong enough to compete with albumin binding so that unconjugated bilirubin accumulates within cells, where it is potentially toxic to cellular functions. On this basis, bilirubin may accumulate in the basal ganglia of the brain in newborn infants with severe neonatal jaundice. In these cases of kernicterus, bilirubin produces permanent neurological damage associated with specific pathological changes.

Because kernicterus can be prevented by exchange transfusion performed before the bilirubin level becomes critical, accurate measurement of the serum bilirubin is of basic importance in the treatment of neonatal jaundice. Although many excellent procedures are available, the microdetermination of serum bilirubin presents certain difficulties in the average clinical laboratory. An accurate procedure, readily performed on small amounts of serum, and simple enough to be done on an emergency basis, is essential for providing proper information.

Procedures based on measurement of the color produced when bilirubin solutions are treated with diazotized sulfanilic acid have produced satisfactory results for many years[3, 8]. General usage is shown by a survey[14], in which over 95 per cent of responding pathologists reported using a method of this type. Direct spectrophotometric measurement of the yellow color of the serum, as described by Shinowara[13] and discussed in Chapters 22B and 22C, is also satisfactory. Solvent partition methods are useful in research[12, 16], and have recently been studied by Stevenson and associates[15]. As yet, a method of this type suitable for routine work has not been devised.

Modified Method of Meites and Faulkner [9]

PRINCIPLE

Diazotized sulfanilic acid in acid solution reacts with bilirubin to produce azobilirubin, which has a lavender color with maximum absorbancy at 570 mμ. The intensity of the color, which is directly proportional to the bilirubin concentration, is measured in the spectrophotometer.

REAGENTS

1. *Acidified methanol.* Two hundred ninety ml of methanol and 25 ml of 1 N hydrochloric acid are transferred to a 500 ml volumetric flask. Distilled water is added to the mark.

2. *Sulfanilic acid.* Two and a half gm of sulfanilic acid are transferred to a 500 ml volumetric flask. About 400 ml of distilled water and 25 ml of 1 N hydrochloric acid are added. The flask is then stoppered and inverted until all the sulfanilic acid goes into solution. Distilled water is added to the mark. This solution is stable.

3. *Sodium nitrite,* (20 per cent w/v). This reagent is stable if kept in a brown bottle in the refrigerator.

4. *Diazo reagent.* This reagent is prepared just before use by mixing 6 ml of sulfanilic acid reagent and 20 μl of sodium nitrate reagent.

5. *Hydrochloric acid,* 0.05 N.

6. *Hydrochloric acid,* 0.4 N.

7. *Standard bilirubin solution.* This solution must be made up fresh just before use and kept in the dark. Using an analytical balance, a precise amount of pure bilirubin between 8 and 10 mg is weighed out and transferred to a 100 ml volumetric flask. About 90 ml of chloroform is added, and the bilirubin is dissolved by inverting the flask while it is wrapped in a dark cloth. Then more chloroform is added to the mark.

8. *Diluted working standard.* This is prepared as described in the standardization procedure.

PROCEDURE

The 12 mm cuvette adaptor for the Coleman Junior Spectrophotometer is provided with metal strips that slide into the adaptor, partly occluding the opening, so that 1.3 ml of liquid may be used for the readings.

A. Total Bilirubin

To a 12 mm cuvette is transferred 1.3 ml of the acidified methanol reagent, followed by exactly 50 μl of serum. If the serum is very jaundiced, only 20 or even 10 μl may be used. After mixing well, the cuvette is allowed to stand at room temperature for at least two minutes. With the spectrophotometer at 570 mμ, and using a 12 mm cuvette filled with distilled water, the galvanometer is adjusted to 100 per cent transmission. For this purpose, the strips described above *must* be in place. The reading from the cuvette containing the sample is made and recorded as R_1. 0.13 ml of recently prepared diazo reagent are added, mixed, and the solution is allowed to stand for at least eight minutes. A second reading, R_2, is taken, using the same water blank. Another reading is obtained five minutes later (total of 13 minutes). If this reading is of the same order as R_2, the latter reading is considered final. If the thirteen-minute reading shows significant increase in absorbancy, additional readings should be taken until maximum absorbancy is reached.

Calculation. The apparent bilirubin concentration for R_1 obtained from the chart is multiplied by 0.9, and the product is subtracted from the concentration found for R_2. If the reading of R_2 is less than 15 per cent transmission, 1.5 ml of acidified methanol are added to the cuvette and mixed. Readings are then repeated as above. The concentration found is multiplied by two and then subtracted from the apparent bilirubin found for R_1 multiplied by 0.45.

B. Direct Bilirubin

This procedure is carried out in the same way as the total determination with the exception that the 0.05 N hydrochloric acid is used instead of the acidified methanol. The reading must be made exactly one minute after adding the diazo reagent.

C. Standardization

Exactly five ml of freshly prepared bilirubin standard are transferred to a 50 ml volumetric flask. The flask is filled to the mark with methanol and the contents are mixed. Of this standard, 1.2, 1.0, 0.8, 0.6 and 0.4 are transferred to 12 mm Coleman cuvettes. Methanol is added to make the total volume in each tube 1.2 ml. .15 ml of 0.4 N hydrochloric acid are added to each tube followed by 0.13 ml of diazo reagent. After at least eight minutes, readings are made at 570 mμ using methanol as a blank, and with the blocking strips in place. Knowing the concentration of the standard prepared and the amount of materials used, a standard curve is plotted on semilogarithmic paper, and a reference chart is constructed. For instance, if exactly 10 mg of bilirubin was weighed out, the absorbancy obtained in the first tube of the dilutions would be equivalent to that of a serum concentration of 24 mg per 100 ml. In our experience, a standard corresponding to a serum concentration of 20 mg per 100 ml usually produces an absorbancy of about 20 per cent transmission.

DISCUSSION

This procedure is based on the Meites-Faulkner[9] modification of the Malloy and Evelyn[8] method. The principles underlying this method have been considered previously[7]. The modification consists of an increase in the concentration of the diazotized sulfanilic acid to produce rapid development of an intense lavender color, intended to produce optimum spectrophotometric readings at relatively normal levels of serum bilirubin. The procedure was designed for the Coleman Junior spectrophotometer, but other spectrophotometers may be used with equal satisfaction under similar conditions.

In our original studies, it was found that serum color development was complete in five to seven minutes after diazo reagent was added and the color was relatively stable. Therefore, an eight-minute waiting period was regarded as being sufficient. Henry and associates have cast doubt on the adequacy of this eight-minute interval, and others have observed an increase in intensity of color between eight and thirteen minutes. In order to guard against the possibility of incomplete color development, a second reading should be made thirteen minutes after addition of diazo reagent. If there is no change from the eight-minute reading to the thirteen-minute reading, color development is complete.

For standardization of this procedure, a chloroform-methanol solution of bilirubin is recommended, although the protein-containing solution advocated by an inter-society group[1] may be used with equal satisfaction. According to the recent studies of Meites and Traubert[10], and confirmed by us, there was no difference in the readings obtained so long as the recommendations of the group were carefully followed. Variations reported by some observers are probably due to the contraction in volume occurring in water-methanol solutions, or may result from the use of other methods which produce a final mixture with less color intensity. The method described here, utilizing a relatively concentrated solution of diazotized sulfanilic acid, produces an intensely colored relatively stable azobilirubin. The intensity of color may be responsible for the ease of standardization with chloroform solutions of bilirubin. The bilirubin used for standardization should have a molecular absorbtivity between 59,100 and 62,300. Newbold and LeBlanc[11] have studied various samples of commercially available bilirubin, and found considerable variation in the quality of the product. Clarke[2] has described methods for purifying bilirubin, and reports a method for obtaining bilirubin of satisfactory quality from human bile.

Lyophilized commercial standards of bilirubin in serum may be used for standardization or quality control. Our experience, like that of Meites and Traubert[10], is that they are satisfactory for the clinical laboratory. These preparations retain their diazo reaction characteristics for at least one week, even when melted and refrozen daily.

REFERENCES

1. A uniform bilirubin standard. Recommendations of the College of American Pathologists Standards Committee. Amer. J. Clin. Path., 39:90-91, 1963.
2. Clarke, J. T.: Purification and analysis of bilirubin. Clin. Chem., 11:681-690, 1965.
3. Ehrlich, P.: Sulfodiazobenzol, ein reagens auf Bilirubin. Cbl. Klin. Med., 4:721-723, 1883.
4. Gambino, S. R., and Di Re, J.: Manual on Bilirubin Assay. Chicago, Commission on Continuing Education, Council on Clinical Chemistry, American Society of Clinical Pathologists, 1963.
5. Henry, R. J.: Fractionation of free and conjugated bilirubins. In Sunderman, F. W. and Sunderman, F. W., Jr.: Hemoglobin — Its Precursors and Metabolites. Philadelphia, Lippincott, 1964.
6. Hogg, C. K., and Meites, S.: A modification of the Malloy and Evelyn procedure for the microdetermination of total serum bilirubin. Amer. J. Med. Techn., 25:271-279, 1959.
7. de la Huerga, J., and Sherrick, J. C.: Measurement of bilirubin in serum. In Sunderman and Sunderman, op. cit.
8. Malloy, H. T., and Evelyn, K. A.: The determination of bilirubin with the photoelectric colorimeter. J. Biol. Chem., 119:481-490, 1937.
9. Meites, S., and Faulkner, W. R.: Manual of Practical Micro and General Procedures in Clinical Chemistry. Springfield, Thomas, 1962.
10. Meites, S., and Traubert, J. W.: Use of bilirubin standards. Clin. Chem., 11:691-699, 1965.
11. Newbold, B. T., and LeBlanc, G.: Physical characteristics of commercial bilirubins. Canad. J. Biochem., 42:1697-1702, 1964.
12. Schachter, D.: Estimation of bilirubin mono- and diglucuronide in the plasma and urine of patients with nonhemolytic jaundice. J. Lab. Clin. Med., 53:557-562, 1959.
13. Shinowara, G. Y.: Spectrophotometric studies on blood serum and plasma: The physical determination of hemoglobin and bilirubin. Amer. J. Clin. Path., 24:696-710, 1954.
14. Shively, J. A.: Evaluation of methodology in

clinical chemistry. Amer. J. Clin. Path., **43**: 505-516, 1965.

15. Stevenson, G. W., Jacobs, S. L., and Henry, R. J.: Determination of bile pigments. IV. Spectrophotometric determination of free and total bilirubin in serum. Clin. Chem., **10**: 95-102, 1964.

16. Valera-Fuentes, B., and Escuries, J.: Nou-velles methodes pour la separation et la dosage des deux bilirubines directe et indirecte du serum. C. R. Soc. Biol., **107**:884-887, 1931.

17. van den Bergh, A. A. H., and Muller, P.: Über eine direkte und eine indirekte Diazo-reaktion auf Bilirubin. Biochem. Z., **77**:90-103, 1916.

Microanalysis of Serum Bilirubin by Direct Spectrophotometry

HARRISON H. LEFFLER, M.D.

INTRODUCTION

In the diagnosis and treatment of jaundice in the newborn, the use of an accurate and reliable method for the estimation of serum bilirubin is most important. The diazo methods in current use are not always reliable. Hemolysis, especially, interferes with their use. The method being presented is accurate, easy to perform, and is not affected by hemolysis.

PRINCIPLE

The absorbancy of the serum is determined in a spectrophotometer at two different wavelengths which give the minimum and maximum densities due to bilirubin and, at the same time, give identical readings with hemoglobin solutions. The difference between the maximum and the minimum densities gives a value which is proportional to the concentration of bilirubin.

REAGENT

Sodium carbonate, 0.1 per cent, is the only reagent used.

STANDARDIZATION PROCEDURES

Before standardizing for bilirubin, it is necessary to select the two desired wavelength settings. This is accomplished as follows: Oxalated blood, 0.02 ml, is transferred to a cuvette containing 5.0 ml of 0.1 per cent sodium carbonate. Readings of this hemolyzed blood are made at 575 mμ and at 455 mμ against a water blank set at 100 per cent transmittance. Since spectrophotometers differ, the second wavelength may have to be adjusted by trial and error until the reading is identical to the reading at 575 mμ. With the author's Spectronic 20, a point halfway between the scale markings for 455 and 460 (λ 457.5 mμ) gave a reading identical to that obtained at 575 mμ. By using these two selected settings, it is now possible to standardize the spectrophotometer for bilirubin without interference from hemolysis.

In subdued light, exactly 10.0 mg of bilirubin are dissolved in 10 ml of 1 per cent sodium carbonate. (Solution should be complete in five to ten minutes and should be used as soon as possible.) To 1 ml of this solution are added 9 ml of distilled water and 10 ml of 0.1 per cent sodium carbonate to give a bilirubin standard containing 1 mg bilirubin in 20 ml, or 5 mg per 100 ml. This diluted standard and fresh non-icteric serum are used to prepare calibration standard. Into matched cuvettes, the solutions are placed as follows:

	Blank	Standard
ml of fresh serum	0.5	0.5
ml of diluted standard	0.0	0.5
ml of 0.1 per cent sodium carbonate	4.5	4.0

This gives a bilirubin standard containing 0.5 mg of bilirubin per 100 ml of 0.1 per cent sodium carbonate in 10 per cent serum.

The density readings of the standard at the selected wavelengths against the serum blank set at 100 per cent transmittance are recorded as follows:

At 457.5 mμ, density (D) = 0.500 and

At 575 mμ, density (D) = 0.000, giving a density difference

Of 0.500 for the concentration of 0.5 mg per 100 ml of solution

The concentration (C) divided by the density (D) gives a constant (K) which is always the same value for the specific cuvette-spectrophotometer combination being used. This constant, when multiplied by the density of the bilirubin solution, gives the bilirubin concentration.

Using microcuvettes with 1-cm light paths for the blank and standard, the following values are obtained:

At 457.5 mμ, the standard density (D) = 0.400 and

At 575 mμ, the standard density (D) = 0.000, or a density difference of 0.400

$$\frac{C}{D} = \frac{0.5}{0.4} = 1.25 = K,$$ the constant obtained when using microcuvettes.

PROCEDURE FOR SERUM USING TEST TUBE CUVETTES

Into a test tube cuvette containing 4.9 ml of 0.1 per cent sodium carbonate

is transferred 0.1 ml of serum. Readings are then made at the two selected wavelengths against a water blank set at 100 per cent transmittance, and the density is recorded. Example:

Density (D) at λ 457.5 = 0.523
Density (D) at λ 575 = 0.051

Density difference   = 0.472

Since the constant K= 1.0, the density difference multipled by the dilution (50) gives the concentration of bilirubin:

0.472 × 50 = 23.6 mg bilirubin per 100 ml of serum

PROCEDURE FOR SERUM USING MICROCUVETTES

Into a microcuvette with a 1-cm light path and containing 0.98 ml of 0.1 per cent sodium carbonate is pipetted 0.02 ml of serum. Readings are made at the selected wavelengths against a water blank set at 100 per cent transmittance. Density readings are recorded, and the concentration of bilirubin is computed as in the following example:

Density (D) at λ 457.5 = 0.4184
Density (D) at λ 575 = 0.0408

Density difference   = 0.3776

With the use of microcuvettes, the constant (K) = 1.25, and the dilution is 50, as with the test tube cuvettes. Since the density difference x K x dilution = concentration of bilirubin,

$0.3776 \times 1.25 \times 50 = 23.6$ mg of bilirubin per 100 ml of serum.

DISCUSSION

The purity of bilirubin used in the standard is very important. The committee appointed to investigate the properties of satisfactory bilirubin gives the following recommendations[1]: When dissolved in chloroform at 25 C and the absorbancy is read at 453 mμ with a cuvette having a 1-cm light path, the bilirubin should give a molecular absorbancy of 60,700 ± 800. Bilirubin having these properties was used to obtain the results presented.

A bilirubin standard made up in serum does not give the same molecular absorbancy. The standard readings made in a microcuvette with a 1-cm light path gave a density of 0.400 for 0.5 mg of bilirubin per 100 ml (5.0 mg per liter). If the concentration is 5.0 gm per liter, then the density obtained would be 400. Since the molecular weight of bilirubin is 584:

In the present method, hemoglobin gives identical readings at the two wave legths. Since no other interfering substance is present in the serum of the newborn, the density difference is due entirely to bilirubin. The degree of accuracy is excellent. In a range of bilirubin concentrations of 0.6 to 2.0 mg per 100 ml, the SD = ±0.03 mg, and, in the range of 3.0 to 8.0 mg per 100 ml, SD = ± 0.06 mg.

If the density reading of 0.7 or greater is obtained, further dilution with 0.1 per cent sodium carbonate is necessary to obtain the proper accuracy.

White et al.[3] show that capillary blood and venous blood give practically the same bilirubin values.

SOURCES OF ERROR

Preparation of the bilirubin standard in subdued light is important. Complete solution in 1 per cent sodium carbonate requires about five minutes. Immediate dilution and reading of the calibration standard should prevent errors in standardization. In this manner, loss of density owing to light exposure is prevented.

Careful and accurate pipetting of serum and reagents should eliminate any further difficulties.

$$\frac{5 \quad (\text{gm per liter})}{400 \quad (D)} = \frac{584 \, (\text{gm mol wt})}{X}$$

X = 46,720 = molecular absorbancy of bilirubin in 10 per cent serum and 0.1 per cent sodium carbonate.

Shinowara[2] determines the constant (K) at each wavelength, and using complex mathematical formulae, makes the necessary correction for interference of hemoglobin.

RANGE OF VALUES

Examination of the cord blood in the newborn infant frequently shows over 3.0 mg of bilirubin per 100 ml without jaundice being evident. When the level exceeds 4.0 mg per 100 ml, jaundice is apt to be present, and further developments should be carefully watched.

REFERENCES

1. A Uniform Bilirubin Standard. Recommendations of the College of American Pathologists Standards Committee. Amer. J. Clin. Path., 39:90-91, 1963.

2. Shinowara, G. Y.: Spectrophotometric studies on blood serum and plasma. Amer. J. Clin. Path., 24:696-710, 1954.

3. White, D., Haidar, G. A., and Reinhold, J. G.: Spectrophotometric measurement of bilirubin concentrations in the serum of the newborn by use of a microcapillary method. Clin. Chem., 4:211-222, 1958.

Alternative Microanalysis of Serum Bilirubin by Direct Spectrophotometry

Adaptation for the Clinical Spectrophotometer

J. DE LA HUERGA, M.D., Ph.D., GEORGE W. SMETTERS, M.D.,
AND JOSEPH C. SHERRICK, M.D.

The direct spectrophotometric measurements of serum bilirubin presents certain advantages in the jaundiced infant. It is a rapid, accurate method which may be performed on small amounts of serum even in the presence of considerable hemolysis. Pigments other than bilirubin, which may interfere with the procedure, are much less common in infants than in adults. The method has the disadvantage of measuring total bilirubin only, so its results are not as helpful in the differential diagnosis of jaundice of the newborn as are those of the diazo methods. Nevertheless, once the cause of jaundice has been established, it is a most useful method for following the course of the infant in an attempt to prevent the development of kernicterus. The main reason that this method has not been more widely used is that, in the past, it was thought to be necessary to employ a spectrophotometer of high resolution and narrow band-width for the determination. The work of Meites and

Hogg[2], however, indicates that the procedure may be readily adapted to clinical spectrophotometers, such as the Coleman Junior and the Bausch and Lomb Spectronic 20.

It is the purpose of this study to present our experience in adapting the direct spectrophotometric measurement of serum bilirubin to several clinical spectrophotometers, and to present a means of constructing a nomogram for the calculation of the results obtained by the use of any spectrophotometer.

PRINCIPLE

This method is based on the observation that bilirubin in serum, when diluted with phosphate buffer, absorbs light at a wavelength of 455 mμ. Hemoglobin also absorbs light at this wavelength. However, hemoglobin also absorbs light at a wavelength of 575 mμ, while bilirubin does not absorb light significantly at this latter wavelength. Thus, by comparing the absorption of light by a serum sample containing both bilirubin and hemoglobin at 455 mμ with that absorbed at 575 mμ, the absorption due to bilirubin may be calculated, and this is proportional to the bilirubin concentration.

Shinowara[3] was the first to apply this principle to the measurement of bilirubin and hemoglobin in undiluted serum and plasma. His method was devised for normal or slightly jaundiced serum. White, Haidar and Reinhold[4] applied the method to the determination of bilirubin in small volumes of serum by dilution with phosphate buffer. The work was performed using the Beckman DU Spectrophotometer, in which the absorption of hemoglobin is the same at 455 as at 575 mμ, thus making the calculations simple.

APPARATUS

Coleman Junior spectrophotometers. Six Model 6C and one Model 6D instruments were used with 12 mm round cuvettes. The wavelengths were calibrated with the didymium filter furnished by the manufacturer.

Bausch and Lomb Spectronic 20 spectrophotometers. Three instruments of this type were used with 13 mm round cuvettes. Calibration of the wavelength was performed using cobalt chloride as recommended by the manufacturer.

Beckman spectrophotometers. One Model B and one Model DU were used with 1 cm square cuvettes having an optical pathway of 10 mm. Calibration of the wavelength was done using a mercury lamp for the 491.6 mμ wavelength.

REAGENTS

1. *Sorenson phosphate buffer,* 0.067 M, pH 7.4. Precisely 0.75 gm of diso-dium phosphate anhydrous (Na_2HPO_4) and 0.18 gm of monobasic potassium phosphate (KH_2PO_4) are dissolved in distilled water in a 100 ml volumetric flask, which is filled to the mark with distilled water. This solution is stable.

2. *Bilirubin solvent.* One ml of 5 N sodium hydroxide is diluted to 100 ml with Reagent 1 (Sorenson buffer).

3. *Bilirubin standard.* This solution must be made up fresh just before use and kept in the dark. Using an analytical balance, a precise amount of pure bilirubin between 15 and 25 mg is weighed out in a 10 ml beaker. Four ml of bilirubin solvent (Reagent 2) are added, and the bilirubin is dissolved by gentle stirring during the next two to four minutes. The mixture is transferred to a 100 ml volumetric flask by repeated rinsing with clear non-hemolyzed pooled serum, and more serum is added to the mark.

Commercial preparations of bilirubin in lyophilized serum have been used for standardization with good results.

4. *Serum blank.* One ml of bilirubin solvent is added to 25 ml of the serum used in Reagent 3.

5. *Hemoglobin standard.* A sample of fresh normal blood is centrifuged and the supernatant plasma is discarded. The cells are then suspended in at least ten volumes of saline and centrifuged. This procedure is repeated twice. The well-packed red cells are then hemolyzed, using sixty volumes of distilled water, by vigorous shaking, and the tube is centrifuged. This will produce a supernatant solution with hemoglobin concentration of approximately 500 mg per 100 ml. The actual content is determined by a standard colorimetric method. The hemolysate is diluted with

TABLE I

	Buffer	Cuvette	Bilirubin Standard
Coleman Junior spectrophotometer	1.8 ml	12 mm round	0.05 ml
Spectronic 20 spectrophotometer	2.5 ml	13 mm round	0.05 ml
Beckman B and DU spectrophotometers	1.0 ml	{1 cm square, {1 ml	0.025 ml

distilled water to give an approximate concentration of 300 mg per 100 ml.

STANDARDIZATION

1. Three of the proper cuvettes for the instrument are labelled "B," "S" and "H," and the proper amount of Sorenson buffer (Reagent 1) is transferred to each. The proper amount of serum blank is added to B; the same amount of bilirubin standard to S; and the same amount of hemoglobin standard to H. The contents are well mixed. For amounts and cuvettes to be used, see Table I.

These dilutions have been selected to produce absorbancy readings of approximately 0.4, the most accurate zone of the spectrophotometers for bilirubin concentration of 15 to 25 mg per 100 ml.

2. At a wavelength of 455 mμ, the spectrophotometer is adjusted to 0 absorbancy with distilled water, and readings of the serum blank, bilirubin standard and hemoglobin standard are obtained and recorded. The absorbancies of the bilirubin standard and hemoglobin standard are corrected by subtracting the absorbancy of the serum blank from each.

3. Similar readings are obtained at 575 mμ.

4. Calculations:

$$\frac{\text{Corrected absorbancy standard bilirubin solution at 455 m}\mu}{\text{Concentration of bilirubin standard in mg per 100 ml}} = Kb^{455} \cdot \text{Absorbancy represents a 1 mg per 100 ml bilirubin solution at 455 m}\mu^{\circ}$$

$$\frac{\text{Corrected absorbancy standard bilirubin solution at 575 m}\mu}{\text{Concentration of bilirubin standard in mg per 100 ml}} = Kb^{575} \cdot \text{Absorbancy represents a 1 mg per 100 ml bilirubin solution at 575 m}\mu^{\circ}$$

$$\frac{\text{Corrected absorbancy standard hemoglobin solution at 455 m}\mu}{\text{Concentration of hemoglobin, mg per 100 ml}} = Kh^{455} \cdot \text{Absorbancy represents a 1 mg per 100 ml hemoglobin solution at 455 m}\mu^{\circ}$$

$$\frac{\text{Corrected absorbancy standard hemoglobin solution at 575 m}\mu}{\text{Concentration of hemoglobin, mg per 100 ml}} = Kh^{575} \cdot \text{Absorbancy represents a 1 mg per 100 ml hemoglobin solution at 575 m}\mu^{\circ}$$

$$\frac{\text{Absorbancy hemoglobin solution at 455 m}\mu}{\text{Absorbancy hemoglobin solution at 575 m}\mu} = R$$

°The absorbancies here refer to the concentration of the original standard or sample solution previous to dilution as in Step one.

These calculations are made to be used later in the calculation of the concentration of bilirubin in the unknown.

PROCEDURE

This procedure is designed for samples obtained in capillary tubes from infants, and should be performed promptly, as it is usually requested on an emergency basis. The sample should be kept in the dark until the analysis is undertaken.

1. The proper amount of Sorenson buffer is transferred to one of the proper cuvettes for the instrument to be used, and the proper amount of serum is added. The contents are well mixed.

For amounts and cuvettes, see standardization, Table I.

2. At a wavelength of 455 mμ the spectrophotometer is adjusted to 0 absorbancy with distilled water, and absorbancy readings of the sample are obtained and recorded.

3. The same sequence is used to obtain readings of the sample at a wavelength of 575 mμ.

4. Calculations:

$$\frac{d^{455} - (R \times d^{575})}{Kb^{455} - (R \times Kb^{575})} = \text{bilirubin concentration in mg per 100 ml}$$

Where: R, Kb^{455} and Kb^{575} are obtained from the standardization of the procedure, and

d^{455} = absorbancy of unknown sample of serum at 455 mμ

d^{575} = absorbancy of unknown sample of serum at 575 mμ

RESULTS

The absorpancies of standard bilirubin solutions containing 20 mg of bilirubin per 100 ml and of standard hemoglobin solutions containing 300 mg of hemoglobin per 100 ml are shown in Table II. These results show that the procedure may be satisfactorily performed on any of the instruments studied, since readings were all in the most accurate range of the spectrophotometer, from 0.38 to 0.46 absorbancy. The significantly higher absorbancies observed in the Beckman and Bausch and Lomb spectrophotometers were compensated by different degrees of dilution. The absorbancy was proportional to the concentration of bilirubin up to levels of 28 mg per 100 ml with the Coleman instruments and even higher with the other instruments.

From Table II it can be seen that there is distinct variation in the R factor, i.e., in the ratio of the absorbancy of hemoglobin at 455 mμ to that at 575 mμ, from one instrument to the next, even among instruments of the same

TABLE II

Instrument	No.[*]	Dilution		Bilirubin (20 mg per 100 ml)		Hemoglobin (300 mg per 100 ml)		"R"
		Buffer (ml)	Serum (ml)	Absorption at		Absorption at		
				455 mμ	575 mμ	575 mμ	455 mμ	
Coleman 6 C	6	1.8	0.05	0.380–0.440	0.019–0.020	0.077–0.090	0.042–0.050	1.8–2.2
Coleman 6 D	1	1.8	0.05	0.390	0.020	0.094	0.053	1.7
Bausch and Lomb	3	2.5	0.05	0.400–0.430	0.018–0.020	0.043–0.046	0.041–0.039	1.05–1.18
Beckman B	1	1.0	0.025	0.456	0.015	0.056	0.056	1.00
Beckman DU	1	1.0	0.025	0.450	0.017	0.050	0.050	1.00

[*]Number of individual instruments of indicated type examined.

make. Since the ratio is all that is necessary in the calculation, and since it is not necessary to know the exact hemoglobin concentration, it is most important to ascertain the exact value of the R factor for the individual instrument to be used. The determination should be done on hemolysates of at least six blood samples and the results averaged. Once this is done, day-to-day variations in the R factor of as much as 20 per cent (more than twice that observed experimentally) produce less than 5 per cent error in concentration of bilirubin.

Another set of experiments was performed to test for the influence of *in vitro* addition of hemoglobin to serum with a high concentration of bilirubin. This was done to rule out the possiblity of interference or chemical reaction between hemoglobin and bilirubin. To study this effect, standard solutions of bilirubin in serum were used to which increasing amounts of a concentrated hemolysate were added. Two 5 ml aliquots of a serum sample containing

20 mg per 100 ml of bilirubin were transferred to two test tubes. To one, 0.5 ml of water was added, and to the other, 0.5 ml of hemolysate containing 7.7 gm per 100 ml of hemoglobin. These two solutions were mixed in different proportions so as to have various samples all containing the same amount of bilirubin (18.2 mg per 100 ml) and from 700 mg per 100 ml down to 0 mg per 100 ml of added hemoglobin. The results obtained are shown in Table III. The results show that there is no interference by hemoglobin, and also show good recovery of bilirubin even at hemoglobin levels much higher than those encountered in actual practice.

DISCUSSION

The choice of a hemoglobin standard of 300 mg per 100 ml was made because this represents a relatively high level of hemolysis, even in samples obtained by faulty technique. Higher concentrations were investigated and it was found that linearity was present at the chosen wavelength up to at least 700 mg per 100 ml.[*]

With some instruments, absorbancy was not directly proportional to concentration of bilirubin at high levels. Since linearity varied from one instrument to the next, the upper limits of linearity should be known for the instrument to be used. This is easily ascertained by using twice the aliquot of bilirubin standard and making successive dilutions with Sorenson buffer (Reagent 1). The absorbancies obtained are then

TABLE III

Hemoglobin Added (mg per 100 ml)	Bilirubin Found (mg per 100 ml)	Percentage of Bilirubin Actually Present[*]
700	19.0	104
600	18.7	103
500	18.7	103
400	18.6	102
300	18.6	102
200	18.2	100
100	18.3	101
50	18.2	100
0	18.2	100

[*]Percentage of bilirubin as measured with the indicated amount of hemoglobin present compared to the 18.2 mg per 100 ml of bilirubin found with no hemoglobin present.

[*]Contrary to bilirubin, the absorption characteristics of hemoglobin are the same when diluted with buffer, serum or water under the conditions of the method.

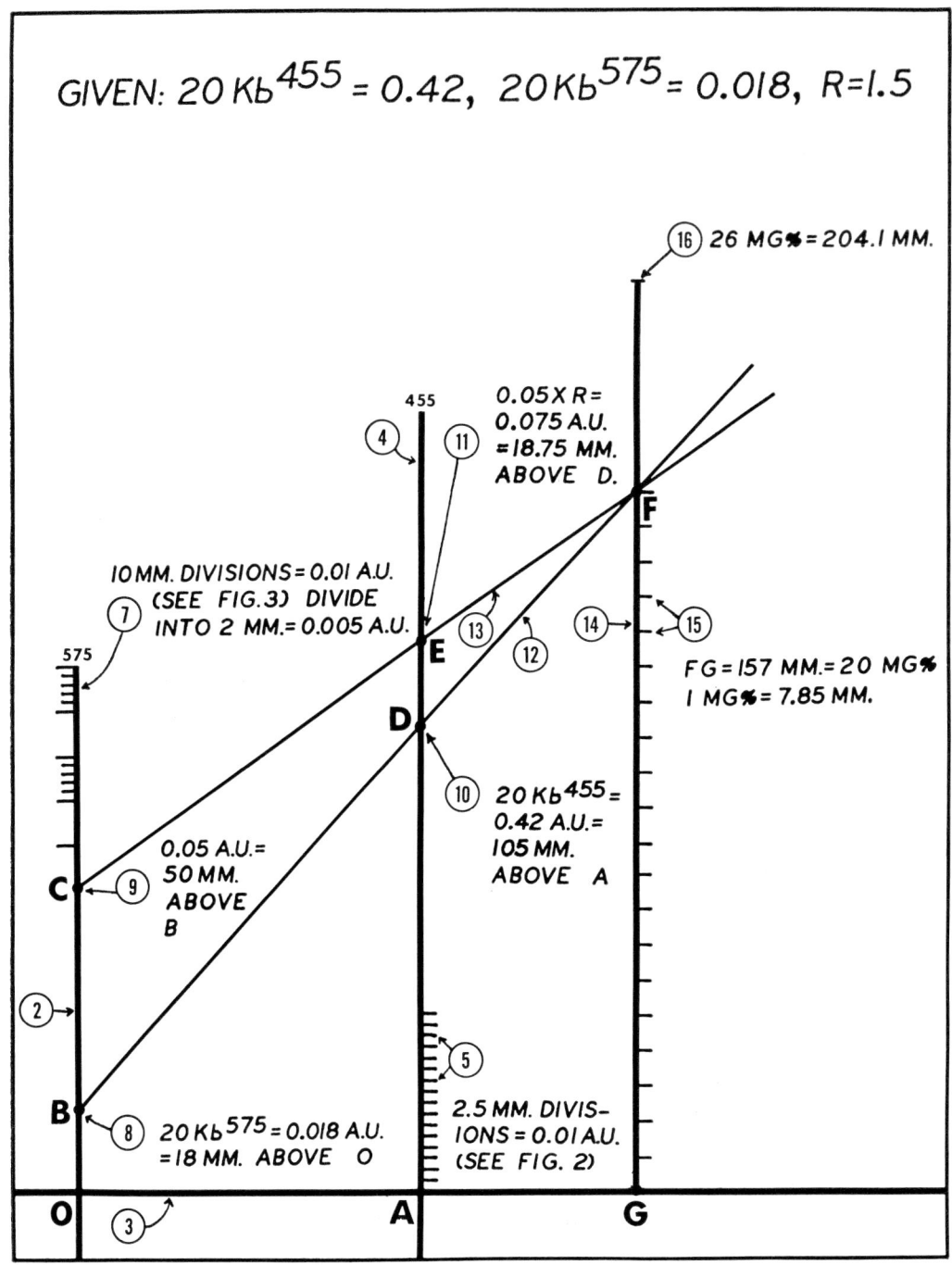

Fig. 1.   Example. Steps (circled numbers) in construction of nomogram for instrument where $20 \times Kb^{455} = 0.42$, $20 \times Kb^{575} = 0.018$ and $R = 1.5$.

plotted against concentration, and the range of linearity is obtained. Should the specimen contain such a high bilirubin level as to be above this range, the contents of the cuvette are diluted by adding an equal volume of buffer, and the results then obtained are multiplied by two.

The simplicity of the method, which involves only the diluting of an aliquot of serum with buffer and two spectrophotometric readings, makes it most rapid and suitable for emergency use. The calculation is obviated by the construction of a nomogram.

INTRODUCTION

Although the spectrophotometric method for the determination of bilirubin in serum is simple and rapid, the calculation is time consuming and tedious. The calculation actually takes more time to perform than the procedure itself. The time consumed and chances of error may be considerably decreased by utilizing a nomogram for the calculation. It is necessary to construct a nomogram for the particular instrument to be used. Once this is done, the calculation may be made promptly.

NOMOGRAPHY[1]

Data: The following data, obtained from the standardization previously described, are used in the construction of the nomogram:

1. *R*, which is the ratio between the ratio between the absorbancy of the hemoglobin standard at 455 $m\mu$ and 575 $m\mu$;
2. *20 Kb^{455}*, which is twenty, multiplied by the factor experimentally obtained in standardization; and

3. *20 Kb^{575}*, which is the absorbancy equivalent to that of a 20 mg per 100 ml bilirubin solution at 575 $m\mu$.

PROCEDURE

1. A sheet of paper is placed so that the long margins are at the sides.
2. A vertical line is constructed parallel to the left-hand margin and 15 mm to the right of it. This line should extend up at least 120 mm from the lower margin. The upper end of the line is labelled "575 $m\mu$."
3. A horizontal line is constructed parallel to the lower margin of the paper and 15 mm above it. The intersection of this line with the vertical line is labelled "O."
4. A second vertical line is constructed parallel to the first vertical line and 80 mm to the right of it (95 mm to the right of the left-hand margin). This line should extend up at least 150

20 x Kb^{455}	"455 mμ" Scale Mm. per 0.01 Absorb. Units	0.9	1.0	1.1	1.2	1.3
0.34	3.0	6	6	8	8	8
0.36	3.0	6	8	8	8	10
0.38	3.0	8	8	8	10	10
0.40	3.0	8	8	8	10	10
0.42	2.5	6	6	8	8	8
0.44	2.5	6	6	8	8	10
0.46	2.5	6	6	8	8	10

Fig. 2. Portion of Table IV illustrating Step 5. When 20Kb^{455} = 0.42, the table shows that there should be 2.5 mm per 0.01 absorbency unit (a.u.) on the "455 mμ" scale.

mm from the horizontal line (165 mm above the lower margin). At its upper end this line is labelled "455 mµ." The intersection of this line and the horizontal line is labelled "A."

5. In the left-hand vertical column of Table IV is located the value of 20 Kb^{455}. In the adjacent vertical column will be found the number of millimeters corresponding to 0.01 absorbancy units on the 455 mµ scale. Segments of this number of millimeters are laid off on the 455 mµ scale, beginning at Point A. This divides the 455 mµ scale into divisions which correspond to 0.01 absorbancy units for the instrument actually used.

6. Located in Table IV is the horizontal line of numbers corresponding to the value of 20 Kb^{455} observed experimentally. The vertical column corresponding to the R value determined

20 x Kb^{455}	"455 mµ" Scale — Mm. per 0.01 Absorb. Units	0.9	1.0	1.1	1.2	1.3	1.4	1.5
								Millimeters
0.34	3.0	6	6	8	8	8	10	10
0.36	3.0	6	8	8	8	10	10	10
0.38	3.0	8	8	8	10	10	10	12
0.40	3.0	8	8	8	10	10	10	12
0.42	2.5	6	6	8	8	8	8	10
0.44	2.5	6	6	8	8	10	10	10
0.46	2.5	6	6	8	8	10	10	10

Fig. 3. Portion of Table IV illustrating Step 6. When 20 Kb^{455} = 0.42 and R = 1.5, the intersection of the "20 KB^{455} 0.42" row and the "R = 1.5" column shows that there should be 10 mm per 0.01 absorbency unit (a.u.) on the "575 mµ" scale.

experimentally is then located. The number in the square at the intersection of this vertical column and the horizontal line is noted. This number is the

TABLE IV TABLE FOR CONSTRUCTION OF NOMOGRAM

20 × Kb^{455}	"455 mµ" Scale — mm per 0.01 Absorb Units	\"575 mµ\" Scale — R Values																
		0.9	1.0	1.1	1.2	1.3	1.4	1.5	1.6	1.7	1.8	1.9	2.0	2.1	2.2	2.3	2.4	2.5
		Millimeters per 0.01 Absorbancy Units																
0.34	3.0	6	6	8	8	8	10	10	12	12	12	12	14	14	14	16	16	16
0.36	3.0	6	8	8	8	10	10	10	12	12	12	12	14	14	14	16	16	16
0.38	3.0	8	8	8	10	10	10	12	12	12	14	14	14	16	16	16	16	16
0.40	3.0	8	8	8	10	10	10	12	12	12	14	14	14	16	16	16	16	16
0.42	2.5	6	6	8	8	8	8	10	10	10	10	12	12	12	14	14	16	16
0.44	2.5	6	6	8	8	10	10	10	10	12	12	12	12	14	14	14	16	16
0.46	2.5	6	6	8	8	10	10	10	10	12	12	12	12	14	14	16	16	16
0.48	2.5	6	8	8	10	10	10	12	12	12	12	14	14	14	14	16	16	16
0.50	2.5	6	8	8	10	10	10	12	12	12	12	14	14	14	14	16	16	16
0.52	2.0	5	5	6	6	8	8	8	8	10	10	10	10	12	12	12	12	14
0.54	2.0	5	5	6	6	8	8	8	8	10	10	10	10	10	12	12	12	14
0.56	2.0	5	6	6	8	8	8	10	10	10	10	12	12	12	12	14	14	14
0.58	2.0	6	6	8	8	8	8	10	10	10	10	12	12	12	12	14	14	14
0.60	2.0	6	6	8	8	10	10	10	10	10	10	10	12	12	12	14	14	14

number of millimeters to be plotted on the 575 mμ scale to represent 0.01 absorbancy units.

7. On the 575 mμ line, segments of this number of millimeters are laid-off, beginning at Point O. This divides the 575 mμ scale into divisions which correspond to 0.01 absorbancy units. Each of these divisions is further subdivided into five equal lengths, each of which corresponds to 0.002 absorbancy units.

8. On scale "575 mμ" a distance above Point O corresponding to the value of 20 Kb^{575} is measured. This new point is labelled "B."

9. On scale "575 mμ" a distance corresponding to 0.05 absorbancy units is measured *above* Point B. This point is labelled "C."

10. On scale "455 mμ" a distance above Point A is measured, corresponding to the value of 20 Kb^{455}. This new point is to be labelled "D."

11. The experimental value of R is multiplied by 0.05. On the "455 mμ" scale a distance is measured corresponding to 0.05 × R absorbancy units *above* Point D. This point is labelled "E."

12. Using a ruler, a line is drawn through Points B and D, extending it almost to the right-hand margin of the paper.

13. Similarly, a line is drawn through Points C and E, extending it until it intersects Line BD. This point of intersection is labelled "F." This corresponds to a serum bilirubin of 20 mg per 100 ml.

14. Through Point F a vertical line is constructed parallel to the two vertical scales and extending from the top of the sheet to meet the horizontal line

at a point; this point is labelled "G." Line FG is labelled "bilirubin, mg per 100 ml."

15. The distance between F and G is measured and divided into twenty equal divisions. Each division represents 1 mg per 100 ml.

16. Above Point F additional segments are marked until the interval in which the instrument obeys Beer's law is covered. This will be about 0 to 28 mg per 100 ml for Coleman spectrophotometers and 0 to 40 mg per 100 ml for other instruments tested.

17. The intervals on the "455 mμ," "575 mμ" and "bilirubin" scales are labelled so that they may be read conveniently.

USE OF THE NOMOGRAM

1. The procedure previously described is followed to obtain absorbancy readings for the unknown serum sample at 455 mμ and 575 mμ.

2. The points corresponding to these readings are located on the respective nomogram scales, and are aligned, using a straight edge.

3. The point of intersection of this line with the "bilirubin" scale represents the mg of bilirubin per 100 ml corrected for the amount of hemoglobin present.

DISCUSSION

The main purpose of this section is to present an easy method for constructing a nomogram from the experimental data actually obtained. Any spectrophotometer may be used if proper dilutions are employed. The variations between different instruments, even of the same make and model, may be marked, so that the values found for R may vary from 1.00 to 2.20. These differences may be exaggerated because two wavelengths are used instead of one. Therefore, determination of the "R" value for the particular instrument to be used must be done accurately.

To facilitate construction of the nomogram, Table IV was prepared using the following considerations: The scale divisions must be separated widely enough to permit discrimination between small differences in absorbancy; the scale modulus for the 575 mμ readings should be such that the point corresponding to 20 mg of bilirubin per 100 ml will be neither too close nor too far from the "455 mμ" scale, so as to minimize errors in aligning the various points; both the "455 mμ" and "575 mμ" scales must be of a size such that the resulting "bilirubin" scale is long enough to permit discrimination between bilirubin concentrations differing by as little as 0.1 ml per 100 ml.

For completeness, Table IV was prepared to include many more conditions than will actually be encountered in practice. The table comprises all values of R from 0.9 to 2.5 and all absorbancies of 20 mg per 100 ml solutions from 0.34 to 0.06. In practice, both extremes should be avoided; if necessary, dilutions should be adjusted to obtain any absorbancy of about 0.4 optical density units for serum samples containing 20 mg of bilirubin per 100 ml. The use of Table II eliminates trial and error methods and simplifies drawing of the nomogram by those who are not familiar with this type of graphical representation.

REFERENCES

1. Levens, S. A.: Nomography. New York, Wiley, 2nd ed., 1959.
2. Meites, S., and Hogg, C. K.: Direct spectrophotomery of total serum bilirubin in the newborn. Clin. Chem., 6:421-428, 1960.
3. Shinowara, G. Y.: Spectrophotometric studies on blood serum and plasma: The physical determination of hemoglobin and bilirubin. Amer. J. Clin. Path., 24:696-710, 1954.
4. White, D., Haidar, G. A., and Reinhold, J. G.: Spectrophotometric measurement of bilirubin concentrations in the serum of the newborn by the use of a microcapillary method. Clin. Chem., 4:211-222, 1958.

Chapter 23

Measurements of Pigments in Amniotic Fluid in Hemolytic Disease of the Newborn

LEON N. SUSSMAN, M.D. AND HOWARD BERK, M.D.

The spectrophotometric analysis of amniotic fluid obtained by transabdominal uterine paracentesis during pregnancy was first reported by Bevis in 1956[1]. Since that time, extensive studies have been done in this area by many workers[2, 3, 4, 5, 6], all of whom have con-firmed and extended the reported findings.

The method consists of examining the amniotic fluid in a spectrophotometer at various wavelengths from 330 mμ to 700 mμ, readings being taken at approximately 10 mμ intervals. Normally, a

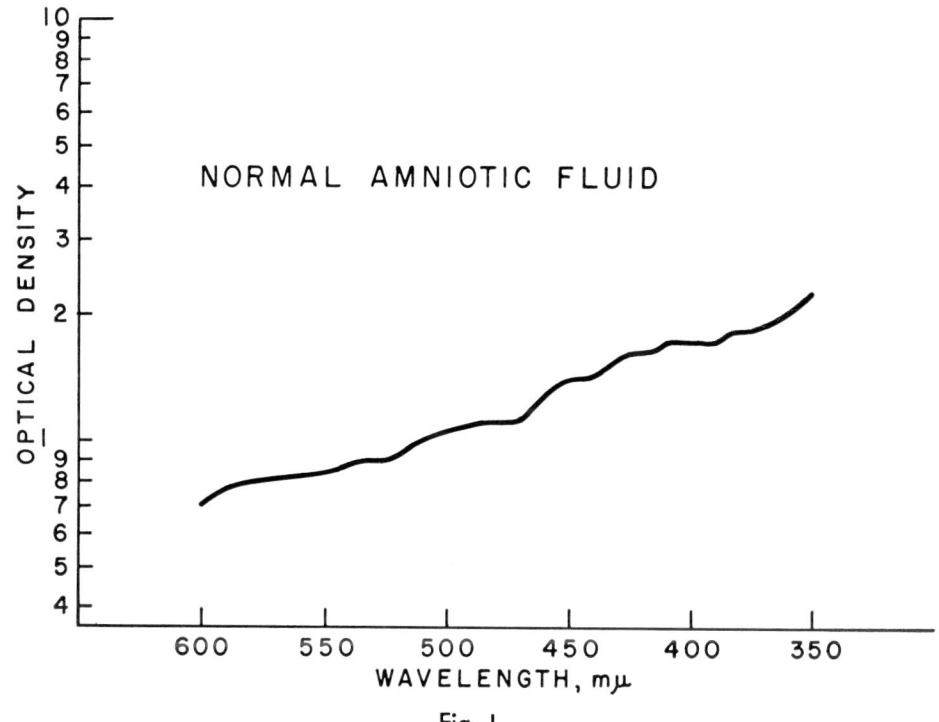

Fig. 1.

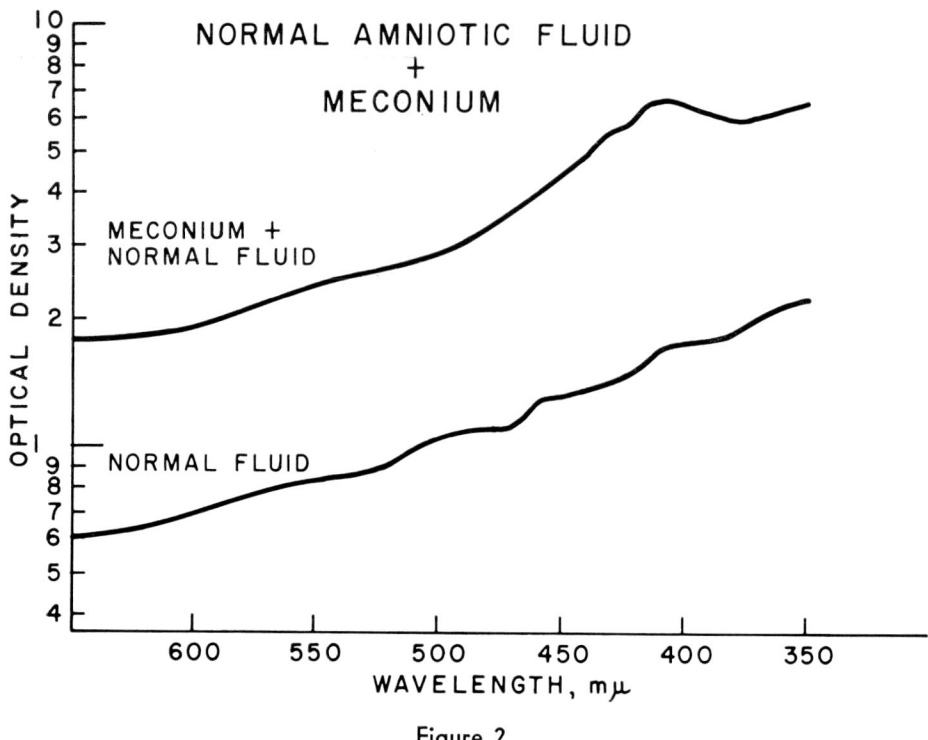

Figure 2.

relatively straight line can be drawn through the observed optical densities when plotted on semilog paper (Fig. 1). In the presence of intrauterine hemolysis of the fetal red blood cells, a deviation from this expected line occurs in the form of a "peak" at 450 mμ. This corresponds to the absorption band for bilirubin and is believed to be caused by "bilirubinoid" pigments.

In the presence of hemolysis in the fetus, the bilirubin that is produced is cleared from the fetal serum by the placenta. The amniotic fluid, which circulates through the fetal gastrointestinal tract, is stained by these bilirubinoid pigments. Since the amniotic fluid is not exposed to the placental circulation, the pigment cannot be excreted, but is retained in increasing amounts as the hemolysis continues. A quantitative relationship has been shown between the height of the amniotic fluid bilirubin "peak" and the level of the newborn cord hemoglobin — thus reflecting in some measure the clinical condition of the neonate.

The presence of numerous other contaminants in the amniotic fluid may interfere with its analysis and therefore must be considered.

TURBIDITY DUE TO VERNIX, DESQUAMATED EPITHELIUM AND MECONIUM

Particulate matter of this nature can usually be removed by prompt centrifugation of the specimen. This must be done, without exposure to light, as soon after the aspiration as possible. Occasionally, the residual turbidity may still prevent passage of the light beam. This can then be accomplished by diluting the specimen with distilled water up to eightfold. (Correction in the calculation of the optical density is made by multiplying the result by the dilution factor.) The effects of the meconium, etc. are shown in Figure 2.

Unhemolyzed Red Cells ("Bloody" Tap)

The presence of placental blood in the amniotic fluid introduces a serious complication, since the accompanying plasma contains bilirubin and may invalidate the optical density at 450 mμ. However, the washed red cells themselves are most useful, especially if they can be identified as fetal cells. The ABO, Rh and Coombs tests can be determined, as well as a percentage of normoblasts and reticulocytes; even sex determination can be performed by

count of the "drumsticks" on the polymorphonuclear cells seen on smears.

Light Sensitivity

Exposure of the amniotic fluid sample to light (especially sunlight) should be as short as possible, since the T½ of bilirubin is measured in minutes. The specimen is therefore kept in a dark test tube or in a light-proof box until examined. At room temperature, the specimen can be kept for several days without effect, providing light is excluded. This permits the mailing of specimens to distant laboratories, if necessary.

Dissolved Oxyhemoglobin

The presence of hemolyzed red blood cells can be shown by characteristic absorption peaks at 415, 540 and 575

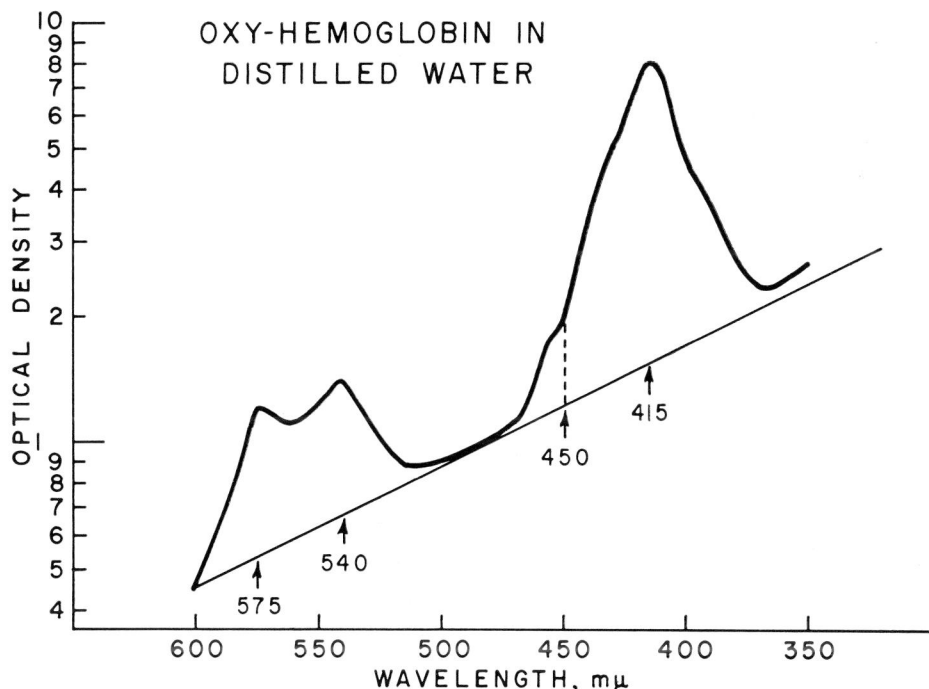

Figure 3.

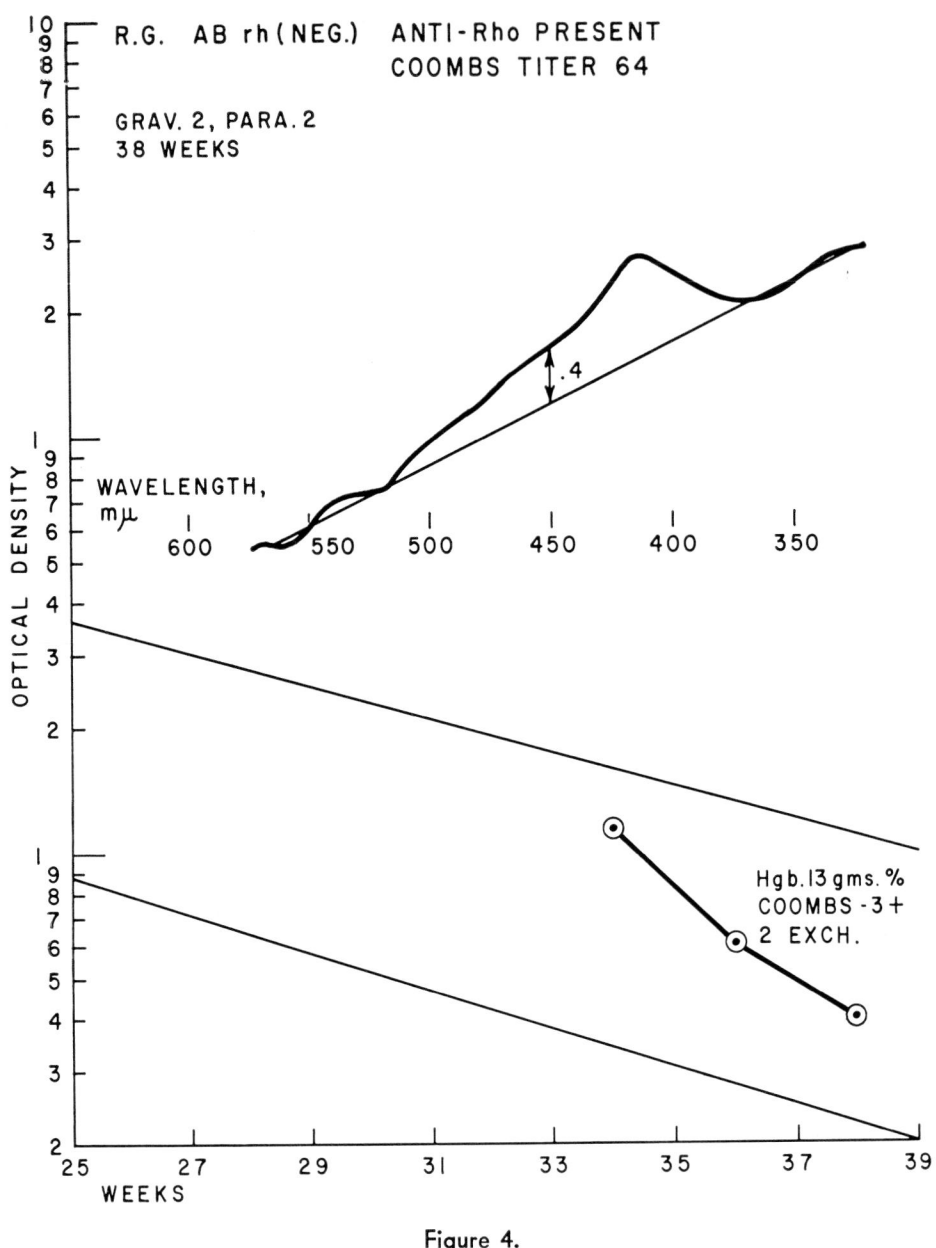

Figure 4.

mμ Figure 3. Liley[4] has shown that the broad base of the oxyhemoglobin peak at 415 mμ may magnify the bilirubin deviation at 450 mμ when both substances are present. Experimentally, he has shown this correction to amount to

5 per cent of the observed optical density at 415 mμ.

DURATION OF PREGNANCY

In normal amniotic fluid, a straight base line can be drawn through the plotted points from 350 mμ to 600 mμ

(Fig. 1). Where a deviation from the expected straight line is found, the amount of the deviation is measured and reported as the difference between the expected and observed curves at 450 mμ (Fig. 4). Liley[3] observed that the normal curve is not linear early in pregnancy, but does become more nearly so as the pregnancy progresses. Thus, limits of normalcy in relation to maturity were established. These were correlated with the clinical condition of the fetus at delivery. He constructed an arbitrary "zone pattern" into which

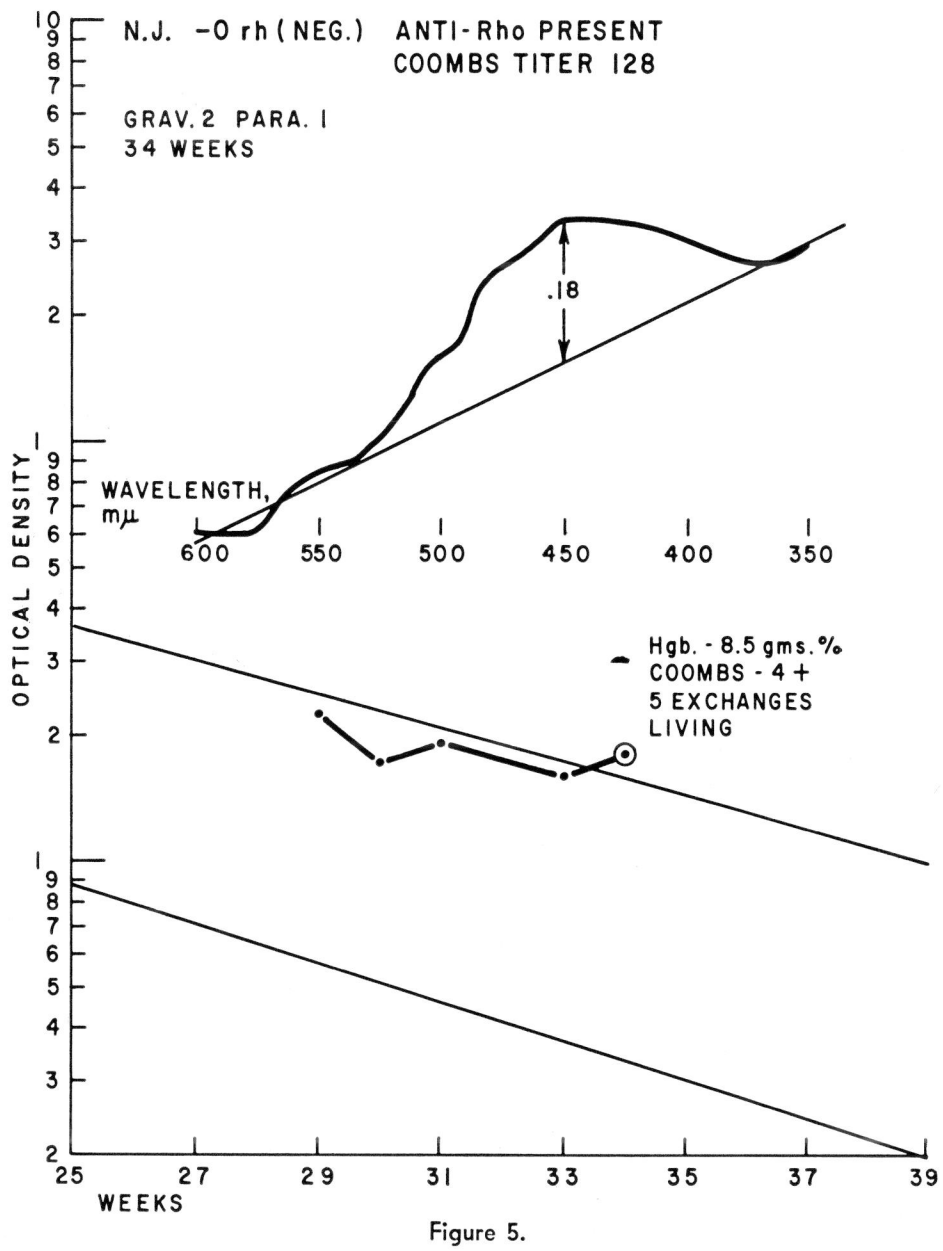

Figure 5.

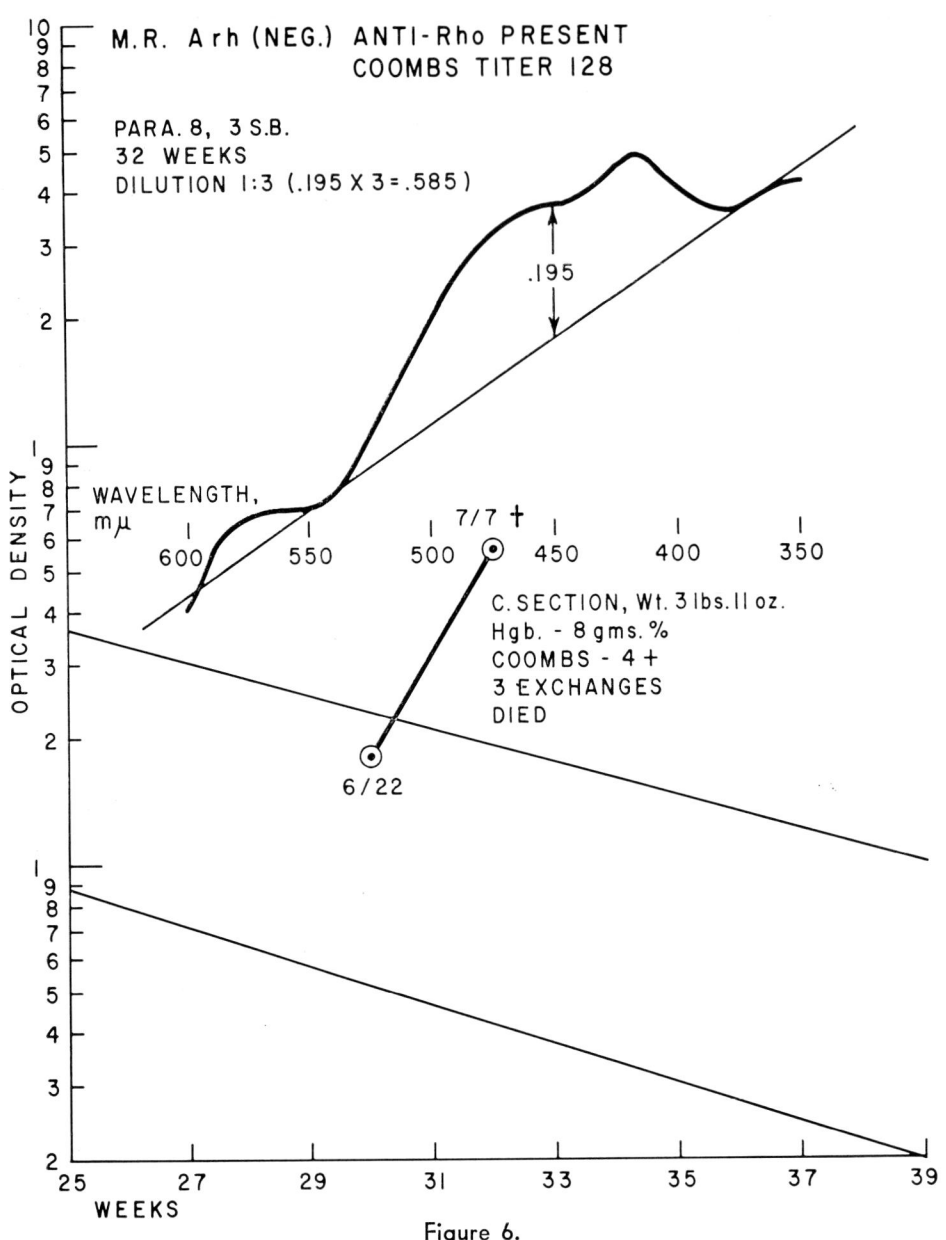

Figure 6.

the deviation of optical density could be plotted against the weeks of pregnancy. The top zone represented severely affected infants where impending intrauterine deaths could be expected. The middle zone represented moderately to mildly affected cases, whereas the lower zone represented mildly or unaffected infants. By successive determination of the spectral absorption curves from repeated taps, it was possible to plot the progress of the disease and thus to determine the optimal time for therapy (Figs. 5 and 6). Thus, the "plot" of the deviation in optical density at thirty-two weeks of pregnancy could be compared with the findings at thirty-four weeks of pregnancy. If the line joining these two points crossed a zone line, for example, from the middle to the top zone, it could be anticipated that the condition of the fetus was deteriorating and that intrauterine death could be expected soon. Such conclusions would lead to prompt delivery in an attempt to salvage the fetus. On the other hand, if the evidence from the progressive taps indicated no worsening of the fetus, a delay in delivery could very well enable the infant to mature and increase the possibility of postnatal survival. It must be emphasized that the optical density absorption is significant only in relation to the duration of pregnancy, and must be plotted in the "zone pattern" for proper interpretation.

CLINICAL INTERPRETATION

Normal. The usual normal curve connecting the readings at variable wavelengths from 350 mμ to 650 mμ is a relatively straight line (Fig. 1). Minor deviations, especially in early pregnancy, are not significant of hemolytic disease. These deviations are more specific after twenty-six weeks of pregnancy.

Affected Infants. An increase in optical density at 450 mμ indicates the presence of bilirubinoid pigments (Fig. 4). The height of the peak, corresponding to the concentration of pigment, gives information relative to the severity of the disease. Clinical correlation of the height of the peak and the postnatal condition of the fetus has been demonstrated by Walker[2] and corroborated by many other observers[5, 6].

Repeated Determinations During Preg- nancy. The value of repeated analysis of the amniotic fluid obtained from sensitized mothers lies in the ability to measure the progression of the disease (Figs. 5 and 6). Changes indicating worsening of the condition of the fetus, such as the peak reaching into the top zone, indicate the need for early delivery or transamniotic intraperitoneal transfusion. On the other hand, evidence indicating no impending disaster can provide the necessary confidence to permit greater fetal maturity with the subsequently better chance of postnatal survival.

CONCLUSIONS

It can be reasonably expected that the information available by the analysis of the amniotic fluid obtained from sensitized mothers will greatly improve the intrauterine management of the affected fetus. If only to differentiate the affected from the unaffected infants and thus permit the latter to develop to full maturity, a sufficient purpose would be served. However, by the use of repeated samplings, it is possible to prognosticate the severity of the disease in the affected fetus. Remedial measures can be taken in attempts to salvage these infants.

An objective basis for determining impending fetal death is available. This information can be used in selected cases for intraperitoneal transfusion, premature delivery and other avenues of therapy that may be proposed.

REFERENCES

1. Bevis, D. C. A.: Blood pigment in haemolytic disease of the newborn. J. Obstet. and Gynaec. Brit. Comm., **63**:68-75, 1956.
2. Walker, A. H. C.: Liquor amnii studies in the prediction of hemolytic disease of the newborn. Brit. Med. J., **2**:376-378, 1957.

3. Liley, A. W.: Liquor amnii analysis in the management of the pregnancy complicated by Rh sensitization. Amer. J. Obstet. Gynec., 82: 1359-1370, 1961.

4. Liley, A. W.: Current concepts, amniocentesis. New Eng. J. Med., 272:731-732, 1965.

5. Crosby, W. M., and Merrill, J. A.: Spectro-photometric analysis of amniotic fluid. Amer. J. Obstet. Gynec., 92:531-561, 1965.

6. Freda, V. J.: The Rh problem in obstetrics and a new concept of its management using amniocentesis and spectrophotometric scanning of amniotic fluid. Amer. J. Obstet. Gynec., 92: 341-374, 1965.

The Immunohematologic Diagnosis of Erythroblastosis Fetalis*

JAMES J. HUMES, M.D., AND JAMES G. HARMELING, M.D.

Since the discovery of the Rh factor by Landsteiner[1] and the establishment of its relationship to erythroblastosis fetalis by Levine[2] in the early 1940's, great strides have been made in the immunohematologic diagnosis of this disease. The advent of exchange transfusion in the 1950's placed emphasis on early diagnosis of this condition. Still further emphasis on early detection has been added by the newer techniques of amniocentesis and intrauterine transfusion. In response to this demand, newer and more sensitive immunologic tests have been developed. This has resulted in the detection of both increased numbers of pregnancies potentially at risk as well as an ever-expanding number of antibodies involved in sensitization.

Anti D continues to be the most common cause of severe erythroblastosis fetalis (Table I). The incidence of sensitization due to this factor is estimated at approximately 1 in 200 of all pregnancies. Of these, about 65 per cent of live-born infants require exchange transfusion. This is an incidence of 1 in 300 pregnancies, certainly not an insignificant figure[3].

Hemolytic disease of the newborn owing to ABO incompatibility carries a similar incidence of 1 in 150 pregnancies. On the other hand, only 1 in 3,000 of these infants ever require exchange transfusions[4].

The immunohematologic diagnosis of erythroblastosis fetalis is dependent in its strictest sense on the demonstration of maternal antibodies attached to the infant's erythrocytes. Of equal importance, however, is the establishment of the presence or absence of a potential for sensitization. Without this, the proper management of the pregnancy and the necessity for early intervention and therapy might be missed. Therefore, the immunohematologic diagnosis of this disease properly begins at the

TABLE I INCIDNCE OF HEMOLYTIC DISEASE OF THE NEWBORN

Due to Anti-Rh:

1 in 200 pregnancies

1 in 300 pregnancies require exchange transfusion

Due to Anti-ABO:

1 in 180 pregnancies

1 in 3000 pregnancies require exchange transfusion

*The opinions or assertions contained herein are the private ones of the authors and are not to be construed as official or reflecting the views of the Department of the Navy or the Naval Service at large.

time of the first prenatal visit. It is here that information as to the risk of sensitization during this or future pregnancies is obtained. Also, the value of further follow up on each individual patient can be ascertained. The initial examination should, of course, contain a complete history, especially relating to numbers and course of past pregnancies and prior transfusions. This may provide valuable information not only as to the possibility of sensitization but to the eventual prognosis of the infant.

The first important immunohematologic test is the accurate grouping and typing of the mother. *The patient's statement as to her own group and type should never be accepted.* The development of more potent antisera has reduced the incidence of error in grouping and typing to less than 1 per cent. Even this small degree of error, however, dictates close attention to such routine physical variants as time and temperature of reaction. The inexperienced technologist may still make an error in grouping, especially in slide testing, if the reaction is allowed to exceed the specified time of one to two minutes. Of greater risk is the mistyping of the Rh factor if the temperature is not optimum for this reaction, namely 37 C. While details of these test procedures are readily available, it is of paramount importance that the manufacturer's directions are always followed explicitly.

The second, extremely important, test that should be routinely performed at this time is the serum antibody screen. Here the maternal serum is reacted against pooled "O" cells which, by selection, contain the largest possible number of antigens attached to their surface.

This is usually obtained by a mixture of R_1r, R_2r and, in some cases, a third cell of type rr. Agglutination of these cells by the mother's serum indicates that an antibody exists.

It is important to remember, however, that this in no way establishes the potential of erythroblastosis fetalis. This agglutination may be caused by a nonspecific antibody, or the antibody involved may be totally unrelated to any antigenic stimulus by the fetus. This may be established only by further testing, as is outlined below.

The results of these initial two procedures will dictate any further steps and may conveniently be placed in five major categories.

1. If the mother's group is A, B or AB, further testing is probably not indicated as far as the ABO system is concerned. While cases of ABO hemolytic disease of the newborn due to anti-A_1 in a group A_2 or B mother and anti-B in group A mothers have been reported, they are so infrequent that further routine testing is impractical.

2. If the mother is group "O," the chance of ABO incompatibility exists. In approximately 20 per cent of all pregnancies, an ABO incompatibility between mother and fetus does indeed exist. However, as mentioned previously, less than 1 per cent of these pregnancies ever develop any evidence, however mild, of hemolytic disease of the newborn. This also raises a question as to the value of prenatal testing for the presence of immune anti-A and anti-B. Such testing has been evaluated in the past, and two thirds of the women who were found to possess these antibodies in their serum prenatally gave birth to completely normal infants[5]. Therefore,

the most effective and simple screening method in such cases is the routine testing of the infant's cord blood by the direct Coombs test. An additional adjunct is the grouping and typing of the father. If he is also group "O," the possibility of ABO incompatibility is excluded (from a scientific point, although not completely from a sociological point).

3. If the mother is Rh positive, the possibility of sensitization to other Rh factors cannot be excluded. Their incidence, however, is again so small that routine testing in the absence of a positive serum screen is impractical.

4. If the mother is Rh negative, further testing is mandatory. The first step in such testing is the genotyping of the father in an effort to obtain two valuable bits of information. First, it will be an aid in determining the most likely potentially offending antigen on the infant's erythrocytes. Second, and perhaps of greatest value, is the information it affords in determining the chances of further pregnancies being affected. If the father is heterozygous, then of course there is a 50 per cent chance that the infant will not be affected. In the event the serum screen is negative, repeat testing at approximately thirty and thirty-six weeks should be performed.

5. If the serum screen is positive, testing of the serum against a battery of selected cells must be carried out. This constitutes the *sine quo non* of the diagnosis in this disease. It is with this test that the specific etiologic antibody is identified. From this identification further therapy may be planned. From this identification some relatively accurate idea of the prognosis may be gar-

nered. The test itself is simple in conception but can at times be complex in execution. This is never more true then when one is dealing with two or more antibodies. Most of the vicissitudes of this procedure are covered in Chapter 24B.

The potential of any panel is limited, but, fortunately, so are the number of antigens that have been encountered in hemolytic disease of the newborn. In Table II are listed the antigens involved

TABLE II   ANTIBODIES ENCOUNTERED IN HEMOLYTIC DISEASE OF THE NEWBORN

Anti-D (Rh_o)	.97.00%
Anti-c (hr')	.00.40%
Anti-E (Rh″)	.00.30%
Anti-c & Anti-E	.00.15%
Anti-C^w	.00.15%
Anti-C	.00.01%
Anti-Le[a, b]	.01.30%
Anti-K	.00.90%
Anti-Fy[a]	.00.19%
Anti-Jk[a]	.00.11%

in this disease and their relative frequency[6].

It may again be noted that anti-D accounts for 97 per cent of all cases of erythroblastosis fetalis due to Rh incompatibility. Of the other Rh factors, anti-c is the next most important, followed by anti-E and then by a combination of anti-c plus anti-E. The remaining antibodies constitute rarities when found in hemolytic disease of the newborn. Of the non-Rh blood groups, the most potent antibody is anti-Kell. Parenthetically, it might be added that Anti-Le a-b is frequently encountered in pregnant women, but naturally constitutes no threat to the infant. Next in frequency is a seemingly ubiquitous, but in fact rarely seen factor, anti-Fy^a. This is followed by anti-Jk^a and then trails off into extremely rare antibodies such as anti-M, Di, etc.

Following identification of the antibody by panel testing, the titer of the antibody should be determined. However, correlation between changing antibody titers and the severity of clinical illness is often poor. Thus, a hydropic infant may be delivered when no rise in antibody titer was detected during pregnancy. Conversely, an unaffected or mildly affected infant may be born after a marked rise in titer. Limitations to the value of titers still persist. However, if certain precautions are followed, they can be useful in the management of hemolytic disease of the newborn. The first and the most important condition is that samples from the previous specimen always be saved frozen and run in parallel with the next specimen. Second, the titration should be ideally carried out using a single cell which contains the specific antigen for the antibody being titered. Third, the reaction characteristics, i.e., time, temperature, media, for the specific antibody should be duplicated as closely as possible during each successive run.

If these precautions are followed, it may still be impossible to predict the severity of the disease. Nevertheless, a persistence of titer should alert the physician to the danger and warrant procedures such as amniocentesis at the appropriate times. Repeat titers are usually obtained at the thirty and thirty-six weeks and perhaps more frequently if indicated.

Finally, a brief consideration will be given to the diagnosis of erythroblastosis fetalis in the newborn infant. The simplest, and yet one of the most useful diagnostic tools in the management of hemolytic disease in the newborn has proved to be the direct Coombs test. This can be performed in minutes, requires the minimum in reagents and materials and yields an answer in the great majority of cases. It should be performed routinely on all newborn cord bloods. If positive, the presence of an antibody on the infant's erythrocytes is confirmed. If negative, of course, ABO incompatibility cannot definitely be excluded. However, the use of the more sensitive tube test, plus reliable positive and negative controls, should aid in detecting a significant number of weakly reacting antibodies[7]. At the same time, ABO forward grouping and Rh typing of the infant's cells should be performed. This will further confirm or deny the possibility of sensitization.

If the direct Coombs test is positive, elution of the antibody from the infant's red blood cells for identification may be necessary[8]. This is especially true when prenatal antibody studies have not been performed or when maternal blood is not available. In the case of ABO hemolytic disease of the newborn, this may be the only diagnostic test in the face of a negative direct Coombs test. It may also prove useful in removing the blocking antibodies from the infant's red blood cells and allowing the true antigenic nature of the erythrocytes to be demonstrated.

Following elution, the eluate is reacted against a panel of known cells for the specific identification of the antibody. In cases of ABO incompatibility the eluate may be tested for the presence of immune anti-A and anti-B against known A or B cells.

In addition to the various immuno-hematologic procedures which have been briefly outlined, base-line hemoglobin, hematocrit, reticulocyte count and bilirubin should be performed and repeated as indicated.

In summary, a simple, step-wise approach has been presented for the immunohematologic diagnosis of erythroblastosis. Routine testing of all prenatal and neonatal bloods by these methods should result in the early and accurate identification of patients at risk from this disease.

REFERENCES

1. Landsteiner, K., and Wiener, A. S.: An agglutinable factor in human blood recognizable by immune sera for Rhesus blood. Proc. Soc. Exp. Biol. Med., 43:223, 1940.
2. Levine, P., Burnham, L., Katzin, E. M., and Vogel, P.: The role of iso-immunization in the pathogenesis of erythroblastosis fetalis. Amer. J. Obstet. Gynec., 42:925, 1941.
3. Mollison, P. L.: Blood Transfusion in Clinical Medicine. Oxford, Blackwell, 3rd ed., 1961, pp. 602-603.
4. Ibid., pp. 655-657.
5. Reepmaker, J., and Van Loghem, J. J.: Anti-A and anti-B immune antibodies in pregnancy. Vox Sang., 3:143, 1953.
6. Bowman, H. S.: Antibodies responsible for hemolytic disease of the newborn — Results of routine screening. A seminar on hemolytic disease. Presented at the 18th Annual Meeting of the AABB, September 14, 1965.
7. Fesco, R., Busch, S., Hanson, M., and Huestis, D.: A simple method of preparing "coated" red blood cells for use as a control in antiglobulin testing. Transfusion, 4:262, 1964.
8. Landsteiner, K., and Miller, C. P.: Serological studies on the blood of primates. II. The blood group in anthropoid apes. J. Exp. Med., 42:853, 1925.

Identification of Antibodies in Erythroblastosis Fetalis*

JAMES J. HUMES, M.D., AND JAMES G. HARMELING, M.D.

INTRODUCTION

In every pregnancy there exists the possibility of an immunologic incompatibility between the mother and the developing fetus. In all pregnancies it is therefore necessary to ascertain this potential as accurately as possible. If it can be determined that this potential exists, further investigations are mandatory to identify the cause of this immunologic incompatibility and to assist the obstetrician and pediatrician in the management of the case.

To determine the possibility of sensitization of the mother by a fetal antigen, the ABO blood group and Rh type must be determined as early as possible for each pregnant woman. In addition, the maternal serum is screened for the presence of circulating antibodies. If the blood group is A, B or AB, and the Rh type is positive, the possibility of maternal sensitization in these systems is remote. If, in addition, the screen for circulating antibodies is negative, further immunologic studies need not be performed.

---

*The opinions or assertions contained herein are the private ones of the authors and are not to be construed as official or reflecting the views of the Department of the Navy or the Naval Service at large.

If, however, the maternal blood is O and/or the Rh type is negative, or the serum screen is positive, there is the possibility of ABO or RH sensitization and further testing as outlined below may be indicated.

The cord blood of all newborns should be tested for the presence of antibodies attached to their red blood cells. If present, these antibodies portend a possible severe hemolysis and the attendant dangers of hyperbilirubinemia. Exact identification of the antibody is therefore important not only as a means of predicting the eventual severity of the hemolysis, but of selecting the *best possible* blood for future transfusion.

PRINCIPLE

The principle underlying the identification of antibodies in erythroblastosis is threefold:

1. To determine if an antibody exists;
2. To determine if the antibody is etiologically related to the erythroblastosis; and
3. To determine the specific identity of the antibody.

These three steps are all dependent upon the combination of the antibody involved with a specific erythrocyte antigen to produce visible agglutination and/or hemolysis. Since the antibodies are usually of the incomplete variety, either a high-protein medium or an antiglobulin serum, or both, are required to produce this reaction. In addition, different antibodies may react optimally at different temperatures and, therefore, these reactions are also carried out at various thermal ranges.

REAGENTS

A. *Pooled O Cells*

Donors for these cells may usually be obtained from laboratory or hospital personnel. Small amounts, sufficient to cover the particular laboratory needs, should be drawn so that the donors may be used at more frequent intervals.

1. Two group O, Rh positive bloods are selected. One type should be R_1r (CDe/cde) and the other R_2r (cDE/cde). At least one should also be Kell (K) positive. Testing for other factors such as Fy^a, JK^a, M, N, S, etc., may be carried out, but the incidence in the random population is such that these antigens should be present on one or the other of the two cells.

2. Blood in appropriate quantities is drawn into ACD solution. (Glycerolization and freezing must be done before the cells are three days old.)

3. Packed red cells are prepared by centrifuging at 2,000 rpm for sixty minutes, and plasma is aspirated.

4. Cell volume is estimated, and, while agitating, one half volume of Solution 1 is added by injection through a 20-gauge needle from a syringe. Solution 1 is allowed to stand for ten minutes and then one half volume of Solution 2

is added to the same tube (e.g., 20 ml of cells; 10 ml of Solution 1 is added, and 10 ml of Solution 2).

5. Solution is allowed to stand thirty minutes, and then aliquots are prepared by delivering 1 ml into 10×75 mm properly labeled tubes; cork and store in deep freeze at -20 C.

Solutions

1. 73.2 ml of Solution 3; 26.8 ml of glycerol.

2. 33.2 ml of Solution 3; 66.8 ml of glycerol.

3. 3.46 per cent tripotassium citrate; 0.60 per cent dipotassium hydrogen phosphate (K_2HPO_4); 0.53 per cent potassium dihydrogen phosphate (KH_2PO_4); *q.s.* to 100 ml with distilled water.

Thawing of Glycerolized Red Cells

1. Cells are warmed in water bath until thawed.

2. Cells are centrifuged at 3,000 rpm for five minutes, and supernatant is aspirated.

3. One volume of 20 per cent glycerol in 3 per cent trisodium citrate (TSC) is added, mixed well, centrifuged for 5 minutes and supernatant aspirated.

4. One volume of 12 per cent glycerol in 3 per cent TSC is added; proceed as in Step 3, but centrifuge only two minutes.

5. One volume of 8 per cent glycerol in 3 per cent TSC is added; proceed as in Step 4.

6. One volume of 4 per cent glycerol in 3 per cent TSC is added; proceed as in Step 4.

7. One volume of 2 per cent glycerol in 3 per cent TSC is added; proceed as in Step 4.

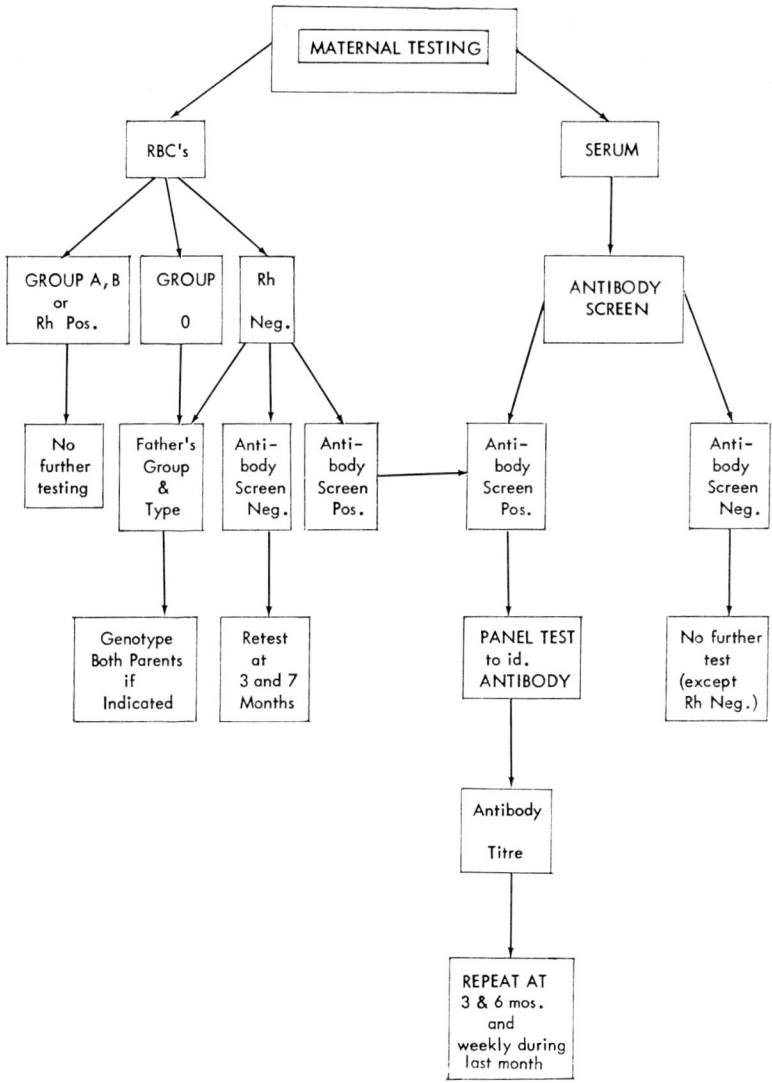

Fig. I

8. Cells are washed four times with normal saline.

9. A 2 per cent suspension is made by diluting with saline.

10. Cells from three donors may be pooled after Step 9 for screening purposes.

SOLUTIONS

Glycerol-trisodium citrate wash solutions are prepared by adding the appropriate amounts and q.s. to 100 ml with distilled water (e.g., 20 per cent equals 20 ml glycerol plus 3 gm TSC; 12 per cent equals 12 ml glycerol plus 3 gm TSC).

2. *Known A and B Cells*

Cells for this purpose may be obtained fresh from available donors or from ACD blood less than three days old which has been stored at 4 C.

1. Cells are tested by standard slide or tube techniques with potent anti-A$_1$, anti-B and adsorbed anti-A sera.

2. The selected A$_1$ and B group bloods are divided into appropriate aliquots for future use.

3. Blood drawn in ACD solution is satisfactory for up to three weeks if stored at 4 C. If longer storage is desired, the cells must be glycerolized and frozen.

4. To use, the cells are thawed and washed four times with normal saline, then re-suspended to a 2 per cent suspension with saline.

C. Additional Reagents

Those reagents listed below are best obtained from commercial sources because of their standardized methods of production which guarantees a much higher degree of uniformity among various lots. Manufacturers' instructions should be rigidly adhered to in their use.

1. *Selected "O" cells;* produced under trade names such as Selectogen, Indentogen, etc.

2. *30 per cent albumin.* The 22 per cent concentration has not been found satisfactory, since, after dilution, a concentration for less than the minimum 19 per cent results.

3. *Anti-human globulin (AHG) serum.* Serum composed of both anti-γ and anti-non-γ globulin fractions is recommended.

4. *Anti-A, anti-B, anti-A, B (Group O) and adsorbed anti-A sera.* Sera must meet National Institutes of Health criteria for specificity and avidity.

5. *Normal saline* (0.85 per cent). May be purchased in two or five gallon lots (Scientific Products).

6. *10 × 75 mm tubes.* The use of disposable tubes has been found to be no more expensive and eliminates contaminated tubes as a source of error.

PROCEDURES

I. Maternal Testing

  A. Grouping and Typing.

    1. The mother's red cells are tested with good grade potent anti-A, anti-B and anti-Rh$_o$(D) serums to determine the group and type. This is done by standard tube or slide methods.

    2. The grouping is confirmed by the use of anti-A,B (group O) serum and by the reverse serum grouping technique.

      a. Anti-A,B (group O) serum is used on the slide or in the tube, utilizing the same methods as for anti-A and anti-B sera. This antiserum will agglutinate cells of group A,B or AB but not group O, and will detect the weakly reacting subgroups of A.

      b. Reverse grouping should be performed in the test tube only.

        (1) 2 per cent suspension of known A$_1$ and B red cells in saline are prepared.

        (2) Two drops of serum under test are added to

each of two tubes.

(3) Two drops of A_1 cells are added to one tube labelled "A," and two drops of B cells are added to the second tube labelled "B."

(4) Incubation at room temperature is allowed for fifteen minutes.

(5) Tubes are centrifuged at 1,000 to 2,000 rpm for one minute.

(6) Suspension is examined for agglutination or hemolysis.

(a) Agglutination in "A" tube only—Group B.

(b) Agglutination in "B" tube only—Group A.

(c) Agglutination in "A" and "B" tubes — Group O.

(d) No agglutination in "A" or "B" tubes —Group AB.

B. Serum Antibody Screen.

1. After thawing, the aliquot of pooled O cells is washed four times with sterile saline and re-suspended to a 2 per cent suspension in saline.

2. Two drops of fresh patient-serum are placed in a test tube.

3. Two drops of the freshly prepared group O test cells are added.

4. Tube is centrifuged thirty seconds at 1,000 to 2,000 rpm and observed for agglutination. (This "immediate spin" reading aids in detecting prozone phenomena.)

5. Incubate one hour at 37 C.

6. Centrifuge for thirty seconds at 1,000 rpm.

7. Cells are re-suspended and observed for agglutination.

8. Cells are washed three times with sterile saline. Following the last wash, the saline is thoroughly drained by holding the tube inverted and wiping the tube mouth with clean gauze.

9. Two drops of anti-human globulin serum are added and mixed well. Tube is centrifuged fifteen seconds at 1,500 to 2,000 rpm.

10. Re-suspension is done gently, and observation made for agglutination.

INTERPRETATION: Agglutination indicates the presence of an antibody in the mother's serum against one of the antigens on the pooled test cells. Specific identification is carried out using selected "O" (panel) cells.

Since antibodies have variable physical reactive characteristics, the test should be repeated at the three optimum temperatures (4 C, 25 C, 37 C) and in saline, albumin and AHG sera before proceeding with the panel testing. This will establish in which medium and at what temperature the test will optimally be performed.

C. Antibody Identification.
1. Numbered tubes are arranged in a rack according to the number of cells in the panel. One tube is added for the patient cell control.
2. Two drops of fresh patient-serum are added to each tube.
3. One or two drops of the panel cells are added to each tube except the control tube.
4. Two drops of patient's cells are added to the control tube.
5. After three to five minutes at room temperature, tubes are centrifuged for thirty seconds at 1,000 rpm. Read for agglutination and hemolysis (immediate spin or other).

6. All tubes are incubated at 37 C for one hour.
7. Tubes are removed and centrifuged thirty seconds at 1,000 rpm. The excess supernatant fluid is expelled, and agglutination and hemolysis readings taken.
8. The cells are washed three to four times with sterile saline and thoroughly decanted after the last wash.
9. Two drops of AHG serum are added to each tube.
10. Tubes are centrifuged for fifteen seconds at 2,000 rpm.
11. Agglutination or hemolysis readings are made.
12. Results are recorded and compared with identification chart which accompanies each cell panel.

D. Antibody Titers. The cells chosen for titration may either be the pooled "O" cells used in the screening test or a specially selected cell which is homozygous for the antibody found in the serum, e.g., R_1R_1 (CDe/CDe) for titration of anti-D (Rh_o) or anti-C (rh^1).
1. A 2 per cent suspension of

TABLE I

Tubes	1	2	3	4	5	6	7	8	9	10
Serum	0.2ml	0.2ml								
Saline		0.2ml	0.2ml	0.2	0.2	0.2	0.2	0.2	0.2	0.2
Transfer			0.2 #2	0.2 #3	0.2 #4	0.2 #5	0.2 #6	0.2 #7	0.2 #8 discard	None
Cells	0.2	0.2	0.2	0.2	0.2	0.2	0.2	0.2	0.2	0.2
Dilutions	1:1	1:2	1:4	1:8	1:16	1:32	1:64	1:128	1:256	

the cells in saline is prepared.

2. Saline, serum and cells are added to each tube according to Table I (pg. 347).

3. NOTE: The 0.2 ml from Tube 9 may be saved in a separate tube to continue dilutions if necessary. A separate 1 ml pipette should be used for each transfer.

4. All tubes are incubated for one hour at 37 C.

5. Tubes are centrifuged at 1,000 rpm for one minute.

6. Agglutination reading made. Begin reading at Tube 10 and proceed downward, since prozon-

ing may prevent agglutination in the lower dilutions.

7. If all tubes are negative, the cells are washed three times with sterile saline and decanted thoroughly after the last wash.

8. Two drops of AHG serum are added to each tube and mixed well.

9. Tubes are centrifuged at 1,000 rpm for one minute.

10. Read for agglutination. Record as the reciprocal of the highest dilution showing definite macroscopic agglutination.

DISCUSSION: In performance of titrations it is extremely important that the serum from the previous titration

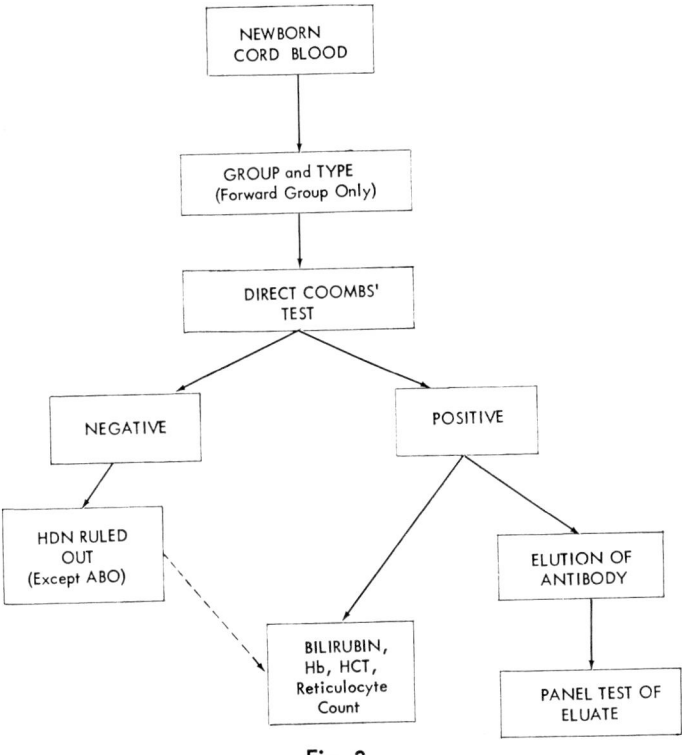

Fig. 2.

be saved frozen and run in parallel with the next specimen. This aids in detecting any variation in titer which may be due to reagent or technical variations and makes changes in titer more meaningful.

II. Newborn Testing. Since antibodies may be present in the mother's serum from causes other than erythroblastosis, their presence is only presumptive evidence of hemolytic disease of the newborn. The testing of the infant's cord red blood cells provides the only truly diagnostic evidence of the disease. Of the tests available, the direct antiglobulin test is by far the most valuable.

A. Direct Coombs' Test.
1. Cord red cells are washed at least four times in sterile saline to ensure the removal of all serum and/or Wharton's jelly.
2. A 2 per cent suspension of the washed cord red cells is prepared.
3. One drop of washed red cells is added to a tube.
4. One to two drops of AHG serum is added.
5. Mix well and centrifuge at 1,000 rpm for one minute.
6. The cells are gently dislodged and read for agglutination.

Discussion: Agglutination indicates the presence of antibodies attached to the red cells. The degree of agglutination may be some help in differentiating ABO from Rh HDN, since the former is characteristically only weakly positive and may be negative while the latter is usually strongly positive.

B. Grouping and Typing.
1. The infant's cord red cells are washed four times in sterile saline.
2. The washed red cells are tested by either standard tube or slide methods, using potent anti-A, anti-B and anti-Rh sera.
3. The grouping is confirmed by the use of anti-A_1B (O) serum.
4. Reverse serum grouping is not carried out, since the level of natural antibodies is usually not sufficiently high until four to five weeks of age.

C. Elution. Several methods of elution are available, namely, either by heat or by alcohol. In our hands, the heat method has been eminently satisfactory and offers the advantages of simplicity and speed.
1. Antibody-coated cells, 0.5 to 1.0 ml, are added to a tube and washed four times with sterile saline.
2. After the last wash, the supernatant saline is decanted as completely as possible.
3. An equal volume of saline is added to the packed, washed cells and mixed well.
4. The tube is placed in a 56C water bath for fifteen minutes and shaken at frequent intervals during incubation.
5. The tube is transferred im-

mediately to centrifuge cups containing water previously heated to 56 C so that the tube does not become cooled.

6. Centrifuge at 2,000 rpm for three minutes.

7. The supernatant (elute) is removed immediately and placed in a clean, properly labeled tube.

DISCUSSION: In addition to elution, two additional techniques useful in antibody identification are available. These tests, while simple in principle, may become very time consuming and complicated and, therefore, will not be detailed in this section.

The first of these is absorption, which is sometimes necessary to identify mixtures of antibodies. Generally, the procedure is based on absorption of serum with cells known not to contain antigens specific for any antibodies intended to be left in the serum and absorption with cells known to contain antigens specific for antibodies which are intended to be removed from the serum. Thus, if two antibodies are present in a serum, one may be removed and the serum retested against a panel for specific identification.

The second technique is the use of enzymes. By their use, reactivity of some systems is enhanced while that of others is apparently destroyed. In appropriate systems the agglutination is generally more rapid and stronger. In addition, this technique may give false positive reactions. Papain, ficin, trypsin and bromelin are some of the commonly employed enzymes. The procedures may be found in appropriate references.

D. Testing for immune anti-A and

B. If the presence of ABO hemolytic disease is suspected, a simple screening test for the presence of immune anti-A and B antibodies in the mother's serum or in the eluate from cord red cells, may be carried out as follows:

1. 0.1 ml of undiluted serum or eluate to be tested is placed in a tube.

2. 0.3 ml of Blood Group Specific Substances A and B are added and mixed, then incubated at room temperature for five minutes. (Manufacturers' instructions for the use of Blood Group Specific Substances A and B should be followed, as they vary among manufacturers.)

3. Two tubes are labelled "A" and "B"; two drops of the neutralized serum are placed in each tube.

4. Two drops of fresh 2 per cent saline suspension of known A_1 cells are added to the tube labelled "A." Two drops of fresh 2 per cent suspension of Group "B" cells are added to the tube marked "B."

5. After mixing well, incubate at 37 C. for thirty to sixty minutes.

6. The indirect anti-globulin test is performed on both tubes.

DISCUSSION: Agglutination following the anti-globulin test indicates the presence of immune anti-A or anti-B.

If the test is positive on the mother's serum, it is not diagnositic, since these antibodies may have been formed in response to antigenic stimuli other than the infant's cells, e.g., immunizations or previous transfusion. If they are found in the eluate of the infant's cells, however, this is confirmatory evidence of ABO hemolytic disease.

Sources of Error: If agglutination takes place prior to the performance of the anti-globulin test, this indicates that the naturally occurring anti-A and B have not been neutralized and the test must be repeated, using 0.6 ml of Blood Group Specific Substance A and B.

E. Antibody Identification.

1. If ABO hemolytic disease is suspected, the test for detection of immune anti-A and B may be carried out as outlined in the previous section.

2. If hemolytic disease due to Rh or other blood factors is more likely, the eluate from the infant's cells is used in place of serum and tested against a panel of selected group O cells.

Sources of Error: Despite the multitude of errors that may be introduced by technical variations, ranging from inexperience to outright laxity, the most common causes of erroneous results are still defects in equipment and materials. In the forefront of these are the wasted time and reagents caused by unclean glassware. Second only to this are errors introduced by contaminated diluents, most commonly saline. Next in line of suspicion are reagents prepared in the laboratory, especially if the personnel preparing

them do so only irregularly. Last, but not least, are defects in commercial reagents and sera. The following list outlines some of the common causes of these defects and where possible, a solution.

1. Glassware. Dirty glassware results only from improper washing and/or storage. The most common cause is incomplete soaking, wherein the very bottom position of the tube is not rinsed, due to placing of the tubes in the rinse solution in an inverted manner. Next is improper brushing. This should be done with a soft nylon brush, and each tube must be thoroughly scoured. After drying, inspection for scratched tubes should be carried out. To obviate these difficulties, disposable tubes are recommended and have been found eminently satisfactory in our laboratory from both a technical and economic standpoint. Storage of tubes, whether reusable or disposable, must be done in a dust-free manner either in an enclosed bin or inverted on pegs.

2. Saline. The saline diluent should be changed frequently and at least once a day. The two or five gallon carboy, available commercially, is packaged in a closed system, and

only the working solution is exposed to possible contamination.

3. Reagents. Meticulous preparation and storage of all reagents is a must. Slight variations in temperature can appreciably affect the storage longevity of both cell and serum reagents. Cell suspensions should always be checked for hemolysis prior to use. Frequently, an additional washing will suffice to render a partially hemolyzed suspension usable. The reactivity of both cell and serum reagents may be checked by the routine use of positive and negative controls as well as an auto-control. Their use cannot be overemphasized.

Commercially prepared typing sera, albumin, anti-human globulin and selected "O" cells should also occasionally be checked. The typing sera can be checked by reacting serial dilutions against appropriate cells. A satisfactory result should be obtained at a dilution of 1:64 at least, and most react well at dilutions of 1:256 or higher. The albumin and AHG may be evaluated by electrophoresis as well as by immunoelectrophoretic methods.

REFERENCES

1. Mollison, P. L.: Blood Transfusion in Clinical Medicine. Philadelphia, Davis, 3rd ed., 1961, pp. 237-246.
2. Technical Methods and Procedures of the American Association of Blood Banks. Chicago, 1960, pp. 63-66, 68-70, 72-74.
3. Laboratory Manual of the Blood Transfusion Service. Toronto, The Canadian Red Cross Society, 4th ed., 1963, pp. 18-23, 26-31, 46-47.
4. Dunsford, I., and Grant, J.: The Anti-Globulin Test in Laboratory Practice. Edinburgh, Oliver and Boyd, 1961.
5. Allen, N. K., and Palmer, J. W.: Hyland Reference Manual of Immunohematology. Hyland Laboratories, 1963, pp. 58-64, 67-68, 76-83, 87-88.
6. Low, B.: A practical method using papain and incomplete Rh antibodies in routine Rh blood grouping. Vox Sang., 5:94, 1955.
7. Pirofsky, B., and Mangum, M. E., Jr.: Use of bromelin to demonstrate erythrocyte antibodies. Proc. Soc. Exp. Biol. Med., 101:49, 1959.

Chapter 25

Blood Grouping Tests for Exclusion of Paternity

LEON N. SUSSMAN, M.D.

INTRODUCTION

The status of the medicolegal application of blood grouping tests for the exclusion of paternity was delineated by the Committee on Medicolegal Problems of the American Medical Association in its reports of 1952 and 1957[2, 6]. The committee accepted only the findings in the ABO, MN and Rh-Hr systems for these purposes; however, in the hands of qualified experts, the use of the other blood groups was permitted. Since many of the states in the United States accept the reports of exclusion of paternity as decisive of the issue, it is most important that such tests be performed in experienced laboratories[3] under the supervision of knowledgeable directors. Such directors should be thoroughly familiar with the variants in the blood factors and the atypical laboratory findings that occasionally present themselves, as well as the laws of genetics which control the inheritance of the genes that determine the blood factors[4, 10, 11, 13, 14].

PRINCIPLES

The fundamental principles in the performance of these tests are related to the laws of heredity and genetics, the techniques of blood grouping and the use of proper and adequate controls. The genetic laws are as follows:

1. A blood factor cannot appear in the red blood cells of a child unless this factor is present in the red blood cells of *either* the father or the mother.
2. A parent, homozygous for any gene which determines a blood factor, must transmit one such gene to *each* of his offspring.
3. A child, homozygous for any gene which determines a blood factor, must have inherited one gene for this factor from *each* of the parents.

The technical principles are as follows:

1. The directions of the manufacturer of the serum used must be followed exactly, since different lots of serum vary in their reactivity, depending on the suspending medium, the time and the temperature of the reaction and on the cell concentration.
2. All blood grouping tests for medicolegal purposes must be performed simultaneously with

known positive and negative controls.

3. All tests must be performed in duplicate, by separate technicians using different lots of serum. The readings of the results and the comparison of the two sets of findings should be done by a third person, if possible.

4. Any discrepancies, differences or indecisive results must be convincingly resolved before reporting, and no doubtful or questionable findings are permitted.

5. Any unresolved problem should be referred to a qualified expert for final study and solution.

6. It is useful if all parties involved in a medicolegal paternity dispute are tested simultaneously, using the same techniques, the same antisera and the same controls under the same conditions.

REAGENTS

The reagents, consisting primarily of antisera, may now be purchased from serum supply firms. However, the well-qualified and experienced serologist usually produces his own testing serums, since in this way he becomes most familiar with its optimum working conditions. The antisera required minimally are: anti-**A**, anti-**B** and O serum (anti-**A** + **B**) for ABO testing; anti-**M** and anti-**N** for MN testing; and anti-**Rh**$_o$, anti-**rh'**, anti-**rh"**, anti-**hr'** and anti-**hr"** for RH-Hr testing. Other testing antisera which may be useful are anti-**K** (Kell), anti-**k** (Cellano) for Kell testing and other special serums such as anti-**hr** (f)[8], anti-**rh**$_i$[7], anti-**Fy**^{a} (Duffy), etc.

In addition, a source of fresh testing cells of known antigen composition must be available for controls. In any large laboratory there will be found, among the personnel, individuals with a sufficient variety of blood factors to provide such testing cells. It is customary to obtain a small amount of blood from such donors at one- to two-week intervals to insure a supply of known controls. These should include A cells, B cells, O cells, as well as O M cells, O MN cells, O N cells and O Rh positive cells, O rh (negative) cells and both heterozygous and homozygous O rh' and O rh" cells. If other special antisera are to be used, the necessary control cells for these systems must be obtained.

Anti-human globulin serum (so-called Coombs serum) from several sources will be necessary. If a particular antiserum requires the enzyme treatment of the cells being tested, it will then be necessary to have the indicated enzyme on hand, either trypsin, ficin, bromelin or papain.

STANDARD SOLUTIONS

Aside from the specific antisera, the only other solution used in the blood grouping laboratory is normal saline solution. This is used to make the required two to five per cent cell suspensions usually required and to wash the testing cells when this is indicated. Distilled water in a blood grouping laboratory is usually unwise, since its erroneous use in place of normal saline leads to confusing hemolysis.

SPECIAL APPARATUS

The apparatus required is usually that found in a blood grouping laboratory. This consists of a 37 C water bath or block, centrifuges (the small rapid centrifuge is indispensible) and the necessary test tube racks and glassware. Usually, special small test tubes (8 mm × 75 mm) or similar sizes are convenient. A low-power microscope completes the needed equipment.

PROCEDURES

In the performance of the tests, the specific directions of the manufacturers must be meticulously followed. This includes careful preparation of the red cell suspension to the suggested concentration, the proper amount of anti-serum, the correct temperature and duration of the reaction, the duration and speed of centrifugation, the Coombs testing of the sensitized red cells, if required, and the need for microscopic reading of the results. All work sheets must contain the reaction of the known controls in every run.

Whenever possible, the tests should be performed on all the involved persons at the same time, using the same antisera, techniques and controls. Since the clearest results are obtained by the use of fresh cells, the tests should be done as soon as possible after the specimens are obtained. Clotted blood specimens are easy to draw, easy to handle and reasonably well preserved for several days at cool (not frozen) temperatures. Specimens sent by mail should be sterile, taken in duplicate for separate mailings and marked "Airmail, Special Delivery, Keep Cool, Do Not Freeze." Any blood grouping laboratory in the United States can thus be reached with a well-preserved blood specimen whenever a consultation or corroboration is required.

All grouping tests are done in duplicate and read by separate observers by the "blind" technique to avoid unconscious bias. This implies that the observer will not be conscious of the identification of the specimen he is reading except for the controls. The results of such separate readings are then compared by the ultimate responsible serologist who proceeds with the interpretation if the findings are in agreement. Doubtful results, conflicts in observation or any other than absolute clear-cut findings are investigated, repeated and, if necessary, may require recall of the persons for repeat testing.

DISCUSSION

The results of the ABO, MN and Rh-Hr blood grouping tests will provide an exclusion of paternity in about 51 per cent of cases where the alleged father is falsely accused[11]. This represents, therefore, the best possible defense to a charge of paternity. It has also been shown that in situations where paternity has been admitted, the tests revealed that in about 18 per cent of cases the so-called "father" is not the true parent[12]. This has led to the statement: "Maternity is a fact, whereas paternity is only an opinion."

It is not only in claims of illegitimacy that blood grouping has medicolegal value. Several cases of "mixed babies" in hospital nurseries have been quickly solved by comparison of the blood groups[15]. In other instances, such as kidnapped children, where the suspect claims the child is her own[15], in cases of fradulent claims of derivative citizenship[9] and in matters of personal identification, blood gouping has been used to resolve problems. In common practice today is the use of blood grouping of blood stains in homicide cases, unidentified bodies and crimes of violence. An additional but less commonly known use is the establishment of a person's blood group from examination of the body secretions, such as sputum, edema fluid, sweat, saliva and even from urine. This is possible in about 80 per cent of individuals, these being secretors of blood group substances. Historically, the blood groups of mummies and body remains have been identified by absorption studies utilizing antisera of particular specificity. Anthropological investigations of population shifts, origin of races and similar genetic studies have been aided by these examinations[5].

The necessity, however, for meticulous attention to the specific details of these procedures, the duplication of all tests and the use of adequate controls demands the attention of the most experienced technologist. The interpretation of the results of the tests requires familiarity with the laws of heredity governing the genes that determine the blood factors. Without such knowledge, the performance of these procedures should not be attempted.

SOURCES OF ERROR

A. Clerical

1. The identification of the parties involved in medicolegal blood grouping investigations is obviously an important matter. Whenever possible, mutual identification accompanied by signatures and fingerprints should be the rule, since these would be most acceptable to the courts. Other methods include photographs taken at the time the blood specimen is obtained, affidavits attesting to the identification of the specimen, if it has been submitted by mail, etc. or the consent of legal representatives of both sides to any other method acceptable to the court.

2. Continuous identification of the specimen from the subject through the laboratory is essential. Pre-labelling of the original test tube with the name and identifying number of each subject establishes a reference control. Thereafter, each tube used is numbered exactly the same. This includes a cell-washing tube, cell-suspension tube and each reacting tube. Approximately thirty such tubes are needed to perform all the tests as follows (all tests done in duplicate):

ABO serum testing—anti-**A**, anti-**B** and O (anti-**A** + **B**)
ABO cell testing — A cells, B cells and O cells
MN cell testing — M cells, N cells
Rh-Hr cell testing — **Rh**$_o$, -rh', -rh", -hr', -hr"

---

3. In the event that an exclusion is found, it is advisable to repeat promptly the particular test involved, by going back to the original specimen to rule out any possibility of error. Occasionally, this may require the reappearance of the parties. If so, this should be demanded and a high index of suspicion be maintained if any failure to cooperate becomes manifest.

B. Technical

1. Failure to follow directions. A constant reminder that each batch of antiserum may require special handling to produce dependable results seems superfluous. Nevertheless, this is a repeated area for blood grouping error. The characteristics of each serum may vary, and the conditions for its maximal reactivity require readjustment. For this reason, most experienced serologists prefer to produce their own antisera

and are thus constantly familiar with their specific behavior.

2. Failure to duplicate. The possibility of clerical and technical error is considerably reduced by the duplicate testing method. Two independently working technicians, using different batches of testing serum, must produce exactly the same result of each test to insure validity. Any differences require immediate investigation to explain the findings. Final readings are best done by a third observor using the "blind" technique, that is, with no knowledge of the identification of the specimens being examined.

3. Failure to control. The high specificity of the rare antisera and the possibility of interfering contaminants make it mandatory that tests be run simultaneously with known positive and

SPECIMEN LETTER A

Physicians' Letterhead

REPORT ON
BLOOD GROUPING TEST
in the matter of

..............................against...........................

Pursuant to an order duly entered in the above entitled action, I proceeded to examine the following named persons on the dates listed below:

Date	Name	Identification

SPECIMEN LETTER B

Physician's Letterhead

Date

......................., Esq.
Clerk of Family Court
52 Chambers Street
New York, New York

Dear ....:

I am herewith submitting results of blood tests performed on .... (alleged father), ... (mother) and .... (child) in reference to paternity dispute of .... *versus* ....

Results of the blood tests follow:

		K	Rh_o	rh'	rh"	hr'	hr"	
.... (alleged father)	O MN	—	+	+	—	+	+	Rh_1rh
.... (mother)	O MN	—	+	—	—	+	+	Rh_o
.. .. (child)	O MN	—	+	+	—	+	+	Rh_1rh

There are no contradictions to the laws of theoretical expectancy in these findings; paternity therefore cannot be excluded.

Respectfully yours,

....

LNS/spr (Trial date   )
cc: , Esq.
                       , Esq.

SPECIMEN LETTER C

Physician's Letterhead

Date

........................., Esq.
Clerk of Family Court
52 Chambers Street
New York, New York

Dear ....:

    I am herewith submitting results of blood tests performed on ....
(alleged father), ... (mother), and ....
(child), in reference to paternity dispute of .... *versus* ....

    Results of blood tests follow:

		K	Rh_o	rh'	rh"	hr'	hr"	
(alleged father)	O MN	—	+	+	—	+	+	Rh_1rh
(mother)	A_1 N	—	+	+	—	—	+	Rh_1Rh_1
(child)	B MN	—	+	+	—	—	+	Rh_1Rh_1

    There are contradictions to the laws of theoretical expectancy in these findings, in that child who is of blood group B must have inherited this factor from one of his parents. Since the child (....................) is of blood group B, whereas the alleged father (.................... ....) is of blood group O and the mother (.................... ....) is of blood group A_1, paternity therefore is excluded.

Respectfully yours,

....

LNS/spr (Trial date   )
cc: , Esq.
              , Esq.

negative control cells. Thus, any "loss of reactivity" of the serum or erratic behavior due to spoilage, contamination or unclean glassware becomes exposed promptly. The control cells should be fresh, reactive and of known antigen content.

C. Immunological

    1. Lack of understanding of the laws of genetics and the rules of inheritance of the blood groups can be a major source of error. The responsible investigator must be thoroughly familiar with these principles in order to apply them profitably.

    2. The use of the more exotic testing serums, such as anti-M^{g1}, anti-hr^8 and anti-rh_i^7, may resolve some cases and thus improve the possibility for exclusion. Familiarity with the potential value of these serums is essential. Where their use is indicated, and if they are not locally available, help should be requested from a consulting serologist, since such laboratories can be reached easily with specimens sent by airmail.

RANGE OF VALUES

    In blood grouping tests for the exclusion of paternity, there can be only two results. The tests are either positive or negative, and no indecisive results are acceptable. The reports must read either: "There are contradictions to the laws of theoretical expectancy in that — —; paternity is therefore excluded"; or "There are no contradictions to the laws of theoretical expectancy; paternity therefore cannot be excluded." (See appended reports.)

Occasionally, the finding of a rare blood factor present in a child and in an alleged father may tempt the serologist to a positive *inclusion* of paternity. Thus, the blood factor rh$_y$ (frequency — 1 in 10,000 Caucasians), present in both child and alleged father, may be strong *presumptive* evidence of filial relationship. This information may be made available to the court, but cannot be submitted as *absolute* proof of paternity. The court may then include this evidence in their final judicial consideration.

REPORTS

The reporting form should not be so detailed or complicated as to confuse, but should summarize the results of the tests and the conclusions drawn from these results. The protocols and work sheets, including the controls, should be filed for reference, as they may be requested at some future date, as with any other legal documents. Examples of typical reports are included as Specimen Letters A, B and C.

REFERENCES

1. Allen, F. H., Jr. Corcoran, P. A., Kenton, H. B., and Breare, N.: M^g, a new blood group antigen in the MNS system. Vox Sang., 3: 81-91, 1958.

2. Davidsohn, I., Levine, P., and Wiener, A. S.: Medicolegal application of blood grouping tests; Bureau of Legal Medicine and Legislation, Committee on Medicolegal Problems. JAMA, 149:699-706, 1952.

3. Law Department: Medicolegal abstracts. Weight to be given to paternity tests in bastardy cases. JAMA, 166:1242, 1958.

4. Marsters, R. W.: Determination of non-paternity by blood groups. J. Forensic Sci., 2:15-37, 1957.

5. Mourant, A. E.: The Distribution of the Human Blood Groups. Springfield, Thomas. 1954.

6. Owen, R. D., Stormont, C., Wexler, I. B.. and Wiener, A. S.: Committee on Medicolegal Problems, medicolegal applications of blood-grouping tests. JAMA, 164:2036-2044, 1957.

7. Rosenfield, R. E., and Haber, G. V.: An Rh blood factor, rh$_i$ (Ce) and its relationship to hr (ce). Amer. J. Human Genet., 10:474-480, 1958.

8. Rosenfield, R. E., Vogel, P., Sanger, R., and Race, R. R.: A "new" Rh antibody, anti-f. Brit. Med. J., 1:975, 1953.

9. Schatkin, S. B., Sussman, L. N., and Yarbrough, D. E.: Blood test evidence to detect false claims of citizenship. New York Law J., 133:110-111, 1955.

10. Sussman, L. N.: Blood grouping tests in disputed paternity proceedings. JAMA, 155: 1143-1145, 1954.

11. Sussman, L. N.: Blood grouping tests in disputed paternity proceedings and filial relationship. J. Forensic Sci., 1:25-34, 1956.

12. Sussman, L. N., and Schatkin, S. B.: Blood grouping tests in undisputed paternity proceedings. JAMA, 164:249-250, 1957.

13. Unger, L. J.: Blood grouping tests for exclusion of paternity. JAMA, 152:1006-1010, 1953.

14. Wiener, A. S.: Blood grouping test in disputed parentage. J. Forensic Sci., 3:139-148, 1956.

15. Wiener, A. S.: Blood grouping tests in disputed maternity. J. Forensic Sci., 4:351-361, 1959.

Chapter 26

Quantitative Aspects of Exchange Transfusion

J. DE LA HUERGA, M.D., Ph.D., GEORGE W. SMETTERS, M.D., AND JOSEPH C. SHERRICK, M.D.

INTRODUCTION

Blood transfusion was not widely used until the early part of the twentieth century, when the demonstration of blood groups by Landsteiner[8], in 1901, and of cross-matching by Hektoen[7] (1907) and Epstein and Otterberg[4] (1908) made the procedure somewhat less hazardous. Exchange transfusion, or exsanguination transfusion as it was called, was first used by Robertson[11] in 1921, in the hope that it might relieve the toxic state of severely burned infants. Bowers and Trattner[2] (1924) successfully employed phlebotomy followed by transfusion in the treatment of a patient with uremia due to acute nephritis. Hart[5], in 1925, was apparently the first to utilize exchange transfusion for what was undoubtedly a case of erythroblastosis fetalis. Hart was called to see a male infant born to a mother who had six successive infants die of neonatal jaundice. This infant became jaundiced on the first day, and a deep orange color by the third day of life. To let Hart tell the story in his own words[5]:

> Since in this case there was no evidence of infection or sepsis it seemed as though the condition must be due to some toxin circulating in the blood which was destroying the liver cells, and as both the parents and I felt that if something drastic was not done at once the child was certainly going to die as the six other previous male babies had done, it was decided to do an exsanguination transfusion after the technique brought out and perfected by the late Dr. Bruce Robertson, in the hope of removing a sufficient amount of toxin to prevent the progress of the disease. The baby was in Group II Jansky. Dr. J. L. MacDonald, of the Hospital for Sick Children, exsanguinated 300 cc of blood from the anterior fontanelle, at the same time transfusing 335 cc of blood into the internal saphenous vein at the left ankle. The transfusion of blood was commenced after 20 cc of blood had been removed, and the transfusion and exsanguination went on synchronously until the required quantity had been used, and we ended by giving the baby 35 cc more than had been removed. In addition, 60 cc of 5 per cent glucose solution were given. The donor was a healthy male not belonging to the family. By the following morning the jaundice was much less intense. It continued to fade so that by the fourth day it had entirely dis-

appeared and the baby seemed much better.

In 1948, Hart[6] reported that the patient was living, healthy and practicing his profession of butcher. In spite of this initial unqualified success, the report apparently was unnoticed for over twenty years.

Following the discovery of the Rh factor by Levine and Stetson[10] (1939) and Landsteiner and Wiener[9] (1940), and the appreciation of its relation to erythroblastosis, the mortality of the disease was reduced by simple repeated transfusion of Rh negative blood. However, many infants still died. Exchange transfusion was reintroduced by Wallerstein[14] (1946) and Wiener and Wexler[15] (1946). The procedure was immediately successful, and has come into widespread use. The mortality of erythroblastosis fetalis has been reduced from about 70 per cent to less than 10 per cent[3].

QUANTITATIVE ASPECTS

In erythroblastosis fetalis, exchange transfusions are performed for two reasons: first, to remove bilirubin from the blood and indirectly from the tissues, second, to eliminate a large part of the child's antigen-coated erythrocytes, which will eventually be destroyed, producing more bilirubin to maintain a high toxic level. The amount of blood to be removed and replaced is thus of considerable significance to the pediatrician, and it is important for him to have a simple accurate means of calculating the volume of donor blood which must be administered to produce a given percentage of replacement. This percentage of replacement must be determined clinically.

These quantitative aspects of exchange transfusion have been studied by Wiener and Wexler[15] (1946). Veall and Mollison[13] (1950) produced a formula for predicting the amount of red cell exchange, and constructed a nomogram, based mainly on hematocrit levels, which facilitates the calculation. Allen and Diamond[1] utilized a formula to calculate the amount of blood replaced. Trossman, Alzofon and Malkin[12] have published a nomogram for the same purpose. This present study, while derived from basic established principles, was designed specifically for application to the newborn infant. Our study was directed at enabling the pediatrician to calculate specific transfusion volumes both rapidly and accurately, for various conditions of weight and percentage replacement.

In order to understand the problems involved in determining the efficiency of exchange transfusion, let us consider the technique most favored in the actual performance of the transfusion. A plastic catheter is inserted into an umbilical cord vein, and is attached to two three-way stopcocks and a 20 ml syringe, arranged in such a way that blood may be withdrawn from the vein, discarded and replaced by an equal aliquot of donor blood. The procedure is repeated until the desired volume of blood has been exchanged. In performing the operation, an attempt is usually made: (a) to keep the amount of blood withdrawn in any step small in relation to the baby's blood volume; (b) to transfer the same amount of blood in and out in each step; and (c) at the end of the procedure to have removed from the child the same amount of blood as has been injected so that his blood volume will be essentially unchanged.

While performing this procedure, the first 20 ml of blood withdrawn are the child's own blood, but starting from the second cycle, the blood removed from the child is a mixture of his own blood plus that which has been injected. Consequently, decreasing volumes of the child's original blood are discarded and increasing volumes of the previously injected donor's blood mixed with it are discarded at the same time. The following will illustrate this in a quantitative manner.

Let us take as an example the case of a child weighing 2 kg. The volume of blood is assumed to be one tenth of

the child's weight, i.e., 0.2 liter or 200 ml. When the first 20 ml of blood have been removed, all this blood is the child's own blood, and at this time the blood volume is reduced to 180 ml. Then this is followed by a 20 ml injection of donor's blood. At this stage, the blood volume returns to the original 200 ml and consists of 180 ml of the child's blood and 20 ml of the donor's blood just injected. The child will then have $180/200 \times 100 = 90$ per cent of its own blood. The conditions after repeating this procedure several times can be seen in Table I, which was obtained from successive calculations. Notice that, up to the seventh cycle, most of the blood

TABLE I

Cycle No.	ml of Child's Blood Removed at this Cycle	ml of Donor's Blood Removed at this Cycle	ml of Child's Blood Remaining at the Completion of this Cycle	Per Cent of Child's Blood Remaining at the Completion of this Cycle	Total ml of Donor's Blood Injected at the Completion of this Cycle
0	0	0	200.00	100	0
1	20.00	0	180.00	90.0	20
2	18.00	2.00	162.00	81.0	40
3	16.20	3.80	145.80	72.9	60
4	14.60	5.40	131.20	65.6	80
5	13.10	6.90	118.10	59.5	100
6	11.80	8.20	106.30	53.1	120
7	10.60	9.40	95.70	47.8	140
8	9.57	10.43	86.13	43.1	160
9	8.61	11.39	77.52	38.8	180
10	7.75	12.25	69.77	34.9	200
11	6.97	13.03	62.80	31.4	220
12	6.28	13.72	56.52	28.3	240
13	5.65	14.35	50.87	25.4	260
14	5.08	14.92	45.79	22.9	280
15	4.58	15.42	41.21	20.6	300
16	4.12	15.88	37.09	18.5	320
17	3.71	16.29	33.38	16.7	340
18	3.35	16.65	30.03	15.0	360
19	3.00	17.00	27.03	13.5	380
20	2.68	18.32	24.35	12.2	400

removed was the child's own blood, but from there on, most of the blood removed is actually the donor's injected blood.

This sequence of events is regulated by the following exponential equation:

$$\frac{\% \ C}{100} = \left[\frac{(100 \times W) - 20}{100 \times W} \right]^{N} \quad (1)$$

In this equation,

N = number of cycles (removal of 20 ml of blood followed by injection of 20 ml of donor's blood)

% C = percentage of the child's blood remaining; conversely (100 − % C) is the percentage of child's blood removed

20 = volume in ml of blood removed and donor's blood injected at each cycle

W = child's weight in kilograms

100 × W = child's blood volume in milliliters

The above equation may be simplified as:

$$\frac{\% \ C}{100} = \left[1 - \frac{1}{5W} \right]^{N} \quad (2)$$

In our example, Equation 2 may readily be shown to be correct by reference to Table I. For instance, the calculated percentage of child's blood remaining after the *third* cycle will be:

$$\frac{\% \ C}{100} = \left[1 - \frac{1}{10} \right]^{3}$$

$$= (0.9)^{3}$$
$$= 0.729$$
$$\% \ C = 72.9$$

This value is the same found in Table I for the third cycle.

Equation 2 may be converted to a logarithmic equation as follows:

$$\text{Log } \% \ C - 2 = N \log \left[1 - \frac{1}{5W} \right] \quad (3)$$

Solving Equation 3 for N, we have:

$$N = \frac{\log \% \ C - 2}{\log \left[1 - \frac{1}{5W} \right]} \quad (4)$$

In Equation 4, N is the number of cycles necessary to produce the desired percentage of replacement, % C. Since each cycle N involves the injection of 20 ml of blood, the total volume of donor's blood injected after N cycles, will be V = 20 N.

Thus, substituting in Equation 4

$$V = \frac{20 \ (\log \% \ C - 2)}{\log \left[1 - \frac{1}{5W} \right]} \quad (5)$$

INVESTIGATIONS

The above equations, strictly speaking, will hold true only when exactly 20 ml of the child's blood is replaced at every cycle with 20 ml of donor's blood. Obviously, accuracy of this degree can seldom be attained in practice. To evaluate the effect of possible variations in technique, two types of investigations were performed. First, using mathematical models and calculating the results according to Equation 5, the conditions were varied in different ways.

For this type of work an automatic calculator was used. Secondly, to supplement the results obtained by calculations, experimental models were devised in which volumetric flasks filled with blood were used. Aliquots of the blood were removed in cycles using accurate pipettes, the blood then being replaced by accurately measured amounts of water. The hemoglobin content of the flask at various cycles was then determined colorimetrically, and the percentage of blood remaining (or conversely removed) was evaluated. The results so obtained were then compared with those obtained from the mathematical model. This type of approach mirrors the conditions prevailing during the exchange transfusion, as performed in the living infant.

EXPERIMENTAL VERIFICATION OF EQUATIONS

To find out if Mathematical Equation 5, derived above, holds true in an experimental model, a 200 ml volumetric flask was filled with blood to the mark. An exchange transfusion was simulated by removing 20 ml aliquots of blood and replacing them with 20 ml aliquots of water until various volumes of water had been injected. The results obtained by hemoglobin measurement in the discarded aliquots were very close to those calculated from Equation 5. After exchanging 200 ml, the analytical result was 100.5 per cent of the calculated one, and, after 300 ml, the analytical result was 95 per cent of the calculated one, thus demonstrating the reliability of the equations mentioned above. These results are well within the limits of error of the hemoglobin analysis.

EFFECT OF SYRINGE SIZE

The effect of syringe size was then studied in a mathematical model. For blood volumes of 100 ,200 and 300 ml, the volume of blood to be transfused for 90 per cent replacement was calculated when exchange was performed in cycles of 10 ml, 20 ml, 30 ml and 40 ml. As can be seen in Table II, the

TABLE II EFFECT OF CHANGING THE AMOUNT OF BLOOD REMOVED PER CYCLE ON THE VOLUME OF BLOOD TO BE TRANSFUSED TO ACCOMPLISH 90 PER CENT REMOVAL OF CHILD'S BLOOD IN CHILDREN WITH BLOOD VOLUMES OF 100, 200 AND 300 ML. CALCULATED DATA.

Syringe Size (ml.)	For Blood Volumes					
	100 ml		200 ml		300 ml	
	ml°	%†	ml°	%†	ml°	%†
10	218.5	105	448.3	102	679.8	102
20	206.4	100	437.1	100	667.1	100
30	193.7	94	425.1	97	655.6	98
40	190.3	92	421.8	96	643.8	96

°Ml to be injected to produce 90 per cent replacement of indicated blood volume.

†Percentage of the total volume to be injected by a syringe of the indicated size compared to the total volume to be injected by a 20 ml syringe.

volume of blood necessary to replace 90 per cent of the original blood decreases slightly as syringe size is increased. The amount of change is not considered significant compared to the effect of the large blood volume shifts produced by the use of large syringes.

EFFECT OF VARYING THE VOLUME EXCHANGED BETWEEN CYCLES

A mathematical model then was calculated to ascertain the effect of varying the volume of exchange fluid at successive cycles from 15 ml to 25 ml, but maintaining a constant volume within the cycle. That is, 15 ml was withdrawn and replaced by 15 ml in the first cycle, 20 ml withdrawn and replaced with 20 ml in the second cycle, 25 ml withdrawn and replaced in the third, 15 ml exchanged in the fourth and so on. The calculations showed that if the total volume of exchange fluid is taken into consideration, the same percentage of removal was accomplished as when uniform cycles of 20 ml were used. Less than 1 per cent difference was introduced by varying the cycle size when from 41 to 88 per cent of the original blood was replaced. This shows that variations in the volume of individual cycles make no difference in the percentage of removal of the child's blood so long as the total volume of blood exchanged is kept constant.

EFFECT OF VARYING THE VOLUME EXCHANGED WITHIN A CYCLE

Another mathematical model was then created in which, at each cycle, the volume of exchange liquid removed was different from the volume injected in the same cycle, and also the volume removed differed in successive cycles. The volumes varied from 15 to 25 ml, and the largest difference in any cycle was of 8 ml. In this particular case, although the volume of blood removed in a particular cycle was different from that of the liquid subsequently injected, the total blood volume at the end of any cycle was kept between 95 and 105 per cent of the original 200 ml. These variations were kept relatively small, because, in an exchange trans-

fusion, it is dangerous to increase or decrease the original blood volume significantly.

An experiment was carried out in the same fashion as in the mathematical model. Using a 200 ml volumetric flask filled to the mark with blood, aliquots were removed and replaced by water. The aliquots of blood removed varied from one cycle to the next. The aliquots of water added were also varied and were different from the volume of blood removed. The total fluid volume at the end was kept equal to that at the beginning. For example, in the first cycle, 25 ml of blood were removed and 18 ml of water injected; in the second, 15 ml removed and 23 injected and so on. The results are compared in Table III with those obtained when 20 ml of blood are replaced with 20 ml of water at each cycle. As can be seen, there is practically no difference in the percentage of blood exchanged, even though the individual volumes within each cycle and from one cycle to the next were deliberately varied.

EFFECT OF THE DEAD SPACE OF THE TRANSFUSION SET

The mathematical approach leading to Equation 5 holds only when precisely 20 ml of blood are removed and 20 ml of donor's blood are transfused. In practice, this cannot be done with exactitude because of the dead space in the catheter, valves and syringe. It is customary to fill the dead space with donor's blood, then to enter the child's vein. When the syringe is retracted to the 20 ml mark and the whole system is filled with blood, the first blood coming into the syringe is the donor's blood present in the catheter and valves.

TABLE III COMPARISON BETWEEN THE REMOVAL OF 20 ML AT EACH CYCLE
FOLLOWED BY INJECTION OF 20 ML OF DONOR'S BLOOD, CHANGING THE
VOLUME OF BLOOD REMOVED IN SUCCESSIVE CYCLES, AND VARYING THE
VOLUME OF BLOOD INJECTED SO THAT IT DIFFERS FROM THE VOLUME OF BLOOD
REMOVED IN THE SAME CYCLE.

Volume of Liquid Exchanged (calculated data)	Per Cent of Blood Remaining		
	Calculated for Equal Cycles of 20 ml	Variation in Cycles	
		Calculated Data	Experimental Data
100 ml	59.0	58.6 (99%)°	not determined
200 ml	35.0	35.6 (102%)°	33.9 (97%)°
300 ml	20.7	20.0 (98%)°	21.2 (101%)°

°Numbers in parentheses are percentages of calculated results in second column represented by experimentally measured volumes.

Thus, not all of the blood in the syringe at this point is the child's blood.

To investigate the effect of the dead space in a commercial transfusion kit this was measured by filling the dead space with blood of known hemoglobin content and then rinsing with a known amount of water. The hemoglobin content of this wash water was then measured, and, by comparison with the original hemoglobin content of the blood, the volume of the space was measured. The total measured dead space was 0.51 ml, most of it present in the plastic catheter. When the blood in the syringe is discarded, the dead space remains filled with child's blood. When the donor's blood is drawn into the syringe, the child's blood remaining in the syringe and in the closest valve is mixed with the donor's blood. When the blood now in the syringe is injected, the first blood that goes into the child is the child's own blood that remained in the dead space beyond the valve closest to the syringe. By making calculations according to these conditions, and assuming that the syringe is accu-

rate, it was found that, in each cycle, 19.49 ml of child's blood are actually removed and 19.44 ml of donor's blood are injected. This very small variation will have no practical significance.

CONCLUSIONS

The following conclusions may be drawn: The only factor of importance in exchange transfusions is the total amount of donor's blood exchanged for the infant blood; the same percentage of removal is accomplished using different volumes of blood between cycles or within a cycle, so long as the total blood volume is kept constant.

NOMOGRAM

To facilitate the application of Equation 5, a nomogram (Fig. 1) has been constructed that shows the volume of donor's blood necessary to replace from 60 to 90 per cent of the child's blood in children of various body weights. To use it, one locates the diagonal line corresponding to the body weight of the child and notes where it intersects the horizontal line representing the per-

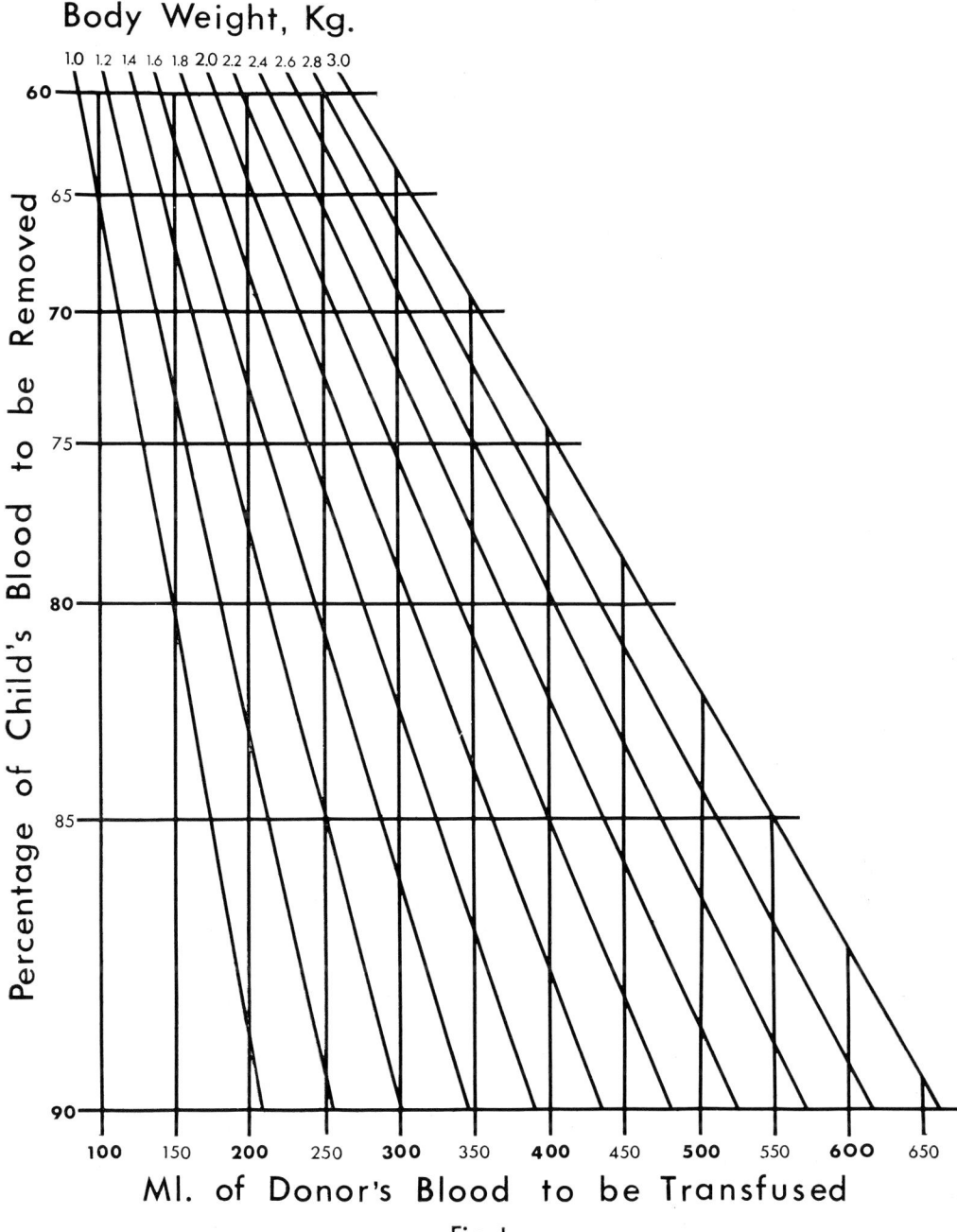

Fig. 1.

centage of blood desired to be removed. The vertical projection of this point of intersection on the bottom scale shows the volume of donor's blood to be used. In practice, visual estimation of this projection is sufficiently accurate, and a straight edge is unnecessary.

The volume of donor's blood, of course, refers to that volume to be injected and equals the volume of blood to be removed in order to maintain the original blood volume. If it is thought necessary to increase or decrease the blood volume, an extra volume of blood may be added or subtracted.

This nomogram has been constructed for infants weighing from 1 to 3 kg, the group most commonly in need of exchange transfusions for erythroblastosis fetalis. Should the infant weigh more than 3 kg, one needs only to divide the child's weight by two, obtain the transfusion volume corresponding to this weight from the nomogram, then multiply this volume by two to find the actual amount of donor's blood to be transfused. For example, for a child weighing 4 kg, requiring 80 per cent replacement, it is easy to see that 620 ml of donor's blood will be necessary.

A review of the nomogram shows several points of interest. For any given percentage of blood removed, the volume of donor's blood to be exchanged is almost directly proportional to the weight of the child. However, there is a significant disproportion between the volume of donor's blood needed and the percentage of child's blood removed. For example, for a child weighing 2 kg, it will be necessary to exchange 430 ml of donor's blood if 90 per cent of the child's blood is to be removed; while, for removal of 80 per cent, only 310 ml will be necessary.

At this point it is also interesting to examine Table I, which shows that, at the end of the fifteenth cycle, when 300 ml of donor's blood has been injected into a 2 kg child, 80 per cent of the blood to be discarded in the sixteenth cycle is donor's blood that was injected in previous cycles. It is obviously undesirable to administer large volumes of

blood, thereby unnecessarily prolonging the procedure without actually removing much of the child's blood. This certainly is true if more than 90 per cent of the blood is to be removed. It might be better, as recommended by some investigators, to remove a smaller percentage at one time by using relatively less donor's blood and later, if necessary, repeat the exchange transfusion.

REFERENCES

1. Allen, F. H., Jr., and Diamond, L. K.: Erythroblastosis Fetalis, Including Exchange Transfusion Technic. Boston, Little, 1957.
2. Bowers, C. A., and Trattner, H. R.: Repeated venesection — blood transfusion in anuria: Report of a case of acute nephritis with anuria. Surg. Gynec. Obstet., 39:229-234, 1924.
3. Daetwyler, A.: Ergebnisse der Nachuntersuchung der ersten hundert in Bern wegen Icterus gravis mit Austauschtransfusionen behandelten Kinder. Helv. Paediat. Acta, 18 (Supp. 12):1-43, 1963.
4. Epstein, A. A., and Ottenberg, R.: A simple method of performing serum reactions. Proc. New York Path. Soc., 8:117-123, 1908.
5. Hart, A. P.: Familial icterus gravis of the newborn and its treatment. Canad. Med. Ass. J., 15:1008-1011, 1925.
6. Hart, A. P.: Exsanguination transfusion in a new born infant in 1925. J. Pediat., 32:760, 1948.
7. Hektoen, L.: Isoagglutination of human corpuscles. J. Infect. Dis., 4:297-303, 1907.
8. Landsteiner, K.: Ueber Agglutinationserscheinungen normalen menschlichen Blutes. Wien. Klin. Wschr., 14:1132-1134, 1901.
9. Landsteiner, K., and Wiener, A. S.: An agglutinable factor in human blood recognized by immune sera for rhesus blood. Proc. Soc. Exp. Biol. Med., 43:223, 1940.
10. Levine, P., and Stetson, R. E.: An unusual case of intra-group agglutination. JAMA, 113:126-127, 1939.
11. Robertson, Bruce: Blood transfusion in severe burns in infants and young children. A preliminary report of the treatment of the toxic shock by blood transfusion — with or without the preceding exsanguination. Canad. Med. Ass. J., 11:774-750, 1921.

12. Trossman, C. M. Alzofon, F., and Malkin, H.: An exchange transfusion nomogram. Amer. J. Dis. Child., **105**:449-452, 1963.

13. Veall, N., and Mollison, P. L.: The rate of red cell exchange in replacement transfusion. Lancet, **2**:792, 1950.

14. Wallerstein, H.: Treatment of severe eryth-roblastosis by simultaneous removal and replacement of the blood of the newborn infant. Science, **103**:583-584, 1946.

15. Wiener, A. S., and Wexler, I. B.: The use of heparin when performing exchange blood transfusion in newborn infants. J. Lab. Clin. Med.. **31**:1016-1020, 1946.

Chapter 27

Collection and Handling of Blood and Urine from Infants

HOWARD QUITTNER, M.D.

INTRODUCTION

No matter how profoundly scientific insight probes the basis and nature of disease, both diagnosis and treatment must be anchored to the sober practical problem of the workable laboratory method. Simply, we are hampered by technical difficulties in obtaining adequate blood and urine specimens from newborns and small children. This obstacle prevents the derivation of large bodies of statistics from newborn populations and limits the practicality of many of the suggested mass screening programs. The scattered population and broad geography of this country requires that collections be made in distant places, and sometimes under sub-optimal conditions. Since only the most elementary procedures are performed in the field, most specimens reach large centers by mail.

When newborns and infants are located in a well-staffed hospital, the technical difficulties of obtaining blood may be resolved by the adept physician versed in the techniques of venipuncture of the femoral, internal jugular or external jugular vein. These locations have almost completely replaced the unrewarding approach to obtaining blood from the antecubital vein or the unwarranted risk of infection present in using the superior sagittal sinus. Venipuncture, even of the femoral vein, is not without hazard, and the expertise required always restricts its use to special situations.

It is thus apparent that most routine specimens will be obtained with a lancet from the deeper dermal area and that they must be collected in suitable containers for transport. The term "skin-stick" is used to indicate that the wound made in this method is of adequate size and depth. Long ago, it was observed that a properly inflicted wound into the dermis would normally bleed spontaneously for about three minutes and that bleeding would be increased if the area had a heat-induced erythema or if the venous pressure were increased. Many individuals have confirmed that dependency of the part also increases the blood flow.

Containerization of the small blood sample can be effected in many ways. Table I enumerates the array of methods employed in most of the recent technology.

If small amounts of whole blood are measured into receiving solutions, suitable corrections must be made through the use of hematocrit values, so that the determined constituent can be reported as a function of the delivered plasma volume. The correction should also account for the plasma trapped with the red cell mass, and the method should establish whether the erythrocytes have contributed additional material to the receiving solution. If not corrected, the normal differences in hematocrit between two newborns may lead to as much as a 50 per cent variation in the result of the analysis when the levels are really identical. The danger of the unknown hematocrit is especially critical when the blood is obtained on filter paper. This potential error limits the filter paper method to qualitative screening procedures and quantitative tests where the difference between normal and abnormal is quite great (e.g., the phenylalanine assay).

Only filter paper and plastic tubes can assuredly survive postal transport. Specially devised containers can protect glass capillary tubes, but these are relatively expensive for mass procedures. Recent advances in glass technology provide numerous in-hospital savings of money and effort. The remarkable uniformity in the internal diameters of capillary tubes allows them to replace micropipettes in many methods. By the addition of single or double scoring to the tubes, it is possible to meter accurate microsamples of serum or whole blood by breaking off precise segments of tubing. This simplified process may entirely eliminate micropipettes.

SPECIAL APPARATUS

1. *Polyethylene tubing*, 0.114 inch O.D., 0.082 inch I.D.,* cut into 6 inch lengths with each end bevelled at a 45-degree angle by a sharp razor blade.

2. *Sterile Bard-Parker Blades* #11 or *Redi-Lance.*†

3. *Hand Sealer Clips* and *Hand Sealer.*‡

4. *Test tubes,* 12 × 100 mm.

5. *Hypodermic needle wires.*

6. *Silicone ointment* (20 or 30 per cent).§

PROCEDURE

1. After cleansing the outer aspect of the heel with antiseptic and drying the area with gauze, a small amount of silicone ointment is rubbed into the area. A puncture of sufficient depth is made with a sterile blade or lancet. The heel must be in a dependent position with relation to the infant at this time. An assistant to the operator is essential

---

*Bel-Art Products, Pequannock, New Jersey, #F = 21852.

†Clay-Adams, Inc., New York, New York.

‡Fenwal Laboratories, Morton Grove Illinois, #BS5 and BS4.

§American Hospital Formulary Service, or Arner Stone Company, Mt. Prospect, Illinois.

if good specimens are to be obtained.

2. The first drop of blood is wiped away. The tubing is held vertically below the level of the puncture wound.

3. The tip of the bevelled edge of the tubing is applied to the blood flowing from the wound. The tubing is allowed to fill for a convenient distance (between 5 to 10 cm). The tip of the tubing should not be wiped through the blood. Capillarity will cause the tube to fill if blood flow is adequate. One centimeter of newborn blood yields 12.5 μl or more of serum.

4. The filled pieces of tubing are placed flat upon a porcelainized metal tray and, after the appropriate number of tubes is collected, a label of identification is placed over them, securing them as a group.

5. The tray is sent to the laboratory, where the specimens are separated, the ends distal to the blood are folded over carefully, the ends inserted into the clips and the tubes sealed with the clamp.

6. A set of tubes is placed clip downward in a test tube, and these are spun for ten minutes at 3000 RCF in a horizontal centrifuge. If the clots do not centrifuge down readily, the tubes can be carefully rimmed with the fine wire and respun.

7. With a sharp razor blade against a white background, the tubes are severed through the serum just above the cell interface.

8. Serum may then be successfully aspirated directly, or expressed from the tubes into pipettes, dilutors, gasometers or autoanalyzers. If a CO_2 analysis is to be done, it is best to use the serum for this purpose immediately after separation from the cells.

DISCUSSION

The use of plastic tubing in the method allows the realization of easy processing and the use of economical materials. For liquid serum samples, sealed plastic tubes represent a sensible container. The bevelled edge of the capillary provides for minimal contact between the flowing blood and the collecting tube.

The sites of preference for skin-stick in the newborn are on the lower extremity. Experience has indicated that the heel is the area of choice, and the small vein behind the internal malleolus is preferred if the procedure is to be done only once. The big toe or the medial arch are also acceptable sites. More important than the site is the often-forgotten fact that bleeding occurs not from capillaries but from arterioles and venules. These are present deeply enough beneath the skin that the lancet should be inserted to a depth of 3 to 4 mm. The lancet should have a width of 2 mm at the skin surface when inserted to its full depth. Proper flow from such a puncture will continue for two to four minutes and yield a specimen of 0.2 ml or more. The use of heat, attention to the dependent position of the bleeding area, and the application of a silicone ointment to the skin, all improve the flow of blood.

SOURCES OF ERROR

Hemolysis is the only significant artefact produced in blood obtained by skin-stick. Michaëlsson and Sjölen[11] emphasize that the fragile nature of the erythrocyte in the newborn period is such that it is extremely difficult to obtain serum with less than 100 mg per

100 ml of free hemoglobin. They also emphasize the use of silicone ointment, collecting tubes of no more than 3 mm internal diameter and no more than 4 mm in external diameter, and freely flowing blood as factors in reducing free hemoglobin. All of these facets of technique are integral parts of the described method. Heparin reduces hemolysis in glass tubes, but it cannot be added readily to plastic tubes. Comparable reductions in hemolysis have been obtained with plastic tubing and serum if a continuous column of blood, free of air bubbles, is obtained.

Urine Collection

INTRODUCTION

Our expanding technology also demands simple methods for the collection of the routine urine specimen. An effective method should be easy to apply and yield a representative specimen. Many of the devices and approaches present in the literature are either complex, barbarous or dangerous, and some embody all of these disadvantages. The practical methods in general use are outlined in Table II. Catheterization or

TABLE II METHODS OF URINE COLLECTION

1. Tube methods
   a. "Strapping" of tubes and funnels[1]
   b. "Rubber finger" tube
   c. Adhesive plastic bag[8]
2. "Midstream-catch method"[1]
3. Gauze-pad method
4. Catheterization
5. Suprapubic aspiration[12]

suprapubic aspiration should be reserved for critical bacteriological studies. The method described here is

modified from a previously described sweat collection technique[5, 6].

SPECIAL APPARATUS

1. *Centrifuge tubes,* round, plastic, 50 ml capacity.
2. *Parafilm closure or polyethylene caps.*
3. *Plastic golf tees,* 43 mm or longer.[*]
4. *Polyethylene sheeting,* 0.0015 inch thick, cut into 6 inch squares.
5. *Gauze pads,* 16 ply, 20 × 12 mesh, 4 inch square, *all gauze,* USP Type VII, one for each anticipated 10 ml of sample to be collected.
6. Plastic bags (Whirl-Pak Bags 9 × 4½ inch.[†]

PROCEDURE

1. The infant is prepared by the nurse between diaperings in the usual manner, making certain that the region of the urethra, perineum and pubic area is clean and dry. Powder is not to be used. The gauze square is placed over the urethral region extending more superiorly than inferiorly, and is backed by the polyethylene sheeting. The materials are held in place by careful application of the diaper. After a suitable period of time, (determined by nursery experience, generally 3 to 4 hours) the diaper is removed, and the moist gauze is transferred to the whirl-pak, which is sealed, a label applied, and transmitted to the laboratory in the same manner as other urine specimens.

2. Two clean dry plastic golf tees are dropped into the centrifuge tube, points downward, and the gauze

---

[*]Plawood Mormac Corp., 10215 Meech Avenue, Cleveland, Ohio.

[†]Scientific Products, Evanston, Illinois, #B1205-18.

pad containing the urine is packed *loosely* into the centrifuge tube above it with a forceps, care being taken to lose none of the liquid. The tube is sealed with parafilm or a plastic cap and is spun for about ten minutes in a balanced horizontal centrifuge at no more than RCF 1000. After centrifugation, the gauze and tees are removed, leaving the urine for analysis.

3. Microscopic examination of the urine sediment may be made by re-centrifuging the urine specimen in the conventional manner.

4. *Caution!* If too great a centrifugal force is used in the extraction period, the gauze will slip past the tees and interfere with effective extraction of the urine.

DISCUSSION

The simplicity of the technique permits the collection of an adequate screening urine specimen by untrained personnel. The use of a simple gauze pad is not an ideal answer to the urine collection problem. Further development of the method is needed to find better absorptive materials. In spite of this, almost quantitative collections of urine can be made if the urinary output does not exceed the absorptive capacity of the gauze. Quantitative collection requires weighing of the gauze and container before and after collection. Evaporation can be minimized by incorporating with the pad a simple electronic warning device which signals that urination has occurred (Fig. 1). Since the expressed urine is representative of the particular sample, a constant fraction (e.g. one third) of each specimen can be pooled. The pooled specimens can be used to determine the twenty-four hour urinary excretory value. With careful cleansing methods, sterile gauze, the warning device and sterile transport containers, material approximating a "clean catch" specimen can be obtained for bacteriologic evaluation.

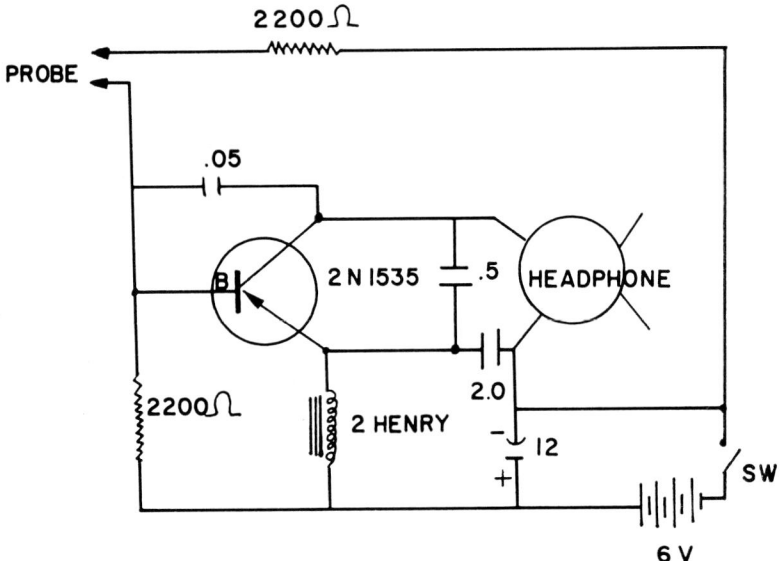

Fig. 1.   Electrical diagram of urination "warning" device.

SOURCES OF ERROR

The microscopic sediment obtained through the use of this method is not reliable. It appears that the cotton fibers traumatize the formed elements during the period of centrifugation-extraction, leading to a low recovery of formed elements. This defect may be corrected in the future by the substitution of a better absorptive material.

RESUME OF CLINICAL INTERPRETATIONS

TABLE III

Urinalysis (247 newborns)	
Insufficient volume	5.7%
"Pathological"	4.3%
"Normal values" (225 newborns)	
Specific gravity	1.002 − 1.004
pH	5.0 − 6.5
Glucose (Clinistix® °)	15.5% positive
Clintest® ° (25 mg per 100 ml)	6.2% positive
Clinistix° & Clinitest° (25 mg per 100 ml)	2.2% positive
Protein (Albustix® °)	6.7% positive
Red blood cells (Hemastix® °, 1+)	

° Ames Company, Elkhart, Indiana.

Table III presents data obtained upon random urine specimens from 247 consective newborns. Some of these specimens were obtained by the mothers in the "live-in" section of the obstetrical suite without nursing or technical assistance. In spite of this, only a small number of specimens were of too small a volume to permit a complete analysis. The reducing substance test was performed by modifying the standard technique so that fifteen drops of urine and no water were used, lowering the screening level to the order of 25 mg per 100 ml.

REFERENCES

1. Boehm, J. J., and Haynes, J. L.: The "midstream catch" in newborn infants. Southern. Med. J., 57:1466-1467, 1964.
2. Cox, F. M., Hull, E. W., and Searcy, R. L.: Laboratory suggestion: A new device for collecting capillary blood. Amer. J. Clin. Path., 39:661, 1963.
3. Davies, J. A. V.: A method of collecting small blood specimens. J. Lab. Clin. Med., 23:1206-1209, 1938.
4. Davison, W. C.: Compleat Pediatrician. Durham, Duke University Press, 6th ed., 1949, p. 185.
5. Dubowski, K. M.: In Measurements of Exocrine and Endocrine Functions of the Pancreas (with a Section on Fibrocystic Disease). Philadelphia, Lippincott, 1951, p. 168.
6. Gibbs, G. E., et. al.: Cystic fibrosis. Postgrad. Med., 22:515-524, 1957.
7. Guthrie, R., and Susi, A.: A simple phenylalanine method for detecting phenylketonuria in large populations of newborn infants. Pediatrics, 32:338-343, 1963.
8. Hill, E. J.: New method for collecting urine samples in infants. Plast. Reconstr. Surg., 22:567-571, 1958.
9. Lewis, S. M., and Benjamin, H.: Break-off capillary tube method for blood counts. J. Clin. Path., 18:689, 1965.
10. Meites, S., and Faulkner, W. R.: Manual of Practical Micro and General Procedures in Clinical Chemistry. Springfield, Thomas, 1962, p. 8.
11. Michaëlsson, M., and Sjölin, S.: Hemolysis in blood samples from newborn infants. Acta Paediat. Scand., 54:325-330, 1965.
12. Nelson, J. D., and Peters, P. C.: Suprapubic aspiration of urine in premature and term infants. Pediatrics, 36:132-134, 1965.
13. Portnoy, J., Brewer, J. H., and Harris, A.: Rapid plasma reagin card test for syphilis and other treponematoses. Public Health Rep., 77:645-652, 1962.
14. Walter, A. R., and Gerarde, H. W.: A rapid semiautomatic system of chemical analysis using true microspecimens. Clin. Chem., 10:509-518, 1964.

Chapter 28

Hematological Norms in Infancy

HERBERT DERMAN, M.D.

Any physician dealing with children must be impressed with the changing values of pediatric physiology which form the background against which the health of his diminutive patient is to be judged. The speed and the extent of the hemodynamic alterations occuring after birth are so remarkable as to require, frequently, the use of general concepts rather than specific numbers. Greater than 20 per cent increases in circulating red cell volume, plasma volume and total blood volume take place in three to five hours after delivery of normal

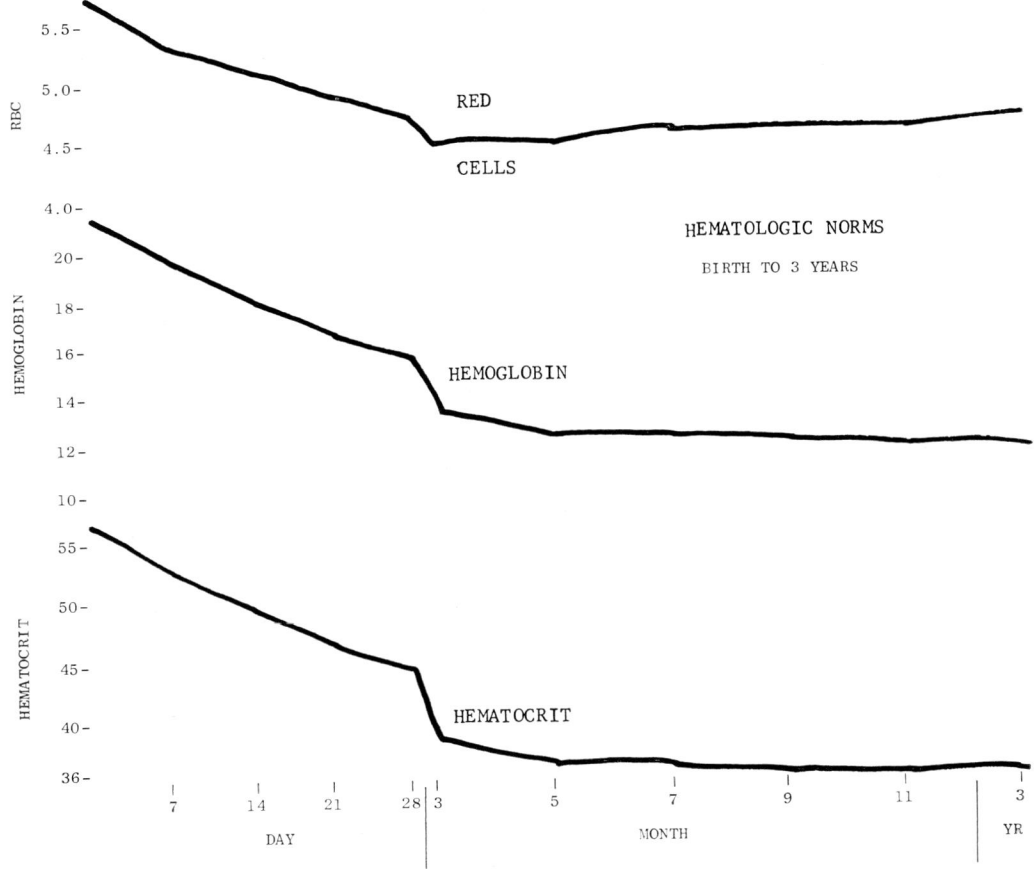

Fig. I.

full-term infants without anesthesia or complication[14]. Considerable respect is therefore warranted for the delicate balance between stimuli and responses which lead these alterations into normal rather than into pathological channels.

cent at birth, drops to 45 per cent at two months, and then stabilizes at 35 per cent through two years of age. All three of these values hold the high birth levels or even increase during the first twenty-four hours of life. Owing to

TABLE I ERYTHROCYTE AND PLATELET VALUES*

Age	RBC	Hgb.	Hct.	Retic.	MCV	MCHC	MCH	MCD	Platelets
	mil/cu mm	gm/100ml	%	% tot RBC	. cu μ	gm/100ml RBC	μμg	μ	000/cu mm
Birth	5.7(4.8-7.1)	21.5(18.0-27.0)	56.6	4.35(2.5 -6.5)	106.0	38.0	38.0	8.6	227(140-290)
1 wk	5.3(4.5-6.4)	19.6(16.2-25.5)	52.7	1.12(0.1 -4.5)	101.0	37.2	37.0		235(150-320)
2 wk	5.1(4.3-6.0)	18.0(14.5-24.2)	49.6	0.67(0.2 -1.5)	96.0	36.3	35.0	8.1	247(163-340)
3 wk	4.9(4.1-6.0)	16.6(13.2-23.0)	46.6	0.63(0.2 -1.3)	93.0	35.6	34.0		267(177-367)
4 wk	4.7(3.9-5.9)	15.6(12.0-21.8)	44.6	0.73(0.1 -1.0)	91.0	35.0	33.0		280(185-390)
3 mo	4.5(3.8-5.8)	13.3(10.8-18.0)	38.9	1.2 (0.5 -3.1)	85.0	34.2	30.0	7.7	315(200-428)
5 mo	4.5(3.8-5.3)	12.4(10.2-15.0)	36.5	1.66(0.9 -2.94)	79.0	34.0	27.0		338(205-465)
7 mo	4.6(3.9-5.3)	12.3(10.0-15.0)	36.2	1.38(0.72-2.3)	78.0	34.0	27.0		340(205-470)
9 mo	4.6(4.0-5.4)	12.1(9.8-15.0)	35.8	1.12(0.65-1.9)	77.0	33.8	26.0		345(210-473)
11 mo	4.6(4.0-5.5)	11.9(8.4-14.9)	35.5	0.97(0.62-1.8)	77.0	33.5	26.0	7.4	345(212-470)
3 yr	4.7(3.8-5.4)	11.7(9.2-15.5)	35.5		78.0	33.0	25.0	7.4	

*Modified from *Handbook of Biological Data*, Table 262'.

RED CELLS, HEMOGLOBIN AND HEMATOCRIT (FIG. 1 AND TABLE I)

The red cell count at birth has a mean value of 5.7 million per cubic millimeter, with a broad range of 4.8 to 7.1 million. The count drops progressively to a mean low of 4.5 million at three months, at which time counts ranging from 3.8 to 5.8 million may be encountered. Thereafter, the red cell count remains at about this level until puberty. Hemoglobin values at birth have a mean of 21.5 gm per 100 ml, with a wide range of 18 to 27 gm. Hemoglobin falls to 15.5 gm at one month and 13.0 gm at three months. It then remains just below 12 gm until the age of two. The mean hematocrit begins at 56 per

their wide range, none of these three measurements is reliable for the diagnosis of anemia during infancy. Even the combination of a hematocrit and a hemoglobin level may fail to show a severe iron deficiency anemia[6]. Of greater value in the diagnosis of iron deficiency is the calculation of the three corpuscular indices: mean corpuscular volume (MCV); mean corpuscular hemoglobin (MCH); and mean corpuscular hematocrit (MCHC).

CORPUSCULAR INDICES

The mean red cell diameter is at life's highest level at life's earliest moments (Fig. 2). The newborn has a red cell diameter of 8.6 μ. The adult level of 7.5 μ is not reached until the end of the

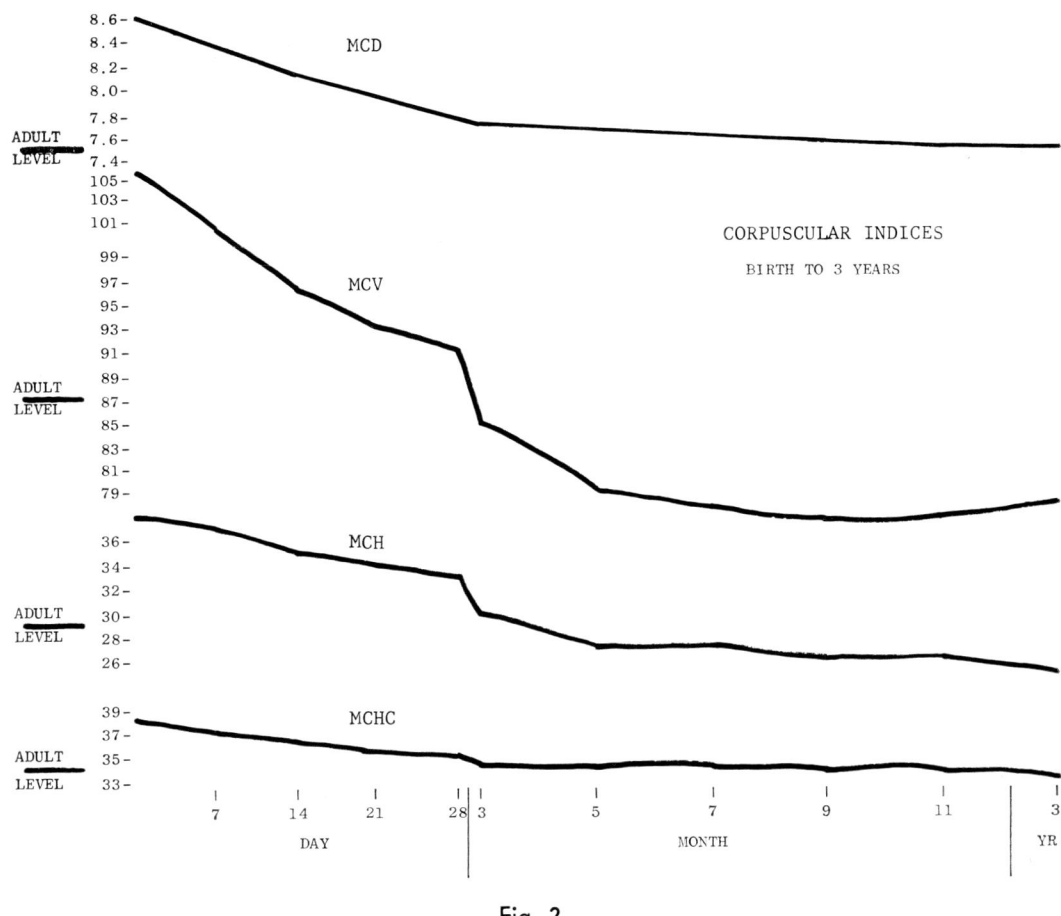

Fig. 2.

first year. The mean corpuscular volume begins high above adult levels at 106 cuμ at three months drops below the adult level of 87, and reaches a low of 77 cuμ near the end of the first year. Adult levels are not again attained until puberty. The mean corpuscular hemoglobin curve begins at 38 $\mu\mu$g, drops to 30 at three months, and levels off between 25 and 27 $\mu\mu$g from the fifth month through the tenth year. The mean corpuscular hemoglobin concentration drops from an initial 38 per cent to be the earliest index to approach the adult value of 34 per cent at three months of age.

PLATELET, LEUKOCYTE AND RETICULOCYTE COUNTS (FIG. 3, TABLE II)

The platelet count is the normal adult value at birth. It rises during the neonatal period to an average of 350,000 per cumm throughout infancy and childhood. The range of platelet counts at different ages reported by different workers and methods is great. The total leukocyte count is high at birth. Within the first twelve hours the count rises from 18,000 per cumm to almost 23,000. It returns to its original level at twenty-four hours of age and then falls abruptly to a mean of 12,000 at one week. During

TABLE II LEUKOCYTE VALUES* (10^3/cu mm; % OF TOTAL LEUKOCYTES)

Age	Total Leukocytes	Neutrophils			Eosinophiles	Basophiles	Lymphocytes	Monocytes
		Total	Band	Segmented				
Birth	18.1(9.0-30.0)	11.0(6.0-26.0)	1.65	9.4	0.4 (0.02-0.85)	0.1 (0.0-0.64)	5.5(2.0-11.0)	1.05(0.4 -3.1)
%	100	61(40-80)	9.1	52	2.2	0.6	31	5.8
12 hr	22.8(13.0-38.0)	15.5(6.0-28.0)	2.33	13.2	0.45(0.02-0.95)	0.1 (0.0-0.50)	5.5(2.0-11.0)	1.20(0.4 -3.6)
%	100	68(40-80)	10.2	58	2.0	0.4	24	5.3
24 hr	18.9(9.4-34.0)	11.5(5.0-21.0)	1.75	9.8	0.45(0.05-1.00)	0.10(0.0-0.30)	5.8(2.0-11.5)	1.10(0.20-3.1)
%	100	61(40-75)	9.2	52	2.4	0.5	31	5.8
1 wk	12.0(5.0-21.0)	5.5(1.5-10.0)	0.83	4.7	0.50(0.07-1.10)	0.05(0.0-0.25)	5.0(2.0-17.0)	1.10(0.30-2.7)
%	100	45(25-65)	6.8	39	4.1	0.4	41	9.1
4 wk	10.8(5.0-19.5)	3.8(1.0- 9.0)	0.49	3.3	0.30(0.07-0.90)	0.05(0.0-0.20)	6.0(2.5-16.5)	0.70(0.15-2.0?)
%	100	35	4.5	30	2.8	0.5	56	6.5
6 mo	11.9(6.0-17.5)	3.8(1.0- 8.5)	0.45	3.3	0.30(0.07-0.75)	0.05(0.0-0.20)	7.3(4.0-13.5)	0.58(0.10-1.3?)
%	100	32	3.8	28	2.5	0.4	61	4.8
12 mo	11.4(6.0-17.5)	3.5(1.5- 8.5)	0.35	3.2	0.30(0.05-0.70)	0.05(0.0-0.20)	7.0(4.0-10.5)	0.55(0.05-1.1?)
%	100	31	3.1	28	2.6	0.4	61	4.8
2 yr	10.6(6.0-17.0)	3.5(1.5- 8.5)	0.32	3.2	0.28(0.04-0.65)	0.05(0.0-0.20)	6.3(3.0- 9.5)	0.53(0.05-1.0?)
%	100	33	3.0	30	2.6	0.5	59	5.0

*Modified from *Handbook of Biological Data*, Table 263*.

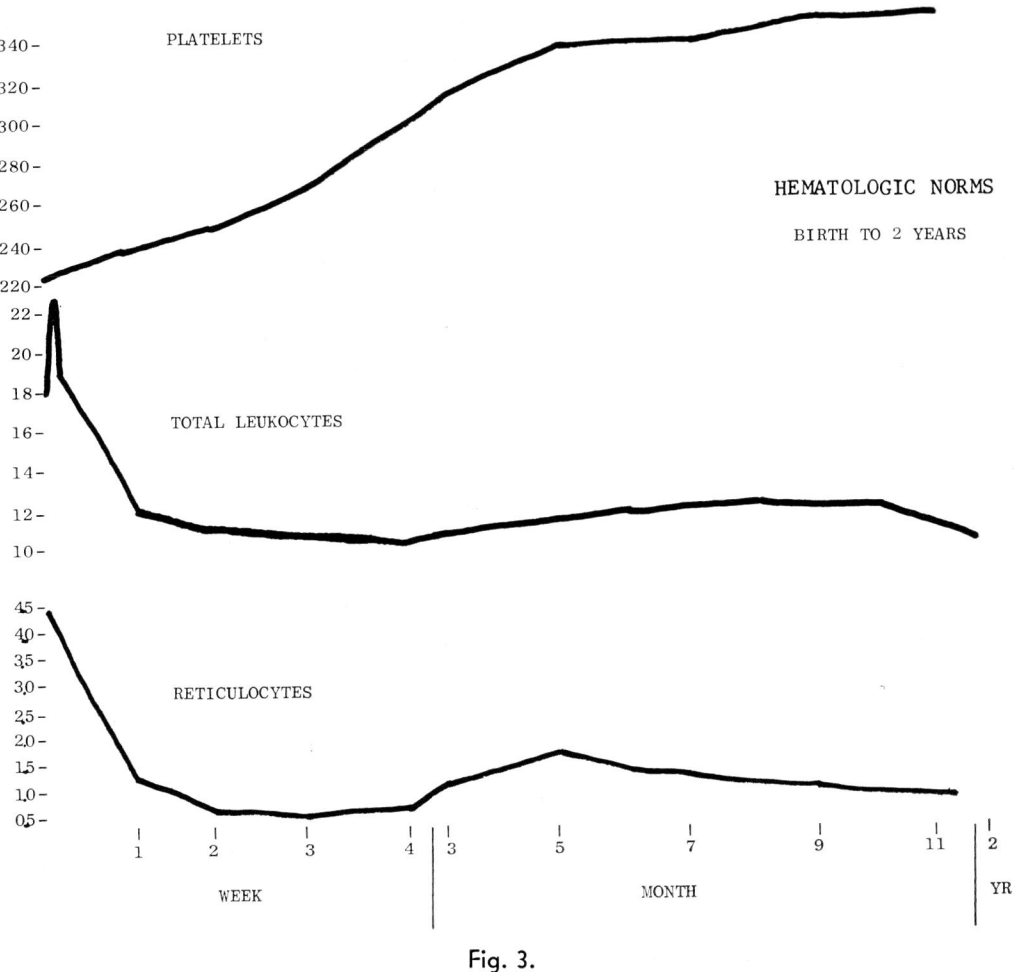

Fig. 3.

the first twelve months counts vary between 5,000 and 20,000, but retain a mean of 11,000 to 12,000 per cumm. During the first six months at least, there is no apparent rhythm to the fluctuation of the leukocyte count which might be attributable to time of day, age, activity or feeding[7]. The neonatal leukocytosis is characterized by neutrophilia up to about 70 per cent. With a drop in the leukocyte count at the first week the neutrophils decrease to 45 per cent, and from then through the fourth year of life, both the absolute and the relative numbers of granulocytes are less than lymphocytes. During the first two weeks of life there is a shift to the left of granulocytes, and monocytes are more numerous than at any other time in childhood. The reticulocyte percentage is almost 4.5 per cent at birth but decreases abruptly to 0.5 per cent or less from the second day to the sixth or eighth week. Reticulocytes again reach a peak at the end of the fourth month, before leveling off at about 1 per cent at the end of the first year. These figures indicate that the rate of production of red cells between the first and fifth to sixth weeks is too low for maintenance of the red cell volume in the presence of an increasing plasma volume.

It is easy to accept the variability of hematologic norms in an organism growing as rapidly as an infant. It is less easy to find parameters by which to measure what is normal or optimal. Zuelzer[18] has colorfully expressed the hemodynamic problem: "Unlike the adult who . . . needs to manufacture new red corpuscles only to the extent of replacing physiologic breakdown at the rate of about 1 per cent per day, the infant, like Alice in Wonderland, must run as fast as he can merely to stay in the same place. In other words, the infantile organism must keep the hemoglobin concentration per unit volume approximately constant while tripling the total blood volume in the first year of life."

BLOOD VOLUME (TABLE III)

Term infants

The average blood volume of normal term infants is given by Brines et al.[3] as 250 to 300 ml. Nomograms have been devised[3] for the prediction of normal plasma and total blood volumes on the basis of height, weight and surface area. Correlations based on weight or surface area are not as dependable as those based on height. Until a height of 130 cm, or the age of puberty, there is no sex difference in blood and plasma volumes.

Several other studies[5, 11, 13, 14] support the average values given by Brines et al. However, the interpretation of any single value in an individual as normal or abnormal is subject to considerable error since the averages are based upon widely scattered individual values. Even the average values fluctuate considerably with time. In one study[14] the mean blood volume of normal full-term infants was 283 ml (87.9 ml/kg) between birth and one hour of age, and 345 ml (107.1 ml/kg) between three and five hours of age. At the sixth day[13] the mean blood volume is 344 ml (110.0 ml/kg), following which there is a gradual drop in the volume: weight ratio until at 14 weeks it is 74 to 83 ml/kg. The mean volume at the end of the first year is

TABLE III   NORMAL VALUES OF NEWBORN

	Birth	One Week
Blood pressure, mm Hg	80/40	92/50
Bleeding time, min (Duke)	(1.5-2.5)	
Clotting time, normal plasma, min	4	4
Clotting time, platelet free plasma, min	5	7
Prothrombin time, venous, % normal	76(37-100)	86(69-100) (5th day)
Volume, blood,* % body wt	9.4(7.2-12.8)	9.6(8-13.8) (3rd day)
Volume, blood,† % body wt	12.2(8-14.9)	12.1(8.2-16.2) (3rd day)
Sedimentation rate,‡, mm/hr	0-2	3–13(12 days–14 yr)

*Early clamped cord.
†Late clamped cord.
‡From Sunderman & Boerner[17].

85.6 ml/kg. Sisson *et al.*[13] have written: ". . . . the assumption of a "normal" blood volume for any infant during the first year is illogical. In addition to the remarkable group variability, blood volume does not remain at nearly as stable a level individually from month to month as it does in the adult."

Blood volume studies have been performed by both the Evans Blue and I[131] labeled human serum albumin methods. Good correlation of results in the newborn may be expected if the blood sample is withdrawn from the infant not more than five minutes after injection of the isotope[9]. With the Evans blue technique the sample may be withdrawn at the usual ten-minute interval after dye injection since it is not eliminated so rapidly from the intra-vascular compartment.

Premature infants

The total blood volume of prematures shows the same variability in mean values as seen in full-term infants[15]. At fifty-two weeks the mean volume is about 10 ml/kg less than that of the term infant.

THE ASSESSMENT OF ANEMIA IN THE FIRST YEAR

There is no relationship between the hemoglobin concentration or the hematocrit and the blood volume. The interpretation of both the hemoglobin and hematocrit values is based on an assumption of "normal" blood volume which cannot be expected during the first year of life. Sisson *et al.*[13] have found 20 per cent of infants to be hypo- or hypervolemic during this period. Therefore, other parameters are necessary to assess anemia in infancy. Two

measurements have been recommended[13], the total hemoglobin mass (gm/kg) and the total red cell volume (ml/kg). The minimal levels for these values in infants of four to fifty-two weeks are 8.0 gm hemoglobin per kg, and 20.0 ml red blood cells per kg. Since more than half the body iron at birth is present as circulating hemoglobin[2] the most reliable estimates of the presence or degree of anemia may be made through these determinations.

There is an unresolved controversy in the pediatric literature concerning the need or desirability of supplementary iron administration in infancy. There is disagreement over the daily iron requirement of full-term infants[12], and evidence has been presented[1, 6, 10] which indicates no reduction has occurred in the incidence of iron deficiency anemias since the introduction of iron-enriched cereals in 1932-1939. Others[4, 16] do not necessarily share the concern for the creation of a "legacy" of hemochromatosis for internists and geriatricians, but there is general agreement that a hemoglobin concentration of 15 gm/100 ml of blood is not necessary for well-being.

REFERENCES

1. Beal, V. A., Meyers, A. J., and McCammon, R. W.: Iron intake, hemoglobin, and physical growth during the first two years of life. J. Pediat., 30:518-539, 1962.
2. Bothwell, T. H., and Finch, C. A.: Iron Metabolism, Boston, Little, 1962, pp. 302-310.
3. Brines, J. K., Gibson, J. G., 2nd, and Kunkel, P.: The blood volume in normal infants and children. J. Pediat., 18:447, 1941.
4. Diamond, L. K.: Letter to the editor. J. Pediat., 31:343-344, 1963.
5. Fashena, G. J., Bates, H. H., and Reid, A. F.: Changes in blood volume in the neonatal period. Amer. J. Dis. Child., 80:510-511, 1950.
6. Guest, G. M., and Brown, E. W.: Erythrocytes and hemoglobin of the blood in infancy

and childhood. III. Factors in variability, statistical studies. A.M.A. J. Dis. Child., **93**: 486-509, 1957.

7. Guest, G. M., Brown, E. W., and Lahey, M. E.: Normal blood values in infancy and childhood. Pediat. Clin. N. Amer. Philadelphia, Saunders, May, 1957, pp. 357-369.

8. Handbook of Biological Data (Ed. by W. S. Spector). Philadelphia, Saunders, 1956.

9. Jegier, W., MacLaurin, J., Blankenship, W., and Lind, J.: Comparative study of blood volume estimation in the newborn infant using I^{131} labeled human serum albumin (ISHA) and T-1824. Scand. J. Clin. Lab. Invest., **16**:125-132, 1964.

10. Lahey, M. E.: Iron deficiency anemia. Pediat. Clin. N. Amer. Philadelphia, Saunders, May, 1957, pp. 481-496.

11. Low, J. A., Kerr, N. D., and Cochon, A. R.: Plasma and blood volume of the normal newborn infant and patterns of adjustment in initial 24 hours of the neonatal period. Amer. J. Obstet. Gynec., **86**:886-892, 1963.

12. Schulman, I.: Iron needs in infancy. J. Pediat., 30:516-517, 1962.

13. Sisson, T. R. C., Lund, C. J., Whalen, L. E., and Telek, A.: The blood volume of infants. I. The full-term infant in the first year of life. J. Pediat., **55**:163-179, 1959.

14. Sisson, T. R. C., and Whalen, L. E.: The blood volume of infants. III. Alterations in the first hours after birth. J. Pediat., **56**:43-47, 1960.

15. Sisson, T. R. C., Whalen, L. E., and Talek, A.: The blood volumes of infants. II. The premature infant during the first year of life. J. Pediat., **55**:430-446, 1959.

16. Smith, N. J., Thatcher, L. G., and Desposito, F. T.: Letter to editor. J. Pediat., **31**:344, 1963.

17. Sunderman, F. W., and Boerner, F.: Normal Values in Clinical Medicine. Philadelphia, Saunders, 1950.

18. Zuelzer, W. W.: Diagnostic principles in pediatric pathology. Pediat. Clin. N. Amer. Philadelphia, Saunders, May, 1957, p. 349.

Chapter 29

Normal Values for Urinalysis in Infancy

HELEN M. FREE, B.S., ALFRED H. FREE, Ph.D., AND
JOSEPH C. SHERRICK, M.D.

There is comparatively little recorded in the literature regarding the results of routine urinalysis procedures in infants. Schaffer[9], in *Diseases of the Newborn*, states, when discussing the value of laboratory tests on newborns, that urine is "not examined as promptly or frequently as it should be." The purpose of this chapter is to present data on results of routine tests and to mention briefly some of the less routine analyses on the urine of infants. For this discussion, examples of routine tests are specific gravity, glucose, total reducing substances, pH, protein, ketone bodies, occult blood, bilirubin and microscopic examination of urine sediment.

During the past few years, urines from more than 400 infants have been tested in our laboratories. Comparisons have been made of observations on the urine of premature and full-term infants. In this discussion, the words, "full term," "newborn" and "term" will be used interchangeably, whereas "premature" will refer to an infant whose birth weight is 2500 gm or less.

SPECIFIC GRAVITY

Throughout all studies, specific gravity was determined with the TS Meter or Goldberg Refractometer. A comparison of results on 67 specimens from prematures with 297 specimens from newborns is shown in Table I.

TABLE I SPECIFIC GRAVITY OF URINE SPECIMENS FROM PREMATURE AND FULL-TERM INFANTS*

Specific Gravity Range	Premature (67 specimens)	Full Term (2 to 4 days old) (297 specimens)
1.005 or less	53	69
1.006 to 1.010	19	24
1.011 to 1.015	9	5
1.016 to 1.020	18	2
1.021 to 1.025	1	0.3
Mean	1.008	1.005

*Numbers represent percentage of total specimens in each column representing each specific gravity range.

It is of interest to note that the great majority of specimens were of specific gravity of 1.005 or less. Seventy per cent of the specimens from premature infants had a specific gravity of 1.010 or less, and 90 per cent of the specimens from newborns fell into this category. It is of interest to note that only two specimens (one in each series) had a specific gravity of more than 1.020. The totally liquid diet of the infant and the expected limitations of the infant kidney contribute to the low specific gravity of these urines. In the newborn series, all specimens were collected between 1 and 7 AM, and infants were two, three or four days old at the time of urine collection.

GLUCOSE AND TOTAL REDUCING SUBSTANCES

All specimens were tested for glucose with one of the "dip-and-read" enzyme test strips. These enzyme tests are specific for glucose but more sensitive than the copper reduction tablet test. The enzyme preparations are so sensitive that they react positively with as little as 0.003 per cent (w/v) glucose in water; their sensitivity in urine is approximately 0.1 per cent. It follows from this that the enzymatic glucose tests are more sensitive in dilute urines than in concentrated urines. This explains the apparent disagreement between the enzyme test and the copper reduction tablet test on 173 specimens from newborn infants shown in Table II. There were sixteen urine speci-

mens which showed a positive enzyme reaction but a negative copper reduction test. These contained small amounts of glucose (less than ¼%). There were twenty specimens which contained ¼ per cent or more total reducing substances which reacted with the tablet test but not with the glucose-specific enzyme test. None of these specimens contained galactose, but this is the type of reaction one would expect with a galactose-containing specimen. Thin-layer chromatography, according to the method of Baron and Economidis[1], was performed on some of these urines and indicated that the reducing substance was lactose. In cases where the concentration of sugar was high enough, the presence of lactose was also confirmed by osazone formation.

The thin-layer chromatography method of Baron using microscope slides in Coplin staining jars is rapid for presumptive identification of sugars, but effective separation of glucose and galactose was not obtained in our laboratory.

TABLE II ENZYMATIC GLUCOSE TEST COMPARED WITH COPPER REDUCTION TEST ON URINE OF NEWBORN INFANTS*

		Copper Reduction Tablet Test	
		Number Negative	Number Positive
Enzymatic Test	Number negative	136	20
	Number positive	16	1

*173 specimens.

TABLE III COMPARISON OF GLUCOSE EXCRETION BY PREMATURE AND FULL-TERM INFANTS

Glucose Result	130 Specimens from Premature Infants (% of total)	297 Specimens from Full-Term Infants (% of total)
Negative	75	93
Less than ¼%	20	6
¼%	5	1

Table III compares the glucose excretion pattern of premature and full-term infants. Glucose in small amounts was found in 25 per cent of specimens from premature infants but in only 7 per cent of the specimens from term infants. These data tend to support the concept proposed by McCance[7] that glomerular filtration is quite rapid in the newborn but that tubular reabsorption is less efficient. Calcagno[3] considers renal function in the young infant to vary quantitatively rather than qualitatively from the renal function of the adult. He reports that the glomerular filtration rate in young infants is 25 to 50 per cent of that of adults and that maximal rate of tubular reabsorption of glucose is only 20 to 35 per cent of the adult range. These typical figures indicate that infants should not be considered simply as miniature adults. The glucose excretion pattern shown in Table III indicates that reabsorption is less in the premature than in the full-term infant.

Table IV indicates that urine from infants appears as likely to contain trace amounts of non-glucose reducing substances as has been reported for adults[4]. The tabulation indicates only 59 negative reactions with Benedict's (which reacts with reducing subtances equivalent to about 1/10% glucose), whereas there were 152 negative reactions with the copper reduction tablet (which reacts with reducing substances equiv-

alent to about 1/4% glucose). In a program to detect galactosuria by concurrent testing with glucose-specific enzyme tests and a copper reduction test, it must be remembered that; (a) non-glucose non-galactose reducing substances may frequently appear in the urine of newborn infants in trace amounts; and (b) the intensity of the enzyme test reaction should not be used to estimate the amount of glucose present.

Other investigators have reported small series of urine specimens showing positive enzyme glucose tests[8] and positive sugars with refined paper chromatography techniques[2].

pH

Measurement of pH was performed as part of one of the combination "dip-and-read" tests. A comparison of pH results on specimens from prematures and from full-term infants is shown in Table V. In both series, the greatest number of urines have a pH of 6. With the series from premature infants, however, the trend is toward the alkaline side. There seems to be no explanation for this trend.

TABLE IV COMPARISON OF BENEDICT'S QUALITATIVE TEST AND COPPER REDUCTION TABLET TEST ON URINES FROM 195 NEWBORNS*

Benedict's Qualtitative		Copper Reduction Tablet	
Reaction	Number of Specimens	Reaction	Number of Specimens
Negative	59	Negative	152
Trace (approximately 1/10%)	85		
1+ (approximately ¼%)	20	¼%	20
2+ (approximately ½%)	7	½%	1
Insufficient quantity of urine	22	Insufficient quantity of urine	24

*Number of urine specimens giving designated reaction.

TABLE V COMPARISON OF pH RESULTS ON 130 URINE SPECIMENS FROM PREMATURE AND 297 SPECIMENS FROM FULL-TERM INFANTS[*]

pH	Prematures (130 specimens)	Full-Term (297 specimens)
5	14	21
6	48	71
7	26	7
8	10	1
9	2	0

[*]Numbers represent percentage of each series.

PROTEIN

Colorimetric protein testing was also done as part of one of the combination "dip-and-read" tests. In Table VI is

TABLE VI URINE PROTEIN EXCRETION OF PREMATURE AND FULL-TERM INFANTS[*]

Protein Result	130 Specimens from Premature Infants	297 Specimens from Full-Term Infants
Negative	45	50
30 mg or less per 100 cc	47	49
100 mg or more per 100 cc	8	1

[*]Numbers represent percentage of each series.

given a comparison of the protein excretion pattern of premature and full-term infants. Both series appear to show about the same type of pattern with the premature infants having an increased incidence of higher protein excretion. In view of the discussion in the glucose section, this is to be expected since the kidneys of the premature infant seem less effective than those of full-term infants. Similar protein excretion reflects the glomerular immaturity of both premature and full-term infants, whereas the greater incid-

ence of glucose excretion in prematures reflects their greater inability to reabsorb.

KETONE BODIES

Of 297 urine specimens from new-borns, 20 gave a slight positive reaction for ketone bodies with the "dip-and-read" nitroprusside test. Some of these reactions could have been caused by inadequate food intake for the short period prior to urine collection.

OCCULT BLOOD

In a series of 195 specimens from new-borns, occult blood testing in the form of a chemical orthotolidine reagent strip test gave reactions tabulated in Table VII. In twenty-nine specimens

TABLE VII OCCULT BLOOD REACTIONS ON 195 URINE SPECIMENS FROM NEWBORN INFANTS[*]

Negative	157
Small	5
Moderate	3
Large	1
Positive after circumcision	29

[*]Number of specimens giving designated reaction.

which gave positive reactions, recent circumcision doubtless was a contributing factor. Seven of the remaining nine positives were obtained on specimens from female infants and could have been due to the menstruation-like vaginal discharge observed in some newborn females. In addition, accidental cord blood contamination during application of the plastic urine collection bag to the infant is a possibility. Of particular interest is the urine specimen from a Negro male infant which gave a "large" occult blood reaction. With such a strong positive chemical test and a specific gravity of 1.016, it was odd that not a single red blood cell or ghost cell could be found with careful examination of the urine sediment. Therefore, the specimen was subjected to myoglobin-hemoglobin immuno-diffusion identification studies. Results indicated that the urine contained a large amount of myoglobin, the source of which was unexplained. The baby was reported to be doing well when discharged from the hospital.

BILIRUBIN

The diazo tablet test results for urine bilirubin on specimens from 287 newborns are shown in Table VIII. There

TABLE VIII DIAZO TABLET TEST
REACTIONS FOR BILIRUBIN ON 287
URINE SPECIMENS FROM NEWBORN
INFANTS*

Negative	247
Trace	26
Small	13
Large	1

*Number of specimens giving designated reaction.

were several trace reactions, as might have been expected. The somewhat stronger reactions were considered by the attending physicians to be due to physiologic jaundice which disappeared without treatment.

MICROSCOPIC EXAMINATION OF URINE SEDIMENT

To prepare urine sediment for microscopic examination, 2 ml of well-mixed urine were placed in a graduated centrifuge tube and centrifuged at 2000

rpm for five minutes. The supernatant was withdrawn to a volume of 0.1 ml and the sediment was re-suspended in this volume. This produces a sediment equivalent to a twenty fold concentration of urine. Appropriate calculations were made in those few cases where smaller volumes of urine were used or where the field was so obscured with this concentration of sediment that it had to be diluted with more of the supernatant. In each examination, 0.02 ml of sediment was placed under a 22 x 22 mm cover glass, and a high-power field magnification of 400x was used. With this system, using previously published calculation[6], multiplying "cells/hpf" by 12,000 gives "approximate number of cells per cc of uncentrifuged urine." Five or ten widely scattered high-power fields from each sediment were examined. This is admittedly not the usual "routine" procedure, but measurement of the volumes of urine and sediment gives more meaning to the number obtained per high-power field.

Table IX presents the average number of cells per high-power field counted

TABLE IX AVERAGE NUMBER OF CELLS
COUNTED PER HIGH POWER FIELD OF
URINE SEDIMENT FROM 286 NEWBORN
INFANTS*

Cells/hpf	RBC†	WBC	Epithelial
None	237	192	146
Less than 5	21	87	81
5-10	3	5	15
11-20	1	2	41
More than 20	1	0	3

*Numbers represent number of urine sediments giving designated results.

†Not included in this tabulation are 23 urines obtained after circumsion which contained red blood cells.

in sediments obtained from urine specimens from 286 newborn infants. Results have been arbitrarily grouped into several categories for summarization. It is obvious that many urines contain epithelial and white blood cells where urines are collected in plastic pediatric urine collectors with no special precautions beyond the normal nursery care given at diaper change.

Other elements of the sediment were not counted, but estimated as few, many, loaded, etc. A summary of the incidence of the important elements of the sediment in this series is shown in Table X. Half of the urines contained

TABLE X SUMMARY OF THE INCIDENCE OF FORMED ELEMENTS IN THE SEDIMENT OF URINE*

Element	Number of Times Found	% of Series
Bacteria	157	56
Epithelial cells	140	49
WBC's	94	33
Uric acid crystals	40	14
RBC's	26†	10
Casts, hyaline	6	3
granular	1	
Oxalate crystals	5	2

*Specimens obtained from 286 newborn infants.
†26 out of 263 since the positive urines from circumcized males are not included.

bacteria; no attempt was made to identify these organisms. The incidence is much higher than that reported by Rhodes *et al.*[8], who found only a few bacteria in 100 fields of sediment from three urines of their series of sixty-seven infants. The incidence of white blood cells in his series (9%) is also much lower.

Most uric acid-containing sediments showed many very large crystals.

SODIUM CHLORIDE

Chloride concentration of the urine was determined by a modification of the Fantus method[5]. To ten drops of urine and one drop of 20 per cent potassium chromate in a test tube, 2.9 per cent $AgNO_3$ is added dropwise until the red silver chromate color persists. Each drop of silver nitrate is equivalent to a urine chloride concentration of 0.1 per cent expressed as sodium chloride. Chloride concentrations of 267 urine specimens from newborns are listed in Table XI. The low chloride

TABLE XI CHLORIDE ESTIMATIONS ON 267 URINE SPECIMENS FROM NEWBORN INFANTS

Chloride Concentrations (as % NaCl)	Number of Urine Specimens Giving Designated Value
Less than 0.1%	113
0.1 to 0.2%	107
0.2 to 0.3%	39
0.3 to 0.4%	5
0.4 to 0.5%	1
0.5 to 0.6%	2

concentrations correlate well with the low specific gravity of urine specimens from newborn infants.

SUMMARY

Data on routine tests have been presented on 130 urine specimens from premature infants and on 297 specimens collected from full-term infants two to four days after birth. Tabulations of results include such routine tests as specific gravity, pH, sugar, protein, occult blood, ketone bodies, bilirubin and microscopic examination of urine sediment. These data have been collected over the past five years and comprise one of the largest known series of infant urine specimens tested with recent methods.

REFERENCES

1. Baron, D. N., and Economidis, J.: Thin-layer chromatography for amino-acids and sugars. J. Clin. Path., 16:484-486, 1963.
2. Bickel, H.: Mellituria, a paper chromatographic study. J. Pediat., 59:641-656, 1961.
3. Calcagno, P. L.: Clinical aspects of renal physiology. In Nelson, W. E.: Textbook of Pediatrics, Philadelphia, Saunders, 8th ed., 1964, pp. 1083-1088.
4. Cook, M. H., Free, A. H., and Giordano, A. S.: The accuracy of urine sugar tests. Amer. J. Med. Techn., 19:283-290, 1953.
5. Fantus, B.: Fluid postoperatively. JAMA, 107: 14-17, 1936.
6. Free, H. M., Free, A. H., and Giordano, A. S.: Studies with a simple test for the detection of occult blood in urine. J. Urol., 75:743-752, 1956.
7. McCance, R. A.: Renal function in early life. Physiol. Rev., 28:331-348, 1948.
8. Rhodes, E. L., Hammel, C. L., and Berman, L. B.: Urinary constituents of the newborn infant. J. Pediat., 60:18-23, 1962.
9. Schaffer, A. J.: Diseases of the Newborn. Philadelphia, Saunders, 2nd ed., 1965, p. 8.

Chapter 30

Normal Values in Clinical Chemistry in Infancy

ROBERT E. ZIPF, M.D., AND RICHARD S. WEGRYN, M.D.

In this chapter are presented, chronologically, normal values in clinical chemistry in premature infants, newborn infants and infants up to the age of two years.

By definition, a premature infant is a live-born infant weighing 2500 gm (5 lb, 8 oz) or less at birth. This definition, in common use, has many inconsistences. Drillein[1] studied the growth of premature infants over a period of five years and noted that 25 to 73 per cent required special care. The IQ was under 100 in 90 per cent. Physical defects, behavior problems and difficulty in training are a few of the medical difficulties described.

The normal values in clinical chemistry are variable, depending upon the degree of prematurity and the ability of the premature infant to accommodate to extrauterine life. The normal values in clinical chemistry in the premature infant appear to be rather consistent, although not agreed upon by all investigators. The values also vary with the chemical methods and techniques.

The newborn infant is well supplied with body water in that the extracellular compartment may constitute up to 35 per cent of body weight. During the first few days of life, there is a loss of excess fluid, which, in the absence of substantial oral intake, generally averages 6 per cent of body weight and may occasionally exceed 10 per cent. When the water loss is excessive, there may be so-called dehydration or inanition changes. Metabolism of the newborn infant favors the aerobic glycolytic pathway so that he is more intolerant to anoxia than the older infant or adult. This relative intolerance to anoxia is one of the characteristics of the newborn, and if oxygenation of the newborn infant does not establish quickly, there may be rapidly developing metabolic acidosis, owing to the accumulation of lactic acid, and respiratory acidosis, owing to a rapid accumulation of carbonic acid.

PREMATURITY

The concentration of carbon dioxide is lower at birth and rises slightly during the first four days of life. Normal values are: serum from venous blood, 20.3 to 31.5 mEq per liter; whole venous blood, 18.0 to 27.0 mEq per liter; arterial blood, 15.5 to 20.5 mEq per liter. Oxygen saturation of venous blood in the infant is 60 to 85 per cent; in the newborn it is 30 to 80 per cent. The oxygen capacity of whole blood is 19 to 22 volumes per cent.[2]

The compilation of work reported by Silverman[3] and Nelson[2] gives some of the readily available normal values (Table I).

TABLE I NORMAL VALUES IN CLINICAL CHEMISTRY IN THE PREMATURE INFANT

Plasma Constituent	Mean
pH	7.3-7.4
Total CO_2 (mEq/liter)	19-21
pCO_2 (mm Hg)	36-37
Protein base binding power (mEq/liter)	11.7-12.8
Chloride (mEq/liter)	100-104
Sodium (mEq/liter)	134-138
Potassium (mEq/liter)	5.4-6.4
Urea (mg/100 ml)	16-22
Total protein (mg/100 ml)	4.8-5.3
Albumin (plasma) (gm/100 ml)	2.9-4.2
Globulin (gm/100 ml)	0.56-1.45

The levels of reducing substances (glucose) have been measured in the blood of newborn infants since 1911. Although an extensive literature exists, there is still disagreement over which levels of blood glucose are normal in the neonate and which are hypoglycemic or hyperglycemic. Much of this confusion results from differences in techniques in collecting, precipitating and analyzing the glucose as well as the duration of fasting before sampling. Most authors agree that the blood glucose in full-term infants tends to decrease during the first few hours of life and only reach levels that would be in the range of the normal adult by one or two weeks of age. During this time, it is not unusual to find levels considered to be hypoglycemic by adult standards. Cornblath and Reisner[4] reported the levels tend to be even lower in premature infants and in infants of diabetic mothers. Measurements of

blood glucose in normal infants revealed that 95 per cent of the determinations exceeded 30 mg per 100 ml in the full-term infant, and 98.4 per cent of the determinations exceeded 20 mg per 100 ml in premature infants. It is apparent that premature infants have significantly less blood glucose at the first hours of life[5, 6] (Table II). In

TABLE II NORMAL VALUES IN CLINICAL CHEMISTRY IN THE PREMATURE INFANT

Day	Blood Glucose Mean	(mg/100 ml) (SD)
1	44.9	± 14.7
2	53.3	± 13.0
3	55.3	± 16.2
4	59.8	± 15.8
5	59.8	± 16.4
6	58.5	± 11.0
7	63.0	± 13.8
8	63.1	± 14.5
9	65.7	± 14.7
10	65.0	± 14.4
11	70.6	± 19.9
12	65.0	± 11.3
13	62.9	± 15.4
14	63.9	± 13.6

the low birth weight neonate, hypoglycemia may be defined as levels of blood glucose below 20 mg per 100 ml. In the full-size infant, blood glucose levels less than 30 mg per 100 ml in the first forty-eight hours of life, and less than 40 to 50 mg per 100 ml thereafter, may be considered hypoglycemic. Many times, there are clear-cut signs and symptoms of hypoglycemia. On the other hand, transiently low levels of glucose without obvious symptoms have been observed in infants of diabetic mothers and in premature infants. Whether or not these levels of glucose without clinical manifestations produce brain damage remains to be elucidated.

NEWBORN INFANT

Under the present-day concept, the enzymes are providing more and more information to the clinician, and the technical methods are less sophisticated and now may be done in many clinical laboratories by routine techniques. Table III shows the enzymes and nor-

for all age groups. The values of LD, ALD and MD in all age groups were higher than those found in adults. The ICD value was high up to one year of age. The most important specific enzymes of striated muscle are myokinase, myosin and creatine phosphokinase. Vassella et al.[10] reported normal

TABLE III Normal Values in Clinical Chemistry Cord Blood
and Infant

Enzymes	Cord Blood (Karmen units)	1 mo-2 yrs (Karmen units)
Aldolase (ALD)	7.5 ± 15.0	3.5- 8.0
Amylase (Somogyi units)		70-20
Copper oxidase (Ravin) ceruloplasmin (O.D. units)	0.14 - 0.57	
Creatinine kinase (CK)0-15 yrs.		3.8
Glutamic oxalacetic transaminase (GOT)	32.0 ± 17.0	24.0-41.0
Glutamic pyruvic transaminase (GPT)	15.0 ± 8.0	13.0-26.0
Glutathione reductase (GR)	39 ± 15	33-77
Isocitric dehydrogenase (ICD)	8.1 + 30	4-7.6
Lactic dehydrogenase (LD)	360 ± 60	215-360
Malic dehydrogenase (MD)	110 ± 25	63-94
Phosphatase (serum alkaline), B.L.B. units	5-15	
Phosphohexoses isomerase (PHI)	105 ± 35	43-95

mal values reported in Karmen units, arranged side by side, in cord blood and infants from one month to two years[6].

The determination of glucose-6-phosphate dehydrogenase yields a normal adult range of 150 to 210 units per 100 ml of red blood cells. Patients with glucose-6-phosphate dehydrogenase deficiency have less than 10 units per 100 ml of red blood cells[7].

Serum enzyme levels have been studied extensively in adults[8, 9]. It is apparent that the enzyme values in diseases of children can be interpreted only with knowledge of the normal levels in the age groups in question. The enzymes (see Table III) GPT and GR were within the normal adult range

values and values in neurological and muscular disorders in children.

Oski and Naiman[11] found no significant difference between red cell reduced glutathione content of the term and premature infants, although both groups had significantly more glutathione than the adult red cell. The mean concentration of red cell glutathione in the premature infant was 89.9 ± 16.9 mg per 100 ml red blood cells; while that of term infants was 89.7 ± 12.5 mg per 100 ml, and the adults 78.8 ± 8.7 mg per 100 ml[11].

It can be noted (Table IVA) that there are only minor differences between premature and full-term infants, except for the albumin, which is relatively higher in the full-term infant[12].

The electrophoretic fractionation of serum protein in infants and children are given in Table IVB[13]. Sunderman

TABLE IVA NORMAL VALUES IN CLINICAL CHEMISTRY IN THE NEWBORN INFANT

Constituent	gm/100 ml
Total protein (from nitrogen)	6.5-7.5
Total protein (from plasma)	5.11-5.70
Albumin (plasma)	3.76-3.79
Globulin	1.34-1.66
γ-globulin	0.7-1.2
Fibrinogen (plasma)	0.2-0.4
Mucoprotein protein (serum)	0.045-0.105
Mucoprotein tyrosine (serum)	0.002-0.0045
Uric acid (serum)	2.0-6.0

and Johnson[13] have reported diminished mean concentrations of total proteins, albumin and γ-globulins during the first year of life, and increased mean concentrations of α-globulins in the second to fourth years of life.[7] The α-globulin fraction carries alkaline phosphatase, lipoproteins, mucoproteins, thyroproteins, pseudoglobulins, C-reactive proteins and complement endpiece. The α_2-globulin is somewhat elevated at birth

and falls to a normal level during the subsequent six months. The β-globulin may also be slightly elevated at birth. This fraction carries lipoproteins, fibrinolysin, isohemagluttins, phospholipids, cholesterol, prothrombin and complement midpiece. Concentrations of γ-globulin at birth are higher than the maternal level, owing to the passive transfer from the maternal circulation. During the ensuing two months, γ-globulin falls to a very low level, and, after two months, the infant is capable of producing γ-globulin, and the serum level gradually rises to reach normal childhood level by about the second year of life.

Amino acid nitrogen values for cord sera ranged from 2.3 to 12.0 mg per 100 ml, with a mean of 7.68 mg per 100 ml[14]. The amino acid values for infants and children, aged six weeks to eleven years, was 3.0 to 7.5 mg per 100 ml, and the mean was 5.01 mg per 100 ml found in this group.

There has been little work done in support of normal values of specific amino acids. As early as 1941, Levine et al.[15]

TABLE IVB ELECTROPHORETIC FRACTIONATIONS OF SERUM PROTEINS IN NORMAL INFANTS AND CHILDREN[13]*

Age Group	No.	Protein Concentrations (gm per 100 ml) (mean ± SD)				
		Total Protein	Albumin	α-Globulin	β-Globulin	γ-Globulin
1st and 2nd months	6	7.03 ± 0.36‡	4.05 ± 0.20‡	0.93 ± 0.12	0.72 ± 0.16	1.32 ± 0.19
3rd to 5th months	6	5.68 ± 0.51§	3.70 ± 0.31§	0.78 ± 0.14	0.55 ± 0.10§	0.65 ± 0.10§
6th to 12th months	6	6.42 ± 0.33§	3.77 ± 0.30§	0.97 ± 0.12†	0.78 ± 0.10	0.90 ± 0.12§
2nd year	6	7.30 ± 0.57	4.09 ± 0.42	1.03 ± 0.18†	0.78 ± 0.14	1.40 ± 0.11
3rd and 4th years	6	7.52 ± 0.47	4.02 ± 0.20§	1.20 ± 0.22§	0.80 ± 0.17	1.50 ± 0.18
5th and 6th years	18	7.28 ± 0.67	4.01 ± 0.32§	0.91 ± 0.16	0.85 ± 0.19	1.52 ± 0.26
7th to 15th years	18	7.17 ± 0.53†	4.06 ± 0.33§	0.86 ± 0.26	0.76 ± 0.30	1.49 ± 0.25
Controls	20	7.51 ± 0.37	4.33 ± 0.28	0.86 ± 0.13	0.86 ± 0.14	1.46 ± 0.23

*Probability values indicate significance of differences from mean values for controls; aged 16 to 30 yrs.
†p = <0.05.
‡p = <0.02.
§p = <0.01.

TABLE V NORMAL VALUES IN CLINICAL CHEMISTRY CONTROLS, CORD BLOOD, AND NEWBORN[*]

Amino Acid	Controls		Cord Blood		Second Day		Fifth Day		Ninth Day	
	Mean	SD	Mean	SD	Mean	SD	Mean	SD	Mean	SD
Tyrosine (Tyr)	0.97	0.39	1.16	0.98	2.50	0.30	2.77	0.91	2.32	1.01
Proline (Pro)	1.88	0.82	1.47	0.27	2.69	1.15	3.28	0.72	3.12	0.93
Lysine (Lys)	3.32	1.33	5.75	1.04	3.23	1.31	3.51	1.16	3.47	1.15
Taurine (Tau)	0.83	0.35	2.04	0.64	1.71	0.66	0.95	0.61	1.02	0.62
Threonine (Thr)	1.40	0.40	3.67	0.86	1.82	0.63	2.16	0.81	1.67	—
Glutamine (Glu)	12.05	4.29	11.81	5.09	11.30	1.70	9.75	2.75	12.53	3.13
Glutamic acid (GA)	1.32	0.96	1.33	0.74	1.79	0.97	1.49	0.55	2.09	1.29
Arginine (Arg)	1.39	0.65	1.84	0.87	1.20	0.62	—	—	1.11	—
Glycine (Gly)	1.14	0.18	1.72	0.41	2.40	0.47	1.77	0.86	1.53	0.54
Alanine (Ala)	2.26	0.69	2.55	0.28	2.75	0.44	2.96	1.05	3.48	1.69
Valine (Val)	2.60	0.37	2.25	0.29	1.54	0.49	2.63	0.88	2.89	0.55
Leucine (Leu)	1.64	0.60	1.28	0.18	0.99	0.45	1.79	0.56	1.97	0.36
Isoleucine (Iso)	1.01	0.35	0.73	0.15	0.63	0.22	0.91	0.32	1.01	0.18
Serine (Ser)	1.14	0.34	1.50	0.39	1.93	0.59	1.90	0.98	1.45	0.50
α-amino-n-butyric acid (AABA)	0.29	0.10	0.40	0.32	0.22	0.13	0.23	0.06	0.29	0.14
γ-amino-n-butyric acid (GABA)	trace	—	0.26	0.14	0.41	0.28	0.20	0.17	0.17	0.11
Methionine (Met)	0.18	0.11	0.29	0.04	0.36	0.15	0.40	0.15	0.36	0.04
Cystine (Cys)	0.50	0.29	0.79	0.05	1.15	0.24	0.94	0.25	0.74	0.23
Cysteic acid (CA)	0.10	0.04	0.17	0.09	0.24	0.14	0.20	0.13	0.16	0.14
Aspartic acid (Asp)	0.17	0.04	0.28	0.20	0.25	0.18	0.17	0.20	0.20	0.11
Citrulline (Cit)	0.41	0.15	0.38	0.24	0.47	0.18	0.39	0.17	0.26	0.14
Ornithine (Orn)	1.29	0.68	1.18	0.17	1.89	0.84	2.03	0.39	1.19	0.45
Phosphoethanolamine (PEA)	trace	—	0.22	0.13	0.17	0.15	0.17	0.11	0.13	0.02
Histidine (His)	1.60	0.19	1.82	1.08	1.41	0.63	1.33	0.99	1.27	0.34
Phenylalanine (Phe)	0.88	0.39	0.92	0.19	0.89	0.87	1.15	0.91	1.16	0.34

[*]Mean (mg/100 ml) and standard deviation of free amino acids of plasma.

in a study on metabolites of tyrosine in the urine, indicated that the concentration of at least this amino acid in early life may differ greatly from values established for children and adults. Ghadini and Pecora[16] (Table V) established by quantitation techniques the concentrations of free amino acids during the first two weeks of life. Since biochemical changes occur prior to birth and may be influenced by prenatal conditions, the related cord blood and maternal blood were studied. The range of variations of the concentrations of free amino acids was small between the cord-blood, full-term and premature groups. The premature group showed a wide range for most amino acids. Tyrosine especially was noted to increase up to the fifty-seventh day of life. Many other free amino acids, such as lysine, taurine and threonine, decreased to base-line values of infancy.

The calcium level (Table VI) depends upon the amount of protein present and the kind of milk fed to the infant. When cow's milk is provided, the concentration of calcium tends to be higher. At birth, the total lipid and lipoprotein concentrations are low. The mean concentration of cholesterol is reported to be 66 mg, per 100 ml; phospholipids, 105 mg per 100 ml; and triglyceride, 33 mg per 100 ml. The

TABLE VI NORMAL VALUES IN
CLINICAL CHEMISTRY NEWBORN AND
INFANT

Constituent	mg/100 ml
Bilirubin (direct)	1.0 or more
Bilirubin (indirect)	0.0-0.3
Calcium	10-12
Cholesterol (total)	50-100
Creatine — creatinine	5-8
Galactose	25-35
Iron (serum)	<80
Lead	0.001-0.003
Lipids (total)	170-450
Non-protein nitrogen	25-40
Phospholipid (lipid P x 25) (plasma)	75-170
Total amino acid	4.3-7.7
Triglyceride	33.0
Urea nitrogen (blood)	8-25
Free fatty acid (μg/liter)	230-380

values for premature infants do not differ from those of full-term. The cholesterol-phospholipid ratio in the newborn is 0.63; in adults the ratio is 0.9[17]. This ratio in the newborn is probably due to the changes in lipoprotein distribution and composition[18]. There is a relative increase in the concentration of α-lipoproteins to that of β-lipoproteins when the values of cord blood are compared with the values in the adult. In adults, the cholesterol-phospholipid ratio in β-lipoproteins is greater than 1.0, whereas in cord blood it is less than 1.0. Gyorgy and Rose et al.[19] showed that the type of formula received by a child influenced the concentration of serum cholesterol; the mean values extended from 95 mg per 100 ml at two weeks to 163 mg per 100 ml at twenty-one to twenty-five weeks. The serum levels of lipoprotein were influenced greatly by the diet. After approximately six days, the concentrations of total lipids approach adult values. The levels of free fatty acid are low at birth and are comparable to the values found in

adults when carbohydrates are metabolized. The plasma unesterified fatty acids (UFA) were 0.27 μEq per ml in the newborn. The UFA plasma level rose rapidly within two hours of birth[20]. Shortly after birth, within six hours, the free fatty acids rise slowly and approaching levels. In the premature infant, the free fatty acids rise solwly and approach the levels of a full-term infant within three to four weeks.

TABLE VII NORMAL VALUES IN
CLINICAL CHEMISTRY IN INFANCY

	mEq/liter
Base (Na + K + Ca + Mg)(serum) (Sunderman et al.)	143-150
Bicarbonate cation binding power (serum)	19.0-30.0
Bicarbonate (standard) (serum)	21.0-25.0
Calcium (serum)	5-6
Calcium (ionized Ca)	2.5-3.0
Chlorides (Cl)	98-106
Magnesium (serum)	1.65-2.5
Phosphorus (inorganic as P)	2.3-3.8
Potassium (serum)	4.1-5.6
Serum protein cation binding power (serum)	15.5-18.0
Sodium (serum)	136-143
Sulfates (inorganic as SO_4) (serum)	0.5-1.0

The total base (Table VII) consisting of sodium, potassium, calcium and magnesium in serum are 143 to 150 mEq/liter as reported by Sunderman[21]. Magnesium sulfate has been employed recently[22] in the treatment of newborns suspected of having hyaline membrane disease. Reportedly, there is poor absorption of this salt from the intestinal tract, but marked increases in serum magnesium have been observed following the use of magnesium sulfate enemas.

Serum chlorides at birth and during early infancy are 6.0 to 10.0 mEq per liter higher than in the older infant[2].

Serum inorganic phosphorus is also higher in infants and in newborn, and an increased level up to 5.0 mEq per liter is considered normal.

Bruch and Weintraub[23] and Widdowson and McCance[24] showed that the concentration of serum calcium decreases after birth. The calcium levels then depend upon the formula fed the baby. In breast-fed infants, the phosphorus falls again, but a cow's milk formula results in an increases in serum phosphorus. The serum calcium is likely to be lower in bottle-fed babies and may fall sufficiently to produce tetany[25].

Protein-bound iodine levels in premature newborns average less than the term newborn; both term newborn and premature levels are below corresponding maternal values at delivery. The thyroxine-binding protein level in premature infants is less than maternal levels, but above the nonpregnant levels. *In vitro* uptake of radioactive triiodothyronine is low in maternal blood, indicating high unsaturated thyroxine-binding protein and indirectly confirming low free thyroxine levels in the mother. T_3-uptake percentages in premature infants are at high normal levels. Mean values for protein-bound iodine in micrograms per 100 milliliters are 3 to 8 in the infant and 6.2 ± 1.3 in cord blood. At two and five days post-delivery, the mean values are 9.3 ± 1.82 and 8.1 ± 1.9, respectively. Russel, Rose and Starr[26] further showed the thyroid-binding globulin in micrograms per 100 millilters to be 29.1 ± 8.1 in cord blood, 26.3 ± 7.67 two days post-delivery and 24.0 ± 6.96 five days post-delivery. The T_3 uptake(per cent labelled $T_3{}^{131}$) was 7.3 per cent in maternal blood, 13.1 per cent in cord blood, 16.4 per cent

two days post-delivery, and 15.9 per cent five days post-delivery. Marks and Man[27] showed that full-term neonates have the highest circulating thyroxine-like iodine concentrations observed during the life span of human (7.2 to 15.2 μg per 100 ml). Elevated butanol-extractable iodine (BEI) concentrations have occurred in neonates over 2500 gm birth weight who required transfusions. Low BEI measurements are noted in some (10%) neonates under 2000 gm birth weight. Perry, Hodgman and Starr[28] showed that the protein-bound iodine (PBI) in cord blood in the smallest infants (less than 1500 gm) was lower than the mother or in infants weighing greater than 1500 gm. The initial rise in the first forty-eight hours and then a gradual fall has been established for premature infants as well as full-term infants. The magnitude of rise was less in the smallest premature infants.

Studies of blood androgens measured as 17-ketosteroids, in newborn premature infants, demonstrated unusually high values in half the cases[29] and normal adult female levels (25 to 125 μg per 100 ml in the others[30]) (Table VIII).

TABLE VIII NORMAL VALUES IN CLINICAL CHEMISTRY IN INFANCY

	mg/100 ml
Acetone bodies (as acetone) (serum)	1-6
α-ketoglutaric acid (blood)	8-10
Amino acid nitrogen	3.5-5.5
Ammonia	0.1-0.3
Bromide (serum)	0.0007-0.001
Cholesterol	70-125
Cholesterol esters	125-180
Citric acid (plasma)	1.6-2.7
Lactic acid	10-20
Lipids, total (2-14 yr) (serum)	490-1000
Protein-bound iodine (serum)	0.003-0.008
17-hydroxycorticosteroids (plasma)	0.01-0.013

The highest values occurred in the first three days of life and detectable levels of blood 17-ketosteroids persisted for five weeks or longer[31]. In contrast, full-term infants demonstrated adult blood levels at birth, but very low or undetectable levels at five days of age.

The normal values for serum ascorbic acid, copper, vitamin A and blood thiamine are given in Table IX.

TABLE IX NORMAL VALUES IN CLINICAL CHEMISTRY IN INFANCY

Ascorbic acid (serum) mg/100 ml	0.4-1.5
Copper (serum) mg/100 ml	0.08-0.235
Vitamin A, (serum μg/100 ml	16-60
Thiamine (blood) μg/100 ml	5.5-9.5

REFERENCES

1. Drillien, C. M.: The incidence of mental and physical handicaps in school-age children of very low birth weight. Pediatrics, **27**:452, 1961.
2. Nelson, W. E.: Textbook of Pediatrics. Philadelphia, Saunders, 8th ed., 1964.
3. Silverman, W. A.: Dunham's Premature Infants. New York, Hoeber, 3rd ed., 1961, p. 543.
4. Cornblath, M., and Reisner, S. H.: Current concepts: Blood glucose in the neonate and its clinical significance. New Eng. J. Med., **273**:378, 1965.
5. Norval, M. A.: Blood sugar values in premature infants. J. Pediat., **36**:177, 1950.
6. Emanuel, B., West, M., and Zimmerman, H. J.: Serum enzymes in disease. XII. Transaminases, glycolytic and oxidative enzymes in normal infants and children. Amer. J. Dis. Child., **105**:261, 1963.
7. Hsia, D. Y.: Inborn Errors of Metabolism. Chicago, Year Book, 1959, p. 332.
8. Lapan, B., and Friedman, M. M. P.: A comparative study of fetal and maternal serum enzyme levels. J. Lab. Clin. Med., **54**:417, 1959.
9. Glendening, M. B., Cohen, A. M., and Page, E. W.: Influence of pyridoxine on transaminase activity of human placenta, maternal and fetal blood. Proc. Soc. Exp. Biol. Med., **90**:25, 1955.
10. Vasella, F., Richterich, R., and Rossi, E.:

11. Oski, F. A., and Naiman, J. L.: Red cell metabolism in premature infants. I. Adenosine triphosphate levels, adenosine triphosphate stability, and glucose consumption. Pediatrics, **36**:104, 1965.
12. Metcoff, J., and Stare, F. J.: The physiologic and clinical significance of plasma proteins and protein metabolites, New Eng. J. Med., **236**:26, 1947.
13. Sunderman, F. W. Jr., and Johnson, M. W.: Studies of the serum proteins: VII. Sucrose gradient electrophoresis. Amer. J. Clin. Path. (in press).
14. Andrews, B. F., Bruton, O. C., and deBaare, L.: Serum amino acid nitrogen in infancy and childhood. J. Pediat., **60**:201, 1962.
15. Levine, S. Z., Gordon, H. H., and Marples, E.: A defect in the metabolism of tyrosine and phenylalanine in premature infants. II. Spontaneous occurrence and eradication by vitamin C. J. Clin. Invest., **20**:209, 1941.
16. Ghadimi, H., and Pecora, P.: Plasma amino acids after birth. Pediatrics, **34**:182, 1964.
17. Jakovcic, S.: Lipid metabolism in the developing fetus and the newborn. Pediat. Clin. N. Amer., **12**:585, 1965.
18. Russ, E. M., Eder, H. A., and Barr, D. P.: Protein-lipid relationships in human plasma. III. In pregnancy and the newborn. J. Clin. Invest., **23**:1662, 1954.
19. Gyorgy, P., Rose, C. S., and Chu, E. H.: Serum cholesterol and lipoproteins in premature infants. Amer. J. Dis. Child., **106**:165, 1965.
20. Van Duyne, C. M., and Havel, R. J.: Plasma unesterified fatty acid concentration in fetal and neonatal life. Proc. Soc. Exp. Biol. Med., **102**:599, 1959.
21. Sunderman, F. W.: Measurement of serum total base. Amer. J. Clin. Path., **15**:219, 1945.
22. Stowens, D.: Hyaline membrane disease, Morbid anatomy, hypothesis of its pathogenesis, and suggested method of treatment. Amer. J. Clin. Path., **44**:259, 1965.
23. Bruck, E., and Weintraub, D. H.: Serum calcium and phosphorus in premature and full-term infants. A longitudinal study in the first three weeks of life. Amer. J. Dis. Child., **90**:653, 1955.
24. Widdowson, E. M., and McCance, R. A.: The effect of food and growth on the metabolism of phosphorus in the newly born. Acta Paediat., **48**:383, 1959.

The diagnostic value of serum creatine kinase in neuromuscular and muscular disease. Pediatrics, **35**:322, 1965.

25. Gardner, L. I., MacLachlan, E. A., Pick, W., Terry, M. L., and Butler, A. M.: Etiologic factors in tetany of newly born infants. Pediatrics, 5:228, 1950.

26. Russell, K. P., Rose, H., and Starr, P.: Further observations on thyroxine interactions in the newborn at delivery and in the immediate neonatal period. Amer. J. Obstet. Gynec., 90:682, 1964.

27. Marks, A. N., and Man, E. B.: Serum butanol-extractable iodine concentrations in prematures. Pediatrics, 35:753, 1965.

28. Perry, R. E., Hodgman, J. E., and Starr, P.: Maternal, cord, and serial venous blood. Protein-bound iodine, thyroid-binding globulin, thyroid-binding albumin, and prealbumin values in premature infants. Pediatrics, 35:759, 1965.

29. Green, O. C.: Steroid metabolism in the fetus and the newborn infant. Pediat. Clin. N. Amer., 12:615, 1965.

30. Davidsohn, I., and Wells, B. B.: Todd-Sanford Clinical Diagnosis by Laboratory Methods. Philadelphia, Saunders, 13th ed., 1963, p. 945.

31. Gardner, L. I., and Walton, R. L.: Plasma 17-ketosteroids of full-term and premature infants. J. Clin. Invest., 33:1642, 1954.

Chapter 31

Recent Advances In Microtechniques In Clinical Chemistry

BERNARD J. KATCHMAN, Ph.D.

The principal reason for the application of micro- or ultramicrotechniques in clinical chemistry is the limited availability of blood or tissue samples for the requisite diagnostic procedures that arise in certain clinical situations.

The factors which determine the amount of sample necessary for analysis are the concentration of the material sought in the sample and the sensitivity of the assay system. From a theoretical point of view, the simplest approach to achieve micro- or ultramicro conditions is to "scale-down" each step of the procedure. For example, if 1 ml of base is required to neutralize 1 ml of acid, then $1 \mu l$ of base is required to neutralize $1 \mu l$ of acid; however, the problems which arise by the application of such a "scaled-down" procedure place certain limitations on theory and necessitate radical changes in laboratory equipment, techniques and the quality of laboratory personnel engaged in micro and ultramicro laboratory analysis. From the practical standpoint, the simplest approach is to "scale-down" only sample size and to increase the sensitivity of the assay to conform with the decrease in sample size. Under these conditions, only the initial sample taken for analysis need be in the micro- or ultramicro range, and the requirement for micropipettes and microtechnique is limited. The subsequent analysis may be performed with glassware, pipettes and equipment usually available in the contemporary clinical laboratory.

CLASSIFICATION

The definition of a microtechnique in clinical chemistry, at least as defined by Meites and Faulkner, is at best artificial and at worst confusing. The factor which actually determines whether a technique to be applied is macro, micro, or ultramicro is the amount of substance sought in a specimen presented for analysis. Although the authors recognize this fact, they then decide to classify upon the basis of the volume of the sample without regard to the concentration of the material sought. Their classification is shown in Table I. While there is a certain

TABLE I SCALE OF MEASUREMENT IN CLINICAL CHEMISTRY

Classification	ml	$\mu l, \lambda$
Macro	0.5-2.0	500-2000
Semimicro	0.1-0.5	100- 500
Micro	0.025-0.1	25- 100
Ultramicro	0.005-0.025	5- 25

semantic simplicity to this classification, it is superficial and should be recognized as such.

In the data presented in this chapter, all the methods are micro or ultramicro, based upon the amount of substance sought in the sample used for analysis; a micromethod is indicative of sensitivity of the assay in the microgram range or microliter sample size range.

BLOOD CARBOHYDRATES

A variety of techniques is available for the microanalysis of blood carbohydrates[1, 26, 29, 31, 51, 55, 64]. This variety is shown in Table II.

Blood alcohol can be determined with as little as 10 μl of capillary blood by means of an enzymatic-pyridine nucleotide coupled reaction[31]. The amount of alcohol in the sample is equivalent to the amount of pyridine nucleotide reduced in the alcohol dehydrogenase catalyzed reaction. The concentration of reduced pyridine nucleotide is measured by reading the absorbancy at 340 mμ in a spectrophotometer. Blood lactate is determined in 20 μl of sample by oxidation of the lactate to aldehyde, which combines with semi-carbazide reagent, and the absorbancy is read in a spectrophoto-

meter[51]. A micromethod for the determination of blood pyruvate is based upon the Fredemann and Haugen method[64]. Serum protein carbohydrate (as hexose) is determined upon 100 μl of serum by means of the color produced in a stabilized resorcinol-sulfuric acid solution[55]. In order to accomplish an oral D-xylose test in infants and children that would permit sequential sampling of blood, a micromethod was developed[29]. The protein, from a 100 μl sample of capillary blood, is precipitated, and the supernatant then reacted

TABLE II BLOOD CARBOHYDRATES

Sample Size ($\mu l, \gamma$)	Tissue	Material Sought	Technique	Ref.
10-150	blood	alcohol	spectrophotometry titrimetry	26, 31
50	blood, urine	acetone bodies	colorimetry	1
20	blood	lactic acid	spectrophotometry	51
100	blood	pyruvic acid	colorimetry	64
100	serum	protein-bound carbohydrate	colorimetry	55
100	blood	D-xylose	spectrophotometry	29

with a 5 per cent solution of p-bromoaniline and heated for ten minutes at 70 C; and the color which develops is read in a spectrophotometer at 520 mμ. Acetone, acetoacetic acid and β-hydroxybutyric acid may be determined simultaneously with 50 μl of capillary blood or urine[1]. Free acetone is separated by diffusion, taken up in an alkaline furfural solution and analyzed colorimetrically. Acetoacetic and β-hydroxybutyric acids are converted to acetone and determined as such.

BLOOD ENZYMES

Most, if not all, blood enzymes may be assayed by techniques that require 100 μl or less of serum or whole blood.

TABLE III   BLOOD ENZYMES

Sample Size (μl, γ)	Tissue	Material Sought	Technique	Ref.
100	serum	alkaline phosphatase	colorimetry	2
100	blood	fibrinolytic activity	colorimetry	9
100	serum	phosphohexose isomerase	colorimetry	17
100	blood	lipoprotein lipase	titrimetry	34

Although only four methods[2, 9, 17, 34] are listed in Table III, these are but a representative few of all the enzyme methods which have been catologued in Bergmeyer's *Methods in Enzymatic Analysis*. The details for sample collection, sample preparation, reagents and instrumental analyses are given in this work. In addition to normal values, the values obtained in various diseased states are listed, and the appropriate conversion factors are presented so that the values obtained by various investigators may be equated.

PROTEINS

Microtechniques[5, 16, 19, 44, 47, 49, 65] are available for the determination of certain proteins in serum and cerebrospinal fluid, as shown in Table IV.

Human serum albumin may be determined with as little as 5 μl of serum by reacting it with vasoflavin in alkaline media[5]. This is a rapid and specific test for albumin. A rapid determination of γ-globulin in a 200 μl sample of serum is effected after the specific precipitation of all serum proteins except γ-globulin by a 0.2 per cent rivanol solution and subsequent determination of the tryptophan content of the supernatant with the Hopkins-Cole reagent[49]. Total protein and γ-globulin can be determined with 300 μl of CSF[19]. CSF is treated with alcoholic zinc sulfate in barbital buffer and the γ-globulin is precipitated. The total protein and γ-globulin content are determined colorimetrically. Prothrombin, proconvertin[44, 47, 65] and thermocoagulable fibrinogen[16] can be determined by clotting time techniques with between 50 to 100 μl of blood or plasma.

HEMOGLOBIN METABOLISM

Techniques for the evaluation of several parameters of hemoglobin metabolism are listed in Table V[30, 33, 50,]

TABLE IV   PROTEINS

Sample Size (μl, γ)	Tissue	Material Sought	Technique	Ref.
5	serum	albumin	spectrophotometry	5
200	serum	γ-globulin	colorimetry	49
50-300	blood, plasma	prothrombin, proconvertin	clotting time	44, 47
300	CSF	γ-globulin and total protein	colorimetry	19
100	blood	thermocoagulable fibrinogen	clotting time	16

TABLE V HEMOGLOBIN METABOLISM

Sample Size ($\mu l, \gamma$)	Tissue	Material Sought	Technique	Ref.
25	plasma	total and direct bilirubin	colorimetry	58
200	serum	free, mono and diglucuronide bilirubins	colorimetry	59
Micro-hematocrit	blood	O_2-Hb	spectrophotometry	33
100-200	serum	unsaturated iron binding	radioisotope	30, 62
200	serum	iron and iron binding capacity	colorimetry	50

[58, 59, 62]. Total and direct bilirubin can be determined with 25 μl of plasma[58], while three separate bilirubin fractions designated as free, mono- and diglucuronide bilirubins require only 200 μl of serum[59]. The oxygen saturation of hemoglobin may be determined rapidly from a microhematocrit and reflectance spectrophotometry[33]. The unsaturated iron-binding capacity of serum can be determined with 100 μl samples and the use of Fe[59, 30, 62]. Iron and iron-binding capacity are determined colorimetrically on 200 μl of serum[50].

LIPID METABOLISM

Micromethods[8, 12, 13, 14, 22, 28, 36, 39, 40, 41, 57] for the determination of total cholesterol, free fatty acids, lipids, phospholipids and triglycerides in serum of humans are listed in Table VI. In addition, micromethods are presented for serum lipoproteins,[53] fecal fat[54], cholesterol, cholesterol esters and phospho-

TABLE VI LIPID METABOLISM

Sample Size ($\mu l, \gamma$)	Tissue	Material Sought	Technique	Ref.
60-500	plasma	free fatty acids	colorimetry titrimetry	12, 14 28, 39
15	serum	lipids and total fatty acids	colorimetry	41
5-20	serum	total cholesterol, lipid phosphorus	colorimetry	36, 57
400	serum	triglycerides, cholesterol, phospholipids	colorimetry	22
10-40	plasma, serum	cholesterol	colorimetry,	8, 13 40
30	serum	high and low density lipoproteins	spectrophotometry	53
1-5 mg	feces	fecal fat	turbidimetry	54
2000	CSF	cholesterol, cholesterol ester, phospholipids	colorimetry	56
2000	plasma, tissue	total and polyenoic fatty acids	titrimetry	38

lipids of cerebrospinal fluid[56] and plasma total and polyenoic fatty acids[38]. The high- and low-density lipoproteins are separated in a capillary tube by use of antiserum specific for lipoproteins of density less than 1.063 gm per ml[53]. Fecal lipid is recovered from 1 to 5 mg of fecal material impregnated and dried on glass fiber paper and assayed turbidimetrically at 650 mμ in aspectrophotometer[54]. Variations in results caused by differences in the content of fecal water circumvented by use of dry weights to express results. By means of silicic acid column chromatography cholesterol, cholesterol esters and phospholipids may be separated from as little as a 20 μg mixture of lipids[56]. The small amounts of lipids found in cerebrospinal fluid require 2 ml of CSF for analysis.

MINERAL METABOLISM

Table VII lists several methods[2, 3, 4, 6, 11, 43, 48, 60, 61, 63] for the detection of micro and ultramicro amounts of mineral elements. The specrofluorimetric analysis of calcium[61] and magnesium[60] require 10 μl and 25 μl of serum respectively. The colorimetric method for copper is

sensitive enough to measure microgram amounts in tissues. The copper complex formed with the reagent oxalydihydrazide-acetaldehyde produces an intense color with a molar extinction coefficient of 23,000 to 23,500. The very small amounts of copper usually found in blood and other tissues necessitate the use of a 1 gm sample. Chloride may be determined with as little as 20 μl of blood or blood fractions[48]. This simple and sensitive method is based upon the spectrophotometric analysis of the triiodide ion which is produced in the reaction mixture.

NITROGEN METABOLISM

Several substances of interest in nitrogen metabolism which may be analyzed by micromethods[18, 24, 27, 32, 46, 52] are tabulated in Table VIII. Blood or urinary NH_3 as the NH_4^+ ion may be detected in microgram amounts by an enzymatic spectrophotometric assay[24]. In this highly specific assay for blood NH_4^+, 1 ml of whole blood is deproteinized with 1 ml of trichloroacetic acid, and 0.4 ml of the supernatant after neutralization with sodium hydroxide is used

TABLE VII MINERAL METABOLISM

Sample Size ($\mu l, \gamma$)	Tissue	Material Sought	Technique	Ref.
50	serum, blood	phosphorus	colorimetry	2, 11
10	serum	calcium	spectrofluorimetry	61
100-200	serum	calcium	colorimetry	43, 63
25	serum	magnesium	spectrofluorimetry	60
250	serum, urine	calcium, magnesium	titrimetry	3
20, 100	serum, blood RBC, plasma	chloride	spectrophotometry titrimetry	6, 48
1000	serum, urine tissues	copper	colorimetry	4

TABLE VIII NITROGEN METABOLISM

Sample Size (μl, γ)	Tissue	Material Sought	Technique	Ref.
10	plasma	amino acids	chromatography	52
100	plasma, urine	NH_3, urea	colorimetry spectrophotometry	24, 32
10	plasma	glutamine, asparagine	colorimetry	46
200	serum	creatinine	colorimetry	27
3000	CSF	keto and amino acids	colorimetry	18

for the assay. Resting, fasting normal blood was found to contain less than 6.8 μg per 100 ml blood. Blood, plasma, urine and other tissue extracts may be analyzed for ammonia, urea and non-protein nitrogen, after appropriate sample workup, by a colorimetric assay[32]. The assay is sensitive in the microgram range and is specific for NH_4^+, in that the color which is formed in the reaction is due to the synthesis of indophenol blue; ammonia is the nucleus for the condensation of reagents that form the indophenol blue. The color is stable for twenty-four hours, and the method is reproducible to ±2 per cent. Glutamine and asparagine may be analyzed in 10 μl of plasma by means of an enzymatic-colorimetric procedure[46]. A simple micromethod for screening newborn infants for primary aminoacidopathies which requires only 10 μl of plasma is reported[52]. Whole blood is collected in heparinized microcapillary tubes, and the plasma is analyzed without prior deproteinization by one-dimensional filter-paper chromatography. Cerebrospinal fluid may be analyzed simultaneously for keto-and amino acids in microgram amounts[18]. For the analysis, 3 to 4 ml of CSF are needed.

VITAMINS AND HORMONES

Vitamins and hormones may be analyzed by a variety of microtechniques[7, 10, 20, 21, 35], as shown in Table IX. The macromethod for protein-bound iodine has been scaled down to a microprocedure with a precision equal to that for the macromethod[35]. A 10 μl capillary blood sample is taken for analysis. The blood protein is precipitated, resuspended in sodium carbonate, ashed and

TABLE IX VITAMINS AND HORMONES

Sample Size (μl, γ)	Tissue	Material Sought	Technique	Ref.
10	blood	protein-bound iodine	spectrophotometry	35
100	blood	carotene and vitamin A	microspectrophotometry	21
50,000	urine	esterone, estradiol, estriol	fluorimetry	20
150	plasma	17-hydroxycorticosteroids	spectrophotometry	7
200	plasma	bradykininogen	guinea pig ileum	10

the iodine determined colorimetrically after reaction with arsenious and ceric ions in solution. Carotene and vitamin A are analyzed in as little as 100 μl of whole blood[21]. After a preliminary fractionation of the blood, petroleum ether extracts are read in a microspectrophotometer in the 300 to 400 mμ range. Urinary estrone, estradiol and estriol in a 50 ml sample may be fractionated after acid hydrolysis by elution from an alumina column with 8 per cent sodium bicarbonate solution. The estrogens are assayed by reading the fluorescence produced after incubation in 80 per cent sulfuric acid for twenty minutes at 80 C[20]. Free 17-hydroxycorticosteroids can be assayed in 150 μl of blood plasma when the concentration is as little as 0.05 μg[7]. Methylene chloride extracts of plasma are partitioned against 0.2 N sodium hydroxide, evaporated to dryness and the residue partioned between benzene and water. The 17-hydroxycorticosteroids are removed from water with methylene chloride, and the concentration determined by reading the color produced by the Porter-Silber reagent in a spectrophotometer.

MISCELLANEOUS MATERIALS

In Table X are listed micromethods for the analysis of drugs and other materials of clinical interest[15, 23, 25, 37, 42, 45]. These materials are usually present in microgram amounts in blood or urine samples taken for analysis and, therefore, sample sizes of 1, 2 or 3 ml or gm are needed for analysis. Normal therapeutic doses of chloridazepoxide range from 10 to 30 mg, and plasma levels are conveniently analyzed by this fluorimetric technique, which is sensitive to 0.25 μg per ml of plasma when 1 ml of plasma is used for analysis[25]. Salicylate is determined in a 100 μl sample of plasma after fractionation of the free and plasma-bound salicylates on a Sephadex-25 capillary column, and subsequent analysis is done with a spectrofluorophotometer[45]. Phenyl-and tolysulfonylurea may be assayed at concentrations between 5 to 26 μg per ml of blood[23]. These substances are extracted with organic solvents at acid pH and converted to azo dyes which are measured in the spectrophotometer. The determination of total body water in children by the use of antipyrine and the dilution principle can be effected with a microtechnique which requires as little as 200 μl of serum per assay[37]. Microgram amounts of antipyrine in plasma may be determined

TABLE X MISCELLANEOUS MATERIALS

Sample Size ($\mu l, \gamma$)	Tissue	Material Sought	Technique	Ref.
100	plasma	salicylate	spectrophotometry	45
500	plasma	hippuric acid	fluorimetry	15
1000	blood	phenyl-and tolyl-sulphonyl urea	spectrophotometry	23
1000	plasma	chlordiazepoxide	fluorimetry	25
2000	urine	silica	colorimetry	42
200	plasma, serum	antipyrine, 4-amino antipyrine	colorimetry	37

from aliquots of protein-free filtrates by nitrosation of the antipyrine and coupling with N(1-naphthyl)-ethylenediamine dihydrochloride to form an azo dye. The concentration of the colored product formed in the reaction is read in a colorimeter at 592 mμ.

DISCUSSION

Most of the recent advances in micro- and ultramicrotechniques are the result of the development of more sensitive assay systems in which, for the most part, conventional laboratory equipment and glassware are utilized. In almost all of the literature of the past five years, only the sample size required for analysis has been scaled down.

Nearly all the blood enzymes of clinical significance have been determined with 100 μl of blood. If necessary, all of these procedures could be modified without too much difficulty to assay 5 to 10 μl of blood. Tissue metabolites may be assayed by means of enzymes and enzyme-pyridine nucleotide linked reactions at the 5 to 10 μl volume of sample.

Colorimetric procedures have been increased in sensitivity by use of reagents with very high molar extinction coefficients or with the use of reagents which fluoresce. The use of fluorescence spectrophotometry instead of conventional spectrophotometry may provide an increase in sensitvity of at least three orders of magnitude.

It is surprising if not disappointing that the strides made recently in instrumental analysis have had so limited an impact upon clinical chemistry. Automated system using x-ray fluorescence, emission or atomic absorption spectro-

scopy are expensive and offer little advantage as microtechniques, in the analysis of mineral elements, over conventional laboratory procedures and equipment now in use. The application of gas chromatography to clinical chemistry has not lived up to expectation.

In the years ahead one may look forward to the development of electrodes which are specific for individual mineral elements and which will operate by means of conventional pH meter assemblies.

The achievement of qualitative and quantitative analysis of biological materials for individual amino acids by gas chromatography has an excellent potential for success.

The separation and quantitation of cholesterol, cholesterol esters, lipids, phospholipids and triglycerides by means of a preliminary separation by thin-layer chromatography and gas chromatography should become a routine clinical laboratory technique.

The application of enzymes as a microchemical technique for the routine analysis of materials of clinical significance has a tremendous potential, and the development of methodology for the incorporation of these techniques into the scheme of clinical laboratory analyses will be a major advance in the future.

REFERENCES

1. Ahola, T., and Somersalo, O.: Microdetermination of acetone bodies in blood and urine. B. A., **46**:790, 1965; Ann. Med. Exp. Fenn.,**41**(3):237-246, 1963.
2. Alimova, M. M.: Micromethod for determining inorganic phosphorus and alkaline phosphatase in serum and inorganic phosphorus in urine. B. A., **46**:23601, 1965; Lab Delo, **6**:346-348, 1964.

3. Beale, R. N., and Bostrom, J. O.: Sensitive methods for the titrimetric microdetermination of biological calcium and magnesium. J. Clin. Path., 16(3):252-255, 1963.

4. Beale, R. N., and Croft, D.: The microdetermination of biological copper with oxalydehydrazide. J. Clin. Path., 17(3):260-263, 1964.

5. Betheil, J. J.: Fluorometric microdetermination of human serum albumin. Anal. Chem., 32:560-563, 1960.

6. Bohuon, C., and Leboeuf, M.: Microdetermination of plasma chloride. Path. Biol. (Paris), 9:21-22, 1961.

7. Bowman, R. E.: Micromethod for determination of free 17-hydroxycorticosteroids in plasma. Fed. Proc., 21(2): 185, 1962.

8. Bowman, R. E., and Wolf, R. C.: A rapid and specific ultramicro method for total serum cholesterol. Clin. Chem., 8(3):302-309, 1962.

9. Byshevskii, A.: Micromethod for determining the fibrinolytic activity of the blood. B. A., 46:23607, 1965; Lab. Delo, 6:340-342, 1964.

10. Diniz, C. R., Carvalho, I. F., Ryan, J., and Rocha E. Silva, M.: A micromethod for the determination of bradykininogen in blood plasma. Nature (London), 192(4808):1194-1195, 1961.

11. Doose, H.: The determination of phosphorus in very small samples of serum. Ultramicromodification of the Fiske-Subbarow method. B. A., 35:6624, 1960. Z. Ges. Exp. Med., 131(6):646-648, 1959.

12. Drysdale, J., and Billimoria, J. D.: A new micromethod for the estimation of serum total fatty acids. B. A., 40:18084, 1962; Clin. Chim. Acta, 5(6):828-833, 1960.

13. Duboff, G. S., and Stevenson, W. W.: An ultramicro method for the estimation of plasma cholesterol. Clin. Chem., 8(2):105-112, 1962.

14. Duncombe, W. G.: The calorimetric microdetermination of non-esterified fatty acids in plasma. B. A., 46:19088, 1965; Clin. Chim. Acta, 9(2):122-125, 1964.

15. Elliot, H., and Walker, III, A. A.: Fluorometric microanalysis of plasma hippuric acid and comparison of hippurate with p-aminohippurate clearances in dogs. Proc. Soc. Exp. Biol. Med., 116(2):268-270, 1934.

16. Georgescv, I., and Herzovi, F.: Micromethod for the determination of thermocoaguable fibrinogen. Pediatria (Bucur), 9(3):283-285, 1960.

17. Gromanshevskaya, L. L., and Mironova, E. M.: Micromethod for determining phospho-

hexose isomerase in serum and its clinical significance in infectious hepatitis. B. A., 46:820, 1965; Lab. Delo, 2:77-80, 1964.

18. Grundig, E.: Separation and microdetermination of keto and amino acids in CSF. B. A., 41:9853, 1963; Clin. Chim. Acta, 7(4):498-505, 1962.

19. Hanok, A.: A micromodification of a method for the measurement of globulin in cerebrospinal fluid and its application in the diagnosis of multiple sclerosis. J. Lab. Clin. Med., 57(1):42-46, 1961.

20. Honda, K.: Fluorometric microdetermination of urinary estrogens by spectrophotofluorometer. Acta Med. Biol. (Niigata), 10(4):323-344, 1963.

21. Karpacheva, V. A.: A micromethod for determination of carotene and vitamin A in whole blood. B. A., 46:37536, 1965; Biull. Eksp. Biol. Med., 58(7):120-121, 1964.

22. Kawade, M.: Microdetermination of lipids in serum, with notes on the estimation of triglycerides. B. A., 42:20776, 1963. Mie. Med. J., 11(3):399-407, 1962.

23. Kern, W.: Chemical microdetermination of phenyl-and tolylsulphonylurea derivatives in blood. Anal. Chem., 35(1):50-53, 1963.

24. Kirsten, E., Gerez, C., and Kirsten, R.: An enzymatic microdetermination of ammonia adopted for extracts of animal tissue and fluids. Determination of the ammonium ion content in blood. Biochem. Z., 337(3): 312-319, 1963.

25. Koechlin, B. A., and D'Arconte, L.: Determination of chlordiazepoxide (librium) and of a metabolite of lactam character in plasma of humans, dogs, and rats by a specific spectroëuorometric micromethod. Anal. Biochem. 5(3):195-207, 1963.

26. Krasnova, A. I., Vishnyak, Y. I., and Kamolov, S. K.: Micromethod for determining alcohol in blood. B. A., 46:830, 1965; Lab. Delo, 8(9):52-56, 1962.

27. Kuroda, N.: A portable micromethod for determining creatinine in blood serum. B. A., 42:584, 1963; Tokushima J. Exp. Med., 9 (1):67-74, 1962.

28. Kvam, D. C., Schmidt, J. G., Riggilo, D. A., and Gallo, D. G.: Colorimetric microdetermination of plasma free fatty acids. J. Pharm. Sci., 53(8):988-989, 1964.

29. Lanzkowsky, P., Lloyd, E. A., and Lahey, M. E.: The oral D-xylose test in healthy infants and children. A micromethod of blood determination. JAMA, 186(5):517-519, 1963.

30. Lee, N. E., and Chiamori, N.: A simple

radioisotopic micromethod for determination of unsaturated iron-binding capacity of serum. B. A., **41**:13388, 1963; Clin. Chim. Acta, **6**(5):624-629, 1961.

31. Leithoff, H., and Chan, S. Y.: An ultramicro method for the enzymatic determination of blood alcohol. B. A., **46**:23625, 1965; Med. Welt, **38**:2011-2015, 1964.

32. Liemann, F.: Microdetermination of ammonia, urea, and residual nitrogen by the indophenol blue reaction. B. A., **46**:5395, 1965; Z. Ges. Exp. Med., **138**(3):191-196, 1964.

33. Loewinger, E., Gordon, A., Weinreb, A., and Gross, J.: Analysis of a micromethod for transmission oximetry of whole blood. J. Appl. Physiol., **19**(6):1179-1184, 1964.

34. Lukasik, S.: Studies on the estimation of lipoprotein lipase activity. A micromethod for clinical and experimental purposes. B. A., **39**:21923, 1962; Arch. Immun. Ther. Exp., **9**(4):847-863, 1961.

35. Malkin, H. M.: An ultramicro protein-bound iodine method on capillary blood. J. Clin. Endocr., **25**(1):28-38, 1965.

36. Markova, M. N., and Pokrovskii, A. A.: Determination of total cholesterol and lipid phosphorus in a micro-drop of serum. B. A., **46**:9955, 1965; Lab Delo, **3**:145-150, 1964.

37. Mendelsohn, D., and Levin, N. W.: A colorimetric micromethod for the estimation of antipyrine in plasma or serum. B. A., **36**: 19590, 1961; S. Afr. J. Med. Sci., **25**(1): 13-18, 1960.

38. Norby, J. G.: Microdetermination of polyenoic fatty acids and total fatty acids in plasma and tissue. Acta Chem. Scand., **15** (3):525-534, 1961.

39. Novak, M.: An ultramicro method for the determination of unesterified fatty acids in blood serum. B. A., **36**:J1362, 1961; Physiol. Bohemoslov., **10**(1):98-100, 1961.

40. Novak, M., and Havlova, M.: Lipoprotein serum fraction in blood from a finger prick. Excerpta Med. **13**(1):128, 1960; Cesk. Gastroent. Vyz., **13**(2):149-152, 1959.

41. Pande, S. V., Kahn, R. P., and Venkitasubramaniam, T. A.: Microdetermination of lipids and serum total fatty acids. Anal. Biochem., **6**(5):415-423, 1963.

42. Paul, J.: Microdetermination of soluble silica in urine. Biochem. J., **77**(1):202-205, 1960.

43. Pfordte, K., and Ponsold, W.: Contribution to the analysis of the calcium of blood serum. III. Communication a micromethod for sera which contain ethylenediamine tetraacetate.

B. A., **44**:17935, 1963; Z. Ges. Exp. Med., **136**(6):543-546, 1963.

44. Phillips, G. E., Luddecke, H. F., Breuchaud, J. S., and Lenahan, J. C.: A micromethod for the determination of prothrombin activity. J. Lab. Clin. Med., **56**(4):659-664, 1960.

45. Potter, G. D., and Guy, J. L.: A micromethod for the analysis of plasma salicylate. Proc. Soc. Exp. Biol. Med., **116**(3):658-660, 1964.

46. Ramadan, M. E. A., and Greenberg, D. H.: An enzymatic micromethod for determination of glutamine and asparagine in blood. Anal. Biochem., **6**(2):144-152, 1963.

47. Reilly, E. B., Goodman, J. R., Perry, A., and Ward, B.: Microdetermination of plasma prothrombin using capillary blood. Amer. J. Clin. Path., **33**(1):92-94, 1960.

48. Rodkey, F. L., and Sendroy, Jr., J.: Microdetermination of chloride in blood, plasma, and cells by spectrophotometric analysis using solid silver iodate. Clin. Chem., **9**(6): 668-681, 1963.

49. Saiffer, A., and Gerstenfeld, S.: A photometric microdetermination of serum γ-globulin with a tryptophan reaction. Clin. Chim. Acta, **7**(2):149-152, 1962.

50. Scarlata, R. W., and Moore, E. W.: A micromethod for the determination of serum iron and serum iron-binding capacity. Clin. Chem., **8**(4):360-369, 1962.

51. Scholander, P. F., and Bradstreet, E.: Microdetermination of lactic acid in blood and tissues. J. Lab. Clin. Med., **60**(1):164-166, 1962.

52. Scriver, C. R., Davies, E., and Cullen, A. M.: Application of a simple micromethod to the screening of plasma for a variety of amino-acidopathies. Lancet, **2**(7353):230-232, 1964.

53. Searcy, R. L., and Berquist, L. M.: Microdetermination of total lipid content of high- and low-density lipoproteins. Excepta Med., **18**(5):2021, 1965; Clin. Chim. Acta 9:(2), 194-196, 1964.

54. Searcy, R. L., Dunn, J. M., Simms, N. M., and Berquist, L. M.: Microanalysis of fecal fat. Amer. J. Clin. Path., **41**(5):477-480, 1964.

55. Sexton, J. S., and Aull, J. C.: An evaluation of a microdetermination of serum protein bound carbohydrate. Amer. J. Clin. Path., **12** (3):320-323, 1964.

56. Shin, Y. S.: Silicic acid column Chromatography for the microdetermination of cholesterol, cholesterol esters and phospholipids from human cerebrospinal fluid. Anal. Biochem., **5**(5):369-377, 1963.

57. Shin, Y. S., and Lee, J. C.: Microdetermination of cholesterol and phospholipid in cerebrospinal fluid and serum by silicic acid column chromatography. Clin. Chem., 8(6): 598-606, 1962.

58. Trzaski, M., and Woytowicz, J.: Micromethod of determination of the total and direct bilirubin in plasma of newborns. B. A., 45: 99111, 1964; Pol. Tyg. Lek., 19(2):795-797, 1964.

59. Vodhailo, S. I.: Use of a simple micromethod for determining three bilirubin fractions in newborns. B. A., 46:878, 1965; Lab. Delo, 2:89-93, 1964.

60. Wallach, D., Hoelzl, F., and Perez Esamadi, M.: Fluorescence techniques in the microdetermination of metals in biological materials. III. Method for complexometric determination of magnesium in small serum samples. Anal. Biochem., 7(1):67-73, 1964.

61. Wallach, D., Hoelzl, F., and Strick, T. L.: Fluorescence techniques in microdetermination of metals in biological materials. II. An improved method for direct complexometric titration of calcium in small serum samples. Anal. Biochem., 6(2):176-180, 1963.

62. Wallenius, G., and Waschewsky, H. J.: Micromethod for determination of unsaturated iron-binding capacity of serum. B. A., 46: 23625, 1965; Acta Soc. Med. Upsal., 68 (3/4):141-146, 1963.

63. Wilkes, W. C.: A comparative study of the Clark-Collip tetrimetric and colorimetric micromethod of Trinder for the determination of calcium in blood serum. Amer. J. Med. Techn., 29(3):121-126, 1963.

64. Witkowski, S., Witkowska, F., and Filipowiezowa, J.: A micromethod for the determination of blood pyruvic acid. B. A., 41: 9248, 1963; Pol. Tyg. Lek., 16(22):828-830, 1961.

65. Yin, E. T., and Senn, H. J.: Micromethod for the determination of the combined activity of factors II and VII (prothrombin and proconvertin). B. A., 36:67088, 1961; Thromb. Diath. Haemorrh., 1959:297-301, 1959.

GENERAL REFERENCES

Bergmeyer, H. U.: Methods of Enzymatic Analysis. New York, Academic Press, 1963.

Meites, S., and Faulkner, W. R.: Manual of practical micro and general procedures in clinical chemistry. Springfield, Thomas, 1962.

Wilkinson, R. H.: Chemical micromethods in clinical medicine. Springfield, Thomas, 1960.

The Determination of Calcium in the Serum of Infants

ROBERT P. MACFATE, Ph.D.

INTRODUCTION

The procedures for the determination of calcium in biologic materials were reviewed[15] at the Seminar on *Evaluation of Thyroid and Parathyroid Functions.* The procedures especially applicable to the determination of calcium in serum were reviewed[16] at the Seminar on *Serum Electrolytes in Clinical Medicine.*

The determination of calcium in the serum of infants must necessarily be a micro- or ultramicroprocedure. Where 0.1 ml (100 μl) of serum can be obtained, some of the usual macroprocedures may be used. However, many of these procedures do not adapt well to samples of less than 100 μl. It is important, therefore, to choose a method in which variable smaller amounts, say from 20 to 100 μl of serum may be used without major changes in the procedure.

Several techniques are reviewed here briefly. These include flame photometry, atomic absorption spectrometry and x-ray spectrometry, as well as the colorimetric and complexometric procedures. The first three techniques require relatively expensive equipment. The latter two are more adaptable to the small laboratory.

EQUIPMENT FOR ULTRAMICROCHEMISTRY

The accuracy of the findings, obtained by the use of ultramicroprocedures, depends to a great extent on how precisely the samples and reagents are measured. Ultramicropipettes and -burettes are key items in successful ultramicrochemistry. A thorough knowledge and a fair amount of experience in their use is necessary.

Knights *et al.*[14] have reviewed the types of this equipment currently available. It is recommended that their paper be studied before introducing into the laboratory ultramicroprocedures or microprocedures using ultramicroequipment.

EMISSION FLAME PHOTOMETRY*

Whereas the flame photometric determinations of sodium and potassium in blood serum have been quite successful,

---

*Gilbert[12] states, in a review of fundamental developments in analysis, that flame photometry has been regarded generally as a branch of emission spectrochemistry. One of the newer techniques in the laboratory, known as atomic absorption spectrometry (or spectroscopy), has been classified with conventional flame photom-

the estimation of the calcium concentration has been more of a problem. The flame spectrophotometry of calcium requires high flame temperatures and a high photodetector sensitivity, due to the fact that the emission spectrum of calcium is relatively weak. These conditions limit the application of this technique for the determination of calcium, since the background and radiation interference is thus exaggerated. Not all commercially available flame photometers are suitable for calcium determinations.

Many ions produce a serious and rather unpredictable interference, especially such strong emitters as sodium and potassium, as well as magnesium. Phosphates and sulfates depress calcium luminosity. Proteins may interfere under certain conditions.

Many variations in procedure have been devised to overcome these interferences. The serum may be diluted with water or organic solvents and used directly. Some procedures isolate the calcium; others remove a part of the interfering materials. Internal and external standards may be used.

Few papers have been published in the past five years on the subject of emission flame photometry for the determination of serum calcium. However, many analysts have adjusted their daily procedures to an available flame photometer and do obtain satisfactory results. Some instruments have been adapted to automation[6].

If it is desired to use emission flame photometry for the microdetermination of serum calcium, it is recommended that the macroprocedure, used for the photometer that is available, be adjusted to the smaller amount of sample. Usually, about 100 μl of serum can be used, diluted 1:50. This will provide sufficient fluid for the test, although readings must be made promptly. Findings are reported to be within 1 to 4 per cent of those obtained by the Clark-Collip method[7].

ABSORPTION FLAME PHOTOMETRY (ATOMIC ABSORPTION SPECTROMETRY)*

Just ten years ago, Walsh[26] showed that the phenomenon of atomic absorption could be applied to the quantitative determination of metals. He found that the measurements of metals by atomic absorption spectrometry are more sensitive than the measurements by emission flame photometry and less subject to interference from other elements.

These findings were confirmed by Willis[29, 30], who found that atomic absorption spectrometry offered the advantages of accuracy, precision, speed of performance and small size of sample.

Zettner and Seligson[31] proposed the use of a special diluent, containing lanthanum chloride, butanol and octanol in 10 N hydrochloric acid, to abolish the effects of absorption depressors. This made it possible to measure calcium directly in diluted serum without prior removal of any serum constituent.

The calcium standard was made from

etry, although it is not emission spectroscopy. Gilbert feels that a clearer differentiation could be made by dividing analytical flame photometry into *emission flame photometry* (conventional flame photometry) and *absorption flame photometry* (atomic absorption spectrometry).

*Refer to the footnote on page 411.

calcium chloride, diluted with a solution containing calcium-free protein, sodium chloride and Sorbistat (Pfizer).

A 1:10 dilution of serum is made. Using the standard solution first to determine that the equipment is in working condition, readings can be made with as little as 1 to 2 ml of unknown dilute solution, thus requiring only from 100 to 200 μl of serum.

In a series of approximately 200 calcium determinations by the above method and by a modified Clark-Collip procedure[10], Zettner and Seligson[31] found that the mean of the Clark-Collip values was 3 per cent higher than the mean of the values obtained by atomic absorption. However, some 15 per cent of the values differed by more than 1 mg of calcium per 100 ml of serum. The authors attributed this to the shortcomings of the Clark-Collip method, claiming greater reliability for the atomic absorption technique.

Sunderman and Carroll[20] proposed the use of a protein-free filtrate of serum. The suggested procedure uses 0.5 ml of serum diluted 1:10 in 10 per cent trichloroacetic acid. The clear supernatant after centrifugation is diluted with an equal volume of strontium chloride solution. These quantities may be reduced so that the analysis may be made on 100 to 200 μl of serum. The standard calcium solution is prepared from calcium chloride diluted with a solution containing stronium chloride, sodium chloride and trichloroacetic acid.

Using the Clark-Collip method[7] for comparison, the means of replicate analyses of calcium by atomic absorption agreed with the means of replicate analyses by the Clark-Collip method

within ±2 per cent.

If the equipment is available for absorption flame photometry, it is recommended that the macroprocedure be adjusted to the use of a smaller sample, within the neighborhood of 100 μl.

X-RAY SPECTROMETRY

Natelson[18] wrote an excellent paper on this technique. In x-ray spectrometry, x-rays impinge on the sample and cause the excitation and emission of the characteristic lines of the spectrum. The rays are collimated by means of parallel nickel plates and directed to a crystal. They are then diffracted, and the selected line is directed to a detector after passing through a second collimator. The detector comprises a counting device, usually a gas-filled or scintillation counter. By rotating the crystal by an angle and the detector by twice that angle, it is possible to scan the spectrum emitted by the sample and feed the signal to a recorder to produce a tracing. When analyzing for a particular element, the detector is locked in a set position and the time required for a preset number of counts is recorded. The time found is a measure of the element concentration in the sample when compared to a curve produced from a series of suitable standards.

Extensive equipment and detailed experience are required. The equipment is expensive, generally cumbersome, and the high voltage may be a problem. In spite of these objections, the technique is most attractive. A simultaneous analysis for Na, K, Cl, Ca and Mg may be made on less than 20 μl of serum. No reagents are needed.

The clinical instrument of the near future will be smaller, possibly occupying no more space than the present recording spectrophotometer. It will probably replace the flame photometer for many of our common analyses.

COLORIMETRIC PROCEDURES

Many colorimetric methods for calcium in serum may be modified to micro- and ultramicroprocedures. Some of these, as commonly used, require only 100 μl of serum. Other methods may be adapted to smaller samples and use made of microcuvettes. The main problem is to not complicate the procedure to the point where the time consumption is too great or the possibility of technical errors too prevalent.

If 100 μl of serum is available, it is recommended that the N-hydroxynaphthalimide procedure of Trinder[22] be used[16].

If less serum than 100 μl is available, complexometric method may be used.

COMPLEXOMETRIC PROCEDURES

Many of the complexometric procedures for serum calcium may be adapted to the use of samples smaller than 100 μl. The most serious problem is the determination of the exact end point of the titrations. A secondary problem is the obtaining of pure and uniform indicators.

A review of chelation techniques[16] has shown that no one method is superior to all others in every respect. The search for the most suitable procedure to be used with ultramicrosamples has been mainly a search for a sensitive and reliable end point.

For the determination of serum calcium with variable ultramicroquantities of serum, from 10 to 100 μl, it is recom-

mended that the method of Wallach and Steck[25] be used. This is an EDTA titration using the specially prepared dye, 2,4-bis [N,N' -di (carboxymethyl) aminomethyl] fluorescein, which forms fluorescent complexes with the alkaline earth metals at alkaline pH.

A number of methods for serum calcium have been suggested using the dye mixture named Calcein[1-5, 8, 9, 11, 13, 17, 19, 21, 23, 27, 28]. Wallach *et al*[24] studied Calcein in detail to determine the nature of the changes in fluorescence occurring upon the addition of metals. They found Calcein to be composed of five chromatographically and electrophoretically distinguishable components. Attempts to isolate pure components from Calcein in good yield proved difficult. They then modified the synthesis to favor the recovery of specific products.

The dye fluoresces between pH 3 and 11 but loses this fluorescence at a pH greater than 11. However, the fluorescence will reappear at high pH on the addition of Ca, Sr and Ba, but not Mg. This fluorescence can then by quenched by EDTA. On this basis, a simple procedure for the microtitration of serum calcium has been devised[25]. (See Chapter 32B.)

BIBLIOGRAPHY

1. Andersch, M. A.: A titration method for the determination of calcium in serum using a new indicator. J. Lab. Clin. Med., 49:486-489, 1957.
2. Appleton, H. D., West, M., Mandel, M., and Sala, A. M.: The rapid determination of calcium in biologic material. Clin. Chem., **5**: 36-44, 1959.
3. Ashby, R. O., and Roberts, M.: A microdetermination of calcium in blood serum. J. Lab. Clin. Med., 49:958-961, 1957.
4. Baron, D. N., and Bell, J. L.: Compleximetric determination of calcium in pathological and

physiological specimens. J. Clin. Path., **12**: 143-148, 1959.

5. Bett, I. M., and Fraser, G. P.: A rapid micro method for determining serum calcium. Biochem. J., **68**:13$_p$, 20$_p$, 1958.

6. Bold, A. M., Hurst, R. J., and McSwiney, R. R.: Automated estimation of sodium, potassium, and calcium using the Eppendorf flame photometer. J. Clin. Path., **18**:240-243, 1965.

7. Clark, E. P., and Collip, J. B.: A study of the Tisdall method for the determination of blood serum calcium with a suggested modification. J. Biol. Chem., **63**:461-464, 1925.

8. Collidge, T. B.: A micro calcium method accurate in the presence of magnesium and phosphate. Anal. Biochem., **1**:93-95, 1960.

9. Diehl, H., and Ellingboe, J. L.: Indicator for titration of calcium in presence of magnesium using disodium dihydrogen ethylenediamine-tetraacetate. Anal. Chem., **28**:882-884, 1956.

10. Elert, B. T.: A comparative study of precipitation time and temperature factors affecting blood and urine calciums. Amer. J. Med. Techn., **20**:263-268, 1954.

11. Fingerhut, B., and Miller, H.: Direct determination of calcium in icteric serum. Clin. Chem., **9**:360-364, 1963.

12. Gilbert, P. T., Jr.: Absorption flame photometry. Anal. Chem., **34**:210R-220R, 1962.

13. Jackson, J. E., Breen, M., and Chen, C.: Fluorometric titration of calcium. J. Lab. Clin. Med., **60**:700-708, 1962.

14. Knights, E. M., Jr., Ploompuu, J., and Whitehouse, J. L.: Developments in ultramicro chemistry. Amer. J. Clin. Path., **36**:203-211, 1961.

15. MacFate, R. P.: The determination of calcium in biologic materials. In Sunderman, F. W., and Sunderman, F. W., Jr. (eds.): *Evaluation of Thyroid and Parathyroid Functions*. Philadelphia, Lippincott, 1963, pp. 180-198.

16. MacFate, R. P.: The measurement of calcium in serum. In Sunderman, F. W., and Sunderman, F. W., Jr. (eds.): *Clinical Pathology of the Serum Electrolytes*, Springfield, Ill., Thomas, 1966, pp. 37-55.

17. Mori, L.: Direct microcomplexometric analysis of calcium in biological materials. Arch. Biochem. Biophys., **83**:552-562, 1959.

18. Natleson, S.: Recent developments in x-ray spectrometry as appied to clinical chemistry. Clin. Chem., **11** *(No. 2 Supp.)*:290-308, 1965.

19. Socolar, S. J., and Salach, J. I.: Microtitration of calcium to visible end point in presence of magnesium. Anal. Chem., **31**:473-474, 1959.

20. Sunderman, F. W., Jr., and Carroll, J. E.: Measurements of serum calcium and magnesium by atomic absorption spectrometry. Amer. J. Clin. Path., **43**:302-310, 1965.

21. Toribara, T. Y., and Koval, L.: Determination of calcium in biological material. Talanta, **7**:248-252, 1961.

22. Trinder, P.: Colorimetric micro determination of calcium in serum. Analyst, **85**:889-894, 1960.

23. Tucker, B. M.: Calcein as an indicator for the titration of calcium with ethylenediamine-tetraacetate. Analyst, **82**:284-285, 1957.

24. Wallach, D. F. H., Surgenor, D. M., Soderberg, J., and Delano, E.: Preparation and properties of 3,6-dihdroxy-2,4-bis-[N,N′ -di-(carhoxymethyl)-aminomethyl] fluoran. Anal. Chem., **31**:456-460, 1959.

25. Wallach, D. F. H., and Steck, T. L.: Fluorescence techniques in microdetermination of metals in biological materials. II. An improved method for direct complexometric titration of calcium in small serum samples. Anal. Biochem., **6**:176-180, 1963.

26. Walsh, A.: The application of atomic absorption spectra to chemical analysis. Spectrochim. Acta, **7**:108-117, 1955.

27. Watson, D., and Rogers, J. A.: Serum calcium determination with 1,2-diaminocyclohexane-N-tetra-acetate. Clin. Chim. Acta, **8**: 168-169, 1963.

28. Wilkins, D. H.: Calcein Blue — a new metal-fluorechromic indicator for chelatometric titrations. Talanta, **4**:182-184, 1960.

29. Willis, J. B.: The determination of calcium in blood serum by atomic absorption spectroscopy. Nature (London), **186**:249-250, 1960.

30. Willis, J. B.: The determination of metals in blood serum by atomic absorption spectroscopy. I. Calcium. Spectrochim. Acta, **16**: 259-272, 1960.

31. Zettner, A., and Seligson, D.: Application of atomic absorption spectrophotometry in the determination of calcium in serum. Clin. Chem., **10**:869-890, 1964.

The Determination of Calcium in 10 to 100 μl of Serum

ROBERT P. MACFATE, Ph.D.

The Procedure of Wallach and Steck[1]

PRINCIPLE

This is a very sensitive EDTA titration using the specially prepared dye, 2,4-bis[N,N'-di(carboxymethyl)aminomethyl] fluorescein. It is one of the components of Calcein. Calcein itself has been used, but is not as sensitive nor as uniform chemically as the prepared dye.

The technique permits the accurate titration of from 10 to 100 μl of serum. A calcium solution is used as a standard.

Extreme care must be taken to prevent contamination with calcium.

SYNTHESIS OF THE DYE

The complete formula is (3,6-dihydroxy fluoran)-2,4-bis[N,N'-di(carboxymethyl)aminomethyl]fluoran[2].

To 6.64 gm (0.02 mole) of fluorescein (C. P., J. T. Baker Chemical Co. or the equivalent) dissolved in 20 ml of 60 per cent ethyl alcohol and 6 ml of 30 per cent NaOH are added 10.6 gm (0.08 mole) of iminodiacetic acid (C.P., Dow Chemical Co. or the equivalent) dissolved in 15 ml of H_2O and 12 ml of 30 per cent NaOH. The mixed solutions are chilled in ice water, and 7.5 gm (0.08 mole) of 37 per cent formalde-hyde (C.P., Baker or the equivalent) are added dropwise with stirring while keeping the temperature at 4 C.

The reaction mixture is warmed in a bath to 70 C and maintained at this temperature for eight hours with stirring.

The mixture is then cooled to room temperature, diluted to 1,000 ml with water, and acidified to about pH 3.5 with 3 N HCl. The copious precipitate of isoelectric compound is filtered off (S. & S. Green Ribbon Paper No. 589 or the equivalent), washed with 2,000 ml of deionized water and air-dried.

The precipitate is extracted repeatedly with 50 ml of hot 70 per cent ethyl alcohol, filtered while hot and cooled slowly. The fine yellow needles which crystallize out are filtered off, dissolved in the minimum amount of 0.01 N Na OH, reprecipitated by 1 N HCl to pH 3.5, and recrystallized three times from 70 per cent ethyl alcohol.

The final product is dried twenty-four hours at 80 C *in vacuo.* The yield will be about 3.8 gm.

REAGENTS

NOTE: Care must be taken in the preparation of all glassware, both for the final analysis and the preparation of reagents. Refer to "Apparatus," below.

1. *Deionized water.* Distilled water is passed through an efficient deionizer and used immediately.

2. *Potassium hydroxide solution, 0.7 M.* Potassium hydroxide solution (Baker's Analyzed Reagent 45 per cent solution or the equivalent) is diluted to 0.7 M according to the amount required for one week. The normality is checked by titration with standard acid. The solution is stored in a heavy-walled polyethylene bottle and is replaced weekly.

3. *Dye solution.* The dye is prepared as given above. A 0.4 mM solution is prepared by adding 26.3 mg of crystalline dye to 50 ml of deionized water in a 100 ml borosilicate volumetric flask. Enough 0.7 M potassium hydroxide is added to dissolve the dye, and deionized water is added to volume. The solution is thoroughly mixed and transferred, in approximately 10 ml amounts, to small polyethylene bottles. These are kept frozen and in the dark, where the dye keeps indefinitely. The dye is stable for at least one month when kept at 4 C, (the usual refrigerator temperature) and in the dark.

4. *Standard calcium solution.* A 4 mM solution of calcium is prepared by transferring 40 mg of calcium carbonate (Baker's Analyzed Reagent or the equivalent) to a 100 ml borosilicate volumetric flask, adding a minimal amount of 0.1 N HCl to dissolve, and diluting to volume with deionized water. The solution is stored in a polyethylene bottle.

5. *Standard EDTA solution.* Disodium ethylenediaminetetraacetate (Geigy Industrial Chemical or the equivalent)

is twice recrystallized and dried for eighteen hours at 105 C. An approximately 10 mM solution is prepared by dissolving 372 mg in 100 ml of deionized water. The solution is stored in a polyethylene bottle.

As required, the EDTA solution is diluted to approximately 2.0 mM or to 0.4 mM prior to use, depending upon the amount of calcium to be determined. The diluted solution also is kept in a polyethylene bottle.

APPARATUS

Extreme care must be taken to prevent contamination. All apparatus, glassware and polyethylene containers are prepared as follows.

Each item is individually washed in detergent, rinsed five times with distilled water, rinsed twice with 0.1 N HNO_3, five times with deionized water, twice with acetone (spectral grade) and air-dried. Care must be taken to avoid dust contamination.

All glassware must be made from borosilicate glass.

The titration burette is a micrometer burette of 2 ml capacity with a capillary tip drawn out to about 1 mm external diameter (Micrometric Instrument Co., SB2, Cleveland, Ohio, or the equivalent).

PROCEDURE

Blood is drawn with plastic disposable syringes and transferred into washed borosilicate centrifuge tubes. The tubes are capped with Parafilm and the blood allowed to clot. After one hour the tubes are centrifugalized for fifteen minutes at 3,000 x g and the serum transferred to washed polyethylene tubes. These tubes, also, are capped with Parafilm to avoid dust contamination and loss by evaporation.

The burette is rinsed twice with EDTA solution. If left unused for more than thirty minutes, it should be rinsed and again filled with fresh EDTA solution. The 2.0 mM solution of EDTA is used for the titration of 50 to 100 μl of serum. For smaller amounts, use the 0.4 mM solution.

Titrations are conducted in 10 ml borosilicate beakers placed on a dark red background and illuminated from the side with a microscope illuminator focused so as to project the filament image into the solution in the beaker.

Two ml of 0.7 M potassium hydroxide solution are added to a 10 ml borosilicate beaker, followed by 10 μl of the dye solution and 10 to 100 μl of serum or standard calcium solution. The mixture is gently swirled, avoiding bubbles and raised by a jack into the light path so that the filament image produces a series of streaks fluorescing bright green.

The burette is lowered so that the tip is just below the surface of the liquid. EDTA solution is added with a gentle circular motion until the fluorescence just disappears and is replaced by gray streaks due to serum turbidity. Some fluorescence returns after a few seconds. After waiting for three to five minutes, add more EDTA solution until the fluorescence again just disappears. Record the burette reading.

The titrations are conducted under ordinary laboratory lighting conditions, although some analysts find that a dimmed room permits greater precision.

Check the molarity of the EDTA solution by titrating against the standard calcium solution with each set of unknowns. This is necessary due to the ease with which EDTA can become contaminated with calcium.

When titrating 10 and 20 μl samples, three or four serial titrations may be carried out in a single reaction mixture without loss of accuracy. When the end point of a titration is reached, another sample of serum may be added and titration continued directly.

CALCULATIONS

1. If the EDTA solution is exactly 2.0 mM in strength, then 1 ml of the EDTA solution will react with 0.08 mg of Ca. If the EDTA solution is not exactly 2.0 mM, then the actual concentration or the Ca equivalent must be determined.

As noted above under "Procedure," the standard Ca solution is titrated. If 0.100 ml of standard Ca solution is used, 0.200 ml of EDTA solution will be required if it is exactly 2.0 mM in concentration. If any other result is obtained, calculate as follows:

$$\frac{0.200}{E} \times 0.08 = A$$

Where: 0.200 = equivalent volume of accurate 2.0 mM EDTA solution for 0.100 ml of standard Ca solution

E = actual number of ml of approximately 2 mM EDTA solution used

0.08 = mg of Ca equivalent to 1 ml of accurate 2.0 mM EDTA solution

A = mg of Ca equivalent to 1 ml of approximately 2 mM EDTA solution

2. To determine the concentration of Ca in the unknowns:

$$\frac{T \times A \times 100}{S} = \text{mg of Ca per 100 ml of serum}$$

Where: T = ml of approximately 2 mM EDTA solution used
A = factor determined in 1, above
100 = 100 ml of serum
S = ml of serum used

3. To convert mg of Ca per 100 ml to mEq per liter:

$$\frac{\text{mg per 100 ml}}{2} = \text{mEq per liter}$$

FINDINGS

There is no interference in this procedure from magnesium, phosphates and heavy metals. Added calcium is recovered quantitatively. The average standard deviation in a series of determinations using 50 μl of serum was ± 1.7 per cent. Using only 10 μl of serum, the precision is less.

REFERENCES

1. Wallach, D. F. H., and Steck, T. L.: Fluorescence techniques in micro-determination of metals in biological materials. II. An improved method for direct complexometric titration of calcium in small serum samples. Anal. Biochem., 6:176-180, 1963.
2. Wallach, D. F. H., Surgenor, D. M., Soderberg, J., and Delano, E.: Preparation and properties of 3,6-dihydroxy-2,4-bis[N,N'-di(carboxymethyl)aminomethyl] fluoran. Anal. Chem., 31:456-460, 1959.

Chapter 33

Laboratory Diagnosis of Renal Disease in Infancy

GORDON W. MELLA, M.D.

The major genitourinary diseases in infancy are infection and obstruction, accounting for almost 90 per cent of clinical problems. Obstructive lesions usually manifest infection at some time[1]. A high index of suspicion is required to alert the clinician to what otherwise might be construed as non-renal symptoms in infants. Classical symptoms are absent in 50 per cent of infants with genitourinary disease (Table I).

TABLE I

ATYPICAL PRESENTING SYMPTOMS OF GENITOURINARY TRACT DISEASE IN INFANCY

Fever
Anorexia
Lethargy
Weakness
Weight Loss or failure to gain
Vomiting
Jaundice
Diarrhea
Dehydration
Abdominal distension and paralytic ileus

Early diagnosis of renal disease in infants or children with proper management will prevent disease in future years. There is some evidence that serious adult disease such as hypertension, azotemia and toxemia of pregnancy may be prevented, and there may be a decrease in prematurity and neonatal mortality[2]. On the other hand, over-diagnosis can be dangerous to the infant. North[3] has shown that 10 per cent of children with a febrile illness had pyuria. If pyuria is used as the sole criterion of urinary infection or if a qualitative urine culture is employed, many febrile infants will be treated as if they are infected. As a result of treating a patient who has had one or two episodes of "pyuria" or insignificant bacteruria, many infants will be subjected unnecessarily to diagnostic studies, i.e., intravenous pyelogram or cystogram.

The purpose of this chapter is to present the clinical and laboratory examinations that a physician can perform in his office or a small outpatient laboratory when he cares for the infant with possible genitourinary disease. This is not to say that the physician is autonomous and does not require support from the clinical laboratory. On the contrary, it is in this field of renal disease that the practicing doctor may be brought further into the laboratory and the clinical pathologist can be brought closer to the patient.

METHODS

PHYSICAL EVALUATION

Any examination of the genitourinary system in the infant properly begins with the initial contact in the neonatal period. Sherwood[4] demonstrated that the kidneys of a newborn may be palpated with ease, and this offers a unique opportunity to evaluate their size and position. Pediatricians have also become aware that minor congenital anomalies, such as abnormally shaped ears, may point toward severe urinary tract abnormalities[5]. To date, about 50 per cent of all types of congenital anomalies are recognized during infancy[6].

Knowledge of the normal infant voiding pattern also enhances the physician's awareness of possible renal disease. The pediatrician may gain information about possible disease during "well baby" checkups by asking the parent about the urinary stream.

URINE COLLECTION

The infant presents an unusual problem in that he generally cannot void on demand, and the amount voided may be too small for the laboratory to analyze. The best urine for analysis is generally the first or second morning specimen. Such specimens offer the most uniform concentration and the most favorable pH to preserve the formed elements. Often, though, the clinical situation will not allow collection at this time, and a random sample will have to suffice.

The "clean catch" urine[7, 8] may be employed with small infants by cleansing the perineum and applying a sterile, plastic urine collector.* The technique, however, will not afford a good midstream specimen. Catheterization may be necessary. Since the infant is rather mobile, a slightly rigid catheter with an elbow bend can be used satisfactorily. Recently, the technique of suprapubic percutaneous needle aspiration of the bladder has been reported with excellent results in adults[9]. This procedure can be easily done in infants with much more ease than catheterization and offers a more reliable specimen.

Small amounts of urine for analysis are sometimes all that may be obtained, and the laboratory must be prepared to extract the maximum amount of information from a minimum volume.

The determination of the refractive index can be made on one drop of urine in order to estimate the specific gravity. Uristix** require only minute quantities for a satisfactory estimate of protein and glucose. One ml of urine may be centrifuged for microscopic examination. Gram staining requires only one drop of urine, and a culture and colony count may be made with 0.01 ml of urine. Therefore, a total volume of only 2 to 3 ml of urine will suffice for most clinical purposes.

MICROSCOPIC EXAMINATION

Observation of fresh urine under the microscope and the use of gram stain are standard procedures for most laboratories, and the techniques used with adult urines are the same as those with infant specimens.

CULTURE

Quantitative urine culture with the use of pour plates is recognized as

---

*Sterilon Corporation, Buffalo 11, N.Y.

**Ames Co., Elkhart, Indiana

being more accurate than surface streaking. However, for a busy hospital the latter procedure may serve effectively for routine purposes. The urine sample, whether collected by catheter, clean midstream or bladder aspiration, is collected in a sterile plastic cup with a sealable lid. In the office or any small laboratory, the urine is mixed, using a sterile platinum loop calibrated to deliver 0.01 ml of urine, and this amount is transferred to the center of a blood agar plate. Without flaming the loop, the drop of urine is quickly streaked evenly over the surface of the agar, and the plate is then incubated for twenty-four to forty-eight hours. The original sample is saved in the refrigerator. Plates may then be examined by the physician at twenty-four and again forty-eight hours. If there is no growth or less than ten colonies on the agar, the plate and the original sample may be discarded. If there is growth of more than ten colonies but less than 300 colonies (a number that can be counted accurately), the plate is sent to a bacteriology laboratory for identification of the organisms, antibiotic sensitivity and serotyping if necessary. If there are more than 300 colonies, the original sample should be diluted 1:10 and 1:1000 to obtain a more accurate colony count.

DISCUSSION

Stansfeld[10] has proposed the use of a counting chamber for the microscopic examination of urine. It remains for each laboratory to standardize upon one technique and to establish its normal values. The presence of abnormal numbers of white cells in the urine does not always mean infection[11]. Table II re-

TABLE II CAUSES OF PYURIA OTHER
THAN INFECTION

Extreme dehydration	Chemical inflammations
Trauma	Vaginal secretions
Febrile states	Pelvic stone
Acute glomerulonephritis	

veals other causes of pyuria. Most significantly, 50 per cent of patients who have bacterial infection may not have pyuria[12]. Therefore, it is mandatory not to rely solely on microscopic examination to make a proper diagnosis of genitourinary disease in an ill infant.

Gram staining of a loop of uncentrifuged urine is a quick method for evaluating the urine of an ill infant. Many times the clinician is faced with an acutely ill baby and is unwilling to await the results of culture before using antibiotic therapy. For the recognition of infection, a single gram stain has an 80 per cent correlation with the results of colony counting. If a second specimen is obtained for gram staining before therapy is started, the correlation may be as high as 96 per cent[13].

The number of bacteria present in a given volume of urine is extremely important. Physicians or clinical laboratories that do only qualitative bacterial cultures on urine are not providing adequate information. Contamination results easily from urethral organisms[14] or from errors in collection or handling the urine specimen. To date, the best effort to differentiate contamination from true bacteruria is a quantitative evaluation of the organisms present.

There is general agreement that more than 10^5 bacteria per ml of urine is indicative of infection in the urine, and less than 10^3 per ml means no infection or is the result of contamination[15]. The

TABLE III RESULTS OF URINE CULTURES OUT-PATIENT LABORATORY U.S. NAVAL HOSPITAL, BETHESDA, 1964-1965

	No Growth ($<10^3$ colonies/ml)		Positive Growth ($>10^5$ colonies/ml)		Indefinite Growth (10^3-10^4 colonies/ml) (10^4-10^5 colonies/ml)			
	No.	Per cent	No.	Per cent	No.	Per cent	No.	Per cent
June	15	57.7	3	11.6	5	19.2	3	11.5
July	36	60.0	12	18.2	8	13.3	4	6.6
August	34	60.7	5	8.7	2	3.6	15	26.8
September	21	48.8	4	9.1	13	30.2	5	11.6
October	36	72.0	2	3.6	5	10.0	7	14.0
November	46	60.5	9	10.4	11	14.5	10	13.2
December	63	67.0	8	7.4	16	17.0	7	7.4
January	64	62.7	6	5.1	24	23.5	8	7.8
February	85	74.6	4	2.9	22	19.3	3	2.6
March	69	66.3	5	4.8	25	24.0	5	4.8
April	51	61.4	8	9.5	17	20.4	7	8.4
May	92	77.3	3	2.5	22	18.5	2	1.7

range between 10^3 and 10^4 colonies per ml is doubtful (probably *does not* mean infection), while the range from 10^4 to 10^5 colonies per ml is also doubtful and probably *does* mean infection. Most surveys state that this doubtful range (10^3 to 10^5) does not represent much of a problem because less than 5 per cent of the cultures fall in this range[16]. More difficulty in this area, however, is experienced in pediatric outpatient departments, as indicated by Table III, which reveals an incidence of 20 to 41 per cent "indefinite" cultures. The most satisfactory way to resolve the uncertainty is to analyze more than one urine specimen. Confidence limits can be increased to 95 per cent or better by culturing two successive "clean catch" urines. If these still offer doubtful or conflicting results, needle aspiration of the bladder should be used to resolve the uncertainty.

REFERENCES

1. The Pediatric Patient 1964. Philadelphia, Lippincott, pp. 93-114.

2. Kass, E. H.: Pyelonephritis and bacteriuria, a major problem in preventive medicine. Ann. Intern. Med., 56:46-53, 1962.

3. North, A., Jr.: Bacteriuria in children with acute febrile illness. J. Pediat., 63:408-411, 1963.

4. Sherwood, D. W., et al.: Abnormalities of the genitourinary tract discovered by palpation of the abdomen of the newborn. Pediatrics, 18:782-789, 1956.

5. Potter, E. L.: Pathology of the Fetus and the Newborn. Chicago, Yearbook, 1952, pp. 363-368.

6. Marden, P. M., Smith, D. W., and McDonald, M. J.: Congenital anomalies in the newborn infant, including variations. J. Pediat., 64:357-371, 1964.

7. Hinkle, N. H., Partin, J. C., and West, C. D.: Diagnosis of acute and chronic pyelonephritis in children. Use of simple spread plate technique for colony counting. Amer. J. Dis. Child., 100:333, 1960.

8. Pryles, C. V., Lüders, D., and Alkan, M. K.: A comparative study of bacterial cultures and colony counts in paired specimens of urine obtained by catheter versus voiding from normal infants and infants with urinary tract infection. Pediatrics, 27:17, 1961.

9. Stamey, T. A., Govan, D. E., and Palmer, J. M.: The localization and treatment of urinary tract infections: the role of bactericidal urine levels as opposed to serum levels. Medicine (Balt.), 44:1-36, 1965.

10. Stansfeld, J. M.: The diagnostic value of pyuria. Pediat. Dig., pp. 47-56, March, 1965.

11. Pryles, C. V.: Round Table — Urinary Tract Infection. American Academy of Pediatrics, Annual Meeting, October, 1964.

12. Riley, H. D.: Pyelonephritis in infancy and childhood. Pediat. Clin. N. Amer., 11:731-758, 1964.

13. Information Please. Gen. Pract., 27:135, 1963.

14. Michie, A. J.: Tips for more dependable urine cultures. Consultant, 32-34, 1964.

15. Kunin, C. M., Southall, I., and Paquin, A. J.: Epidemiology of urinary tract infections. New Eng. J. Med., 263:17, 817-823, 1960.

16. West, C. D., and Holland, N. H.: Round Table — Urinary Tract Disease. American Academy of Pediatrics, Annual Meeting, October, 1965.

Chapter 34

Laboratory Diagnosis of Respiratory Diseases in Infancy*

A. M. MARGILETH, M.D.*

The changing pattern of medical practice, with an increasing number of non-hospitalized patients, a myriad of therapeutic agents and the necessity to minimize and prevent adverse drug reactions, has placed an increasing responsibility on the clinician and on the outpatient laboratory to diagnose and treat, appropriately and expeditiously, each patient's illness. Clinicians are developing greater interest in the laboratory diagnosis of acute respiratory disease of infants. In order to utilize more effectively the laboratory facilities, it behooves the physician to develop some skill in performing simple bacteriologic procedures and, at the same time, to learn some of the pitfalls thereof and the proper interpretation of the results.

In the early 1950's, the infant with acute tonsillitis, otitis media or pneumonia was hospitalized; during the past five years, however, a physician seldom admits these children. This has occurred because of better methods of diagnosis, i.e., laboratory data, x-rays and use of

specific antibiotics which may be administered at home by intelligent parents.

The major concern of physicians is the prevention of suppurative and non-suppurative complications of bacterial and viral infections. He must be alert in his recognition of the symptoms of subclinical streptococcal infections to prevent rheumatic fever[1]. Although the majority of respiratory infections in children are primarily due to viruses[2], their complications are infrequent (Table I). There is no effective antiviral agent, and antimicrobial therapy when utilized is usually ineffective unless bacterial complications occur[3, 4].

PEDIATRIC OUTPATIENT LABORATORY METHODS[5, 6]

A single throat specimen is taken on a cotton swab from each patient with a respiratory illness. This is immediately rotated upon a small area of the human blood agar plate. A sterile tube containing a small quantity of nutrient broth serves as a receptacle for the swab and is refrigerated for twenty-four to forty-eight hours, pending determination of the findings on the culture plate. If β-hemolytic streptococci are found,

---

*The views expressed herein are those of the author and are not to be construed as official nor necessarily reflecting those of the Medical Department of the Navy or the Naval Service at large.

then fluorescent antibody studies are done after incubation of the broth for four to six hours.

All blood agar plates are streaked with a wire loop within two hours, and two short stabs are made in the heavy and light growth areas to enhance subsurface hemolysis of the red blood cells by oxygen labile streptolysin "O." This method greatly facilitates the reading of β-hemolysis and also readily differentiates α-hemolysis, especially when there are fewer than ten β-hemolytic colonies. Plates are incubated at 37 C for twenty-four hours. Neither increased carbon

TABLE I MAIN ORGANISMS CAUSING ACUTE RESPIRATORY DISEASE IN INFANTS AND CHILDREN

Adenoviruses:
   Types 1-7, 14, 21

Bacteria:
   Hemolytic streptococci
   H. influenzae
   Pneumococci
   Staphylococci

Common Cold Viruses:
   Coryza virus
   ECHO 4, 8-11, 20, 28
   Rhinovirus

Picornavirus:
   Coxsackie A 9, 21
   Coxsackie B 1-5
   Rhinovirus
Mycoplasma pneumoniae:
   Eaton agent

Myxoviruses:
   Influenza, A, B, C,
   Parainfluenza 1, 2, 3
   Measles virus
   Respiratory syncytial virus

Pox Viruses:
   Herpes simplex
   Varicella

TABLE II TOTAL ENT CULTURES OBTAINED FROM ALL PATIENTS AND THEIR CONTACTS DURING THE STUDY — NUMBER OF PATIENTS WITH β-HEMOLYTIC STREPTOCOCCI AND INCIDENCE FOR EACH YEAR

Fiscal Year	ENT Cultures	β-Hemolytic Streptococcus	
		Number	Per Cent
1958-59	622	39	5.6
1959-60	3294	1126	34
1960-61	4828	528	11
1961-62	7612	628	9
1962-63	5243	150°	2.6
1963-64	3582	226°	6.3
1964-65	7296	447°	6.1
	32477	3144	9.7

°Group A β-hemolytic streptococcus.

dioxide tension nor candle jars are used.

Plates are read each morning at eighteen to twenty-four hours, and again after incubation for forty-eight hours. A hand magnifying lens is used. Gram stains are rarely done. In uncertain cases, subcultures are done, or a repeat culture is taken. Colonies of β-hemolytic streptococci are counted, and pure subcultures are tested for sensitivity to Taxos A bacitracin disks. In plates showing predominate growth of pneumococci, verification is made with Taxos P optichin disks. All β-hemolytic staphylococci are tested for coagulase reaction, and plates showing a significant growth of Escherichia, Aerobacter or Klebsiella colonies and other gram negative organisms are further identified with special media and biochemical reactions. The characteristic pungent odors of *Echerichia coli*, *Proteus* and the *Pseudomonas* species are helpful in early identification.

In selected patients, i.e., severe (Class A) pharyngitis[5], paired sera are drawn for ASO titers; a CBC and sedimentation rate are done, as are a urinalysis and cultures of urine specimens. Nasopharyngeal cultures, using cotton-tipped aluminum wires are done in this latter group and in instances of patients with pneumonia and otitis media. A few cultures are taken from the ear and the trachea. Viral cultures are not done. The ASO titers are determined by the method of Rantz and Randall. A rise in titer of three tubes or more is considered significant.

In most instances, children with pharyngitis are not treated with antibiotics until after culture determinations are made, usually forty-eight to seventy-two hours later. Treatment consists of one injection of benzathine penicillin G when Group A streptococci are isolated. Specimens from family contacts are cultured when Group A β-hemolytic streptococci are isolated. A daily log is maintained in which is recorded pertinent information necessary to assure that every patient or contact with a positive culture for Group A streptococci has been so notified.

RESULTS

During the past seven years, over 36,000 ENT specimens for cultures have been taken. About 10 per cent have been positive for β-hemolytic strepto-

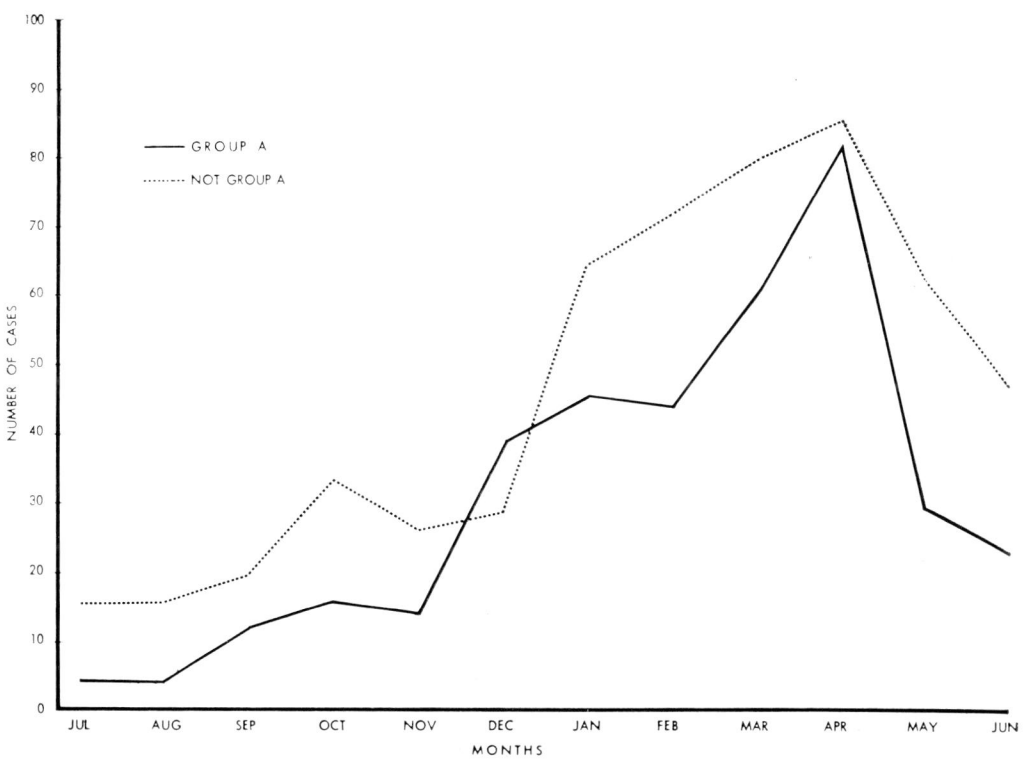

COMPARISON OF GROUP A TO NOT GROUP A BETA HEMOLYTIC
STREPTOCOCCUS IN A, B, C, D PHARYNGITIS, JULY 1964 THROUGH JUNE 1965

Fig. 1.

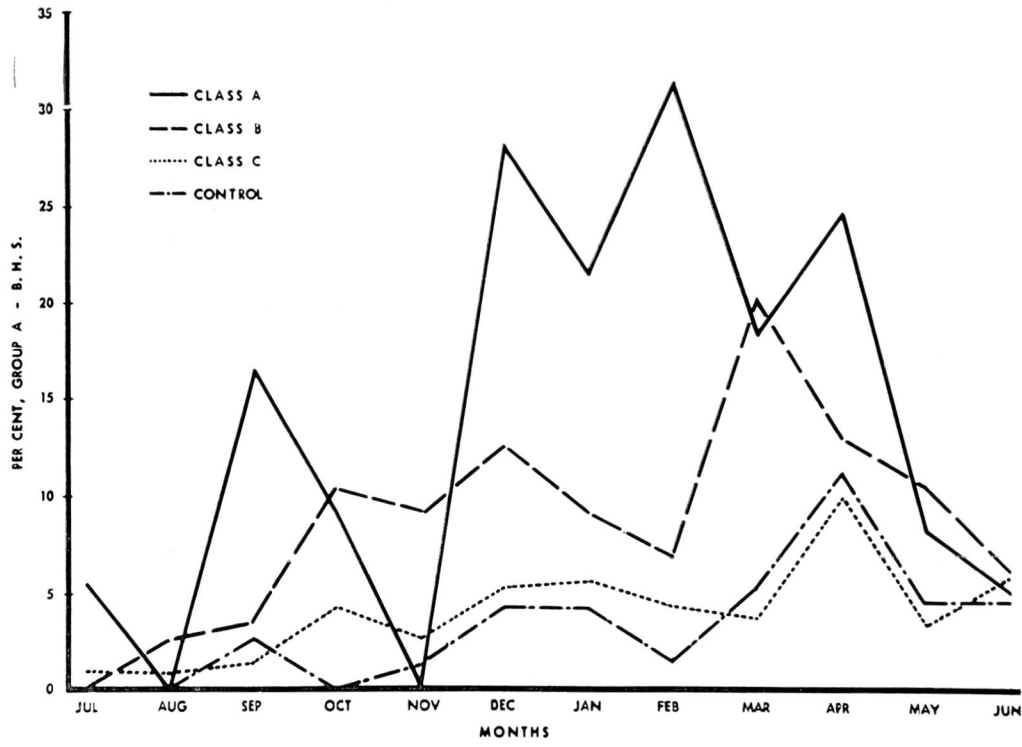

MONTHLY INCIDENCE OF GROUP A BETA HEMOLYTIC STREPTOCOCCUS FOUND IN
THREE TYPES (A, B, C) PHARYNGITIS AND CONTROL, JULY 1964 THROUGH JUNE 1965

Fig. 2.

coccus. Most of the children were under ten years of age. The use of Taxos A disks for grouping of streptococci was initiated in 1962. The number of patients with Group A β-hemolytic streptococci compared with those not Group A during the past year are shown in Figure 1. During non-epidemic periods, a greater number of non-group A streptococci was found[7]. Figure 2 shows the correlation and higher incidence of Group A streptococci found in severe pharyngitis[5] (Class A and B) compared with a low incidence in mild pharyngitis (Class C) or in throats appearing to be normal (Class D – control) during the last fiscal year, July, 1964-1965. Figure 3 depicts the monthly incidence

of Group A β-hemolytic streptococci cultured from contacts in the family and specimens from the total number of contacts cultured. During the summer and fall months, only non-group A β-streptococci were recovered. In the spring, however, about 10 per cent of the contacts were found to carry Group A streptococci in significant numbers, i.e., over five to ten colonies per plate.

COMMENT

It is most difficult for the clinician to diagnose streptococcal pharyngitis in an infant[6, 8]. This is particularly true in patients with mild pharyngitis. This group constitutes the largest number seen in daily outpatient practice. Since

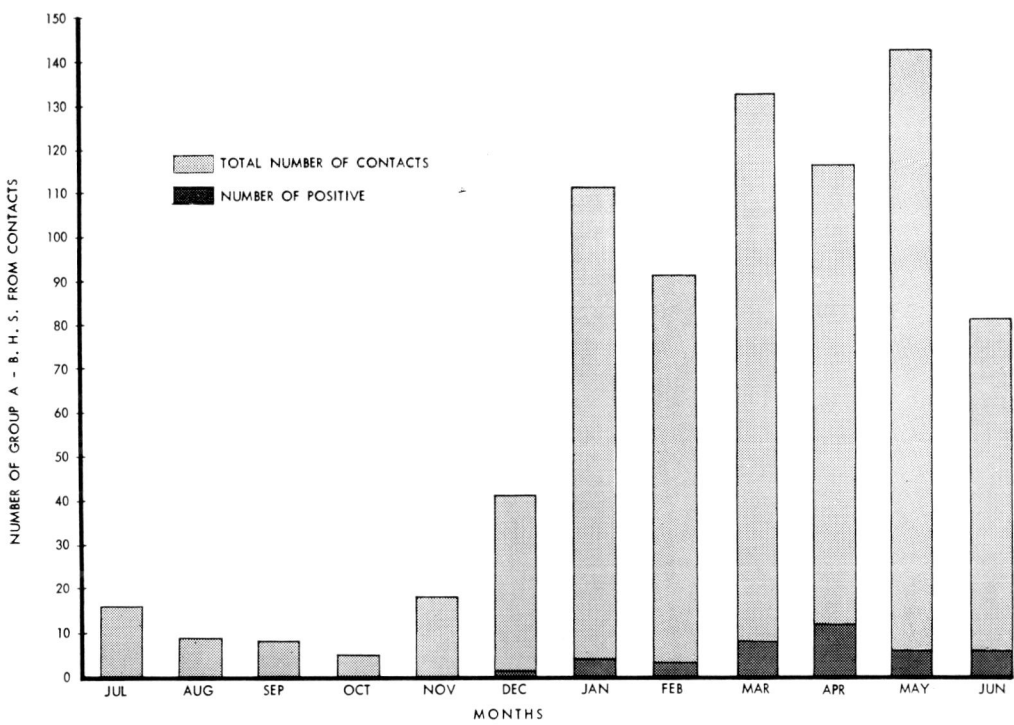

MONTHLY INCIDENCE OF BETA HEMOLYTIC STREPTOCOCCUS
CULTURED FROM CONTACTS, JULY 1964 THROUGH JUNE 1965

Fig. 3.

many believe that bacteria other than β-hemolytic streptococci are rarely an etiology of pharyngitis, the absence of this bacteria is an excellent guide to withholding of antibiotic therapy. If Group A streptococci are found in significant numbers (over 5 to 10 colonies per plate), or if a heavy growth of pneumococci or possibly certain gram negative bacilli are isolated, then the clinician can be guided as to proper therapy. Exudative non-streptococcal pharyngitis is commonly associated with isolation of an adenovirus[3], a Coxsackie virus[8] or glandular fever.

Rapid, accurate identification of bacteria in the throat culture is important in the acutely ill infant; however,

a delay of twenty-four to forty-eight hours is infrequently life-threatening, and will do little harm if treatment is given within seven or eight days[9]. Much more important is the fact that most respiratory infections are viral in origin, and the clinician should withhold specific therapy pending the laboratory report. The most useful aspect of the practice of office bacteriology in the outpatient department is that the clinician can himself observe, usually within eighteen hours, that the culture is a common flora in over 90 per cent of the cases. By the forty-eighth hour, in many instances, the patient is showing improvement on symptomatic therapy. It is gratifying for the senior physician to observe the younger physician using fewer antibiotics and to experience the questioning by parents for the expressed need for an antibiotic in instances two or three days later when the culture is positive for Group A streptococci. The reading of the urine culture (colony counts) in the OPD laboratory has also diminished over-treatment of potential urinary tract infections[10].

ERRORS IN OPD* BACTERIOLOGY

Several of these errors have been mentioned heretofore. A common problem has been the difficulty of obtaining sheep cells for routine use in preparation of blood agar plates. Many investigators[6, 7, 11–14] have found that sheep blood agar greatly facilitates the reading of large numbers of plates, namely, the sheep blood agar causes α-hemolytic organisms to appear greener rather than the bland appearance or lack of green hemolysis as when human blood agar is used. This has resulted, unfortunately, in the erroneous reporting of many cultures as positive for β-hemolytic streptococci. Human blood may fail to differentiate many colonies of β-hemolytic streptococci which are weakly hemolytic. Also, Hemophilius hemolyticus is inhibited by sheep's blood, thereby avoiding the necessity of gram stains.

Direct swabbing of the blood agar plate to allow quantitation[6, 7, 14] of bacteria is essential to the clinician, since many believe that a patient with less than five colonies of Group A streptococci does not require treatment. This is particularly true if the person is an asymptomatic contact and has not had a recent respiratory infection. If selective or inhibitive broths are used for incubation or transportation of media, and, especially if more than 0.5 ml of broth is used, quantitation of streptococci will be difficult if not impossible due to overgrowth of other bacterial inhabitants of the throat. Moffet[13] reported that few patients (3 %) with negative cultures will have a rise in ASO** titer. Patients with exudative pharyngitis and over ten colonies of typeable Group A streptococci will have a significant titer rise in over 85 per cent of the cases. Immediate antibiotic therapy usually suppresses or delays the ASO** response[15].

Precaution must always be taken that plates are not contaminated. This problem has occurred rarely, especially since plates often lay on the physician's desk before use for several hours at room temperature. Under such circumstances, contaminated plates have been detected easily. False positive grouping of A β-hemolytic streptococci may occur if too concentrated (over 0.2 units) bacitracin disks are used. This is true particularly if β-hemolytic staphylococci should have been subcultured erroneously on the grouping plate. False-negative A disk grouping may occur if the Taxos bacitracin disk is old[6], or if the worker inadvertently errs in reading a mixed flora subculture, for example, α-streptococcus on human blood agar.

Other laboratory tests, such as the ASO titer, are most helpful in the detection of recent streptococcal infection, but time factors limit their usefulness for everyday practice. They are also valuable in ascertaining antibody rise in patients with negative throat cultures. It is known that ASO titer rise may occur with Group C or G streptococcal

---

*OPD = Outpatient department

**ASO = Anti-streptolysin O

infections. Such organisms may appear α-hemolytic around surface colonies[16]. Total leukocyte and differential counts are helpful if the values are normal, since acute bacterial infections, especially streptococcal, invariably produce an elevation of values. However, a WBC over 15,000 per cu mm or a shift to the left, or both, in differential count may occur in acute viral infections. Gram stains of throat smears in infants are not helpful. However, those obtained from discharges of the nose, ear and tracheal aspirates may be very helpful. It is always valuable to repeat the culture in cases of contamination, lost specimen, no growth, poor streaking techniques or overgrowth of common flora, and especially the gram negative bacilli in infants. The accessibility and daily morning reading of plates by the clinician overcomes most of these problems which, in a large central bacteriology laboratory with its overload of work, often cannot be circumvented.

One of the greatest errors that the practice of OPD bacteriology avoids is a shortage of trained personnel in the main laboratory. This is frequently seen in many hospitals which do not have a teaching program, or it may occur over a two- or three-day weekend or perhaps due simply to illness or vacation schedules of the well-trained personnel. The absentee factor may present a very real technical problem in fluorescent antibody identification. Also, it is difficult to make quantitative determination of the streptococci with immunofluorescent techniques[7].

SUMMARY AND CONCLUSIONS

Introduction of bacteriological methods is the single most important test used in the diagnosis of respiratory disease in the infant. Establishment of an outpatient bacteriology laboratory has greatly reduced the use of antibiotics in the treatment of respiratory infections. Despite the increasing number of broader spectrum antibiotics available each year, many physicians are relying more and more on the bacteriological findings prior to institution of specific therapy. Much of this program depends upon the availability of culture materials and on the simplicity of the methods used to identify the various organisms cultured from specimens swabbed from the respiratory tract. Practice of office bacteriology has been most valuable in the management of clinic patients.

1. Clinical diagnoses and bacteriological findings are correlated.
2. The physician's ability to manage respiratory infections appropriately is improved.
3. Direction for judicious use of proper antibiotic is provided.
4. Adverse drug reactions are minimized.
5. Education for both parents and physicians is provided.
6. Doctor-parent relationship are enhanced.
7. A continuous epidemiological survey is provided.

REFERENCES

1. Czoniczer, G., Lees, M., and Massell, B. F.: Streptococcal infection. New Eng. J. Med., 265:951-952, 1961.
2. Chanock, R. M., and Parrott, R. H.: Acute respiratory disease in infancy and childhood. Pediatrics, 36:21-39, 1965.
3. Garrow, D. H.: Acute respiratory infections in childhood. Brit. Med. J., 1:297-299, 1965.
4. Baernstein, H. D., Jr., Trevisani, E., Axtell, S., and Quilligan, J. J., Jr.: Mycoplasma

pneumoniae (Eaton atypical) in children's respiratory infections. J. Pediat., 66:829-837, 1965.

5. Mella, G. W., and Margileth, A. M.: Office bacteriology. A practical therapeutic guide. Med. Ann. D.C., 33:487-491, 1964.

6. Markowitz, M., and Kuttner, A. G.: Rheumatic Fever. Philadelphia, Saunders, 1965, pp. 15, 137, 206.

7. Smith, T. B.: Clinical application of immunofluorescence. J. Bact., 89:198-204, 1965.

8. Moffet, H. L., Cramblett, H. G., and Smith, A.: Group A streptococcal infections in a children's home. Pediatrics, 33:11-17, 1964.

9. Feinstein, A. R., and Spagnulo, M.: Sore throats, streptococcal infections and prevention of rheumatic fever. J. Chronic Dis., 15: 623-633, 1962.

10. Mella, G. W.: Personal communication.

11. Margileth, A. M., and Museles, M.: The value of office bacteriology in the diagnosis of streptococcal pharyngitis. Milit. Med., 128:871-880, 1963.

12. Markowitz, M.: Cultures of the respiratory tract in pediatric practice. Amer. J. Dis. Child., 105:12-18, 1963.

13. Moffet, H. L., Cramblett, H. G., and Black, J. P.: Group A streptococcal infections in a children's home. Pediatrics, 33:5-10, 1964.

14. Breese, B. B.: The use of cotton-tipped swabs as a simple method of transporting cultures of beta hemolytic streptococci. Pediatrics, 36:599-603, 1965.

15. Denny, F. W., Perry, W. D., and Wannamaker, L. W.: Type-specific streptococcal antibody. J. Clin. Invest., 36:1092, 1957.

16. Feller, A. E., and Stevens, D. A.: Sheep blood agar for isolation of Lancefield groups of beta hemolytic streptococci. J. Lab. Clin. Med., 39:484, 1952.

Chapter 35

Spectrophotometric Determination of Blood Oxygen Saturation in Infancy

KURT M. DUBOWSKI, Ph.D.

INTRODUCTION

The oxygen saturation of whole blood is commonly defined as the fraction of hemoglobin present in the form of oxyhemoglobin, expressed in per cent, i.e.,

$$\text{blood oxygen saturation} = \%\ HgbO_2 = \left[\frac{[HgbO_2]}{[\text{total Hgb pigment}]} \right] \times 100 \qquad (I)$$

Its rapid and accurate determination has become of increasing importance with extended use of diagnostic cardiac catheterization, the development of advanced cardiovascular surgery techniques, and with increased emphasis on and greater sophistication in the experimental study of cardiovascular diseases. The measurement of the oxygen saturation of the blood is often termed "oximetry," and may be carried out on isolated blood specimens during or after withdrawal from various sites in the vascular system by so-called cuvette methods, or on blood circulating in a particular tissue or organ, often the pinna, of an intact animal or human patient.

Oximetry finds its most frequent application, in infancy and early child-hood, in the differential diagnosis of cyanotic congenital heart disease, usually in conjunction with cardiac catheterization. Cyanotic congenital heart disease in infancy most commonly involves transposition of the great vessels and the hypoplastic left-heart syndrome; less often involved are tricuspid valve atresia, tetralogy of Fallot, and other anomalies. The differential oxygen saturation of the blood samples obtained sequentially from the several heart chambers, the inferior and superior venae cavae, and the pulmonary artery and aorta are of great diagnostic significance, revealing the changes in blood oxygenation which result from the blood flow through false passages, and thus providing clues to location and nature of any structural defects. In studying pathologic shunts, oxygen saturations are commonly measured in samples of pulmonary vein and artery blood and (in the presence of left-to-right shunt) of mixed venous blood from that part

TABLE I METHODS FOR MEASUREMENT OF BLOOD OXYGEN SATURATION

Principle	Method or Technique	Investigators	
Computation from O_2 dissociation curves	measurement of blood pO_2, pH and temperature	Severinghaus	1958
Direct gasometry	manometric measurement of O_2 content and capacity	Van Slyke & Neill	1924
Differential spectrophotometry	direct tissue oximetry	Wood & Geraci	1949
	cuvette microspectro-photometry	Gordy & Drabkin	1957
	reflection-spectrophotometric oximeter	Polanyi & Hehir	1960
	absorption-spectrophotometric oximeter	Siggaard-Andersen et al.	1962
	in-vivo fiberoptics hemo-reflection	Gamble et al.	1965

of the heart immediately proximal to the site of the shunt[1].

In studying frankly cyanotic infants, an early basic decision is usually required to differentiate between congenital heart disease and respiratory distress, whether primary or secondary to central nervous system involvement. Blood oxygen saturation measurements are always a vital part of this diagnostic evaluation because of the urgency of the situation and the rapidity with which the results of oximetry can be provided. Less often, blood oxygen saturation is determined in infancy and childhood in the diagnosis of hemato-logical disorders, such as erythrocytosis or anemia, or in the presence of methemoglobinemia, particularly that secondary to chemical intoxication.

Of the less common clinical applications of oxygen saturation measurements, an interesting instance is to monitor the adequacy of brain oxygenation and thereby to minimize the incidence of cerebral dysfunction during cerebrovascular surgery[2]. As suggested by these authors[2], oximetry has usefulness in the general fields of neurology and neurosurgery and in the evaluation of cerebral oxygenation states as they relate to altered consciousness.

TABLE II METHODS FOR ESTIMATION OF BLOOD OXYGEN TENSION

Principle	Technique	Typical Method	
Computation from O_2 dissociation curves	measurement of blood O_2 saturation, pH, and temperature	Severinghaus	1958
direct microtonometry	bubble analysis for O_2	Riley et al.	1945
Electrometric measurement	potentiometric measurement with dropping Hg electrode	Bartels	1951
	amperometric measurement with bare Pt electrode	Mochizuki & Bartels	1955
	polarographic pO_2 electrode	Clark	1956
	in-vivo polarographic pO_2 electrode	Liston	1958

The blood oxygen saturation can be ascertained by three different principles, shown in Table I. Computation from the oxygen dissociation curve requires knowledge of the oxygen tension, pO_2, which can, in turn, be determined as shown in Table II. Historically, the most commonly employed method to determine blood oxygen saturation in the past was through direct gasometry or the other methods of measuring blood oxygen content shown in Table III, applied to anaerobically collected whole blood specimens before and after saturation with oxygen. The respective values for blood oxygen were then inserted into an equation of the form:

pigments (or establishment of their concentration ratios) in a single solution without need for separation of the components. Analysis of such mixtures depends on the fundamental principle that the spectrophotometric absorbances, at suitable wavelengths, of separate components in a single solution are additive, in the absence of chemical or interfering physical reaction[3]. Each hemoglobin pigment has a different and characteristic absorptivity (= specific absorbance, specific extinction coefficient) at any suitable wavelength. Further, the absorbance attributable to each substance in solution, with monochromatic light, is proportional to the con-

$$\text{blood oxygen saturation} = \% \text{ HgbO}_2 = \left[\frac{\text{Vol. } \% \text{ HgbO}_2 \text{ content}}{\text{Vol. } \% \text{ HgbO}_2 \text{ capacity}} \right] \times 100 \, (\text{II})$$

to obtain the saturation value.

Spectrophotometric methods for the determination of blood oxygen saturation have substantial theoretical and practical advantages over gasometry and other current methods, exemplified by the applicability of spectrophotometry to the rapid, direct and accurate quantitation of two or more hemoglobin

centration of that substance. In oximetry, the existence of only the two pigment system oxyhemoglobin: ("reduced") hemoglobin is usually assumed. The methods then involve absorbance measurements at two wavelengths of suitably diluted, buffered and hemolyzed blood. The *percentage composition* of this two-pigment mixture can be

TABLE III METHODS FOR MEASUREMENT OF BLOOD OXYGEN CONTENT

Principle	Technique	Typical Method	
Direct gasometry	volumetric measurement	Van Slyke & Stadie	1921
	manometric measurement	Van Slyke & Neill	1924
	microvolumetric measurement	Roughton & Scholander	1943
	micromanometric measurement	Natelson & Menning	1955
Electrochemical analysis	polarographic pO_2 measurement of blood/H_2O-displaced O_2	Awad & Winzler	1961
Gas chromatography	gas-solid chromatography	Chambliss & Nouse	1962
Mass spectrometry	vacuum extraction and mass spectrography	Patrick *et al.*	1954
Polarography	amperometric measurement with dropping Hg electrode	Neville	1960

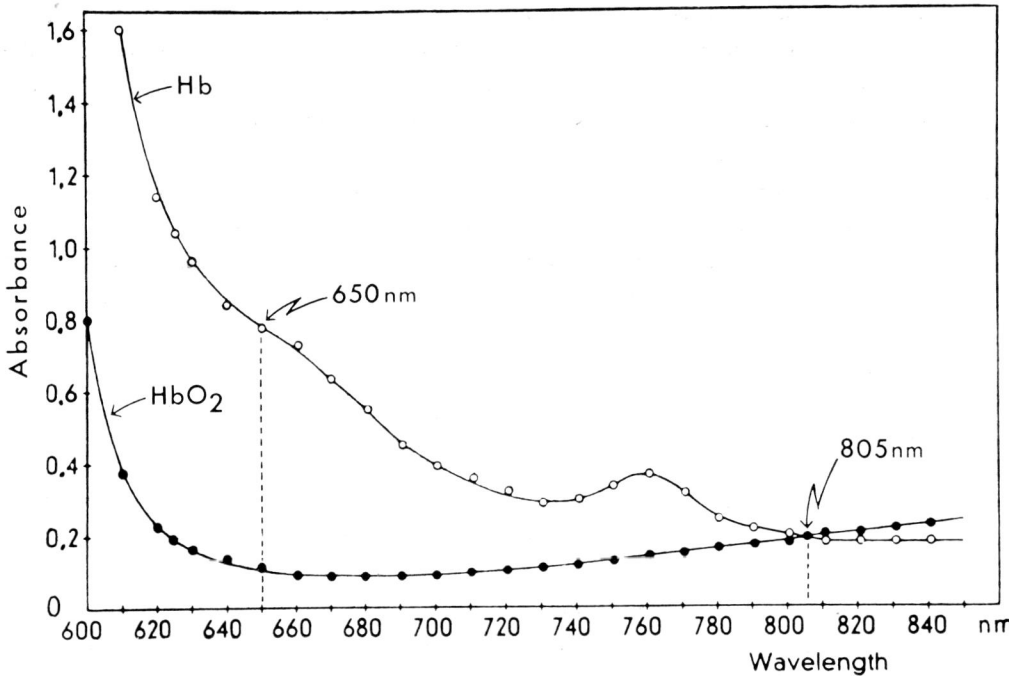

Fig. 1. Absorbance spectra of equal concentrations of oxyhemoglobin and (reduced) hemoglobin in hemolyzed whole blood. Modified from Falholt[10].)

determined from the ratio of the total absorbances of the mixture at each of two suitable wavelengths.

The procedure to be described for spectrophotometric measurement of the oxygen saturation of withdrawn blood samples is based on the methods of Gordy and Drabkin[4], Nahas[5], Deibler, Holmes, Campbell and Gans[6], and Johnston, Holtkamp and Eve[7]. It combines the characteristics of reliability, rapidity and simplicity desirable in practical clinical laboratory methods with the necessary accuracy and precision for investigative applications.

PRINCIPLE

The percentage composition of a two-component mixture can be determined from the ratio of the mixture absorbances at two suitable wavelengths. For the two-pigment system oxyhemoglobin: hemoglobin in hemolyzed blood, where the quotient A_1/A_2 (in which $A_1 =$ absorbance at wavelength 1 and $A_2 =$ absorbance at wavelength 2) of oxyhemoglobin is X and the quotient A_1/A_2 for hemoglobin is Y, any mixture of the two pigments will have an A_1/A_2 value between X and Y, depending on the relative concentration of the pigments. Therefore, the composition of any unknown mixture of these two pigments can be determined by calculation from the observed A_1/A_2 ratio for the unknown mixture and previously observed values of A_1/A_2 for various known mixtures of the two pigments, or from the observed A_1/A_2 ratio of the unknown mixture and a previously prepared calibration curve or computation aid, such as a nomogram, slide rule or table.

The relation between oxygen saturation and the A_1/A_2 ratio is linear throughout its entire range.

While, theoretically, the measurements can be made at any two suitable wavelengths, the absorbance of blood pigments is very great in the visible spectrum region, especially in the green and blue region where $HgbO_2$-Hgb isosbestic points are located. This necessitates use of very thin pigment layers, requiring special cuvettes of 0.01 cm depth or less, which are expensive and technically difficult to manipulate and to clean rapidly. Absorbance of blood pigments is lower in the near infrared region of the spectrum, permitting use of thicker pigment layers with consequent advantages of cuvette economy and handling simplicity. Further, as shown by Marsh[8], with such "thick layers" of approximately 0.1 cm of undiluted or moderately diluted blood, it is unnecessary to prevent exposure of the solution above the light path to air, if measurements will be performed within ten minutes.

The pertinent portion of the oxyhemoglobin and hemoglobin spectra are illustrated in Figure 1. Absorbance measurements are made at 650 mμ and 805 mμ. The latter is an isosbestic point for oxyhemoglobin and hemoglobin, utilization of which simplifies the solution of the two necessary simultaneous equations to the form:

Since the ratios A_{650}/A_{805} for hemoglobin and A_{650}/A_{805} for oxyhemoglobin are relatively independent of hemoglobin concentration and are constant for any given set of experimental conditions, their actual values determined in the laboratory undertaking this analysis can be substituted in Equation III to yield the following working equation (using typical[9] values as examples):

$$\% \, HgbO_2 = 100 \times \left[\frac{3.97 - A_{650}/A_{805}}{3.47} \right] (IV)$$

With anaerobic handling, the whole blood specimen is hemolyzed and moderately diluted with an anionic detergent, Triton X-100, in borate buffer solution. A portion of the resulting solution is anaerobically transferred to a cuvette of narrow light path (approximately 0.1 cm), and absorbance measurements are made at 650 mμ and 805 mμ with a suitable spectrophotometer, using essentially monochromatic light. The ratio A_{650}/A_{805} is calculated, and the corresponding blood oxygen saturation is read directly from a previously prepared calibration curve.

REAGENTS

1. *Hemolyzing reagent*: Triton X-100[*], 5 per cent v/v in 0.1 M sodium

---

[*]Rohm & Haas Co., Philadelphia, Pennsylvania, 19105. Laboratory quantities of Triton X-100 are available from Hartman-Leddon Co., Inc., Philadelphia, Pennsylvania, 19143.

$$\% \, HgbO_2 = 100 \times \left[\frac{A_{650_{Hgb}}/A_{805_{Hgb}} - A_{650}/A_{805}}{A_{650_{Hgb}}/A_{805_{Hgb}} - A_{650_{HgbO_2}}/A_{805_{HgbO_2}}} \right] (III)$$

Where: Hgb = totally reduced blood

HgbO$_2$ = totally oxygenated blood

$\dfrac{A_{650}}{A_{805}}$ = ratio of absorbances for the unknown mixture borate. The 0.1 M sodium borate solution is prepared by dissolving 38.1 gm of reagent grade sodium borate, $Na_2B_4O_7$ • $10H_2O$, in distilled-demineralized water and adjusting the volume to 1 liter. Fifty ml of Triton X-100 are then dissolved with the aid of a magnetic stirrer (avoiding shaking to minimize foaming) in 0.1 M sodium borate, and the volume adjusted to 1 liter. This reagent is stable at room temperature for at least one year.

2. *Hemolyzing-reducing reagent:* 2.5 gm of purified sodium hydrosulfite, $Na_2S_2O_4$, are dissolved in 2.5 ml of hemolyzing solution (reagent 1) in a closed centrifuge tube. The solution is centrifuged, and the supernatant is used with minimal exposure to air. This reagent should be freshly prepared on the day of use.

3. *Heparin sodium,* sterile solution, 1,000 units/ml.

4. *Sodium chloride,* 0.9 per cent w/v. Ninety gm of reagent-grade sodium chloride, NaCl, are dissolved in distilled-demineralized water and the volume adjusted to 1 liter. The reagent is indefinitely stable at room temperature in the absence of microbiological contamination.

SPECIAL APPARATUS

1. *Beckman Model DU or DU-2 spectrophotometer,* with dual thermo-spacer set for temperature control of cell compartment, tungsten lamp, photomultiplier and red-sensitive (600-1000 $m\mu$) phototube; or equivalent high resolution spectrophotometer capable of operating in the near infrared region.

2. *Nahas Lucite Cuvette*,* Model

NAC-22, sample chamber width 0.10 cm; or special 1 mm silica cells† with adapters for cuvette holder; or standard 10 mm silica cells with silica spacers for 1 mm light path.‡

3. *Needle, hypodermic,* 23-gauge, 3 in. The needle is sheathed with polyethylene tubing** (Catalog No. PX025), which projects beyond the tip to protect the cuvette chambers from scratches.

4. *Stopcocks,*** Three-Way, Catalog No. MS02, sping clip Ayer type, female Luer-Lok to male Luer slip plus female Luer-Lok side connection.

5. *Syringes,*** glass, Yale Luer-Lok tip, Catalog No. 2TL, 2 cc; or equivalent. (Syringes with lock tips are preferred to glass or plastic syringes without this feature).

6. *Syringe caps,*** metal, Catalog No. 425A. (Satisfactory substitutes can be made by removing the needle shaft from a hypodermic needle and closing the needle opening with solder).

7. *Tonometer.* Commercial thermostated tonometers§ are available A satisfactory and economical substitute can be improvised from a 500 ml or 1000 ml borosilicate glass bottle with a polyethylene or Teflon-lined cap, horizontally rotated at 5 to 10 rpm on a "bottle roller" device placed in a 37 C incuba-

---

*Waters Corporation, Electro-Medical Instrument Division, P.O. Box 288, Rochester, Minnesota.

†Catalog No. 9116-M10, Arthur H. Thomas Co., Philadelphia, Pennsylvania, 19105.

‡Catalog No. 9199-D40, Arthur H. Thomas Co., Philadelphia, Pennsylvania, 19105.

**Becton, Dickinson and Co., Rutherford, New Jersey.

§Catalog No. P-3600 Swirl Tonometer, Warren E. Collins, Inc., 555 Huntington Avenue, Boston, Massachusetts, 02115; Catalog No. 137-A Tonometer, Instrumentation Laboratory, Inc., 9 Galen St., Boston, Massachusetts, 02172.

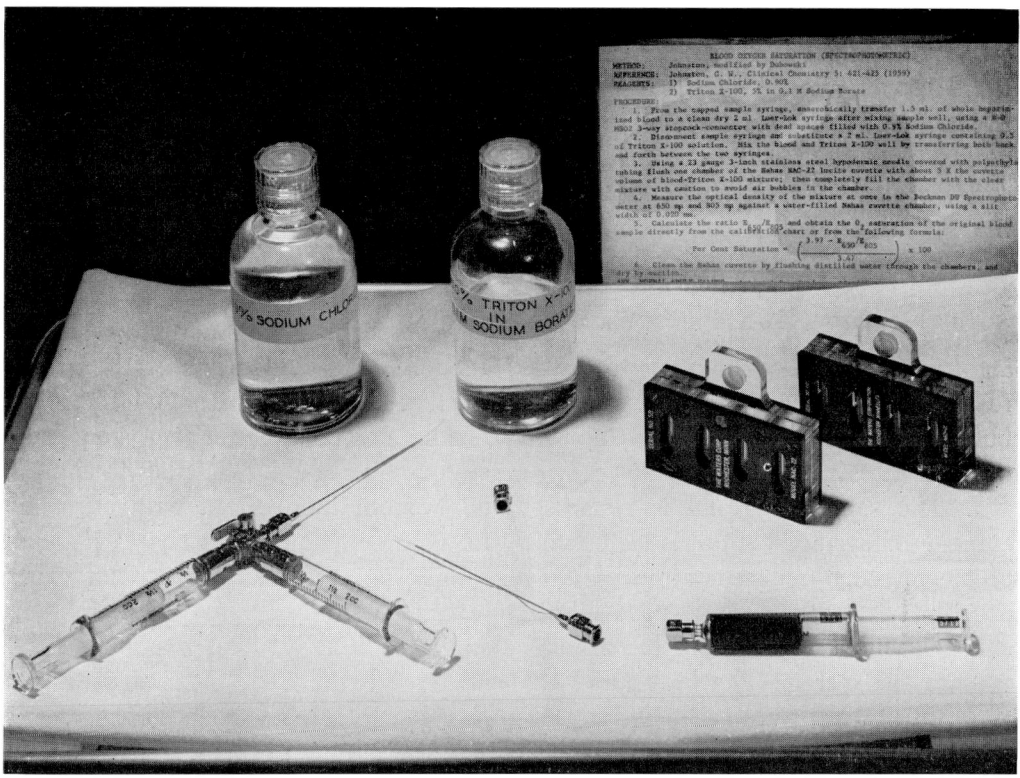

Fig. 2.   Nahas cuvettes and materials for spectrophotometric measurement of blood oxygen saturation.

tor. A small Lapidary Tumbler‡ can serve as the "bottle roller."

The Nahas cuvette and associated equipment are illustrated in Figure 2.

PROCEDURE

A. Collection and Preparation of Specimens

1. Venous or arterial blood can be analyzed, the nature of the sample depending upon the physiological information desired. Sample (2 ml) syringes are prepared by filling the dead space of syringe and needle with sterile heparin sodium solution, using aseptic technique. A convenient volume of

blood, preferably at least 1 ml, is drawn into the sample syringe with gentle suction to avoid air space creation or foaming, and the sample is sealed by impaling a soft rubber stopper on the needle. The syringes are properly identified to indicate origin and sequence of sampling.

2. The blood samples are at once immersed in an ice bath and should be analyzed as soon as possible, but not more than one hour after withdrawal.

3. Immediately prior to analysis, each sample syringe is removed from the ice bath, dried and gently but thoroughly rotated both along its axis and end-over-end to mix the whole blood specimen adequately. No mercury is used in the syringes.

‡Catalog No. F9G1412, Sears, Roebuck & Co., Kansas City, Missouri, 64127.

B. Analysis

1. A 2 ml syringe with attached three-way stopcock is prepared by filling the dead spaces of syringe and stopcock with 0.9 per cent sodium chloride solution. Into it is transfered anaerobically a convenient volume (e.g., approximately 1 ml) of whole blood from the sealed, well-mixed sample syringe, transferring the sample back-and-forth slowly several times to assure removal of a representative aliquot. Any bubbles formed are immediately ejected through the stopcock.

2. The sample syringe is removed, and a 2 ml syringe containing a volume of hemolyzing reagent approximately one third that of the blood used is substituted, with care to avoid introducing air into the system. The blood and the hemolyzing reagent are well mixed by gently transferring both back-and-forth between the two syringes repeatedly until hemolysis and complete mixing have occurred; less than one minute suffices. Finally, the entire mixture is left in one syringe, the empty syringe removed, and the 3-in polyethylene-sheathed needle attached to the three-way stopcock male Luer slip.

3. After a few drops of the sample mixture have been expelled to fill the needle, one chamber of the Nahas lucite cuvette is filled by flushing it continuously from the bottom with five times its volume (approximately 0.08 ml) of sample mixture, absorbing the excess mixture with cellulose wipes or gauze sponges. Finally, the chamber is left filled with the clear mixture, with cau-

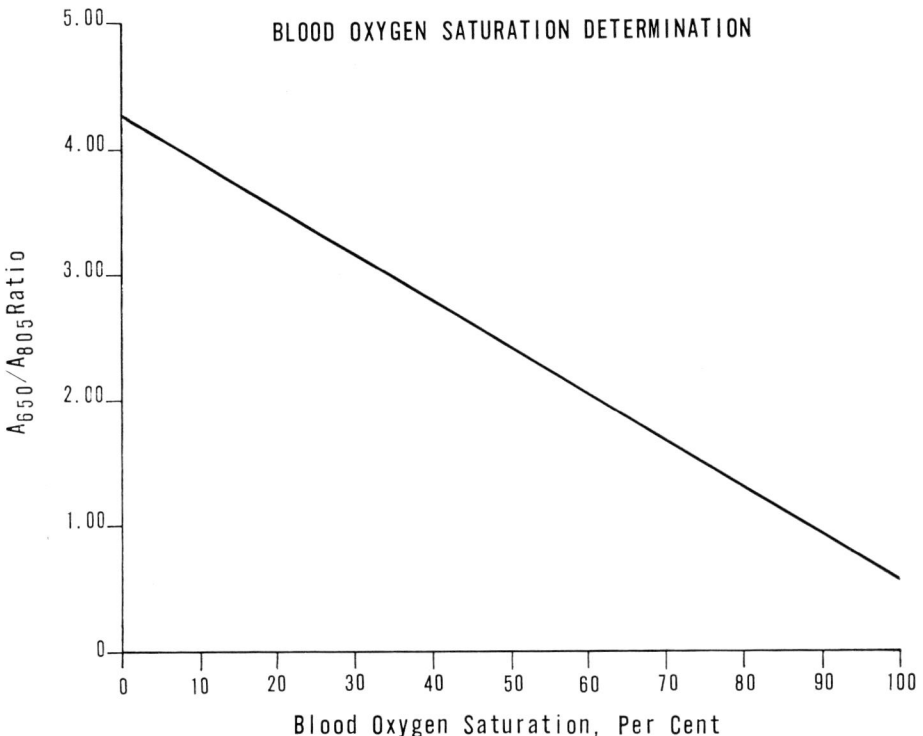

Fig. 3. Typical calibration curve for the spectrophotometric determination of blood oxygen saturation by measurement at 650 and 805 mμ.

tion to avoid air bubbles in the chamber. The process is repeated with other blood specimens if more than one sample is to be analyzed. Three samples can be accommodated in the four-chamber Nahas cuvette.

4. Another chamber of the Nahas cuvette is filled with hemolyzing reagent as a photometric reference solution.

5. The absorbance of each sample mixture is measured at once in the spectrophotometer at 650 and 805 mμ, employing the hemolyzing reagent as a "blank" photometric reference solution. To assure adequate monochromaticity, the slit of the spectrophotometer is adjusted to a width of 0.015 to 0.02 mm, which corresponds to spectral band width of 2.5 to 3 mμ. All measurements are made at a temperature between 25 and 27 C; the spectrophotometer sample compartment is water-cooled as required.

6. The value A_{650}/A_{805} is calculated for each sample mixture, and the blood oxygen saturation of the original blood specimen is read directly from the previously prepared calibration curve of HgbO$_2$ percentage *versus* A_{650}/A_{805} ratio (Fig. 3).

7. The Nahas cuvette is cleaned by flushing it successively with distilled water, mild detergent (e.g., 1% Haemo-Sol* solution), and again distilled water. It is then dried with suction. All organic solvents must, of course be avoided.

C. Preparation of Calibration Curve

Since the relation between blood oxygen saturation and the A_{650}/A_{805} ratio is linear, only two calibration points are needed to establish a calibration

---

*Meinecke & Co., Inc., P.O. Box 6882, Baltimore 4, Maryland.

curve. It is simplest to employ 0 and 100 per cent oxyhemoglobin samples for the two calibration points, and this is universal practice. The success and reliability of spectrophotometric oxygen saturation measurements depend in considerable measure upon the care with which this calibration is performed, and this, in turn, is dependent upon properly prepared 0 and 100 per cent HgbO$_2$ samples.

1. The 100 per cent HgbO$_2$ blood specimen is prepared by completely saturating a fresh whole blood specimen obtained from a healthy subject, preferably a nonsmoker who is not taking drugs, with oxygen in a tonometer. Heparin or EDTA is used as the anticoagulant. A 1000 ml screw-capped reagent bottle is thoroughly cleaned, dried and flushed of room air with a humidified mixture of 94.5 per cent oxygen + 5.5 per cent carbon dioxide. Approximately 10 ml of whole blood are placed into the horizontal bottle, more humidified oxygen-carbon dioxide is added, and the bottle stoppered. The bottle is then rotated about its long (horizontal) axis for three consecutive ten-minute periods, using a "bottle roller" aparatus in a 37 C incubator. After the first and second ten-minute rotation periods, humidified oxygen-carbon dioxide is again passed into the bottle to displace completely the existing atmosphere.

2. The 0 per cent HgbO$_2$ blood specimen is prepared by reducing completely a fresh whole blood specimen by a combination of tonometry and chemical hemoglobin reduction. Deoxygenation of approximately 10 ml of whole blood is carried out by the tonometry technique described above (C.1), sub-

TABLE IV TYPICAL A_{650}/A_{805} RATIOS FOR FULLY OXYGENATED AND FULLY REDUCED BLOOD

Investigator	Reference	Deter-minations	A_{650}/A_{805} Ratio	
			100% HgbO₂	0% HgbO₂
Deibler et al.	6	11	0.491 ± 0.008 (SD)	4.229 ± 0.100 (SD)
Gambino et al.	12		0.43	4.55
Gambino	11		0.46	4.47
Jacobs	9	20	0.58 ± 0.067	4.01 ± 0.145
Johnston	9	17	0.50 ± 0.06	3.97 ± 0.06
Polanyi and Hehir	13		0.43	4.45

stituting humidified helium, carbon dioxide or air-free nitrogen gas (each containing 5.5% carbon dioxide) for the oxygen previously used.

3. The fully oxygenated and fully reduced blood specimens are analyzed immediately after preparation. A convenient aliquot (approximately 1 to 2 ml) of each specimen is drawn into a 2 cc sample syringe, the dead space of which is filled with heparin solution or 0.9 per cent sodium chloride, using a long (5 to 6 in.) needle to avoid unnecessary exposure of the prepared blood to air.

4. The 100 per cent HgbO₂ specimen is analyzed as outlined in Section B, above, using the hemolyzing reagent, while the 0 per cent HgbO₂ specimen is similarly analyzed with use of the freshly prepared hemolyzing-reducing reagent.

5. The entire analysis of both the 0 and 100 per cent HgbO₂ blood specimens should be performed at least in duplicate, beginning with different fresh blood specimens. The replicate A_{650}/A_{805}

ratios obtained should coincide within 5 per cent.

Typical A_{650}/A_{805} ratios for fully oxygenated and fully reduced blood are shown in Table IV.

6. In some circumstances, it may be possible to obtain freshly drawn arterial blood specimens from normal adult subjects breathing 100 per cent oxygen or to obtain blood from the arterial side of a pump oxygenator in use. Such specimens can be utilized as 100 per cent HgbO₂ calibration samples[7].

Figure 3 is a typical calibration curve for this procedure in the author's laboratory.

D. Calculations

The blood oxygen saturation of the unknown blood specimen can be calculated from the ratio of absorbance at 650 mμ to absorbance at 805 mμ by equations III and IV, which must be modified to reflect the A_{650}/A_{805} values found for fully oxygenated and fully reduced blood in the laboratory undertaking the analysis.

Example:

1. *Calibration values found for A_{650}/A_{805}*:

$$100\% \ HgbO_2 = 4.27$$
$$0\% \ HgbO_2 = 0.51$$

2. *Unknown values found*:

$$A_{650} = 0.077$$
$$A_{805} = 0.102$$
$$A_{650}/A_{805} = 0.755$$

3. *% HgbO₂ formula*:

$$\% \ HgbO_2 = 100 \times \left[\frac{4.27 - A_{650}/A_{805}}{3.76}\right] \tag{V}$$

4. *% HgbO₂ of sample*:

$$\% \ HbO_2 = 100 \times \left[\frac{4.27 - 0.755}{3.76}\right] \tag{VI}$$

$$= 93.5$$

DISCUSSION

Spectrophotometric methods for measurement of oxygen saturation, exemplified by this procedure, offer many theoretical and practical advantages over gasometry and other procedures. Since the absorbance ratios depend upon the *relative* concentrations of the two pigments, the blood need not be precisely diluted, nor the total hemoglobin content determined. Considerable time is therefore saved, compared with gasometry, since all measurements are carried out on a single dilution of the unknown blood sample. The spectrophotometric values are totally independent of dissolved oxygen in the blood and do not require correction for this factor, which affects gasometrically determined blood oxygen values to a variable extent, being greater in the saturated samples than in others[14]. Although approximate dilution of the blood sample suffices, two factors limit the usable dilution range. The most accurate measurement range of most photometric instruments is between absorbances of 0.1 to 0.7[15], and the

blood dilution should preferably be sufficient to result in absorbance readings within this range. However, Anderson and Sekelj[16] found that errors in spectrophotometric oxygen saturation measurements increased when the hemoglobin concentration was 8 gm per 100 ml or less. Consequently, blood of normal hemoglobin content should be diluted not more than one quarter or one third, to maintain the hemoglobin content of the final sample solution at about 10 gm per 100 ml or more; and blood with abnormally low or high hemoglobin concentrations should be diluted appropriately to maintain this same final hemoglobin content.

The general spectrophotometric principle described above can be applied to spectrophotometric measurements in various spectral regions. The HgbO₂-Hgb isosbestic point at 805 mμ is particularly convenient and appropriate because it permits use of reasonably wide light paths with resultant practical advantages. When an isosbestic point serves as one of a pair of wavelengths for simultaneous measurements, the other should obviously be characterized by a wide difference in specific absorbance of the two forms of hemoglobin in order to increase the precision of the analysis. Several suitable wavelengths in the red region of the visible spectrum and in the near-infrared region satisfy this requirement. The nature of the spectra of hemolyzed oxygenated and reduced blood[4, 10] dictates a choice above 630 mμ in the light of the requirements for a relatively wide light path and for absorbances within the limits of minimal photometric error. Hickam and Frayser[14] employed measurement at 660 mμ, an isosbestic point for hemoglobin and methemoglobin, where there is a wide absorbance difference between oxyhemoglobin and hemoglobin. Johnston et al.[7] chose 650 mμ for measurement because of a slightly greater difference in absorbance by hemoglobin and oxyhemoglobin than at 660 mμ and its greater ease and assurance of wavelength setting in the spectrophotometer. Maas et al.[17] measured hemolyzed blood at 655 and 795 mμ, having experimentally found the isosbestic point to be 797 ± 2 mμ. They ascribe the lower isosbestic point value they found to their method of producing reduced hemoglobin, equilibration at 38 C for one hour with humidified oxygen-free nitrogen containing 5 per cent carbon dioxide without use of chemical reducing agent, and to the fact that they produced hemolysis at pH 7.4 with a phosphate-buffered Sterox SE Solution. The 655 mμ wavelength was chosen in preference to 650 mμ because the former value is nearer the isosbestic point of hemoglobin and methemoglobin, given by them as 657.5 mμ. The commonly employed 650 mμ wavelength is an isosbestic point for oxyhemoglobin and carboxyhemoglobin, which could lead to error from the presence of carboxyhemoglobin. Obviously, this is a minimal risk in infants and children, but care should be taken to avoid such maneuvers as determination of the diffusing capacity of the lungs by the steady-state CO method within twenty-four hours prior to spectrophotometric oxygen saturation measurements. A narrow-band spectrophotometer with good spectral resolution is required to achieve the potential for precision and accuracy of the spectrophotometric procedures. Generally, photomultipliers are needed for measurements at the lower wavelength at the narrow slit widths necessary for monochromaticity.

The exact cuvette light path length is not a significant factor in this method, although the general limits described should be adhered to in order to remain within the desirable absorbance range. Several commercial cuvettes are available with light paths of approximately 0.1 cm and can be successfully used in this procedure. Silica cuvettes and cuvette spacers or appropriate plastics are preferable to those of Corex or borosilicate glass, since the Triton X-100 solution causes rapid etching of the latter. Mercury causes many unnecessary complications in spectrophotometry as well as in blood sampling[18], and its use is best avoided completely. It is not needed in syringes to effect adequate remixing of blood samples. Other anionic detergents can be used as hemolyzing agents, e.g., 20 per cent Sterox SE[17]; all are greatly preferable to saponin.

Accurate and precise calibration of the procedure is fundamental to reliability, and requires both an optically well-adjusted spectrophotometer and proper preparation of fully oxygenated and fully reduced blood specimens. Successful tonometry requires thin film formation during gas exposure, since concentration gradients form across thick blood layers or films. Temperature control is also important for precise tonometry, and resort is usually had to elevated temperatures e.g., 37 C, which are comparatively easy to achieve and maintain with simple apparatus. Oxygen must be used for tonometry of the fully oxygenated blood sample instead of the commonly employed room air because the oxygen tension of room air changes with temperature, barometric pressure and humidity, and further, at 37 C, even with a maximum room air pO_2 of 160 mm Hg, 100 per cent blood oxygen saturation cannot be achieved with room air alone[19]. The equilibrating gases are saturated with water vapor to prevent water loss from the blood film during prolonged tonometry at the elevated equilibration temperature. To assist in maintaining the blood at its physiological pH during equilibration, gas mixtures containing 5.5 per cent carbon dioxide are preferred (the readily obtainable 95% O_2 + 5% CO_2 is adequate for oxygenation).

The spectrophotometric measurements can be converted into blood oxygen saturation values by calculation or by various graphical computation aids, such as charts, nomograms, slide rules, etc. The linear nature of the calibration curve makes its use probably the simplest and most satisfactory method for obtaining the results rapidly and accurately, as suggested by Nahas[20]. The principle of obtaining oxygen saturation

values from sequential or simultaneous spectrophotometric measurements at two fixed wavelengths lends itself well to design of a specialized single-purpose instrument, and several such instruments have been developed for analysis of isolated samples, mostly as direct reading oximeters. In 1962, Siggaard-Andersen, Jorgensen and Naeraa[21] suggested use of alternate freezing and thawing to hemolyze packed erythrocytes in capillary tubes, subsequently measuring the absorbance of the hemolysate in an ungraduated hemocytometer employed as an ultramicrocuvette. Subsequently, Siggaard-Andersen and Sorensen constructed a special interference filter photometer[22], employing wavelengths of 600 mμ and 505 mμ and capable of utilizing the hemocytometer-cuvette. The instrument became available commercially in 1965* in slightly modified form, and uses sliding interference filters and a sensitive micro-ammeter calibrated in absorbance units to measure the absorbance at 598 and 505 mμ of blood hemolysates in a special hemocytometer cuvette of 0.1 mm light path[23]. Specimen requirements are reduced to 10 μl for a single analysis.

In 1949, *reflection oximetry* was described by Brinkman and Zijlstra[24], and an instrument† was subsequently marketed, in which blood oxygen saturation is empirically correlated with the intensity of light of 600-700 mμ diffusely reflected from a thick layer of unhemolyzed blood by means of a calibration curve. While this instrument required

---

*Radiometer Type OSM1 Oxygen Saturation Meter, London Co., Westlake, Ohio, 44091.
†Hemoreflector MO 1, P. J. Kipp & Zonen, Delft (Holland), available from Fisher Scientific Co., Pittsburgh, Pennsylvania, 15219.

frequent empirical calibration, utilized only one wavelength and tended toward large errors at low oxygen saturation levels, it had the advantage of eliminating the blood hemolysis step and required only a 0.5 ml sample for a single analysis. These inherent advantages of reflection oximetry were successfully exploited by Polanyi and Hehir[25], who developed a new self-contained, direct-reading reflection oximeter. Their instrument* isolates two wavelengths, 650 and 805 mμ by means of interference filters, and measures the ratio of the light reflected at these two wavelengths from an unhemolyzed undiluted whole blood sample by means of vacuum phototubes and a bridge circuit, displaying the result on a potentiometer scale calibrated in per cent oxygen saturation. The instrument determines absolute values for oxygen saturation and is independent of light intensity, temperature, cell size, shape and origin, and hemodilution. Measurements can be made within one minute, but a 2 ml blood sample was required for the original macro-oximeter. In late 1965, therefore, a modified micro-oximeter† was released, which requires only a 0.2 ml whole blood sample, gaining the added sensitivity from a reduced light filament image and gas phototubes, and permitting use of smaller blood samples collected by skin puncture. Gambino et al.[12] compared the results of oxygen saturation measurements employing the macro- and micro-reflection-oximeters

on arterial and capillary blood samples, respectively, with the results of arterial blood oxygen saturation measurements by a spectrophotometric transmittance method using 805 and 650 mμ. They found excellent correlation, reporting a standard deviations for both collection and measurement techniques of ±0.2 per cent for the macro-oximeter and ±0.6 per cent for the micro-oximeter, with respective maximum deviations between duplicates of 0.5 per cent and 1.5 per cent.

The need for rapid and reliable methods for blood oxygen saturation measurements, simpler and faster than the classical Van Slyke gasometry, was greatly accentuated by the multiplicity of samples encountered in cardiac catheterization and in modern experimental procedures. While the spectrophotometric methods meet this need well, the place held by the manometric technique of Van Slyke and Neill[26] as the classical "standard" or reference method has resulted in each new spectrophotometric method being compared with the Van Slyke and Neill method. It has been universally concluded from such studies[5, 6, 8,10, 14, 16, 20, 27–36] that the spectrophotometric methods yield results similar and comparable to those obtained with the Van Slyke techniques and that they are at least as accurate and reliable as the latter. Typically, for the spectrophotometric method employing measurements at 650 mμ and 805 mμ, the standard deviation of spectrophotometric oxygen saturation determination results is ±0.6 per cent[6]; and the mean difference between blood oxygen saturation results obtained by the spectrophotometric and the Van Slyke gasometric methods is 0.3 to 3.0

---

*Catalog No. 10800 Macro-Oximeter, American Optical Co., Medical Division, Chelsea, Massachusetts, 02150.

†Catalog No. 10850, Micro-Oximeter, American Optical Co., Medical Division, Chelsea, Massachusetts, 02150.

per cent[5, 6, 8, 9, 16] in various laboratories. The larger differences are probably attributable to difficulties with the gasometric techniques, as demonstrated by the excellent agreement of spectrophotometric results with those of other physical methods, e.g., a mean difference of 0.9 per cent from results calculated from polarographic measurement of oxygen tension[27]. It is general experience that the spectrophotometric methods yield higher oxygen saturation results than the Van Slyke and Neill gasometric method[5, 6, 8, 9, 31, 34], that the manometric technique tends to yield systematically low values[5, 6], probably mainly explained by the inactive hemoglobin normally present in human blood, and that under optimal conditions the blood oxygen saturation can be determined spectrophotometrically with an accuracy of 1 per cent[8].

Among the greatest advantages of the spectrophotometric methods for oxygen saturation are their rapidity and simplicity. Duplicate analyses of a blood sample are readily performed in five minutes by the procedure outlined, so that twelve specimens can be analyzed in duplicate per hour by a single analyst.

The utility of the spectrophotometric cuvette methods for diagnostic applications in infancy and childhood is greatly increased by the recent instrumental and methodological developments making analysis of micro and ultramicro specimens practical. It has been established for many years that the blood oxygen *content* of capillary blood obtained from the fingertip is identical to that of arterial blood[37-39]. Agreement between blood oxygen *saturation* values of simultaneously sampled arterial and capillary blood has also been amply documented[12, 17, 21, 38, 40, 41], typical mean capillary-arterial differences ranging from 0.0 to − 0.3 per cent. It is consequently universally agreed that blood from such "capillary" sites as the hyperemic earlobe or fingertip can be substituted for arterial blood in oxygen saturation measurements. Modified collection and analysis procedures[17, 21, 40, 41] permit analysis of specimens in the 30 to 50 μl range, with special small-volume cuvettes. Such capability is particularly useful, of course, in pediatric practice in following changes in oxygen saturation produced by exercise or by surgical therapy, when it may be desirable to obviate the need for arterial punctures.

SOURCES OF ERROR

Significant error can arise from improper collection and preparation of blood. The blood sample should be collected with special attention to maintenance of anaerobic conditions. Tightly fitting syringes are necessary, and individually ground glass syringes are superior to those with interchangeable barrels and plungers. Plastic syringes are otherwise satisfactory, but lack the security of a locking Luer tip, which greatly expedites rapid manipulation without disconcerting disconnections. With the small-dimension cuvettes employed, foreign substances such as mineral oil or mercury are troublesome; it is therefore advisable to employ only heparin solution or the hemolyzing reagents to fill the needle and syringe dead spaces. Foaming should obviously be avoided in collecting and transferring blood specimens.

While keeping the blood samples in an ice bath for a period up to one hour has been found not to cause any significant change in the oxygen saturation results[35], it is preferable practice to analyze each specimen as soon as possible after it is drawn. There is some evidence that hemolyzed blood specimens do undergo changes resulting in altered absorbance readings at unpredictable rates[6, 30, 35]. This may be the result of slow conversion of oxyhemoglobin to reduced hemoglobin in hemolyzed blood specimens. Errors from this source can be avoided by prompt measurement of the blood specimens after they are hemolyzed — certainly within seven to fifteen minutes[6, 30]. Once the hemolyzed blood has been placed into the cuvette, moderate speed is essential to avoid eventual interference from the diffusion of atmospheric oxygen into the cuvette which may occur after ten to fifteen minutes[8].

It is obvious that the spectrophotometer must be properly adjusted with respect to wavelength and absorbance in the spectral region used in these measurements. Prior to initial calibration of the procedure, the spectrophotometer should be checked for accuracy of the wavelength and the photometric scales by means of a mercury light source and Bureau of Standards photometric filters, and any necessary adjustments performed. The checks should be repeated periodically, since the original calibration will remain valid only if the wavelength and photometric scales remain unchanged at the calibration points. Spectrophotometric circuit stability is essential, and an appropriate warm-up period always must be observed despite the briefness of the actual analysis.

The spectrophotometric procedure is based in part on the assumption that only oxyhemoglobin and (reduced) hemoglobin are present in the hemolyzed blood solution. While normal blood contains only small quantities of methemoglobin and carboxyhemoglobin[42], both are capable of interfering if present in significant concentrations. Measurements at 660 mμ instead of 650 mμ can avoid possible errors from presence of methemoglobin at some sacrifice in sensitivity of the method, 660 mμ being an isosbestic point for hemoglobin and methemoglobin. Since 650 mμ is an isosbestic point for oxyhemoglobin and carboxyhemoglobin, the measurement is subject to error from significant HbCO concentrations in the blood. This is not a common problem in the situations requiring oxygen saturation measurements, particularly in children, but suggests that experimental subjects and patients should refrain from smoking prior to oxygen saturation measurements. Employing a reagent "blank" as the reference solution for the spectrophotometric readings is satisfactory in the absence of significantly elevated bilirubin and plasma lipid levels. The normal contributions of plasma to the spectrophotometric measurements at 650 and 805 mμ can be ignored; but if the plasma bilirubin and plasma lipids are known or believed to be elevated, plasma diluted with hemolyzing reagent in the same ratio as the whole blood specimen should be employed as the photometric reference solution.

Care in the preparation of the 0 and 100 per cent oxyhemoglobin samples is vitally important to proper calibration of the procedure. It is difficult to achieve 100 per cent HgbO$_2$ saturation without careful tonometry at controlled temperatures. Lack of consistency in the A_{650}/A_{805} ratios obtained with several different blood specimens after saturation indicates probable failure to obtain full saturation. Full hemoglobin reduction is easier to achieve, but all gases employed for tonometry should be saturated with water vapor to prevent plasma water loss during the equilibration process, and care should be taken to maintain adequate mixing of plasma and cellular elements prior to and during sampling in order to minimize the common tonometer problem of disproportionate adherence of plasma to the glass walls of the tonometer.

RANGE OF NORMAL VALUES

In normal adult subjects breathing room air, the spectrophotometric method outlined was found to yield a mean *arterial* blood oxygen saturation of 98.7 per cent (SD $\pm$ 0.6)[6]. In the author's laboratory, the mean *arterial* blood oxygen saturation of normal adult subjects breathing room air at an elevation of 800 ft above sea level was found by the procedure described to be 97.8 per cent (range – 93.2 to 100). The corresponding mean *venous* blood saturation was found to be 60.8 per cent (range – 44.0 to 87.1). These values are close to the corresponding blood values obtained by manometric gasometry: *arterial* blood 96.2 per cent (range – 93.5 to 97.5), *venous* blood 61.8 per cent (range – 55.3 to 70.7)[43].

Oxygen saturation of "arterialized" capillary blood from the warmed earlobe, analyzed by the ultramicrospectrophotometric procedure, was found to differ from that of blood from the brachial artery by an average of only 0.1 per cent[7]. Other studies cited above have confirmed that "arterialized" capillary blood from the warmed earlobe is essentially identical to arterial blood in oxygen saturation.

REFERENCES

1. Behrendt, H.: Diagnostic Tests in Infants and Children. Philadelphia, Lea & Febiger, 2nd ed., 1962, pp. 403-405.
2. Clauss, R. H., Hass, W. K., and Ransohoff, J.: Simplified method for monitoring adequacy of brain oxygenation during carotid-artery surgery. New Eng. J. Med., **273**:1127-1131, 1965.
3. Drabkin, D. L.: Spectroscopy: Photometry and spectrophotometry. In Glasser, Otto (ed.): Medical Physics, Vol. II. Chicago, Year Book, 1950, pp. 1039-1089.
4. Gordy, E., and Drabkin, D. L.: Spectrophotometric studies. XVI. Determination of the oxygen saturation of blood by a simplified technique, applicable to standard equipment. J. Biol. Chem., **227**:285-299, 1957.
5. Nahas, G. G.: A simplified Lucite cuvette for the spectrophotometric measurement of hemoglobin and oxyhemoglobin. J. Appl. Physiol., **13**:147-152, 1958.
6. Deibler, G. F., Holmes, M. S., Campbell, P. L. and Gans, J.: Use of Triton X-100 as a hemolytic agent in the spectrophotometric measurement of blood O_2 saturation. J. Appl. Physiol., **14**:133-136, 1959.
7. Johnston, G. W., Holtkamp, F., and Eve, J. R.: The spectrophotometric determination of the oxygen saturation of blood. Clin. Chem., **5**:421-425, 1959.
8. Marsh, J. B.: Note on results with present optical method in comparison with those by gasometric technique. J. Biol. Chem., **227**:297-299, 1957.
9. Johnston, G. W., and Jacobs, S. L.: Oxygen saturation of blood. In Seligson, D. (ed.): Standard Methods of Clinical Chemistry, Vol. 4. New York, Academic Press, 1963, pp. 183-189.
10. Falholt, W.: Blood oxygen saturation determined spectrophotometrically. Scand. J. Clin. Lab. Invest., **15**:67-72, 1963.
11. Gambino, S. R.: Unpublished data. Cited in Instruction Manual for the 10850 Micro-Oximeter. Chelsea, Medical Division, American Optical Co., 1965, p. 13.
12. Gambino, S. R., Goldberg, H. E., and Polanyi, M. L.: A micro method for determination of oxygen saturation by means of reflec-

tion spectrophotometry. Amer. J. Clin. Path., **42**:364-367, 1964.

13. Polanyi, M., and Hehir, R.: Unpublished data. Cited in Instruction Manual for the 10850 Micro-Oximeter. Chelsea, Medical Division, American Optical Co., 1965, p. 13.

14. Hickam, J. B., and Frayser, R.: Spectrophotometric determination of blood oxygen. J. Biol. Chem., **180**:457-465, 1949.

15. Archibald, R. M.: Criteria of analytical methods for clinical chemistry. Anal. Chem., **22**: 639-642, 1950.

16. Anderson, N. M., and Sekelj, P.: Studies on the light transmission of nonhemolyzed whole blood. Determination of oxygen saturation. J. Lab., Clin. Med., **65**:153-166, 1965.

17. Maas, A. H. J., Zuijdgeest, and Kreukniet, J.: Microspectrophotometric determination of the haemoglobin oxygen saturation in arterialized capillary blood. Clin. Chim. Acta, **9**:236-240, 1964.

18. Buxton, J. T., Hewitt, J. C., Gadsden, R. H., and Bradham, G. B.: Metallic mercury embolism. JAMA, **193**:573-575, 1965.

19. Dittmer, D. S., and Grebe, R. M. (eds.): Handbook of Respiration. Philadelphia, Saunders, 1958, pp. 72-73.

20. Nahas, G. G.: Spectrophotometric determination of hemoglobin and oxyhemoglobin in whole hemolyzed blood. Science, **113**:723-725, 1951.

21. Siggaard-Andersen, O., Jorgensen, K., and Naeraa, N.: Spectrophotometric determination of oxygen saturation in capillary blood. Scand. J. Clin. Lab. Invest., **14**:298-302, 1962.

22. Siggaard-Andersen, O.: The Acid-Base Status of the Blood. 2nd ed., Baltimore, Williams & Wilkins, 1964, pp. 106-107.

23. Instruction Manual—Type OSMI Oxygen Saturation Meter. Copenhagen, Radiometer, 1st ed., 1965.

24. Brinkman, R., and Zijlstra, W. G.: Determination and continuous registration of the percentage oxygen saturation in small amounts of blood. Arch. Chir. Neerl., **1**:177-183, 1949.

25. Polanyi, M. L., and Hehir, R. M.: New reflection oximeter. Rev. Sci. Instr., **31**:401-403, 1960.

26. Van Slyke, D. D., and Neill, J. M.: Determination of gases in blood and other solutions by vacuum extraction and monometric measurement. J. Biol. Chem., **61**:523-573, 1924.

27. Danzor, L. A., and Cohn, J. E.: A new cuvette for the spectrophotometric measurement of hemoglobin saturations. J. Lab. Clin. Med., **63**:355-358, 1964.

28. Feinberg, H., and Mary Alma, S.: Spectrophotometric determination of blood oxygen content. J. Lab. Clin. Med., **55**:784-789, 1960.

29. Fish, R. G., and Lee, M. R.: Technical and experimental errors in the spectrophotometric determination of oxygen saturation. J. Clin. Path., **16**:476-478, 1963.

30. Holling, H. E., MacDonald, I., O'Halloran, J. A., and Venner, A.: Reliability of a spectrophotometric method of estimating blood oxygen. J. Appl. Physiol., **8**:249-254, 1955.

31. Holmgren, A., and Pernow, B.: Spectrophotometric measurement of oxygen saturation of blood in the determination of cardiac output. A comparison with the Van Slyke method. Scand. J. Clin. Lab. Invest., **11**: 143-149, 1959.

32. Nahas, G. G.: Dosage spectrophotométrique rapide de l'hémoglobine et ed l'oxyhémoglobine. J. Physiol. (Paris), **47**:867-881, 1955.

33. Refsum, H. E., and Sveinsson, S. L.: Spectrophotometric determination of hemoglobin oxygen saturation in hemolyzed whole blood. Scand. J. Clin. Lab. Invest., **8**:67-70, 1956.

34. Roos, A., and Rich, J. A.: Spectrophotometric determination of oxyhemoglobin saturation and oxygen content of blood. J. Lab. Clin. Med., **40**:431-435, 1952.

35. Tsao, M. U., Sethna, S. S., Sloan, C. H., and Wyngarden, L. J.: Spectrophotometric determination of the oxygen saturation of whole blood. J. Biol. Chem., **217**:479-488, 1955.

36. Verel, D., Saynor, R., and Kesteven, A. B.: A spectrophotometric method of estimating blood oxygen using the Unicam SP 600. J. Clin. Path., **13**:361-363, 1960.

37. Lundsgaard, C., and Moller, E.: Investigations on oxygen content of cutaneous blood (so-called capillary blood). J. Exp. Med., **36**:559-573, 1922.

38. Lilienthal, J. L., and Riley, R. L.: On determination of arterial oxygen saturations from samples of "capillary blood." J. Clin. Invest., **23**:904-906, 1944.

39. Hultgren, H. N., and Hackett, A. J.: Determination of oxygen content of capillary blood in congenital heart disease. Pediatrics, **6**:93-97, 1950.

40. Naeraa, N.: Remarks on the clinical use of an oxygen saturation micromethod. Scand. J. Clin. Lab. Invest., **16**:45-48, 1964.

41. Torjussen, W.: Oxygen saturation in capillary blood. Scand. J. Clin. Lab. Invest., **17**: 505-507, 1965.

42. Dubowski, K. M.: Measurements of hemoglobin derivatives. In Sunderman. F. W.,
and Sunderman, F. W., Jr. (eds.): Hemoglobin
Its Precursors and Metabolites. Philadelphia,
Lippincott, 1964, pp. 49-60.

43. Dittmer, D. S. (ed.): Biological Handbooks:
Blood and Other Body Fluids. Washington,
FASEB, 1961, p. 169.

Serum Enzyme Alterations in Skeletal Muscle Diseases of Childhood

HAROLD M. PRICE, M.D. AND CARL M. PEARSON, M.D.

In some myopathic conditions, certain enzymes which normally reside within skeletal muscle fibers escape in excess quantities from the membranous confines of the diseased fibers to appear in abnormal amounts in the blood serum. Measurement of the levels of these serum enzymes has come to be one of three major diagnostically useful laboratory tools in many primary disorders of muscle. The other two are electromyography and the muscle biopsy[15].

The value of serum enzyme determinations was first suggested by Sibley and Lehninger in 1949[20]. While carrying out measurements of the activity of the enzyme aldolase in patients with various diseases, these workers noted an increase of the enzyme in the serum in two patients with muscular dystrophy. Since then, results of extensive investigations have been published by Schapira *et al.*[17] and many others on the serum levels of aldolase and several other enzymes in various muscle disorders. The enzymes found to be of greatest diagnostic value are the creatine phosphokinase (CPK)[5, 9], aldolase, the

transaminases (SGOT and SGPT)[6, 10] and lactic dehydrogenase (LDH)[17]. On the other hand, not all serum enzymes are increased in dystrophy and other myopathies, as pointed out by Dreyfus and Schapira[4]. Hence, such enzymes as alkaline and acid phosphatases, dipeptidases, cholinesterase and desoxyribonuclease are all normal.

Creatine phosphokinase is one of the most sensitive biochemical indicators of primary muscle disease, especially muscular dystrophy[5, 9]. It is also one of the most specific of the enzymes, normally being found in appreciable quantities only in skeletal muscle, heart muscle and brain tissue, whereas the other enzymes are more widely distributed in the tissues of the body[17]. Therefore, liver disease, pulmonary infarction and hemolysis do not produce confusing serum elevations of CPK activity. Although present in brain tissue, cerebral infarction almost never affects the serum level of this enzyme[17, 25]. The only significant source of conflict is in heart disease, particularly in the case of a myocardial infarction[8].

Aldolase, because it was the first

enzyme noted to be elevated in muscular disorders, has been the most extensively studied. For example, various conditions, such as hypoxia, which are known to increase membrane permeability, also show loss of aldolase from skeletal muscle[24]. Since aldolase occurs in very high concentrations in the sarcoplasm, its leakage into the serum from damaged muscle fibers has shown it to be a sensitive indicator of selected primary muscle disorders. Its serum levels are markedly elevated in polymyositis and almost as significantly elevated as CPK in Duchenne muscular dystrophy[1, 6, 12, 13, 17]. The most common source of conflict in the interpretation of aldolase elevations is in clinical conditions in which liver damage is present. Eventually it may be possible to avoid this source of error by measuring fructose-1-phosphate aldolase (which is almost specific for liver), in addition to the more usual fructose-1-6-diphosphate aldolase which is routinely analyzed[17].

When either CPK or aldolase determinations are not available, the next

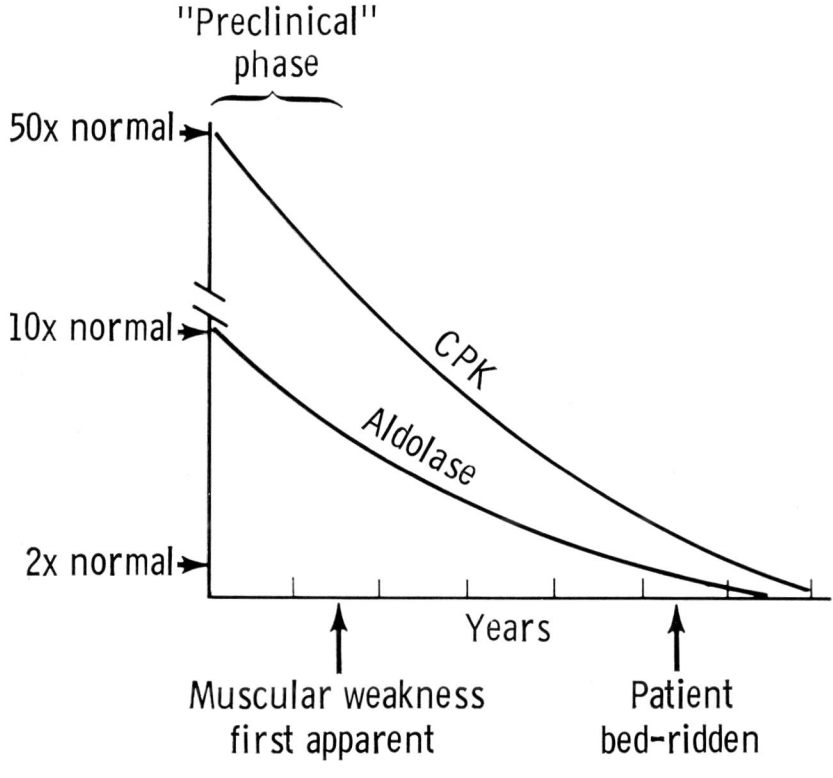

Fig. 1. General trend of serum levels of CPK and aldolase in "typical" case of Duchenne dystrophy. Serum transaminase and LDH values usually parallel aldolase curve. The serum enzyme values are most markedly elevated prior to the advent of clinically detectable muscular weakness. In the end stages of the disease, the CPK values often remain slightly elevated while the other serum enzyme values become normal.

most useful measurements of serum enzymes are those of the transaminases and lactic dehydrogenase. Like aldolase, they are also found in other tissues, but the serum levels of these enzymes in muscular dystrophy are usually less elevated and more variable[4, 12, 17]. The transaminases, however, are often as useful as aldolase and more so than CPK in evaluating cases of polymyositis[13].

DUCHENNE TYPE OF MUSCULAR DYSTROPHY

The most progressive and most common of the muscular dystrophies is the Duchenne type[12, 25]. This type is clinically manifested in the male and very rarely in the female, with onset often in the first five years of life, being transmitted usually as a sex-linked recessive character and, in rare instances, as an autosomal recessive trait. The usual course of the disease is one of relentless, rapid progression of muscle weakness, without arrest, leading to confinement in bed within ten years of onset, and death from a combination of extreme wasting and superimposed infection in the second decade. An occasional "benign" form of the disease may be seen in which the onset is later in life and the patient may retain some ability to walk twenty-five or thirty years after the onset.

The concentrations of the serum enzymes are greatest in the early stages of dystrophy and fall toward normal as the disease progresses (Figs. 1, 2 and 3)[4, 12, 17, 25]. Creatine phosphokinase values are usually elevated to the greatest extent, not uncommonly reaching levels greater than fifty times normal in the very early phases of the disease. The aldolase determination is the next

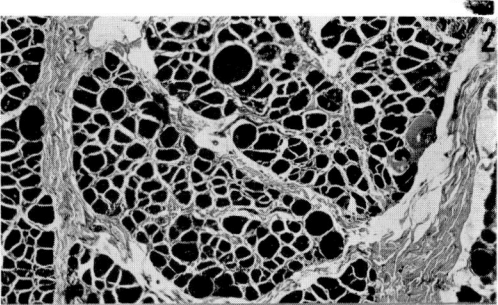

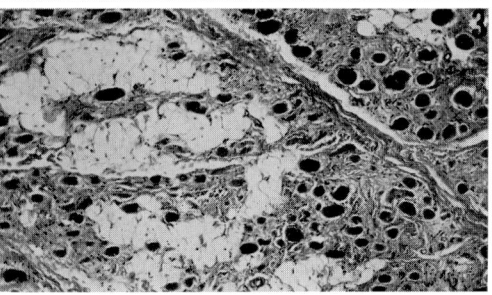

Fig. 2. Cross-section from the muscle biopsy of a five-year-old male with early clinical evidence of Duchenne pseudohypertrophic muscular dystrophy. There is an abnormal random variation in size of muscle fibers and slight endomysial connective tissue proliferation. These are features consistent with an early dystrophy. The serum CPK was forty times normal; aldolase ten times normal; transaminase eight times normal; and LDH five times normal. Masson trichrome stain; x 100.

Fig. 3. Typical histologic appearance in advanced stages of Duchenne dystrophy. There is prominent endomysial fibrosis and fat replacement. This ten-year-old child was bedridden with marked clinical evidence of muscle weakness. The CPK level was two to three times normal; all other serum enzyme values were normal. Hematoxlin and eosin stain; x 55.

most sensitive test, then the serum transaminases and lactic dehydrogenase. In the end stages of the disease, when ambulation becomes impossible, the CPK may remain slightly elevated, but the serum levels of the other enzymes are usually normal.

DETECTION OF PRECLINICAL DUCHENNE DYSTROPHY

The very high enzyme activities observed in the early clinical phases of muscular dystrophy led to the discovery that these biochemical sensors are also valuable diagnostic tools for the preclinical detection of this disease[4, 12]. Elevated enzyme values have been noted in a number of normal-appearing brothers of dystrophic boys. These apparently healthy siblings developed typical features of dystrophy within a short period (months to 1 to 3 years) after the enzyme elevations were found[12]. In a few, the preclinical period lasted for as long as six years, despite early evidence on muscle biopsy of the histopathologic characteristics of dystrophy in these children[11, 12].

DETECTION OF THE CARRIERS OF SEX-LINKED DUCHENNE DYSTROPHY

Reports of various investigators have now shown that serum enzyme measurements may be used to detect the female carriers of sex-linked Duchenne dystrophy[3, 12, 17, 18, 22, 23, 25]. Creatine phosphokinase has proved to be by far the most sensitive and specific enzyme indicator of these heterozygous carriers. The elevation of this enzyme in the carriers, however, is usually quite moderate in comparison to the levels reached in patients with the active disease.

Theoretically, all *known* carriers of the disease should show increased enzyme values, and approximately 50 per cent of all *possible* carriers (or female children of known carriers) should have elevated levels. In practice, results from various laboratories have demonstrated increased serum CPK activity in 60 to 90 per cent of *known* carriers and 33 to 50 per cent of *possible* carriers. The reason that female carriers of an x-chromosome trait can manifest partial disease has been attributed to the phenomenon of x-chromosome mosaicism[14]. Multiple serum CPK determinations taken after complete bed rest, during normal activity and after strenuous exertion appear to increase the precision of detecting the carriers[18, 22, 23].

Other abnormalities have also been demonstrated in female carriers. Electrical excitability studies of muscle have shown that the absolute refractory period is usually reduced[2], and muscle biopsies have sometimes revealed focal histopathologic changes[12, 25]. These techniques are obviously more difficult to perform on a routine basis, but could play a secondary role to enzyme determinations in genetic counseling where detection of the heterozygous female carrier of the Duchenne dystrophy gene is desirable.

OTHER TYPES OF MUSCULAR DYSTROPHY

In the limb-girdle type of muscular dystrophy, the CPK and aldolase are usually elevated in the early stages of the disease. The serum levels are, however, not usually as high as in Duchenne dystrophy, and the CPK determination is the more likely to be abnormal[12, 17, 25].

Serum enzyme levels are usually normal in the slowly evolving *facio-scapulo-humeral* variety of dystrophy. Occasionally, the CPK is moderately elevated early in the disease[12, 17, 25].

Most data indicate that the serum enzyme values are in the normal ranges in the rarer forms of muscular dystrophy, namely, the ocular type and the distal type[12, 17, 25].

POLYMYOSITIS

As in Duchenne dystrophy, serum enzyme values are also commonly elevated in polymyositis and dermatomyositis[1, 4, 6, 13]. Polymyositis is a degenerative inflammatory disease of skeletal muscle that results usually in proximal weakness, often in conjunction with dysphagia, weakness of the anterior neck muscles and, sometimes, weakness of the respiratory musculature. Childhood polymyositis usually has an associated typical skin rash, thus classifying it as dermatomyositis; however, the disease is less frequently found in children than in adults. Most of the experience gained in the measurement of serum enzymes has been in the adult cases; however, serum enzyme patterns in the childhood variant are probably not too dissimilar.

The serum enzyme elevations in polymyositis generally parallel the severity of the disease[1, 6, 13]. In the acute form, the serum enzyme values are usually very high, whereas in the more protracted cases, slightly elevated or even normal values may be found. In contrast to the dystrophies, the aldolase is a much more sensitive indicator of

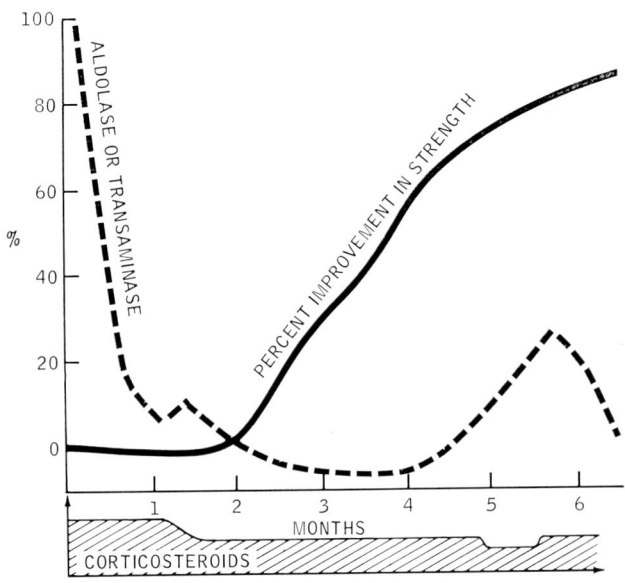

Fig. 4.   Serum enzyme pattern and clinical course of a patient with acute polymyositis on corticosteroid treatment over a six-month period. Dosage of corticosteroids was gradually lowered as the patient improved clinically. Notice latent period, six to eight weeks after start of therapy, before muscle strength improved. In this delay period, however, the serum aldolase and transaminase levels began to decline after the first two to three weeks. The gradual rise of the serum enzymes between the fifth and sixth month indicated that the corticosteroids were being reduced too rapidly and that a clinical relapse would follow if the dosage of the medication was not adjusted accordingly.

active disease than the CPK. The transaminases (GOT and GPT) are usually as useful an index of myopathic abnormalities as the aldolase in polymyositis. Creatine phosphokinase levels are unpredictable in this disease. They are relatively moderately elevated in comparison to the levels of that enzyme as found in dystrophy. They are usually proportional to the other enzymes.

Serum enzyme determinations have also been found useful in assessing the effects of corticosteroid treatment in polymyositis (Fig. 4)[6, 13]. Serial measurements of any enzyme whose serum level was initially found to be raised may be used. Following the administration of the initial high doses of corticosteroids there is often a latent period of six to eight weeks before muscle strength improves. Clinical improvement can be expected after this long latent period if serum enzyme levels begin to decline within two to three weeks after the corticosteroids are started. If the serum enzyme levels do not drop, it is often a sign that the corticosteroid dosage is inadequate and should be increased. Also, during the course of therapy, when the corticosteroid dosage is being lowered, a subsequent rise in serum enzyme values will usually precede a clinical relapse by several weeks, thus serving as a useful warning sign in the therapeutic management of the case.

Occasionally, the differential diagnosis between polymyositis and muscular dystrophy may be difficult in a child who has a slow and insidious onset of proximal muscle weakness without characteristic dermal lesions. In this situation a muscle biopsy is often a more helpful diagnostic test than serum enzyme determinations[15]. In general, however, both diagnostic procedures as well as the electromyogram complement each other in the final assessment of the patient.

OTHER NEUROMUSCULAR DISORDERS

Abnormal serum enzyme values do not occur in disorders in which muscle weakness and wasting are secondary to a neurogenic lesion[4, 6, 10, 17]. Even in acute neurogenic atrophy, such as acute and extensive poliomyelitis, the levels are normal[10]. Enzyme levels, therefore, may assume an important role in the differential diagnosis between muscular dystrophy or polymyositis and a neurogenic atrophy.

In myotonic dystrophy the increase in serum enzymes is moderate and inconstant[4, 12, 17]. Conflicting reports have appeared in patients with myopathies secondary to thyrotoxicosis or hypothyroidism. Generally, the levels are normal[6, 17]. No abnormal levels have been encountered in myasthenia gravis or steroid myopathy[6]. Moderate to very high elevations have been seen in paroxysmal myoglobinuria, crush injuries, surgical trauma and after excessive exercise in untrained individuals[6, 17].

"FLOPPY INFANT" SYNDROME

The syndrome of congenital or infantile hypotonia is usually attributed to one of the following disorders: Werdnig-Hoffmann disease (which results in a neurogenic atrophy)[7]; benign congenital hypotonia[21]; congenital muscular hypoplasia[21]; congenital muscular dystrophy[7, 21]; central-core disease[19]; or nemaline myopathy[16]. The muscle biopsy is usually the most useful diagnostic aid in this group of myopathic abnormalities[7, 15]. Serum enzyme levels can only be expected to be elevated in relatively rare, congenital muscular dystrophy, and then only mildly in degree.

REFERENCES

1. Barwick, D. D., and Walton, J. N.: Polymyositis. Amer J. Med., **35**:646-660, 1963.
2. Caruso, G., and Buchthal, F.: Refractory period of muscle and electromyographic findings in relatives of patients with muscular dystrophy. Brain, **88**:29-50, 1965.
3. Chung, C. S., Morton, N. E., and Peters, H. A.: Serum enzymes and genetic carriers in muscular dystrophy. Amer. J. Hum. Genet., **12**:52-66, 1960.
4. Dreyfus, J. C., and Schapira, G.: Biochemistry of Hereditary Myopathies. Springfield, Thomas, 1962.
5. Ebashi, S., Toyokura, Y., Momoi, H., and Sugita, H.: High creatine phosphokinase activity of sera of progressive muscular dystrophy. J. Biochem. (Tokyo), **46**:103, 1959.
6. Fowler, W. M., and Pearson, C. M.: Diagnostic and prognostic significance of serum enzymes. II. Neurological diseases other than muscular dystrophy. Arch. Phys. Med., **45**:125-130, 1964.
7. Greenfield, J. G., Cornman, T., and Shy, G. M.: Prognostic value of muscle biopsy in "floppy infant." Brain, **81**:461-484, 1958.
8. Hess, J. W., MacDonald, R. P., Frederick, R. J., Jones, R. N., Neely, J., and Gross, D.: Serum creatine phosphokinase activity in disorders of heart and skeletal muscle. Ann. Intern. Med., **61**:1015-1028, 1964.
9. Okinaka, S., Kumegi, H., Ebashi, S., Sugita, H., Momoi, H., Toyokura, Y., and Fujie, Y.: Serum creatine phosphokinase activity in progressive muscular dystrophy and neuromuscular diseases. Arch. Neurol. (Chicago), **4**:520-525, 1961.
10. Pearson, C. M.: Serum enzymes in muscular dystrophy and certain other muscular and neuromuscular disorders. I. Serum GOT. New Eng. J. Med., **256**:1069-1075, 1957.
11. Pearson, C. M.: Histopathological features of muscle in the preclinical stages of muscular dystrophy. Brain, **85**:109-120, 1962.
12. Pearson, C. M.: Muscular dystrophy. Review and recent observations. Amer. J. Med., **35**:632-645, 1963.
13. Pearson C. M.: Patterns of polymyositis and their responses to treatment. Ann. Intern. Med., **59**:827-838, 1963.
14. Pearson, C. M., Fowler, W. M., and Wright, S. W.: X-chromosome mosaicism in females with muscular dystrophy. Proc. Nat. Acad. Sci. U.S.A., **50**:24-31, 1963.
15. Pearson, C. M., and Price, H. M.: Muscle biopsy: why? how? and when? Hosp. Med., **4**:34-38, 1966.
16. Price, H. M., Gordon, G. B., Pearson, C. M., Munsat, T. L., and Blumberg, J. M.: New evidence for excessive accumulation of Z-band material in nemaline myopathy. Proc. Nat. Acad. Sci. U.S.A., **54**:1398-1406, 1965.
17. Schapira, G., and Dreyfus, J. C.: Biochemistry of progressive muscular dystrophy. In Bourne, G. H., and Golarz, M. N. (eds.): Muscular Dystophy in Man and Animals. New York, Hafner, 1963, pp. 48-87.
18. Schapira, F., Demos, J., Schapira, G., and Dreyfus, J. C.: The value of serum enzyme determinations in the identification of dystrophic carriers. Conference on Experimental Primary Myopathies and their Relationship to Human Muscle Diseases. N.Y. Acad. Sci., November 18-19, 1965.
19. Shy, G. M., and Magee, K. R.: A new congenital nonprogressive myopathy. Brain, **79**:610-621, 1956.
20. Sibley, J. A., and Lehninger, A. L.: Aldolase in serum and tissues of tumor-bearing animals. J. Nat. Cancer Inst., **9**:303-309, 1949.
21. Walton, J. N. (ed.): Disorders of Voluntary Muscle. London, Churchill, 1964.
22. Walton, J. N., and Pennington, R. J. T.: Studies of human muscular dystrophy with particular reference to methods of carrier detection. Conference on Experimental Primary Myopathies and their Relationship to Human Muscle Diseases, op. cit.
23. Wilson, K. M., Evans, K. A., and Carter, C. O.: Creatine kinase levels in women who carry genes for three types of muscular dystrophy. Brit. Med. J., **1**:750-753, 1965.
24. Zierler, K. L.: Diffusion of aldolase from rat skeletal muscle. An index of membrane permeability. Amer. J. Physiol., **190**:201-205, 1957.
25. Zundel, W. S., and Tyler, F. H.: The muscular dystrophies. New Eng. J. Med., **273**:537-601, 1965.

Measurement of Serum Creatine Phosphokinase and Aldolase

Serum Creatine Phosphokinase (Modified Method of Duma and Siegel [1])

WELLS R. MOOREHEAD, Ph.D., AND JON V. STRAUMFJORD, JR., M.D., Ph.D.

INTRODUCTION

Creatine phosphokinase (CPK) is localized almost exclusively in skeletal and cardiac muscle cells. In the muscle cell, CPK catalyzes the phosphorylation of creatine by the following reversible reaction:

$$\text{creatine} + \text{ATP} \rightleftharpoons \underset{\text{CPK}}{} \text{creatine phosphate} + \text{ADP}$$

The level of serum creatine phosphokinase (SCPK) has been observed to be significantly elevated in many patients suffering from muscular disorders[1-3].

PRINCIPLE

Serum is incubated for thirty minutes at 37 C in a medium containing creatine phosphate and ADP. If SCPK is present in the serum, ADP is phosphorylated and free creatine is liberated. The reaction is stopped by the addition of p-hydroxymercuribenzoic acid, and the serum proteins are precipitated with NaOH and $ZnSO_4$. The precipitate is subsequently removed from the supernatant liquid by centrifugation. Alkaline a-naphthol and diacetyl are added to the supernatant liquid, and the mixture is incubated at 37 C for twenty minutes. In an alkaline medium, free creatine reacts with a-naphthol and diacetyl to produce a reddish color which is measured at 540 mμ.

REAGENTS

1. *Buffer*, 0.5 M. Into a 100 ml volumetric flask is transferred 3.4 gm of imidazole. Magnesium sulfate heptahydrate, 0.370 gm (0.015 M) and mercaptoethanol, 0.42 ml (0.06 M) are also added to the same volumetric flask. The material is dissolved and diluted to volume with distilled water. The pH is adjusted to 6.8 with acetic acid.

2. *Phospocreatine*, 0.015 M. Into a 100 ml volumetric flask is transferred 0.5 gm of disodium phosphocreatine

tetrahydrate. It is diluted to volume with distilled water and stored frozen if it is not to be used at once.

3. *Adenosine diphosphate*, 0.008 M. Into a 100 ml volumetric flask is transferred 0.4 gm of monosodium adenosine-5'-diphosphate dihydrate. It is diluted with distilled water and stored frozen if it is not be used at once.

4. *Premixed substrate*. Reagent solutions 1, 2, 3 (100 ml of each) are added to a flask containing 100 ml of distilled water and thoroughly mixed. The pH is adjusted to 6.8 by adding either dilute HCl or dilute NaOH. The premixed substrate is then poured into small bottles (about 25 ml per bottle) and stored frozen. Unused portions of the premixed substrate may be refrozen and reused until there is evidence of creatine in the blank.

5. *p-Hydroxymercuribenzoic acid*, 0.03 M. Into a 100 ml volumetric flask is placed 1.02 gm of p-hydroxymercuribenzoic acid. To this is added 25 ml of 1 N NaOH. Mixing is carried out until the material dissolves. One N HCl is added until a slight but permanent precipitate is formed which persists with shaking. Upon dilution to volume with distilled water, the precipitate should dissolve and the solution should be clear.

6. *Sodium hydroxide*, 0.5 N. Into a liter volumetric flask is placed 20.0 gm of NaOH pellets. The material is dissolved and diluted to volume with distilled water.

7. *Zinc sulfate heptahydrate*, 0.348 M. Into a liter volumetric flask is transferred 100.0 gm of $ZnSO_4 \cdot 7H_2O$. The material is dissolved and diluted to volume with distilled water. The zinc sulfate solution is adjusted so that titra-

tion of equal volumes of 0.5 N sodium hydroxide and zinc sulfate just gives a pink color using phenolphthalein as indicator.

8. *Stock alkali*. Into a 1 liter volumetric flask are transferred 60 gm of NaOH and 128 gm of Na_2CO_3. The material is dissolved in distilled water and diluted to volume.

9. *a-Naphthol*. Just before use, 0.8 gm of a-naphthol is dissolved in 10 ml of stock alkali solution and filtered.

10. *Diacetyl* (2,3-butandione). To 100 ml of distilled water is added 0.05 ml of diacetyl.

STANDARD SOLUTIONS

Standard creatine (1.7 μ moles per ml). To a 100 ml volumetric flask is added 25.3 mg of creatine monohydrate which is subsequently dissolved in distilled water and diluted to volume.

PROCEDURE

One ml of premixed substrate is added to each test tube (*test, reagent blank and standard*). Then, to the *test* is added 0.1 ml of serum; to the *reagent blank* is added 0.1 ml of distilled water; and to the *standard* is added 0.1 ml of standard creatine (1.7 μ moles per ml.). After mixing, each tube is immediately placed in a water bath and incubated at 37 C. for exactly thirty minutes. The reaction is stopped by adding 0.5 ml of the p-hydroxymercuribenzoate solution and mixing thoroughly. Next, 0.5 ml of the NaOH solution is added followed by 0.5 ml of the $ZnSO_4 \cdot 7H_2O$ solution. Mixing is again carried out, and the tubes are then centrifuged at high speed for at least fifteen minutes. To 0.5 ml of supernatant liquid, 1.0

ml of the freshly prepared a-naphthol solution is added and mixed. Next, 0.5 ml of the diacetyl reagent is added and thoroughly mixed. Each tube (*test, reagent blank* and *standard*) is then incubated in the water bath at 37 C. for twenty minutes to develop the color.

After color development 3 ml of water are added to each tube, mixed, decanted into a small colorimeter tube, and measured at 540 mμ.

The calculation is as follows:

$$\text{units} = \frac{\text{reading of test}}{\text{reading of standard}} \times 1.7 \times 2 = \mu \text{ mole creatine}$$

formed per milliliter of serum per hour (1 unit = 1 μ mole creatine formed per milliliter of serum per hour at 37 C).

DISCUSSION

Normally, SCPK levels are low, but SCPK levels are generally elevated in patients suffering from disorders affecting muscle tissue.

The outlined procedure provides a relatively simple and rapid method for measuring SCPK levels. Since CPK is localized almost exclusively in skeletal and cardiac muscle cells, this method serves as a rather specific diagnostic tool for determining whether or not muscle injury has occurred.

Reference serums can be stored frozen for as much as two months with little or no loss in SCPK activity.

SOURCES OF ERROR

Since this is an enzymatic reaction, the period of incubation must be measured accurately if correct results are to be obtained. The reaction will proceed at a reduced rate at room temperature, so it is essential that incubation be started as soon as the serum is added to the premixed substrate.

RANGE OF VALUES

Normal range = 0.3 to 3.0 units.

RESUME OF CLINICAL INTERPRETATIONS

The practical clinical application of serum creatine phosphokinase is chiefly limited to the differential diagnosis of musculoskeletal disease and myocardial infarction.

Significant elevations of SCPK activity (approximately 5 to 50 times upper limit of normal) have been reported for all types of progressive muscular dystrophy with most pronounced increases in the Duchenne type[3]. The extent of the elevation of SCPK is related to the time-activity of the disease. As the muscular dystrophy progresses, a gradual decrease in SCPK is noted. Patients with myotonic dystrophy motor neuron disease, poliomyelitis, polyneuritis and myasthenia gravis have normal or insignificant elevations.

The increase in SCPK activity associated with myocardial infarction approximates eight times the upper limit of normal one to three days after onset of pain[1]. The elevated activity often remains for six to ten days following infarction. Increased SCPK has also been reported with dissecting aortic aneurysms.

Increased SCPK activity has also been reported with hypothyroidism[4]. The extent of elevation appears to be related to duration of hypothyroidism. The activity of SCPK returns to normal when the patient becomes euthyroid. Not all hypothyroid individuals demonstrate increased SCPK activity, but, if elevated in an individual patient, it is a helpful adjunct to diagnosis and judging therapeutic response.

REFERENCES

1. Duma, R. J., and Siegel, A. L.: Serum creatine phosphokinase in acute myocardial infarction. Arch. Intern. Med., 115:443-451, 1965.

2. Hughes, B. P.: A method for the estimation of serum creatine kinase and its use in comparing creatine kinase and aldolase activity in normal and pathological sera. Clin. Chim. Acta, 7:597-603, 1962.

3. Okinaka, S., et. al.: Serum creatine phosphokinase activity in progressive muscular dystrophy and neuromuscular diseases. Arch. Neurol. (Chicago), 4:520-525, 1961.

4. Craig, F. A., and Ross, G. R.: Serum creatine-phosphokinase in thyroid disease. Metabolism, 12:57-59, 1963.

Serum Aldolase (Modified Method of Friedman and Lapan [6])

INTRODUCTION

Aldolase is an enzyme normally found in low concentration in serum, but in high concentration in most tissues of the body. It takes part in the intermediary breakdown of glucose at the level of fructose-1,6-diphosphate into glyceraldehyde-3-phosphate and dihydroxyacetone phosphate. Elevation in serum aldolase levels have been reported in various disorders including myopathies[3], acute myocardial infarction[4] and prostatic cancer[1, 2].

PRINCIPLE

Serum is incubated for sixty minutes at 37 C in a medium containing fructose-1,6-diphosphate. The reaction is as follows:

tone phosphate and glyceraldehyde-3-phosphate. This prevents the disappearance of the reaction products due to the presence of other enzymes in the serum. The presence of iodoacetate also inhibits the action of glyceraldehyde-3-phosphate dehydrogenase.

The reaction products are hydrolyzed at room temperature with alkali to the corresponding trioses. Next, the trioses are converted to 2,4-dinitrophenylhydrazones upon the addition of 2,4-dinitrophenylhydrazine. Then, after making the mixture alkaline, the characteristic color of the phenylhydrazones is formed.

REAGENTS

1. *Fructose-1,6-diphosphate*, 0.05 M. Exactly 0.22 gm of fructose-1,6-diphosphate (sodium salt) is weighed and

$$\text{fructose-1,6-diphosphate} \xrightleftharpoons{\text{aldolase}} \begin{array}{c} \text{dihydroxyacetone phosphate} \\ + \\ \text{glyceraldehyde-3-phosphate} \end{array}$$

Hydrazine is also present in the reaction mixture to combine with the products of the forward reaction, dihydroxyace-

made up to 10 ml with distilled water. This solution should be stored frozen.

2. *Hydrazine*, 0.56 M. Exactly 7.28

gm of hydrazine sulfate are suspended in 50 ml of distilled water and adjusted to pH 7.4 with NaOH. The solution is then diluted to 100 ml with distilled water. This solution may be stored at room temperature.

3. *γ-Collidine buffer*, 0.1 M. Exactly 1.21 gm (about 1.32 ml) of γ-collidine (2,4,6-trimethylpyridine) is dissolved in 50 ml of distilled water. The pH is adjusted to 7.4 with HCl, and the solution is diluted to 100 ml with distilled water. The buffer is stored in the refrigerator.

4. *Iodoacetic acid*, 0.002 M. Exactly 40 mg of iodoacetic acid are dissolved in 50 ml of distilled water, adjusted to pH 7.4 with dilute NaOH, and diluted to 100 ml with distilled water. It is stored in the refrigerator.

5. *2,4-Dinitrophenylhydrazine.* Exactly 0.1 gm of 2,4-dinitrophenylhydrazine is dissolved in 100 ml of 2N HCl. The solution should be protected from light and stored in the refrigerator.

6. *Sodium hydroxide*, 0.75 N. Thirty gm of anhydrous sodium hydroxide are dissolved in distilled water and diluted to 1 liter.

7. *Trichloroacetic acid*, 10 per cent. Ten gm of trichloroacetic acid are dissolved in 50 ml of distilled water and diluted to 100 ml.

STANDARD CURVE

For preparing the standard curve, a standard stock solution of dihydroxyacetone is prepared by dissolving 200 mg of dihydroxyacetone in 100 ml of distilled water. The stock solution of 2 mg per ml is kept in the refrigerator for forty-eight to seventy-two hours to complete depolymerization[5]. The following concentrations (mg per ml) of dihydroxyacetone are then prepared from the stock solution and distilled water: 0, 0.2, 0.4, 0.6, 0.8, 1.0, 1.2, 1.4, 1.6, 1.8 and 2.0 mg per ml.

In preparing the standard curve, the procedure is the same as that used for serum except that 1 ml of the various concentrations of dihydroxyacetone is substituted for 1 ml of serum. After color development, the various standard concentrations for dihydroxyacetone are read in a photometer at 540 mμ.

Friedman and Lapan[6] have defined the "dihydroxyacetone unit" as the amount of color developed by 0.01 mg of dihydroxyacetone under the conditions of their procedure. Consequently, the standard curve has a range from 0 to 200 dihydroxyacetone units.

PROCEDURE

The reactants are added to a test tube in the following order: 1.0 ml of collidine buffer; 1.0 ml of serum; 0.25 ml of hydrazine; 0.25 ml of iodoacetate; and 0.25 ml of fructose-1,6-diphosphate substrate. Fructose-1,6-diphosphate is omitted from the blank during incubation. The sample and blank are incubated for sixty minutes at 37 C, and the reaction is stopped by the addition of 5 ml of 10 per cent trichloroacetic acid. Fructose-1,6-diphosphate, 0.25 ml, is now added to the blank. The tubes are then centrifuged until the supernatant liquid is clear.

The supernatant liquid from the sample and blank are then treated as follows: to 1.0 ml of supernatant liquid is added 1.0 ml of 0.75 N NaOH, and it is left at room temperature for ten minutes. Then 1.0 ml of 2,4-dinitrophenylhydrazine is added, and both the sample and the blank are incubated at 37 C for sixty minutes. Finally, 7.0 ml of 0.75 N NaOH are added, and each tube is thoroughly mixed. After five minutes the material is decanted into a colorimeter tube and read at 540 mμ. All tubes should be read within fifteen minutes after the addition of NaOH, for the color that is produced fades with time.

Serum aldolase activity is determined from the standard curve.

DISCUSSION

Normally, the concentration of serum aldolase is low, but it may be greatly elevated in patients suffering from tissue damage. Aldolase is present in many body tissues in high concentration. As a result, the study of this enzyme can not pinpoint specifically the site of tissue damage.

SOURCES OF ERROR

As in all enzymatic reactions, the period of incubation must be measured accurately if correct results are to be obtained. The color produced is not stable and must be read not later than fifteen minutes after it is developed. Since the activity of aldolase is relatively greater in erythrocytes and platelets, hemolysis will give spuriously high values.

RANGE OF VALUES

Normal range = 6 to 20 dihydroxy-acetone units.

RESUME OF CLINICAL INTERPRETATIONS

Increased serum activity of aldolase has been considered one of the most useful biochemical tests for the differential diagnosis of skeletal muscular disease. Activities of serum aldolase from two to fourteen times the upper limit of normal have been reported with progressive muscular dystrophy. The most pronounced alterations are associated with the Duchenne type. Significant increases have not been reported with myotonia dystrophy, motor neuron disease, poliomyelitis or myasthenia gravis. Thus, serum aldolase provides useful information for the differential diagnosis of muscle disease. The specificity of aldolase for myopathies, however, appears to be less than serum creatine phosphokinase, as significant elevations of aldolase have been reported associated with neoplasia and liver disease[9]. Since serum creatine phosphokinase differentiates muscular disease, as well as aldolase, it would appear to be the current method of choice[9].

The normal values for aldolase during the childhood period are slightly higher than for adults. This is most pronounced in the neonatal period, when the normal values are approximately twice that of adults[7]. It is also of interest that the serum activity of fructose-1 phosphate aldolase is moderately decreased, and fructose-1 phosphate aldolase is not detected in children with Tay-Sachs' disease[8].

REFERENCES

1. Baker, R., and Govan, D.: The effect of hormonal therapy of prostatic cancer on serum aldolase. Cancer Res., 13:141-146, 1953.
2. Baker, R., et. al.: Biological titration of diethylstilbestrol against activity of prostatic cancer: Effect on serum aldolase. J. Clin. Endocr., 13:383-391, 1953.
3. Dreyfus, J. C., Schapira, G., and Schapira, F.: Biochemical study of muscle in progressive muscular dystrophy. J. Clin. Invest., 33:794-797. 1954.
4. Volk, B. W., et. al.: The serum aldolase level

in acute myocardial infarction. Amer. J. Med. Sci., **232**:38-43, 1956.

5. Beck, W. S.: Determination of triose phosphates and proposed modifications in the aldolase method of Sibley and Lehninger. J. Biol. Chem., **212**:847-857, 1955.

6. Friedman, M., and Lapan, B.: Serum aldolase in the neonatal period: Including a colorimetric determination of aldolase by standardization with dihydroxyacetone. J. Lab. Clin. Med., **51**:745-752, 1958.

7. Emanuel, B., West, M., and Zimmerman, H. J.: Serum enzymes in disease. Amer. J. Dis. Child., **105**:261-264, 1963.

8. Volk, B. W., Aronson, S. M., and Saifer, A.: Fructose-1 phosphate aldolase deficiency in Tay-Sachs' disease. Amer. J. Med., **36**:481-484, 1964.

9. Okinaka, S., et. al.: Serum creatine phosphokinase activity in progressive muscular dystrophy and neuromuscular diseases. Arch. Neurol. (Chicago), **4**:520-525, 1961.

Chapter 37

Clinical Indications for Cytogenetic Investigations

ROBERT C. NORTHCUTT, M.D.

In so young a laboratory specialty as clinical cytogenetics, no definite rules regarding the indications for chromosome studies have been established, and numerous factors may play a part in the decision to perform such a study. Although a relatively time-consuming procedure, it may provide unique advantages in obtaining useful clinical information which cannot be acquired by other means. In addition to research applications into the behavior of the chromosomes under a variety of experimental conditions, the cytogenetic techniques are becoming more widely available as clinical tools.

Although having some of the characteristics of a standard laboratory test in producing numbers, X's, Y's and a photograph of the patient's chromosome, a chromosome analysis is in actuality a diagnostic procedure akin more to a biopsy or autopsy. It is a pathological examination requiring the direct attention of a qualified professional person, and the decision to perform such a study should be in the hands of this individual.

Little *contra*indication exists to performing a chromosome analysis, since usually only a blood sample is required, which should not present a problem of inconvenience or discomfort to the patient. What are the indications? In other chapters of these proceedings are presented many of the specific "chromosomal" syndromes with which a working knowledge is extremely important to provide a competent consultation[5, 7, 9]. On occasion, the clinical findings may be misleading, or the pathologist is confronted with a situation which is not typical of a defined syndrome. As with all diagnostic procedures, questions must be asked regarding the usefulness of the results obtained. Little would be added to the management of an individual with multiple severe birth defects, but since the possibility of a hereditary chromosomal defect may exist, the study may be indicated. The value of positive information here lies in more intelligent family counseling in regard to recurrence or risk in subsequent children and perhaps to prognosis. At other times, due to intercurrent complications, a well-known disease may manifest itself in an unusual manner. To avoid more time-consuming or hazardous procedures, the cytogenetic studies may provide the necessary diagnostic information.

A "wish to know" or "academic interest" has provided the impetus for most studies done to date, and from such experience almost all our guidelines to the most productive employment of cytogenetic investigation has been obtained. This also, if reasonable, remains an indication. The following brief case presentations will be used to illustrate some of these considerations.

Case I, D.E.E.

The patient, a 2-month-old male infant was referred to the outpatient department of the U.S. Naval Hospital for confirmation of a clinical diagnosis of mongolism. The child was the product of an uncomplicated pregnancy, labor and delivery, and weighed 6 lbs, 10 oz at birth. The mother at the time of delivery was 22 and the father 24 years of age. A clinical diagnosis of mongolism was made shortly after birth on the basis of facies, simian lines, short 5th metacarpals, a cardiac murmur and hypotonia.

Chromosome analysis was performed on the patient and both parents; no siblings were available for study. The patient had forty-six chromosomes with what was felt to be a D/G or 13-15/21 translocation type of mongolism. The mother had only forty-five chromosomes, but also exhibited the translocation chromosome. The father's karyotype was normal.

This case represents an example from an ongoing survey of infants with mongolism born to young mothers. The survey is being done in cooperation with the Department of Pediatrics at the U.S. Naval Hospital in Bethesda. These children are studied because of the known higher incidence of translocation type familial mongolism born

to young mothers under twenty-five than to those over thirty-five years of age[8]. This study was performed partly on the basis of investigational interest and partly to provide more informative family counseling, and the parents were more intelligently advised of the probability of having additional mongol children. With this particular translocation (D/G or 13 15/21), the probability of the marriage to produce a mongol offspring is about 25 to 30 per cent if the carrier parent is the mother and about 5 per cent if the father[8]. This case illustrates the higher-risk type of marriage.

Case II, B.B.L.

The patient was a 7 lb male infant born at 36 weeks gestation complicated by intermittent vaginal bleeding from the 12th week. This was the third pregnancy for this 28-year-old Korean mother and 30-year-old Caucasian father; the first two pregnancies produced healthy normal children. This delivery was spontaneous and conducted under saddle block anesthesia with a total duration of 5 hours, 55 minutes, the early stages of labor being managed with scopalamine and meperidine. At birth, regular unassisted respiration was delayed for 3 to 5 minutes, but hypoxia was prevented. Muscle tone at birth was considered poor, with facies suggestive of mongolism, but not entirely typical. Complete physical examination upon admission to the nursery confirmed these findings. No murmur was present, and, except for the extremities and facies, the examination was essentially normal. No simian crease or high triradii were present in the palms, but short 5th metacarpals and clinodactyly of the 5th fingers were noted. Neurological examination at that time was normal. X-ray examination of the chest was normal, and hand films confirmed the clinical impression of hypoplastic 5th metacarpals.

Because of the suspicion of mongolism and the absence of reliable clinical findings, a chromosome analysis was performed. A chromosome number of forty-seven was found, with an extra chromosome in the small acrocentric group which was compatible with a 21-trisomy. Followup outpatient visits revealed more typical mongol features, and the clinical syndrome is now apparent.

This represents a case with suspect but inconclusive findings at the time of study for the clinical diagnosis of mongolism. The finding of a trisomy in the small acrocentric group consistent with 21 trisomy, and subsequent clinical observations of mental retardation confirmed the diagnosis. The potential confusion which might result from such a child of Oriental parentage as in this situation provides an example of the value of the cytogenetic study of such patients.

Case III, L.L.H.

The patient, an 18-year-old Caucasian female was admitted for evaluation of secondary amenorrhea. History reveals a thelarche at age 10 years, pubarche at age 11, and irregular menses beginning at age 13 and continuing for two years. The patient had reached her present height of 58 inches by age ten with no subsequent growth.

Outpatient evaluation, two years prior to this admission, was essentially negative including a chromatin positive vaginal smear. She was placed on estrogen-progesterone cyclic therapy and regular menstruation resulted.

Three months prior to admission this regimen was discontinued and amenorrhea ensued.

The patient's general medical history was noncontributory and physical examination was that of a normal postpubertal female exhibiting only short stature.

X rays revealed a normal bone maturation without osteoporosis. PBI, urinary steroids and routine laboratory studies were all within normal limits. Urinary gonadotrophins were significantly elevated.

Buccal smear examination was chromatin negative on two occasions; a repeat vaginal smear was chromatin positive. Cytogenetic analysis revealed a mosaic chromosome complement with two cell lines, one 45/XO, the other 46/XX. Final diagnosis was probable gonadal dysgenesis with chromosomal mosaicism. Further mosaicism with a third karyotype 47/XXX was postulated but was not found.

It is well known that mosaicism is frequently seen in cases of gonadal dysgenesis[1, 3, 9] and that the clinical presentation may appear to be modified by the presence of multiple cell lines. A confusing diagnostic problem existed with conflicting mucosal smear reports until the chromosome analysis provided an explanation for this inconsistency.

Case IV, A.W.B.

The patient, a healthy 15-year-old female, was referred by a gynecologist by whom she had been seen for primary amenorrhea. Examination revealed a normal teenage female except for vaginal hypoplasia. A family history revealed the patient to be the oldest of four children (all girls), but no similar history could be elicited in the family background. The testicular feminization syndrome was suspected, and it was for this reasons that cytogenetic consultation was requested. A buccal smear was performed on the patient and her three siblings, all of which were chromatin positive. The patient's karyotype was that of a normal female.

Following the descriptions of the testicular feminization syndrome and its associated male sex chromosome complement[4], gynecologists became quite aware of the high probability of this syndrome in "all female" sibships and in cases of vaginal hypoplasia. Here both bits of leading information were present, and the chromosome analysis and buccal smear examinations proved to be useful negative information.

Case V, C.H.W.

A 34-year-old white male presented himself for a followup evaluation for leukocytosis and a biologic false-positive serology. Positive physical findings on admission revealed only mild splenomegaly and a low-grade fever. Hemograms and bone marrow examinations were interpreted as compatible with either a leukemoid reaction or chronic myelogenous leukemia. Chest film showed no evidence of active pulmonary disease, but parenchymal calcifications were present. Skin tests were positive for histoplasmin and tuberculin. The leukocyte alkaline phosphatase was normal and the white blood cell count was 40,000 to 50,000 per cu mm. Sputum smears and cultures were positive for M. tuberculosis. Documentation of the patient's wife having active tuberculosis was obtained subsequently. The patient was begun on INH,PAS and streptomycin with a subsequent fall in the white count to 30,000 per cu

mm. At this time, a bone marrow was obtained for chromosome analysis, and the Philadelphia chromosome (Ph^1) was found in over 80 per cent of suitable cells.

After two months of anti-tuberculous therapy, the WBC rose to 110,000 per cu mm, and patient then was placed on Myeleran therapy. Subsequent sputum cultures have reverted to negative. The leucocyte count is being maintained at a level of 20,000 to 30,000 per cu mm.

Without the bone marrow examination for the Philadelphia chromosome, diagnosis of the leukemia would have been delayed, although only several weeks in this particular case. Prior to the description and definition of the Ph^1 chromosome[2], the differentiation of a leukemoid from a leukemic reaction was difficult, and the simultaneous diagnosis of chronic myelogenous leukemia and tuberculosis required either treatment of the tuberculosis with the failure to observe a return to normal of the hematologic status or to follow the patient until the development of full-blown clinical leukemia with the white blood count rising to the 80,000 per cu mm range.

DISCUSSION

The role of chromosome analysis in the aforementioned cases has been presented to illustrate certain rather specific situations in which the techniques have been clinically valuable. Unfortunately, such definite situations do not always exist, and the physician responsible for the studies must, following a review the clinical findings with the clinician, determine whether the effort, time and expense involved will provide useful information. The commitment to study a patient may also result in studying several family members.

Case I, a family study, serves to emphasize the use of chromosome studies in selected populations of high risk as a screening technique. The probability of obtaining diagnostic information may be as high as 16 per cent in mongolism if mosaicism is also sought[2]. The indications for study in this case fell into a previously determined protocol which, as time goes on, is becoming part of the routine studies at medical centers. In addition to pointing out the problem of mongolism in a child of Oriental parentage, Case II serves to illustrate the use of cytogenetic studies in the newborn period using little modification of the peripheral blood leukocyte technique when only small quantities of blood are available. (The author has obtained adequate cultures of heart blood from an 87 gm abortus using less than 0.5 ml of whole blood).

The final three cases are examples of the use of the reasonably predictable alternative cytogenetic findings in selecting these patients for study. Enough information was available and the possible cytogenetic findings as they might contribute to the patient's diagnosis and management could be discussed prior to study. Case III is a case of early secondary amenorrhea in a short but otherwise normally developed young girl. The possible karyotypes other than a normal one were those associated with atypical Turner's syndrome[1, 3], and the ones found were highly probable. Although the diagnosis of chronic myelogenous leukemia would have been made

in due time, more careful observations of the patient's hematology were made following diagnosis. Anti-leukemic therapy was readily instituted as the clinical indications arose. Testicular feminization carries with it the hazard of increased incidence of malignancy of the undecended testes. Ultimately, it would require a laporatomy for prophylactic castration and subsequent hormonal replacement therapy. Abdominal exploration in Case IV was thus avoided.

REFERENCES

1. CourtBrown, W. M., Harnden, D. G., Jacobs, P. A., Maclean, N., and Mantle, D. J.: Abnormalities of the Sex Chromosome Couplement in Man. Privy Council, Medical Research Council, Special Report Series No. 305. London, HMSO, 1964, pp. 161-179.
2. Day, R. W., Wright, S. W.: Down's syndrome at young maternal ages: Chromosomal and family studies. J. Pediat., 66:764-769, 1965.
3. Engel, E., and Forbes, A. P.: Cytogenic and clinical findings in 48 patients with congentally defective or absent ovaries. Medicine (Balt.), 44:135-164, 1965.
4. Jacobs, P. A., Baikie, A. G., CourtBrown, W. M., Forrest, H., Roy, J. R., Stewart, J. S., and Lennox, B.: Chromosomal sex in the syndrome of testicular feminisation. Lancet, 2:591-592, 1959.
5. LaPolla, J. J.: The cat cry syndrome and other chromosomal aberrations in the newborn. Proc. Ass. Clin. Sci., 1965.
6. Northcutt, R. C.: The Role of Cytogenetics in the Field of Mental Retardation and Birth Defect. Presented 29 October, 1965, to American Association on Mental Deficiency, Mid-Eastern Region IX, Annual Meeting, Washington, D. C.
7. Nowell, P. C.: Chromosomal abnormalities in the childhood leukemias; the Philadelphia chromosome. Proc. Ass. Clin. Sci., 1965.
8. Peterson, C. D., and Luzzatti, L.: The role of chromosome translocation in the recurrence risk of Down's Syndrome. Pediatrics, 35:463-469, 1965.
9. Ross, G. T.: Cytogenetics in clinical endocrinology of infancy. Proc. Ass. Clin. Sci., 1965.

Chapter 38

Cytogenetics in Clinical Endocrinology of Infancy and Childhood

GRIFF T. ROSS, M.D., Ph.D., AND J. H. TJIO, Ph.D.

INTRODUCTION

Endocrinopathies known to be associated with abnormalities of chromosome number and morphology (abnormalities of the karyotype) are rarely if ever evident clinically during infancy and childhood, since most of these present as hypogonadal states. However, many of the anomalies of growth and development associated with karyotypic abnormalities may be observed in infants and children under circumstances in which an endocrinopathy enters into the differential diagnosis. Studies of the chromosomal constitution of accessible cells from such patients are an essential part of clinical evaluation.

Methods used, indications for investigation and limitations of usefulness of cytogenetic studies in patients suspected of having endocrine disease in the pediatric age group will be considered in this chapter.

METHODS

The objective of all methodology in cytogenetic studies is an adequate amount of material suitable for evaluation. This is no less true for those whose interest is purely diagnostic than for those whose objective is purely investigative. For both the clinician and the investigator, it is important to remember that evaluation of nuclear sex and study of the karyotype constitute only a part of a complete cytogenetic study. Requirements for a complete study have been considered elsewhere[15].

METHODS USED IN DETERMINING NUCLEAR SEX

Polymorphonuclear Leucocytes

Nuclear appendages called drumsticks can be seen in polymorphonuclear leucocytes in stained films of peripheral blood[3]. These occur with greater frequency in cells containing two or more X-chromosomes than in cells containing only one X-chromosome[12]. For the inexperienced, differentiation of drumsticks from other appendages is difficult. In addition, the percentage of cells having nuclei with such an appendage is low, so that careful examination of large numbers of cells is required. Therefore, this procedure is not recommended and will not be discussed in detail.

Nuclei of Other Cells

The study of chromatin masses of chromocenters found in interphase (not dividing) nuclei of cells from somatic tissues constitutes the basis for the evaluation of nuclear sex. The material usually studied consists of stained spread films of exfoliated epithelial cells from buccal mucosa[13]. In such preparations, one looks for a morphologically distinct chromatin mass, most commonly located at the periphery of the nucleus, called a Barr body. A Barr body is thought to represent a portion of an X-chromosome which remains condensed and coiled after other chromosomes in a set have uncoiled to resume metabolic activities.

Barr bodies are present in a nucleus in numbers equal to the number of X-chromosomes present in excess of one. In a normal female with an XX sex chromosome set, a Barr body is found in more than 20 per cent of nuclei examined, and the nuclear sex is said to be chromatin positive. In contrast, in normal males with an XY sex chromosome set, no Barr bodies are found, and the nuclear sex is said to be chromatin negative.

Chromatin positive nuclear sex cannot be equated with an XX, nor can chromatin negative nuclear sex be equated with an XY sex chromosomal constitution of cells in every case. For example, in our laboratory, patients with chromatin positive nuclear sex have been found to have such diverse sex chromosomal sets as XXY, XO/XX, XO/XX/XXX and XO/XXX. Similarly, chromatin negative nuclear sex has been found to be associated with XO, XO/XY, XO/XYY, XO/XY/XYY and XO/XX set chromosomal karyotypes.

In view of the variable expression of nuclear sex in relation to sex chromosomal constitution, reliance on studies of nuclear sex alone may be misleading. In addition, nuclear sexing does not reflect abnormalities of chromosomes other than sex chromosomes and, therefore, cannot be relied upon when abnormalities of autosomes are suspected. However, when repetitive evaluation of nuclear sex produces results which are not consonant with findings expected on the basis of genital sex, an abnormality of number or morphology or type of sex chromosomes is found when the karyotype is determined.

METHODS USED IN DETERMINING CHROMOSOME NUMBER AND MORPHOLOGY (KARYOTYPE)

Recovery and Preparation of Cells for Study

Direct preparations of dividing cells in bone marrow aspirates provide excellent material for rapid evaluation of the karyotype in neonates and infants. In our laboratory, the method of Tjio and Whang[21] has been found to be useful. Frequently, however, only small numbers of metaphases are obtained, so repeated studies may be necessary.

Cultures of lymphocytes from peripheral blood using the technique of Moorhead et al.[14] provide larger numbers of metaphases suitable for study. Optimally, 5 to 10 ml of peripheral blood obtained by venepuncture are used. However, smaller amounts of whole blood obtained via percutaneous stab wounds may be cultured successfully without preliminary separation of cellular components[1].

Cultures of stromal cells from explants of solid tissue fragments by the method of Tjio and Puck[20] have provided ample material for study whenever surgical biopsy material is available. Small fragments of skin obtained under local anesthesia can be cultured successfully.

Variability in the chromosomal constitution of cells derived from various tissues in the same individual coupled with variability due to technological artefacts make repetitive study desirable, regardless of the source of tissue or the preparative method utilized.

Determination of Karyotype

Once a sample of sufficient numbers of metaphases suitable for study has been obtained, chromosomes are counted and morphology assessed simultaneously. Photographs of representative cells are prepared in duplicate. From one photograph, chromosomes are cut out individually and arranged in pairs according to the Denver classification, using either numerical (1-22) designations for individual pairs or alphabetic (A-G) designations for groups of autosomes[8]. The sex chromosomes are designated as X and Y. The remaining photograph and the paired chromosomes are mounted so that a permanent record of the karyotype is produced.

INDICATIONS FOR STUDY
Congenital Malformations

Musculoskeletal System

Congenital malformations of sufficient severity to be appreciated clinically in the neonate should lead the physician to suspect chromosomal abnormalities, and studies of the karyotype may be of diagnostic usefulness. For example, a short neck with low-set hairline and low-set ears, loose folds of skin about the neck, short metacarpals, short metatarsals with hammertoes and cubitus valgus are not uncommonly seen in such entities as arthrogryposis, Klippel-Feil syndrome and Ullrich's syndrome, in all of which the karyotype is normal. Similar stigmata associated with chromosomal abnormalities are frequently encountered in Turner's syndrome[11], the XXXXY syndrome[4] and many of the syndromes of autosomal trisomy[17, 18].

Malformations associated with autosomal anomalies generally result in greater morbidity than those associated with sex chromosomal abnormalities. The clinical expression of these latter is frequently so mild as to escape detection until delayed puberty or short stature lead to more detailed examination.

Genitourinary System

Congenital malformations of the genitoruinary system, particularly of the genital tract, of a degree sufficient to prevent sex determination by inspection present problems in differential diagnosis and treatment. For example, the differential diagnosis of iodiopathic male pseudohermaphroditism from female pseudohermaphroditism due to congenital adrenal hyperplasia or other hormonal influences during gestation can be made on the basis of studies of sex chromosomal constitution.

Optimally, decisions as to the sex of rearing should be made in the first two years of life and appropriate therapy instituted in patients with anomalous external genitalia. It is worthy of emphasis that, while knowledge of the chromosomal sex should not be the sole determinant of the sex of rearing of such infants, it may dictate the timing of further diagnostic and therapeutic measures.

SHORT STATURE

In our experience, failure to grow is the most common basis for reference of patients with sex chromosomal abnormalities prior to the age of puberty. Patients in whom short stature is the most impressive feature to physical examination present problems in differential diagnosis. Primordial dwarfism, (either panhypituitarism or isolated growth hormone deficiency), hypothyroidism (either primary or secondary), pseudohypoparathyroidism and its variant, pseudo-pseudohypoparathyroidism, and Laurence-Moon-Biedel syndrome represent a few of the syndromes which must be differentiated from gonadal dysgenesis. The karyotype is usually normal in all of these except gonadal dysgenesis, where a sex chromosomal aberration is invariant.

It should be mentioned, however, that the pathophysiologic basis for failure to grow in these patients remains unknown. Hence, a diagnosis of sex chromosomal abnormality does not exclude the possibility of a coexistent endocrinopathy, and appropriate studies should be performed.

OLIGOPHRENIA

Oligophrenia may be associated with either sex chromosomal or autosomal aberrations. Both autosomal and sex chromosomal abnormalities have been observed in the same patient, particularly in patients with Downs' syndrome (Trisomy G or 21)[7, 10].

Mental retardation is frequently associated with polysomy of the sex chromosomes, e.g., XXYY[16], XXXY[6] and XXXXY[4] in phenotypic males and XXX[5], XXXX[2] and XXXXX[9] in phenotypic females. Mental retardation is also common in male Turner's syndrome (even with normal male karyotype)[20], but rare in Turner's syndrome associated with female external genitalia and sex chromosomal abnormalities[11].

In contrast, to the variable incidence of oligophrenia in association with sex chromosomal aberration, virtually all patients in whom autosomal trisomy has been observed have been mentally retarded. While mental retardation is not always associated with chromosomal aberrations, in our opinion, the clinical evaluation of the oligophrenic patient is incomplete until chromosomal studies have been done.

LIMITATION OF USEFULNESS OF CHROMOSOMES STUDIES

CYTOGENETIC AND CLINICAL CORRELATIONS

The similarity in clinical manifestations among patients with the same autosomal abnormality is truly remarkable in view of the genetic heterogeneity of the species. For example, Trisomy

D^{17}, Trisomy E^{18}, Trisomy G^{10}, etc. can be suspected on clinical grounds alone. Chromosomal studies are diagnostic, and the clinical consequences are usually predictable.

In contrast, the sex chromosomal constitution of tissues is not predictable with similar accuracy on the basis of clinical signs and symptoms. Further, prior to the age of puberty, knowledge of the sex chromosomal constitution of tissues does not permit complete accuracy in predicting either the degree of gonadal differentiation or the extent of gonadal function[15].

Such variability in expression of sex chromosomal abnormalities *vis à vis* gonadal development and function makes visualization and biopsy of the gonads essential to the complete evaluation of the patient. The information thus obtained provides the basis for rational management in such areas as hormone replacement therapy and surgical procedures which may be required for correcting defects incompatible with the elected sex of rearing.

METHODOLOGY

The usefulness of chromosomal studies can never arise above the adequacy of methods employed. An inadequate study is not only useless but also potentially damaging to the welfare of the patient, particularly if the strategy of clinical management is based upon it.

Chromosomal studies are subject to similar if not greater limitations than determination of hemoglobin or blood glucose, for example. Few clinicians would put ultimate reliance on a single determination of hemoglobin or blood glucose, yet many are inclined to regard results of a single evaluation of chromosome number and morphology on a limited sample as definitive.

Criteria of adequacy with respect to number of metaphases studied, number of tissues studied, etc, are indubitably variable, as even casual review of the published literature will indicate. Suffice it to say that repetitive studies, numerically adequate to minimize the artefacts inherent in preparative methods, are as pertinent to this area as to any other in clinical pathology. Studies of chromosomes, when properly done and cautiously interpreted, constitute a significant addition to the diagnostic techniques available to physicians.

SUMMARY AND CONCLUSIONS

Studies of chromosomal number and morphology are useful in the diagnostic evaluation of anomalies of growth and development in infants and children. These are particularly valuable when an endocrinopathy enters into the differential diagnosis.

Methods of preparation of cells for chromosomal study, some indications for study and some limitations on the interpretation of results have been discussed.

REFERENCES

1. Arakahi, D. T., and Sparkes, R. S.: Microtechnique for culturing leucocytes from whole blood. Cytogenetics (Basel), **2**:57-60, 1963.
2. Carr, D. H., Barr, M. L., and Plunkett, E. R.: XXX sex chromosome complex in two mentally defective females. Canad. Med. Ass. J., **84**:131-137, 1961.
3. Davidson, W. M., and Smith, D. R.: Morphological sex difference in polymorphonuclear neutrophil leucocytes. Brit. Med. J., **2**: 6-7, 1954.
4. Day, R. W., Levinson, J., Larson, W., and Wright, S. W.: An XXXXY male: Case report and review. J. Pediat., **63**:589-598, 1963.

5. Day, R. W., Larson, W., and Wright, S. W.: Clinical and cytogenetic studies on a group of females with XXX sex chromosome complements. J. Pediat., **64**:24-33, 1964.

6. Ferguson-Smith, M. A., Thuston, A. W., and Handmaker, S. D.: Primary amentia and micro-orchidism associated with XXXY sex chromosome constitution. Lancet, **2**:184-187, 1960.

7. Hamerton, J. L., Gianelli, F., and Polani, P. E.: Cytogenetics of Down's syndrome (mongolism) I. Data on a consecutive series of patients referred for genetic counselling and diagnosis. Cytogenetics, **4**:171-185, 1965.

8. Human Chromosome Study Group: A proposed standard system of nomenclature of human mitotic chromosomes. J. Hered., **51**: 214-221, 1960.

9. Kesaree, N., and Wooley, P. V.: Phenotypic female with 49 chromosomes, presumably XXXXX: Case report. J. Pediat., **63**:1099-1103, 1963.

10. Lejeune, J., Gautier, M., and Turpin, R.: Le mongolisme, premier example d'aberration autosomique humaine. Ann. Genet. (Paris), **1**:41-49, 1959.

11. Lindsten, J.: The Nature and Origin of X Chromosome Aberrations in Turner's Syndrome: A Cytogenetical and Clinical Study of 57 Patients. Uppsala, Almquist and Wiksell, 1963.

12. Mittwoch, U.: Sex chromatin. J. Med. Genet., **1**:50-76, 1964.

13. Moore, K. L., and Barr, M. L.: Smears from the oral mucosa in the detection of chromosomal sex. Lancet, **2**:57, 1955.

14. Moorhead, P. S., Nowell, P. C., Mellman, W. J., Gatlips, D. M., and Hungerford, D. A.: Chromosome preparations of leucocytes cultured from human peripheral blood. Exp. Cell. Res., **20**:613-616, 1960.

15. Ross, G. T., and Tjio, J. H.: Cytogenetics in clinical endocrinology. JAMA, **192**:977-986, 1965.

16. Schlegel, R. J., Aspillage, M. J., New, R., and Gardner, L. I.: Studies on a boy with XXYY chromosome constitution. Pediatrics, **36**:113-119, 1965.

17. Smith, D. W., Patan, K., Therman, E., and Inhorn, S. L.: A new autosomal trisomy syndrome: Multiple congenital anomalies caused by an extra autosome. J. Pediat., **57**:338-345, 1960.

18. Smith, D. W., Patan, K., Therman, E., and Inhorn, S. L.: The no. 18 trisomy syndrome. J. Pediat., **60**:513-527, 1962.

19. Steiber, D. D., Mellman, W. J., Bongiovanni, A. M., Eberlein, W. R., and Leboeuf, G.: Turner's syndrome in the male. J. Pediat., **58**:321-329, 1961.

20. Tjio, J. H., and Puck, T.: Genetics of somatic mammalian cells. J. Exp. Med., **108**:259-268, 1958.

21. Tjio, J. H., and Whang, J.: Chromosome preparation of bone marrow cells without prior in vitro culture or in vivo colchicine administration. Stain Techn., **37**:17-20, 1962.

Chapter 39

Chromosome Abnormalities in the Childhood Leukemias

PETER C. NOWELL, M.D.

The chromosomes of the childhood leukemias have not been as extensively investigated as have those of the adult leukemias, but enough data have been accumulated to permit some generalizations. This chapter is not intended as a comprehensive review, but rather as a brief summary of the major findings to date, with some thoughts on their possible significance and some suggestions for further work.

TECHNICAL CONSIDERATIONS

Even more than in studies on adults, chromosome investigations in the childhood leukemias have been plagued by technical problems. Attempts to obtain dividing leukemic cells from cases of acute childhood leukemia by means of leukocyte cultures have been almost universally unsuccessful. Not only are many cases aleukemic or sub-leukemic with very few neoplastic cells in the circulation, but even when immature cells are available for culture, they rarely grow well in vitro[21]. Occasionally, leukocyte cultures are useful in confirming doubtful observations in the bone marrow, but in such cases it is essential that the cultures be grown without phytohemagglutinin so that proliferation of non-leukemic lymphocytes does not confuse the picture.

Generally, satisfactory chromosome studies in the childhood leukemias require direct preparations made from bone marrow, without culture, and with only brief, if any, exposure to colchicine in vitro[21]. Even with such material, however, problems are common. The leukemic metaphases are very frequently of poorer technical quality than are non-leukemic mitoses in the same preparation. The chromosomes of the leukemic cells are commonly "fuzzy" and poorly separated, making accurate counts difficult and karyotype analysis almost impossible[16]. Unless this fact is recognized, only the technically good, non-leukemic metaphases in a mixed population may be counted, and a leukemic stemline may be overlooked.

Such difficulties undoubtedly led to erroneously negative reports in some early chromosome studies on the childhood leukemias, including some personal cases[9], and an attempt has been made, in the summaries that follow, to evaluate the data presented in terms of these technical limitations.

ACUTE CHILDHOOD LEUKEMIA

It now appears well substantiated that the vast majority of the typical cases of acute childhood leukemia, whether diagnosed as "lymphoblastic," "myeloblastic" or "stem-cell," show chromosome abnormalities[16, 19]. Generally, the leukemic population consists of a single clone or stemline of cells in which all members show the same chromosome change. These changes are not constant from case to case, and the childhood leukemias have been remarkable for the extreme deviation from normal which frequently occurs. Thus, while the chromosome abnormalities in the acute leukemias of adults almost always consist of the gain or loss of only one or two chromosomes, in the acute childhood disease, stemlines in the triploid and tetraploid range have been frequently reported[16, 19, 21, 23].

Not only are the stemlines in the childhood leukemias extremely abnormal, but also they appear to be remarkably stable. Additional changes superimposed on the original alteration have been observed late in the course of some cases; but, in other instances, the same abnormality has been shown to persist unchanged from the early untreated stages of the disease through several cycles of remission and relapse[19]. During remission, the leukemic population may be reduced in numbers to a point where it is no longer detectable and only normal mitoses are found, but it appears again at the next relapse. The normal metaphases observed in remission are not leukemic cells in which the chromosome pattern has reverted to normal, of course, but are simply proliferating non-leukemic hematopoietic cells which are suppressed again when relapse occurs.

With the exception of the extra chromosome 21 in mongolism, which will be discussed separately, the chromosome abnormalities in the acute childhood leukemias, as in all tumors, are limited to the neoplastic cells and are not present in the normal tissues, hematopoietic or otherwise. No particular chromosomes or groups of chromosomes are uniquely involved, although some studies[19] have suggested that alterations occur more frequently in Chromosome Groups C (nos. 6-12), D (13-15) and G (21-22) than in the other groups. Several cases of acute myeloblastic leukemia in children have been reported in which there was a single extra C-group chromosome[7, 24], a finding also reported in some adults with myeloproliferative disorders. In general, those acute childhood leukemias diagnosed as "myeloblastic" seem to show less extensive chromosome rearrangements than do the "lymphoblastic" and "stem-cell" varieties, but, as with nearly all mammalian neoplasms studied to date, no variety has been characterized by a specific chromosome pattern. Furthermore, it is noteworthy that occasional cases of acute childhood leukemia, apparently adequately studied, show no detectable chromosome anomalies at all[16, 23, 24].

CHRONIC GRANULOCYTIC LEUKEMIA

Chromosome studies by several workers[5, 18] have helped to confirm the occurrence in children of two forms of chronic granulocytic leukemia (CGL). The so-called "adult" type is remarkably similar to the same disease in adults, including the very low level of leukocyte alkaline phosphatase and also the presence of the Philadelphia chromosome (Ph[1]) in the leukemic cells. This abnormal chromosome, a number 21 with approximately half of its longer arm missing, is a nearly constant finding in adults with typical CGL[16], and has also been present in the leukemic cells of every child thus far studied with the adult form of the disease, including one only two and one half years old[4].

In contrast, both the clinical findings and the chromosome findings in the second form of CGL occurring in children, the so-called "infantile" or "juvenile" form, differ markedly from the picture in adults. This entity usually occurs in younger children than does the adult form and is characterized by hematologic findings more "subacute" than "chronic." The total white cell count tends to be lower with more immature forms; thrombocytopenia and lymphadenopathy are prominent early; and splenomegaly is not as marked. Response to therapy is less favorable and, as a result, survival time is shorter.

Although the leukocyte alkaline phosphate is reduced, as in the adult form, chromosome studies of the leukemic cells in these infants have failed to reveal the Ph[1] chromosome. Instead, the cytogenetic findings have been variable and usually minor, without any consistent pattern emerging. In two of four cases studied by Reisman and Trujillo[18], there were no chromosome changes, and in the other two cases, an extra chromosome, a minute, was present. Hardisty et al.[5] reported on two cases in which the only demonstrable alteration was a possible increase in condensation of one G-group chromosome.

Thus, the chromosome findings in chronic granulocytic leukemia of childhood have certainly helped to substantiate the clinical impression that this diagnosis really includes two distinct disease entities.

CONGENITAL AND NEONATAL LEUKEMIA

Very few children with these rare clinical entities have had adequate chromosome studies done on the leukemic cells. Several early cases were reported as showing no chromosome abnormalities, but since only leukocyte cultures (with phytohemagglutinin) were investigated, it is possible that the metaphases examined were not neoplastic. Surprisingly, however, even in those few children in which the bone marrow has been studied there have been very few abnormalities. LeJuene[11] did observe a stemline with fifty-four chromosomes in a mongol child with congenital leukemia, but Honda et al.[7], in a similar case, initially found only three of fifty-one marrow cells abnormal, with an extra C-group chromosome in addition to the expected trisomy for chromosome 21. This child developed a spontaneous remission which lasted for more than a year, and when fatal relapse eventually occurred, the abnormal stemline with the extra C-group chromosome then predominated in the blood and bone marrow. Hungerford[8] described a rapidly fatal case of leukemia in a three-month-old infant (not strictly in the neonatal period) in which both blood and marrow were examined and no abnormal stemline was found. Currently, in this laboratory, a child is being followed who developed acute leukemia at the age of three weeks. Over a period of fifteeen months, chromosome studies on direct marrow preparations were made on six occasions, including four separate relapses despite extensive chemotherapy. Until the sixth examination, no evidence of an abnormal stemline was detectable, although a total of 111 counts and ten analyses were made. After fifteen months, with the child again entering relapse, a clone of abnormal cells with forty-seven chromosomes was found, comprising 16 per cent of the dividing cells examined (11 of 69), with the extra chromosome in group G. This case will be reported in detail elsewhere[1].

Although the data are extremely sparse and in many cases unsatisfactory, the absent or minor chromosome changes in neonatal and congenital leukemia, as compared with the marked alterations in the usual childhood leukemias, represent an intriguing observation which certainly warrants more study.

Mongolism and Leukemia

Childhood leukemia is much more frequent in mongolism than in the general population[6]. An extra chromosome 21 is present in all tissues of mongol children, whether or not they have leukemia. In those with leukemia, there may be additional chromosome abnormalities, limited to the neoplastic leukocytes. As in the usual childhood leukemias, these alterations are of a clonal nature, varying from case to case, and in some instances there is no abnormality at all, beyond the expected trisomy 21[16, 17]

Thus, the only consistent chromosome change in the leukemic cells of mongols is the extra chromosome 21 present in all mongol tissues, and the fact that it is probably this same chromosome which is altered in chronic granulocytic leukemia (the Ph[1]), and occasionally in other leukemias, has led to speculation concerning a possible genetic locus controlling leukocyte (or myeloid) homeostasis on chromosome 21. The characteristic immaturity of granulocytes ("shift-to-the-left") in mongols, as well as the occurrence of transient reactions closely resembling congenital leukemia in these children[10] lends weight to this hypothesis. Furthermore, the reduced leukocyte alkaline phosphatase in chronic granulocytic leukemia and the less constant increase in this enzyme in mongols may be related to alterations in granulocyte life span. Taken together, these data suggest that chromosome 21 is important in the development of leukemia of mongols, but more specific conclusions will have to await techniques for definitely identifying not only individual human chromosomes, but also sites of specific genetic loci within those chromosomes.

The increased propensity for leukemia in mongols is also observed, to a lesser extent, in other members of their families, especially siblings. Since mongolism results from chromosome alterations, and the cells of childhood leukemia usually show chromosome changes, a common mechanism underlying both diseases has been postulated, perhaps the action of a familial gene leading to nondisjunction or other chromosome rearrangements. Such a gene does appear to operate in certain families, as well as in lower organisms, increasing the frequency of clinical syndromes resulting from nondisjunction, and perhaps increasing the frequency of neoplasms as well[6, 7, 13–15].

The role of prenatal genetic factors in human leukemia is perhaps best substantiated by the extremely high rate of concordance for leukemia in monozygous twins[12]. Unfortunately, no chromosome studies have yet been reported on the leukemic cells of these individuals, but such data would obviously be of great interest.

DISCUSSION

The significance of the accumulated data on the chromosome alterations in the childhood leukemias can be conveniently considered from two aspects: Contributions which these findings have made to our basic understanding of the nature and etiology of the neoplastic process; and practical applications of these observations at the clinical level.

BASIC CONCEPTS OF LEUKEMIA

In most cases of childhood leukemia, the neoplastic cells show marked chromosome alterations which have conferred sufficient selective advantage on the cells bearing them to permit their outgrowth as a dominant stemline. These changes apparently represent somatic mutations, since they are limited to the leukemic cells. Whether these *demonstrable* mutations, the chromosome alterations, represent the initiating event in the neoplastic process, or whether they are secondary phenomena (perhaps superimposed on submicroscopic initiating point mutations) remains unknown. Reisman *et al.*[17, 19] have favored the former view, feeling that the remarkable stability of clonal aberrations throughout the course of many acute childhood leukemias was a strong argument for considering them as initiating phenomena. Others[2] have preferred to consider these visible changes as secondary, finding it difficult to explain how genetic alterations varying so markedly from case to case could produce the same clinical disease in different individuals. This view does not reject a somatic mutation concept of etiology, but, based on the consistent occurrence of the Ph^1 chromosome in adult chronic granulocytic leukemia, suggests that other forms of leukemia may have similarly consistent initiating aberrations which are simply too small to be detected by present techniques.

This argument cannot be resolved with available methods, and perhaps of more immediate importance is the fact that, whether primary or secondary, at the time the disease is diagnosed, the cells of acute childhood leukemia have undergone extensive and extremely variable genetic alterations. These cannot be considered as normal cells in an abnormal environment, nor do they show any consistent genetic change which one might hope to attack with a single therapeutic agent.

Perhaps immuno-therapy, directed at these genetically altered cells is a more promising approach, or else prevention of the disease subsequent to identification of the etiologic agent(s). Unfortunately, the chromosome alterations observed in most childhood leukemias do not provide evidence for or against any postulated cause. It is now recognized that viruses and various chemicals, as well as ionizing radiation, can break human chromosomes[14]. The chromosome alterations observed in the leukemic cells may simply be indicative of a common pathway by which any of these diverse agents can produce neoplasia.

It is of interest that some of the acute childhood leukemias show the most marked chromosome alterations of any of the human leukemias, since this form of the disease has been considered the prime candidate for a human viral tumor, with an RNA virus similar to those producing the murine leukemias as a likely suspect[20]. Chromosome studies in animal tumors, however, have shown that those due to RNA viruses have less frequent and less marked chromosome alterations than do those due to DNA viruses, chemicals or radiation[15]. This observation may argue against an RNA virus as the cause of most acute leukemias in children.

On the other hand, the lack of extensive chromosome changes in human congenital and neonatal leukemia may favor the idea of an RNA virus etiology. Admittedly, the cytogenetic data on these entities are extremely scanty, and since most congenital and neonatal leukemia is apparently "myeloblastic," a variety which shows less chromosome changes in older children than the "lymphoblastic" or "stem-cell" types, this factor might help explain the minimal findings to date. Also, the truly neoplastic nature of some cases of "congenital leukemia," particularly in mongols, is in doubt[7, 10], and it has even been suggested that some of these early leukemias might in fact represent graft-versus-host reactions against the infant of implanted maternal lymphocytes, although our findings[1] and those of Hungerford[8] of *male* leukemic cells in two cases of neonatal leukemia in male infants would argue against this concept. Obviously, additional, technically adequate chromosome studies in congenital and neonatal human leukemia are needed.

PRACTICAL APPLICATIONS

Chromosome studies in acute childhood leukemia have occasionally been of diagnostic value. In the early stages, particularly when the disease is subleukemic or aleukemic, demonstration of an abnormal stemline in the bone marrow may help to confirm the diagnosis[16]. Of course, failure to demonstrate an abnormality does not rule out the presence of leukemia.

If additional work indicates that most congenital and neonatal leukemias do show aberrations, chromosome studies might help to distinguish these entities from leukemoid reactions occurring in the same age groups. However, the meager data presently available suggest that some true leukemias in these children do not show chromosome changes.

From a prognostic standpoint, chromosome studies in the childhood leukemias are of limited value. Certainly the demonstration of the Ph[1] chromosome in a case of chronic granulocytic leukemia in a child, confirming the presence of the adult form of the disease, would permit the expectation of a longer and more indolent course than in the infantile form without the Ph[1] chromosome. However, reports on the prognostic value of chromosome studies in the acute childhood leukemias have, thus far, been contradictory. Sandberg et al.[22] noted that cases with near-tetraploid cell lines responded favorably to therapy, while Fitzgerald et al.[3] felt that such cases often showed a poor response. Obviously, as in many other aspects of the chromosome studies in childhood leukemia, firm conclusions must await further investigations.

SUMMARY

In acute childhood leukemia, whether occurring in normal children or in mongols, the leukemic cells usually show chromosome abnormalities, frequently extensive. The changes are clonal in nature and often are remarkably stable throughout the course of the disease. Although the data are very scanty, chromosome alterations seem much less marked in congenital and neonatal leukemia than in the acute leukemias of older children. Chronic granulocytic leukemia in children comprises two entities, an adult form with the Philadelphia chromosome, and an infantile form, clinically more subacute, with variable, minor changes.

The data indicate that the neoplastic cells of most childhood leukemias have undergone extensive and inconstant genetic changes, making a specific therapeutic approach difficult. More information is needed on the chromosomes of congenital and neonatal leukemia, to help assess the fundamental nature of these entities, and on the diagnostic and prognostic value of chromosome studies in all forms of childhood leukemia.

REFERENCES

1. DePratti, V. J.: Observations on neonatal leukemia: Long-term survival with persistent normal chromosomes. In preparation.
2. Editorial. Chromosome changes in leukemia. New Eng. J. Med., 270:635-636, 1964.
3. Fitzgerald, P. H., Adams, A., and Gunz, F. W.: Chromosome studies in adult acute leukemia. J. Nat. Cancer Inst., 32:395-417, 1964.
4. Fortune, D. W., Lewis, F. J. W., and Poulding, R. H.: Chromosome patterns in myeloid leukemia in a child. Lancet, i:537, 1962.
5. Hardisty, R. M., Speed, D. E., and Till, M.: Granulocytic leukemia in childhood. Brit. J. Haemat., 10:551-566, 1964.
6. Holland, W. W., Doll, R., and Carter, C. O.: The mortality from leukemia and other cancer among patients with Down's syndrome (mongols) and among their parents. Brit. J. Cancer, 16:177-186, 1962.
7. Honda, F., Punnett, H. H., Charney, E., Miller, G., and Thiede, H. A.: Serial cytogenetic and hematologic studies on a mongol with trisomy-21 and acute congenital leukemia. J. Pediat., 65:880-887, 1964.
8. Hungerford, D. A.: Chromosome studies in human leukemia. I. Acute leukemia in children. J. Nat. Cancer Inst., 27:983-1011, 1961.
9. Hungerford, D. A., and Nowell, P. C.: The chromosome of acute childhood leukemia (Abstract). Proc. Amer. Ass. Cancer Res., 3:236, 1961.
10. Lahey, M. E., Beier, F. R., and Wilson, J. F.: Leukemia in Down's syndrome. J. Pediat., 63:189-190, 1963.
11. LeJuene, J.: Constitution d'un clone a 54 chromosomes au cours d'une leucoblastose congenitale chez une infant mongolienne. C. R. Acad. Sci. (Paris), 258:1195-1197, 1963.
12. MacMahon, B., and Levy, M. A.: Prenatal origin of childhood leukemia. New Eng. J. Med., 270:1082-1085, 1964.
13. Miller, R. W.: Down's syndrome (mongolism), other congenital malformations and cancers among the sibs of leukemic children. New Eng. J. Med., 268:393-407, 1963.
14. Nichols, W. W.: Relationships of viruses, chromosomes, and carcinogenesis. Hereditas (Lund), 50:53-80, 1963.
15. Nowell, P. C.: Chromosome changes in primary tumors. Progr. Exp. Tumor Res., 7, 83-103, 1965.
16. Nowell, P. C., and Hungerford, D. A.: Chromosome changes in human leukemia and a tentative assessment of their significance. Ann. N.Y. Acad. Sci., 113:654-662, 1964.
17. Reisman, L. E., Mitani, M., and Zuelzer, W. W.: Chromosome studies in leukemia. I. Evidence for the origin of leukemic stemlines from aneuploid mutants. New Eng. J. Med., 270:591-597, 1964.
18. Reisman, L. E., and Trujillo, J. M.: Chronic granulocytic leukemia of childhood: Clinical and cytogenetic studies. J. Pediat., 62:710-723, 1963.
19. Reisman, L. E., Zuelzer, W. W., and Thompson, R. I.: Further observation on the role

of aneuploidy in acute leukemia. Cancer Res., 24:1448-1456, 1964.

20. Rowe, W. P.: A survey of the tumor virus problem from an epidemiologic standpoint. Cancer Res., 25:1277-1282, 1965.

21. Sandberg, A. A., Ishihara, T., Crosswhite, L. H., and Hauschka, T. S.: Chromosomal dicotomy in blood and marrow of acute leukemia. Cancer Res., 22:748-756, 1962.

22. Sandberg, A. A., Ishihara, T., Kikuchi, Y., and Crosswhite, L. H.: Chromosomal differ-

ences among the acute leukemias. Ann. N.Y. Acad. Sci., 113:663-716, 1964.

23. Sandberg, A. A., Ishihara, T., Miwa, T., and Hauschka, T. S.: The in vivo chromosome constitution of marrow from 34 human leukemias and 60 nonleukemic controls. Cancer Res., 21:678-689, 1961.

24. Weinstein, E. D., and Weinstein, A. W.: Chromosomal abnormalities in children with leukemia (Abstract). J. Pediat., 63:473-474, 1963.

Chapter 40

The Cat Cry Syndrome and Other Chromosomal Aberrations in The Newborn: A Clinical Review*

J. J. LA POLLA

INTRODUCTION

Human genetics was probably first emphasized in 1891 by Hansemann[16]. In 1921, Painter's[38] classic work gave the diploid number of chromosomes in man as forty-eight in both sexes: twenty-three pairs of autosomes plus an X- and Y-chromosome in the male and twenty-three pairs of autosomes plus two X-chromosomes in the female. However, in 1956, Tjio and Levan were able to make consistent and verified counts of forty-six chromosomes in lung tissue taken from abortuses. (Fig. 1 and 2 show the human male and human female karyotype.) With the improvement of cytogenetic technique, considerable interest has been aroused among clinicians in the study of human genetics. Since Lejeune[26] demonstrated in 1959 a specific chromosomal abnormality in mongolism, chromosome patterns have been discovered in a variety of clinical disorders.

Large-scale screening studies suggest that approximately 0.4 to 0.6 per cent of all live-born Caucasians bear a chromosomal abnormality[34, 36]. Until a systematic and detailed chromosome analysis is done on a large number of newborns, the true incidence of chromosomal aberrations will not be known. It should be noted that most of the cases reported have involved Caucasian populations. This may not reflect other ethnic groups. Elevated maternal age is associated with an increased incidence of the various trisomies in man (based on the data of Penrose). Non-Caucasian mothers generally bear children at a younger age. The role of environmental influences, such as radiation exposure, socio-economic factors or disease in the parents, needs further study in evaluating the frequency of chromosomal abnormalities.

The purpose of this chapter is to present a clinical survey of chromosomal aberrations during the neonatal period. More pediatricians are making the diagnosis of chromosomal aberrations in the nursery. It is very important to make an early clinical diagnosis and to obtain chromosome analysis. Good genetic

*Opinions expressed herein are those of the author and do not necessarily reflect the views of the Navy Department or the Naval Service at large.

advice requires certainty about diagnosis. In Down's syndrome of the translocation type, early diagnosis and chromosome analysis of the parents is most essential. Translocation chromosomes are important in genetic counseling because they may be transmitted from generation to generation, independent of maternal age[52]. The chromosomal aberrations discussed in this paper will be those in which a routine physical examination is enough to establish a clinical impression which should lead to subsequent chromosome analysis. Each of these syndromes can be suspected by competent nursery personnel. A part of the discussion will

pertain to one of the newly established chromosomal entities — the *cat cry syndrome* or "cri du chat" first reported by Lejeune[30] in 1963. The classification of each syndrome is based on the terminology of chromosome classification according to Patau[39] and in full accord with the London report[32].

THE "CRI DU CHAT" (CAT CRY) SYNDROME

This recently recognized chromosomal aberration is now well substantiated in the literature[2, 13, 27, 28]. It involves a deletion of a portion of the short arm of a chromosome in the 4-5 group[29] (Fig. 3). Autoradiographic techniques

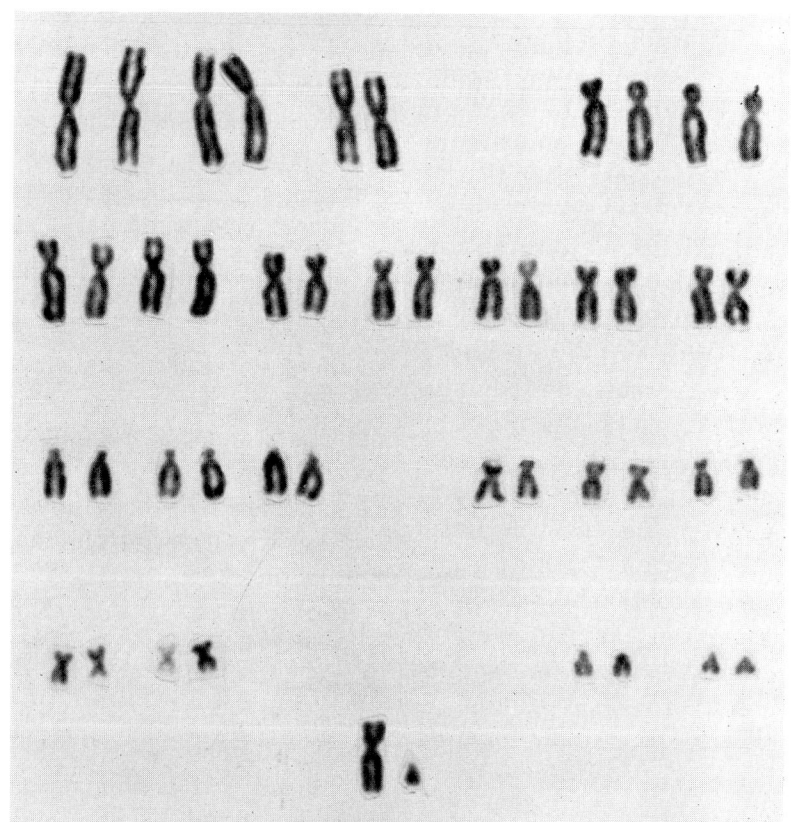

Fig. I. The karyotype of a normal human male. Classification according to Patau[39].

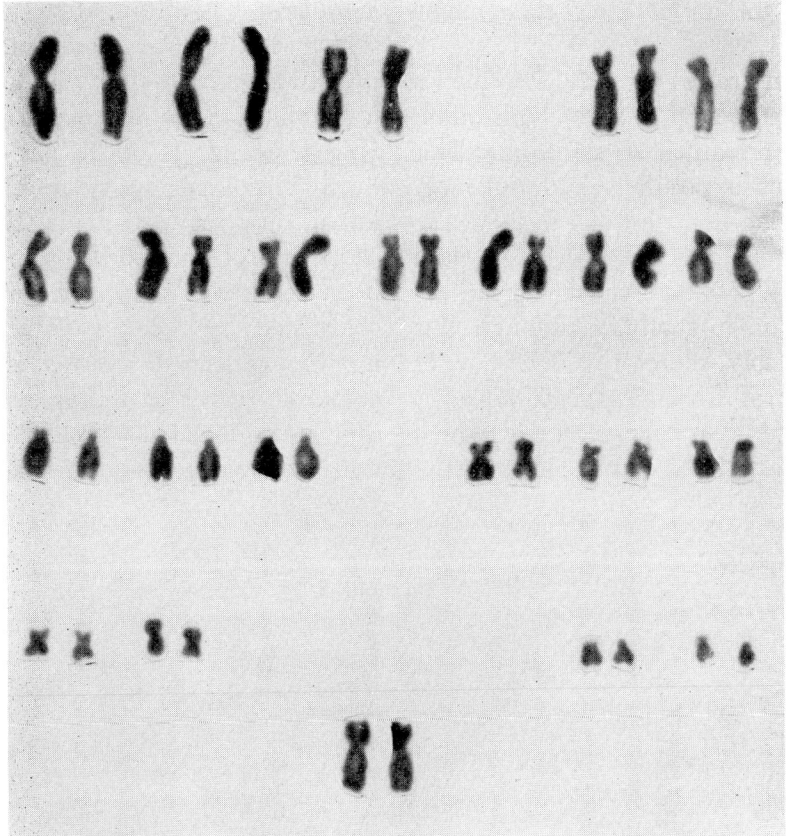

Fig. 2. The karyotype of a normal human female. Classification according to Patau[39].

have defined the deletion as belonging to Chromosome 5[12, 41]. This syndrome has a characteristic which should always alert the physican — the strange, characteristic cat cry. The cry, however, becomes less characteristic as the child grows older[37, 45, 56]. The plaintive tonality seems first to disappear, although the prolonged, high-pitched quality may linger. It should be distinguished from the high-pitched cry associated with severe neurologically retarded infants. It is very difficult to describe in words the actual character of the cry. A recording is available to physicians upon specific request to Dr. Neil MacIntyre, Department of Anatomy, Western Re-

serve University, School of Medicine, Cleveland, Ohio, 44106.

Besides the cry, there are other features commonly associated with this syndrome. These are: severe mental retardation; growth retardation; microcephaly; rounded face, hypertelorism; oblique palpable fissures; epicanthus; low-set ears; micrognathia; and strabismus[8, 33, 48, 49]. (Figs. 4 and 5). Dermatoglyphic analysis performed on Lejeune's cases revealed transverse palmar creases and an axial triradius in the t' position. Cases of deletion of Chromosome 5 have the same features common to other chromosomal aberrations, including the basic feature of failure to thrive[1, 5, 20, 46]. The cry alone is unique.

Bieg and Steele[3] recently described a ring chromosome 5 in a newborn infant with the "cri du chat" syndrome. This patient had a peculiar, kitten-like cry noted on the first day of life. She also had microcephaly, hypertelorism with oblique palpebral fissures, epicanthal folds and micrognathia. Although this case probably represents deletions of both arms of Chromosome 5, it seems no different than other cases in which there is a partial deletion of only the short arm. The fact that this syndrome, which is definitely compatible with life, is associated with the deletion of a significant portion of an autosome is interesting, since it has generally been considered that such deletions are lethal. Several patients with missing short arm of one Chromosome 18 have been reported[4, 14, 54, 55]. The phenotypic expression has been variable and the number of cases reported small. The possibility exists that they could represent an undetected balanced translocation. Lejeune has established evidence

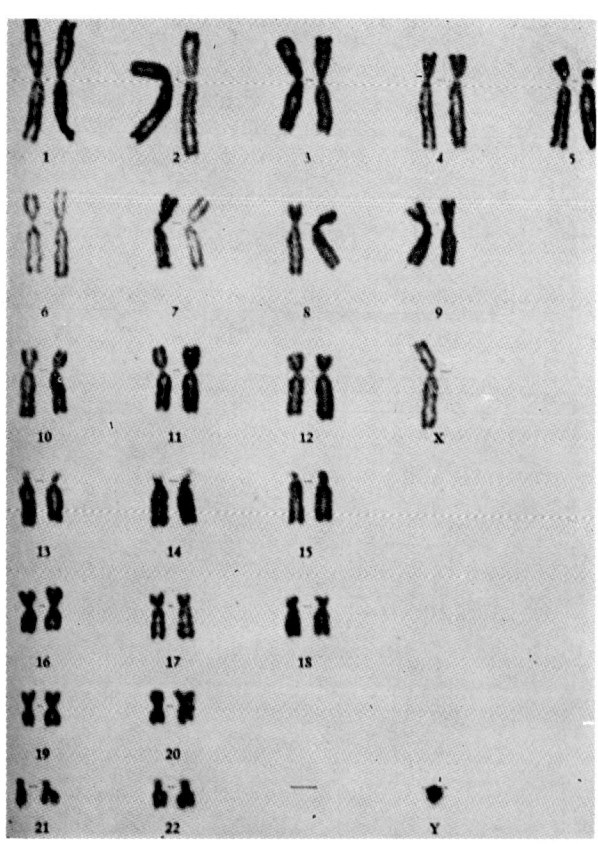

Fig. 3. The karyotype of a patient with the cat cry syndrome. (From Lejeune, J., and others: Partial deletion of the short arm of Chromosome 5. Individualization of a new pathologic state. Sem. Hop. Paris, No. 25, April, 1964. Courtesy of Dr. Lejeune.) Note the deletion of the short arm of Chromosome 5.

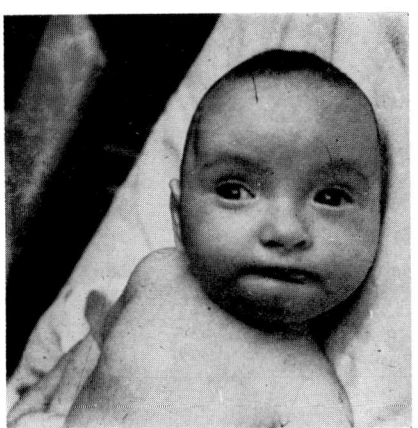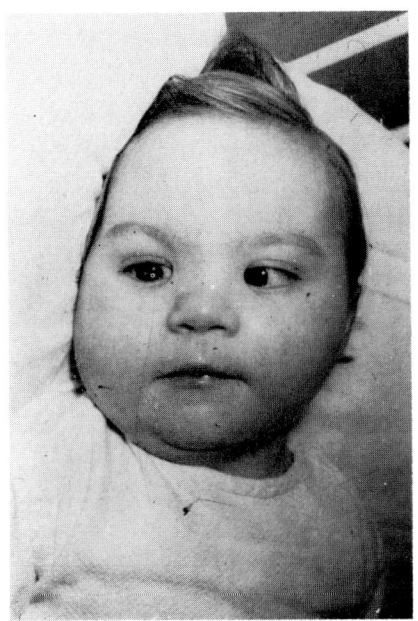

Fig. 4. Two of the original patients described by Lejeune with the cat cry syndrome. Note the rounded faces, hypertelorism, oblique palpebral fissures, epicanthus and micrognathia. (From Lejeune, J., and others: Partial deletion of the short arm of the chromosome 5. Individualization of a new pathologic state. Sem. Hop. Paris, No. 25, April, 1964. Courtesy of Dr. Lejeune.)

from one of his cases that the deletion of Chromosome 5 is a true deletion and not a balanced translocation[27].

Most infants with the cat cry syndrome are of small birth size. The role of maternal age has not been established in this syndrome. There is also little information as to the role of prenatal factors. The ratio of males to females seems to be equal.

TRISOMY G, (DOWN'S SYNDROME)

In 1866, Langdon-Down described a series of English patients with mental retardation who had a resemblance to each other. They all had certain "Oriental" features, and he therefore named the condition mongolism. More recently, this condition has been called Down's syndrome to avoid the connotations of the word mongolism. More appropriately, this syndrome is referred to as Trisomy G_1 denoting the chromosome which is in triplicate in the first recognized G trisomy syndrome. (Fig. 6). In 1959, Lejeune[26] interpreted the extra chromosome as being Chromosome 21. There is, however, current evidence that the extra chromosome in trisomy G_1 is

Chromosome 22 and that this syndrome should be called trisomy 22[58].

The clinical diagnosis of trisomy G_1 can be established within the first postnatal week. The length of gestation is usually to term. Birth weights, in general, are smaller than for other neonates of similar lengths of gestation. According to Hall[15], there are certain

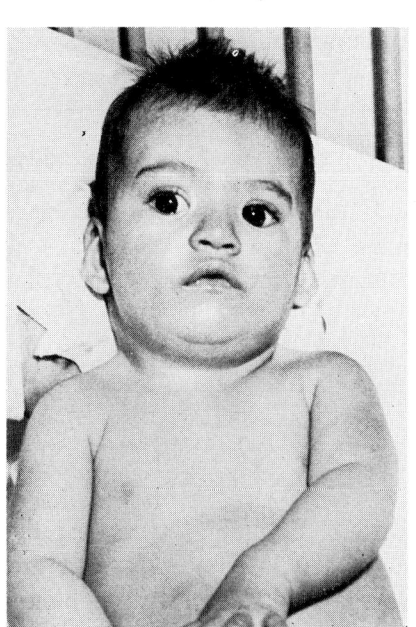
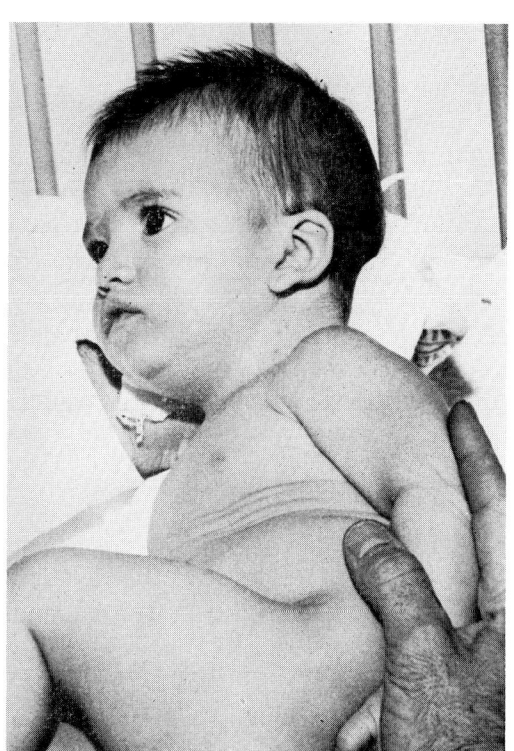

Fig. 5. Patient at age four months with the cat cry syndrome. This patient was one of the first described in the American literature. Note the striking resemblence with Lejeune's patients. (From McIntyre, N., and others: The "cat cry" syndrome. Amer. J. Dis. Child., 108:538-42, 1964. Courtesy of Dr. McIntyre.)

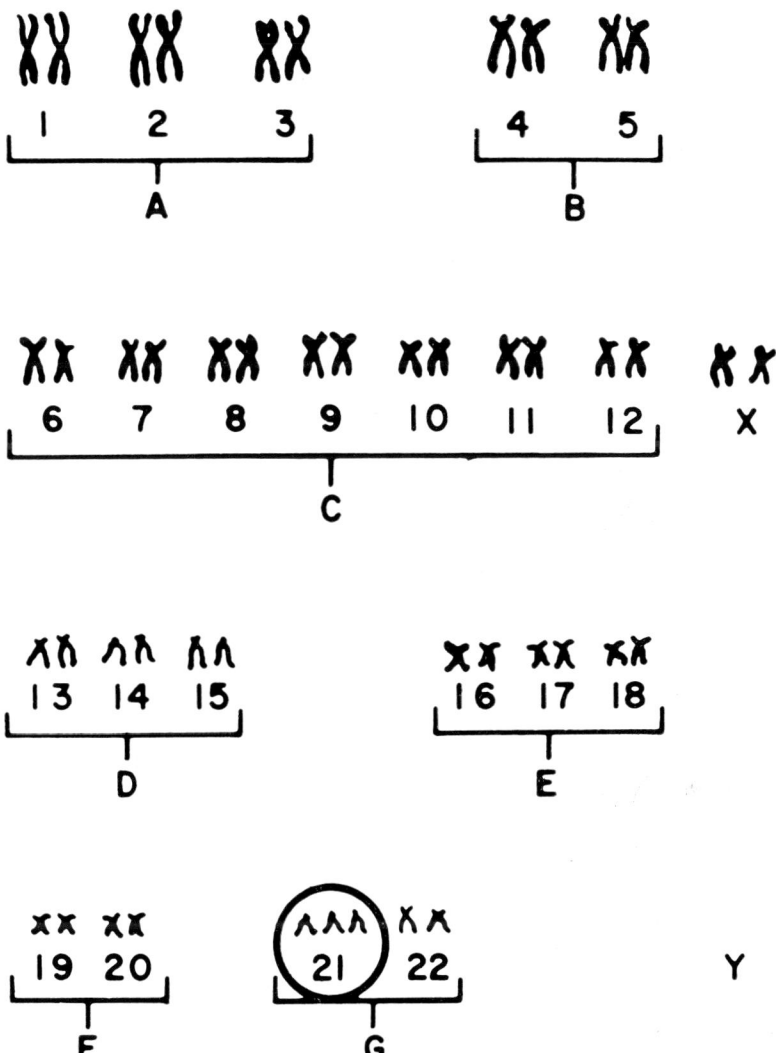

Fig. 6. The karyotype of a patient with standard Trisomy G₁. Note that current information from Patau[39] places the extra chromosome in the number 22 position rather than the conventional number 21 position as described in this karyotype. (Karyotype courtesy of The Pediatric Patient—1964, Lippincott.)

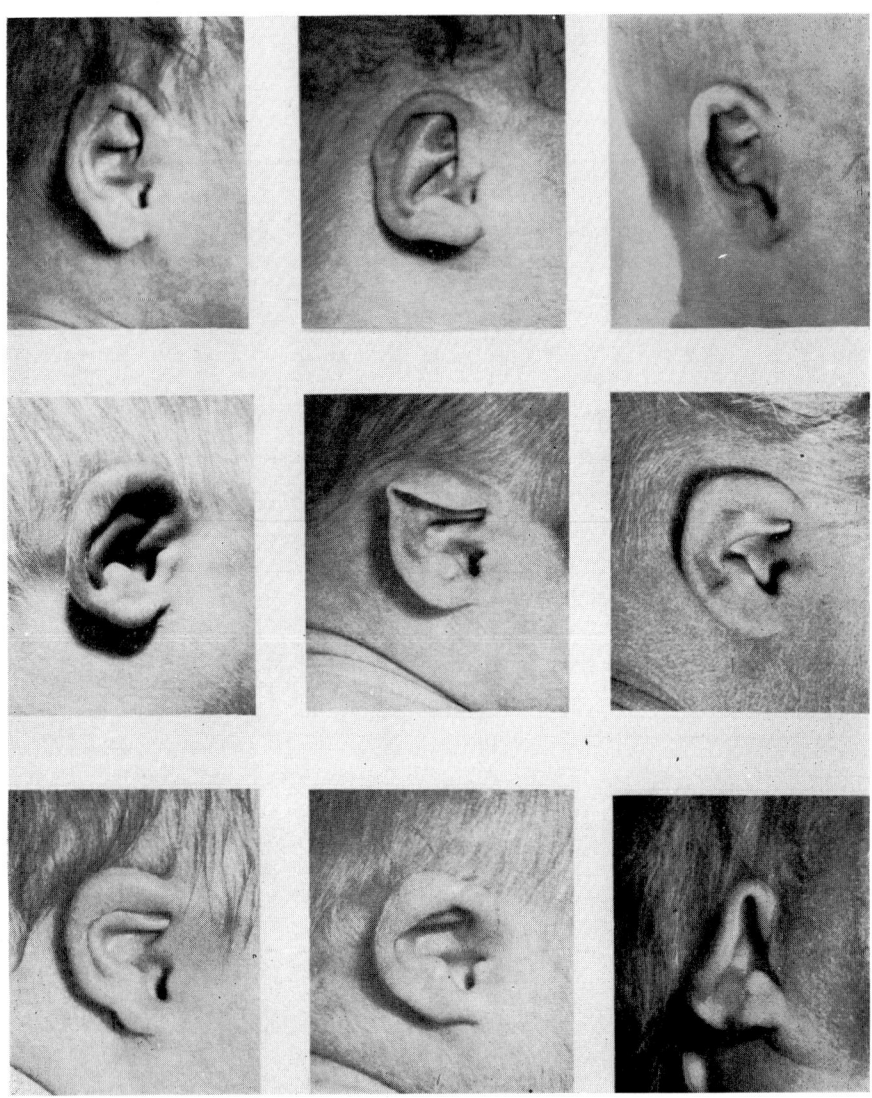

Fig. 7.   Different ear types from newborns with Trisomy G₁ syndrome. (From Hall, B.: Mongolism in newborns. Acta Paediat. (Suppl.), 154:1964. Courtesy of Dr. Hall.

"cardinal signs" of trisomy G_1. These include: lack of Moro reflex; muscle hypotonia; flat facial profile; oblique palpebral fissure; abnormal external ear (Fig. 7); abundant neck skin; four-finger line, hyperflexibility; dysplastic pelvis (found by x ray); and dysplastic middle phalanx of fifth finger (found by x rays). In Smith's[50] experience, the only consistent defect in the newborn has been hypotonia. This also has been our experience.

There are other defects which should be noted: brachycephaly; flat occiput, epicanthal folds; hypertelorism; furrowed tongue; narrow high palate; a short nose; short neck (Figs. 8 and 9); short broad hands; short incurved fifth finger (Fig. 10); clinodactyly; a gap between the great and second toe; speckling of the iris (so-called Brushfield spots), disastasis recti, and unusually small penis in the male.

In making the diagnosis of trisomy G_1, Hall felt that his "cardinal" signs were the easiest to appraise. Most of the signs occurred in low frequency in the normal newborn. Many of the structural defects are minor in type. The clinician should be reluctant to attach too much significance to these minor defects, since any one of them may be found in the normal. It has been reported that, after examination of 4,412 newborn babies, the incidence of at least one minor defect in a baby was found to be 14.7 per cent[36]. However, the occurrence of more than one minor defect in a baby was rare, and only twenty babies (.05%) were found to have three or more associated minor defects. Brushfield spots have been discovered in 17.0 per cent of newborns[36].

The dermatoglyphics of the hands in

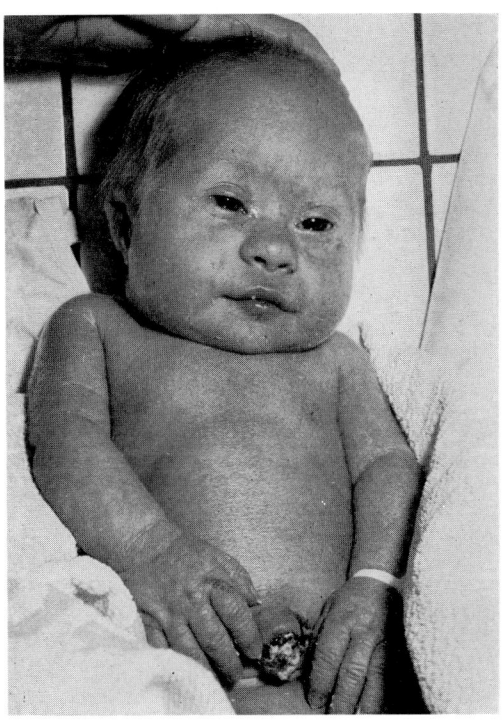

Fig. 8.   Photograph of a newborn patient with Trisomy G_1. Note epicanthal folds, hypertelorism, broad hands and umbilical hernia. (From Hall, ibid. Courtesy of Dr. Hall.)

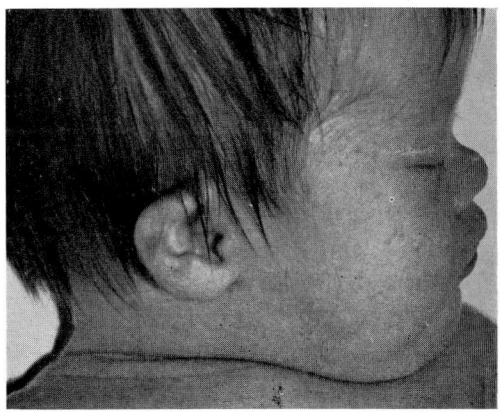

Fig. 9.   Profile of a patient with Trisomy G_1. Note low-set, characteristic ears with the helix overfolded and the rounded form of the pinna. Also note the short nose and short neck. (Official Navy Photograph, U.S. Naval Hospital, St. Albans, N.Y.)

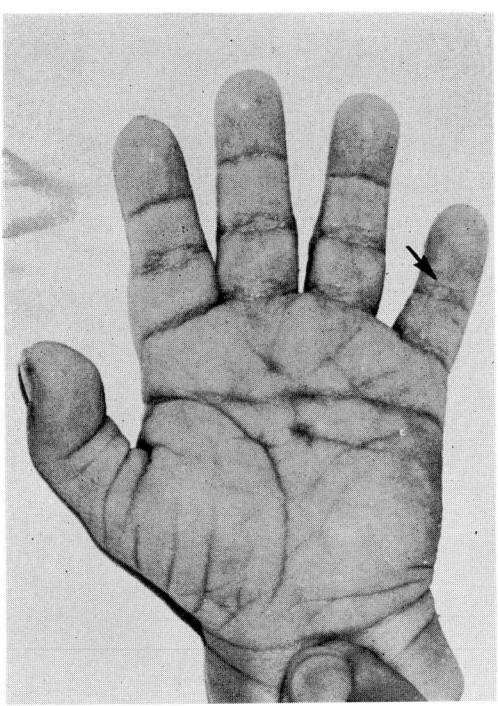

Fig. 10. Photograph of hand of a patient with trisomy G_1. Note the Simian crease (single crease across the palm extending past the bases of the four fingers) and the single crease on the fifth finger (arrow). The general appearance of the hand is short and broad. (From Uchida, I., and Soltan, H. C.: Evaluation of dermatoglyphics in medical genetics. Pediat. Clin. N. Amer., 10:No. 2, May, 1963. Courtesy of Dr. Uchida and the Saunders Company.)

trisomy G_1[53] reveal, besides the Simian or four-fingered line (Fig. 10), a high axial triradius, an increased number of ulnar loops; a radial loop on the fourth finger and a single distal crease on the fifth finger. An arch tibial or a small loop distal is the characteristic pattern of the hallucal area of the sole. (The reader is referred to Uchida's article[53] for a better understanding of dermatoglyphics.)

There are certain congenital heart diseases associated with trisomy G_1. These are atrioventricular communis and ventricular septal defect. There is found in less than 10 per cent of the patients an associated tetralogy of Fallot. Heart disease is found in less than 50 per cent of most cases.

Penrose[42] found the incidence to be 1 per 636 to 776 Caucasian births. trisomy G_1 has been found in Orientals and Negroes, and there is no reason to believe it is restricted to only a few races. Approximately 80 per cent of the mothers of trisomy G_1 children have been over thirty-five years of age at the time of birth. Most of the affected children have had regular or primary non-disjunction type of trisomy G_1. Among trisomy G_1 babies born to younger mothers, a variety of genotypes have been reported[6, 42]. However, a great majority of these are of the standard type. We have recently observed ten trisomy G_1 patients referred to our hospital in the past year with parents under age twenty-five (3 of these were under age 20), and all were standard trisomy G_1.[24]

TRISOMY 18 SYNDROME

In 1960, Edwards[9] and Patau[40] simultaneously described a new syndrome associated with the presence of an extra group E chromosome, now considered to be chromosome 18 (Fig. 11). The adverse effect of the extra 18 autosome is quite severe, and anomalies can occur in almost every organ system. Newborns with this chromosomal aberration can best be described as presenting a pitiable appearance. Their cry is feeble and even kitten-like in quality and must, at times, be carefully discerned from the "cri du chat."

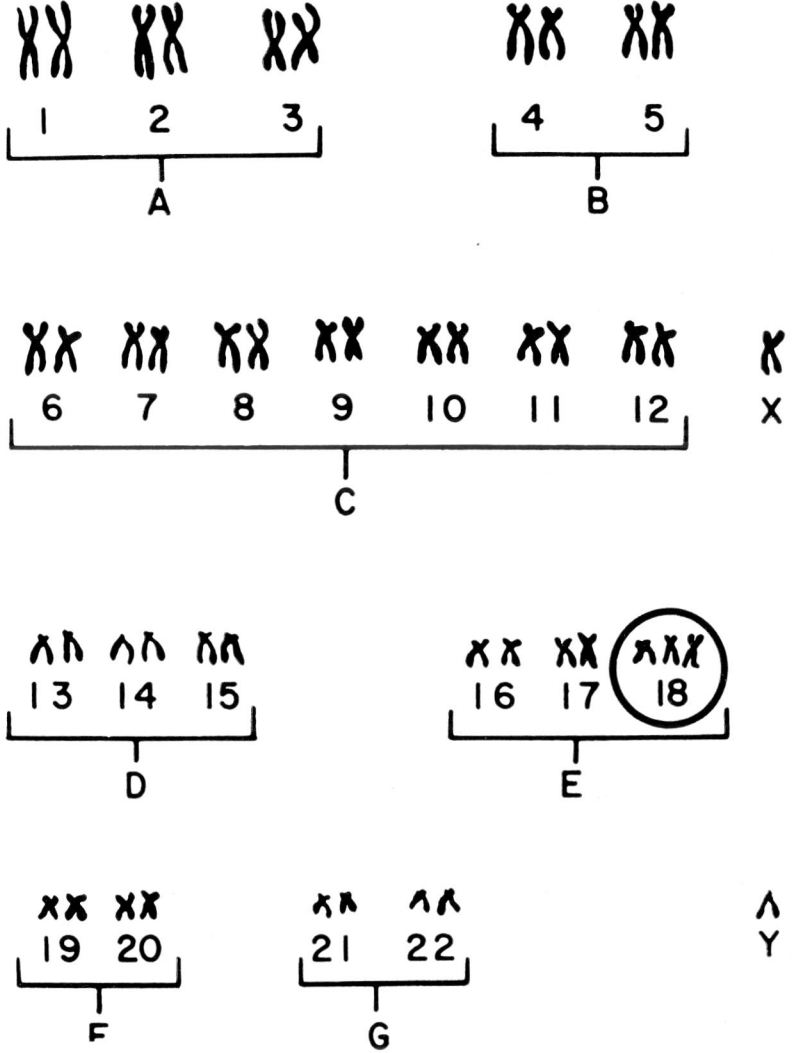

Fig. 11.   Karyotype of a patient with the Trisomy 18 syndrome. Note the extra chromosome 18. Classification according to Patau[39]. (Karotype courtesy of The Pediatric Patient—1964, Lippincott.)   For karyotypes of other genotypes referred to in this article, readers are referred to Smith[50].

Markedly altered time of gestation is a frequent abnormality. According to Smith[52], a gestation of forty-two weeks or more occurred in 36 per cent of the patients reported. Maternal weight gain in pregnancy is low, the placenta small, and polyhydraminos often is present. There is approximately a 3:1 female to male ratio[17]. It is estimated that the incidence of this syndrome is 0.23 per 1000[36].

The most constant features are: small birth weight (average 5 lbs, 2 oz in reported cases); failure to thrive (Fig. 12); dysplastic low-set ears (Fig. 13); neurological retardation; flexion de-

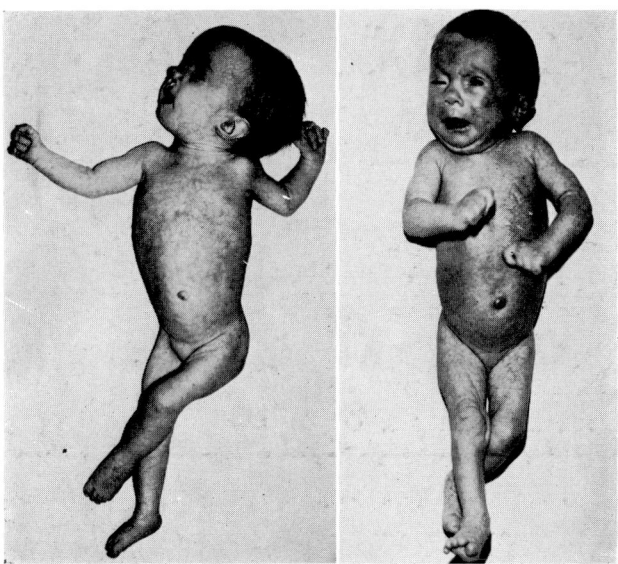

Fig. 12.   Patients with the 18 trisomy syndrome.   A. seven months old; B. ten months old. Note the appearance of failure to thrive. (From Smith, D. W., and others: The no. 18 trisomy syndrome. J. Pediat., Vol. 60. Courtesy of Dr. Smith and C. V. Mosby Company.)

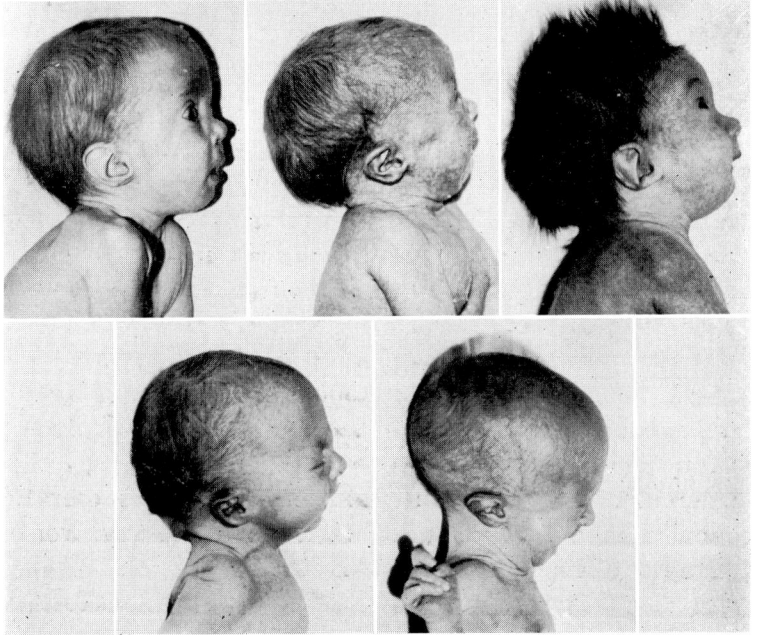

Fig. 13.   Profiles of patients with the 18 trisomy syndrome. Note the small mandible, prominent occiput and dysplastic low-set ears. (From Smith, ibid. Courtesy of Dr. Smith and C. V. Mosby Company.)

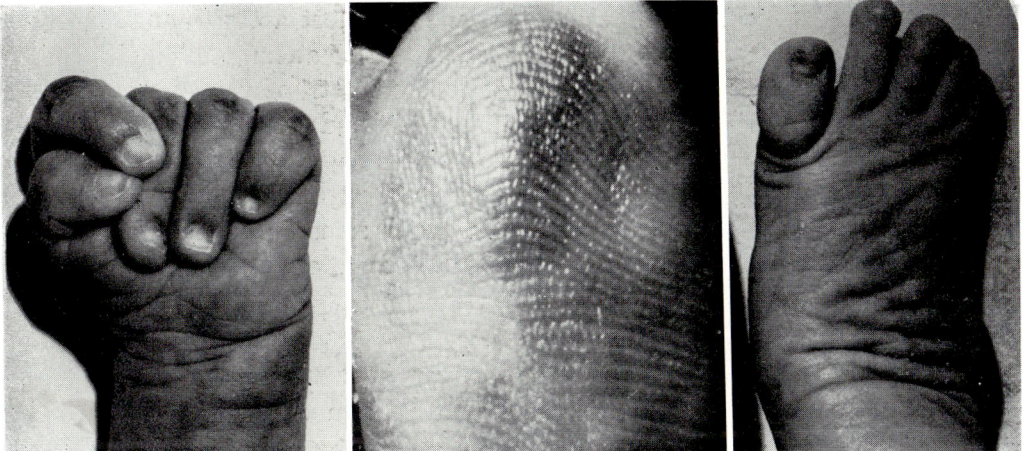

Fig. 14.   Several of the common anomalies in the 18 trisomy syndrome. A. The unusual position of the fingers with hypoplasia of fifth fingernail; B. The low arch dermal
pattern on digit; C. Dorsiflexed hallux and hypoplasia of toenails. (From Smith, D. W.:
Autosomal abnormalities. Symposium on Congenital Defect. Amer. J. Obstet. Gynec.,
90:No. 7, Part 2, 1964. Courtesy of Dr. Smith and C. P. Mosby Company.)

formities of the fingers with an unusual
and very characteristic overlapping of
the index finger in extension (Fig. 14);
small mandible, prominent occiput (Fig.
15); and hypertonicty. Other findings
which have been reported are: single
umbilical artery; Meckel's diverticulum,
heart defects (most common are interventricular septal defects and patent
ductus arteriosus); dorsiflexed hallux
and hypoplasia of toenails (Fig. 14);
small pelvis; limited hip abduction; foot
deformities, such as rocker bottom and
equinovarus (Fig. 16); short sternum;
urinary tract anomalies (especially
horseshoe kidneys); eventration of the
diaphragm; heterotopic pancreatic tissue; and retarded bone age[47]. The low
arch dermal pattern on the digits (Fig.
14), as well as single creases on the
fifth finger, four-finger lines (Simian
crease) on the palms and absent distal
flexion creases on fingers other than the
fifth, have all been noted on dermato-

glyphic patterns of the patients[53].

These individuals have a short life
span and usually die early in infancy
of pneumonia, heart failure or chronic
debilitating diseases. The mean paternal
and maternal ages are elevated, but
the mean maternal-paternal age difference is significantly reduced, and,
according to Yunis[57], this suggests that
it is mainly elevated maternal age which
is etiologically significant. Simple trisomy of number 18 chromosome is the
most frequently observed pattern, although a number of genotypes have
been observed, namely double trisomies,
translocation and Trisomy 18 syndrome,
and mosaicism. Occasionally, one finds
an infant presenting with many features resembling those found in Trisomy
18, but normal chromosomes are found.
It may be that, in these cases, occult
mosaicism occurs or that a fragment or
segment of chromosome goes undetected. When suspected, every available

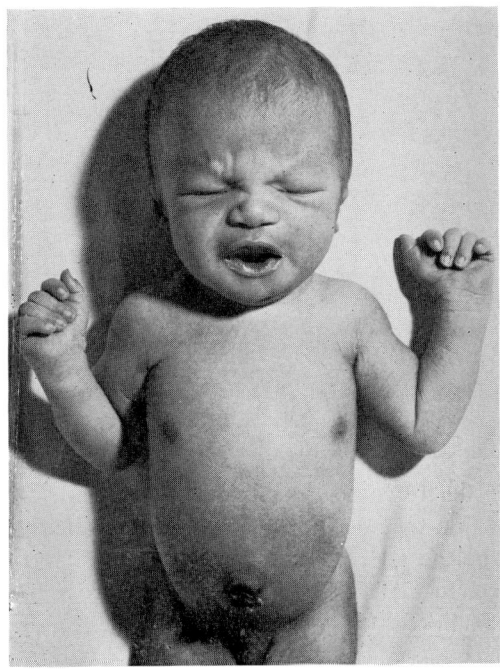

Fig. 15.   Photograph of a two-week-old infant with Trisomy 18 syndrome. Note the prominent occiput and characteristic position of the fingers. There is also evident an umbilical hernia and widespread nipples. Official Navy Photograph. U.S. Naval Hospital, St. Albans, N.Y.)

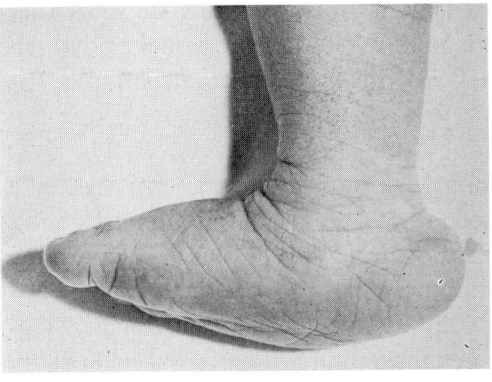

Fig. 16.   The characteristic rocker-bottom deformity of the foot noted in the Trisomy 18 syndrome. There is obvious posterior prominence of the heel. (Official Navy Photograph. U.S. Naval Hospital, St. Albans, N.Y.)

means to detect a chromosome aberration should be attempted. The diagnosis of autosomal trisomy is of great value in the affected infant's prognosis. Most authorities agree that little can be accomplished by attempting to correct the major somatic malformations. This is also true of the next autosomal trisomy.

THE TRISOMY D_1 SYNDROME

The pattern of anomalies associated with the trisomy D_1 syndrome was probably first described in the literature as cases of arhinencephaly[23]. The association of this disorder with an extra chromosome in the D or 13-15 group (Fig. 17) was first reported by Patau[40]. At the present, the chromosomes of the D group cannot be morphologically identified as pairs 13, 14 or 15. It has become customary to refer to this syndrome as trisomy D_1, since it was the first described trisomic condition of the D group.

Of the autosomal trisomies, this has the most grotesque associated anomalies. It has been rarely reported in the literature; papers submitted are usually simply case reports. This may be because babies with this syndrome die early in infancy or because it goes undetected as a chromosomal aberration by the clinician. Most of these newborns are probably classed as monstrosities. There is a very wide variation in the somatic anomalies of this syndrome. In this author's experience, anomalies of the face, head and brain seem to be the most constant. The incidence has been reported as 0.45 per 1000 newborns[36]. There are more affected females than males, and the mean maternal age is consistently elevated.

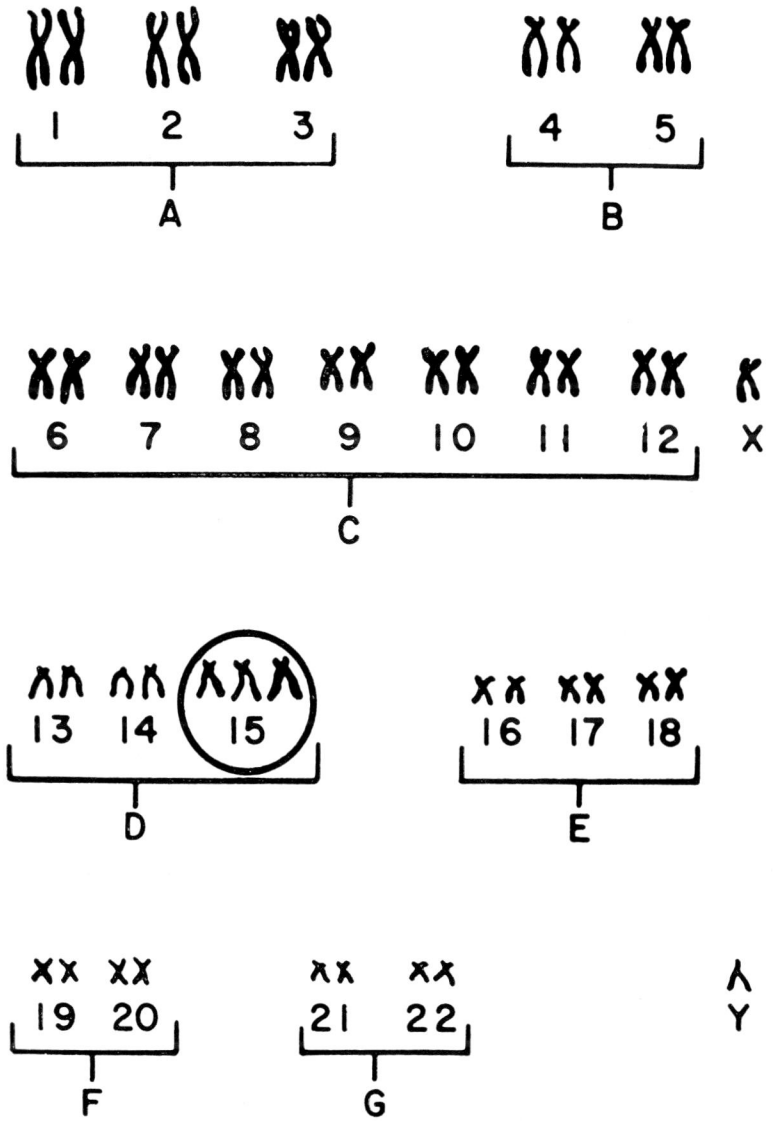

Fig. 17. Karyotype of a patient with the trisomy D₁ syndrome. Classification according to Patau[39]. For karyotypes of other genotypes referred to in this article the reader is referred to Smith[50].

The most common clinical findings are: arhinencephaly; psychomotor retardation; sloping forehead; eye defects (colobomata are most common); cleft palate and lip (Figs. 18 and 19); polydactyly and/or syndactyly; capillary hemangiomata (usually over the forehead); and heart defects (most commonly, interventricular septal defects). The variation in cleft palate and lip is wide, and some reported cases in the literature presented without this defect.

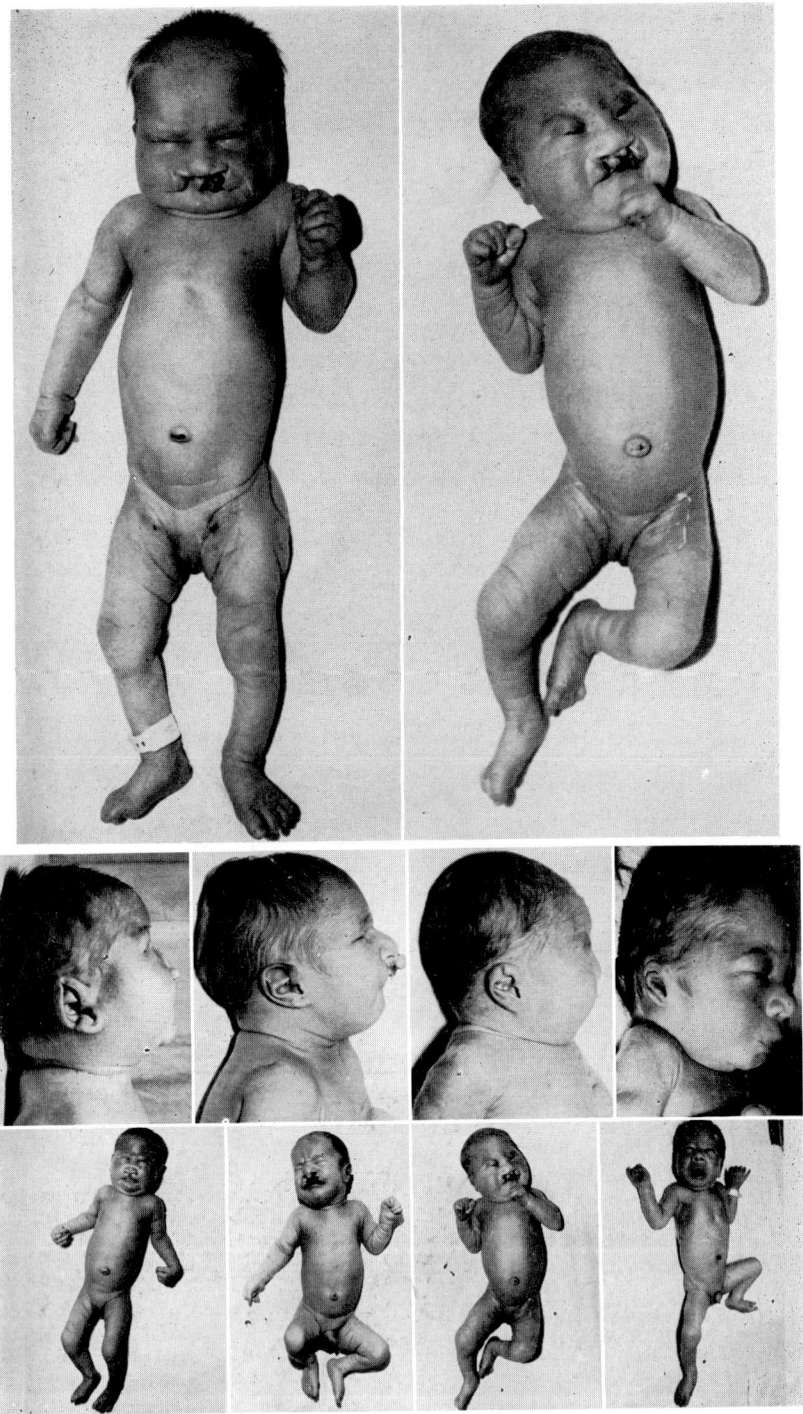

Fig. 18 and 19. Infants with the D_1 trisomy syndrome. Note sloping forehead, eye defects and cleft palate and lip. (From Smith, D. W.: The no. 18 trisomy and d_1 trisomy syndromes. Pediat. Clin. N. Amer. 10:No. 2, May 1963. Courtesy of Dr. Smith and the Saunders Company.)

Apneic spells are common, especially in infants who survive the newborn period. Smith[51] has noted several common anomalies in the D₁ trisomy: namely, flexion of fingers, narrow hyperconvex fingernails, and polydactyly, abnormal scrotum, posterior prominence of heel and midline occipital scalp defects (Fig. 20). Gerald has also noted the fact that midline occipital scalp defects are common. This is a feature which can be observed in the newborn and, when associated with other of the reported anomalies, should quickly arouse the suspicion of the staff.

Other findings reported are: low-set malformed ears; deafness; abnormal calcification of the skull; bicornuate uterus; accessory spleens; retroflexible thumbs; urinary anomalies (hydronephrosis, double pelvis and polycystic kidneys); incomplete rotation of the colon; large gall bladder; umbilical hernia; and cryptorchidism. Dermatoglyphic studies have revealed a high incidence of horizontal palmar creases, a high axial triradius on the palms and on arch fibular in the hallucal area on the sole[53]. Huehns[18] found specific neutrophile abnormalities in a series of trisomy D₁ patients.

Primary nondisjunction is the most common mechanism of trisomy D₁. Other genotypes have been described; among these are partial D₁ trisomy, Translocation D₁ and mosaicism. Recently, Juberg has described a premature female newborn with a ring-D chromosome and multiple congenital anomalies.

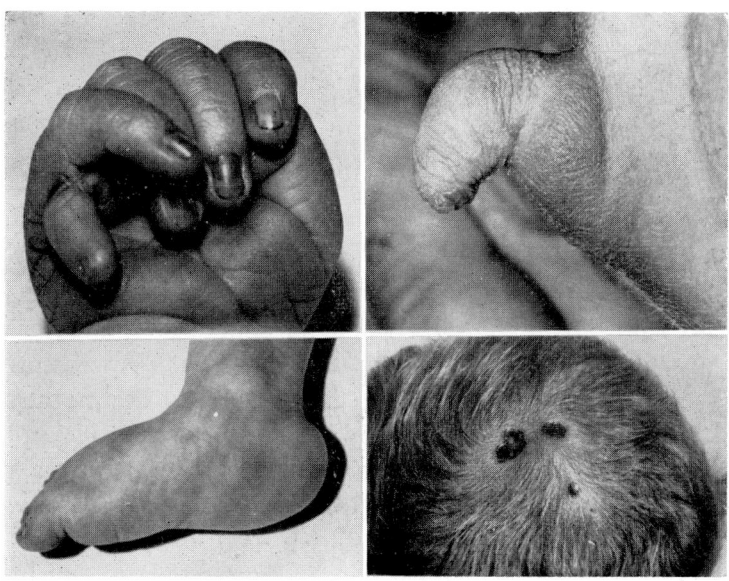

Fig. 20. Several common anomalies in the D₁ trisomy syndrome. A. Flexion of fingers, narrow hyperconvex fingernails, and polydactyly; B. Abnormal scrotum; C. Rocker-bottom foot; and D. Midline occipital scalp defects. (From Smith, Autosomal abnormalities, op. cit. Courtesy of Dr. Smith and the C. V. Mosby Company.)

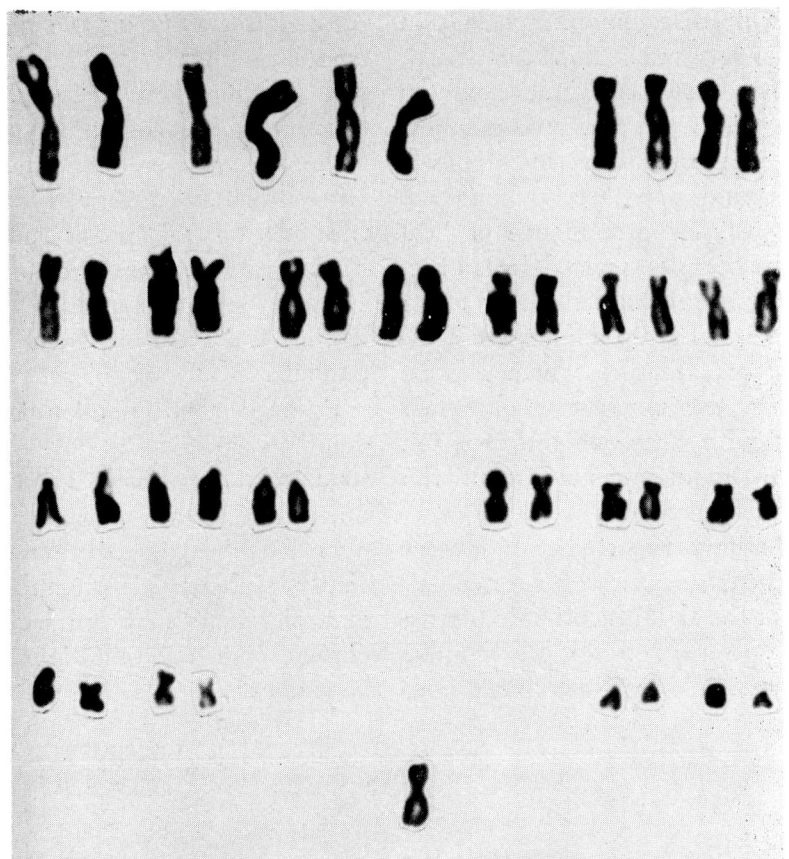

Fig. 21.   Karyotype of patient with Bonnevie-Ullrich-Turner syndrome. Note only one member in the sex chromosome group, i.e., X monosomy. Classification according to Patau[39].

SEX CHROMOSOME ABERRATIONS — BONNIVIE-ULLRICH-TURNER'S SYNDROME

In 1938, Turner described a syndrome in postpuberal females associated with short stature, sexual infantilism, cubitus valgus and webbed neck. In 1959, Ford[10] described forty-five chromosomes and XO karyotype in a fourteen-year-old girl with short stature, primary amenorrhea and absence of secondary sex characteristics. However, X-monosomy can be clinically suspected in the newborn. The use of sex chromatin tests has made it possible to identify XO individuals reliably after the third day of life. This syndrome occurs in 0.4 per 1000 female birth[34]. About 80 per cent of these girls have sex chromatin negative cells[44] with an XO chromosomal pattern (Fig. 21). The remainder of these patients have been reported as bein chromatin positive with either XX pattern, an isochromosome or ring X chromosome[19, 31]. Various types of mosaicism may also occur.

In the newborn, Turner's syndrome is more correctly called Bonnevie-

Ullrich syndrome. This syndrome consists of congenital lymphangiectatic edema of the hands and feet, with cutis laxa and numerous other anomalies (Fig. 22). It was considered a separate entity until recently, when it was noted by Grumbach that the majority of these patients had negative sex chromatin

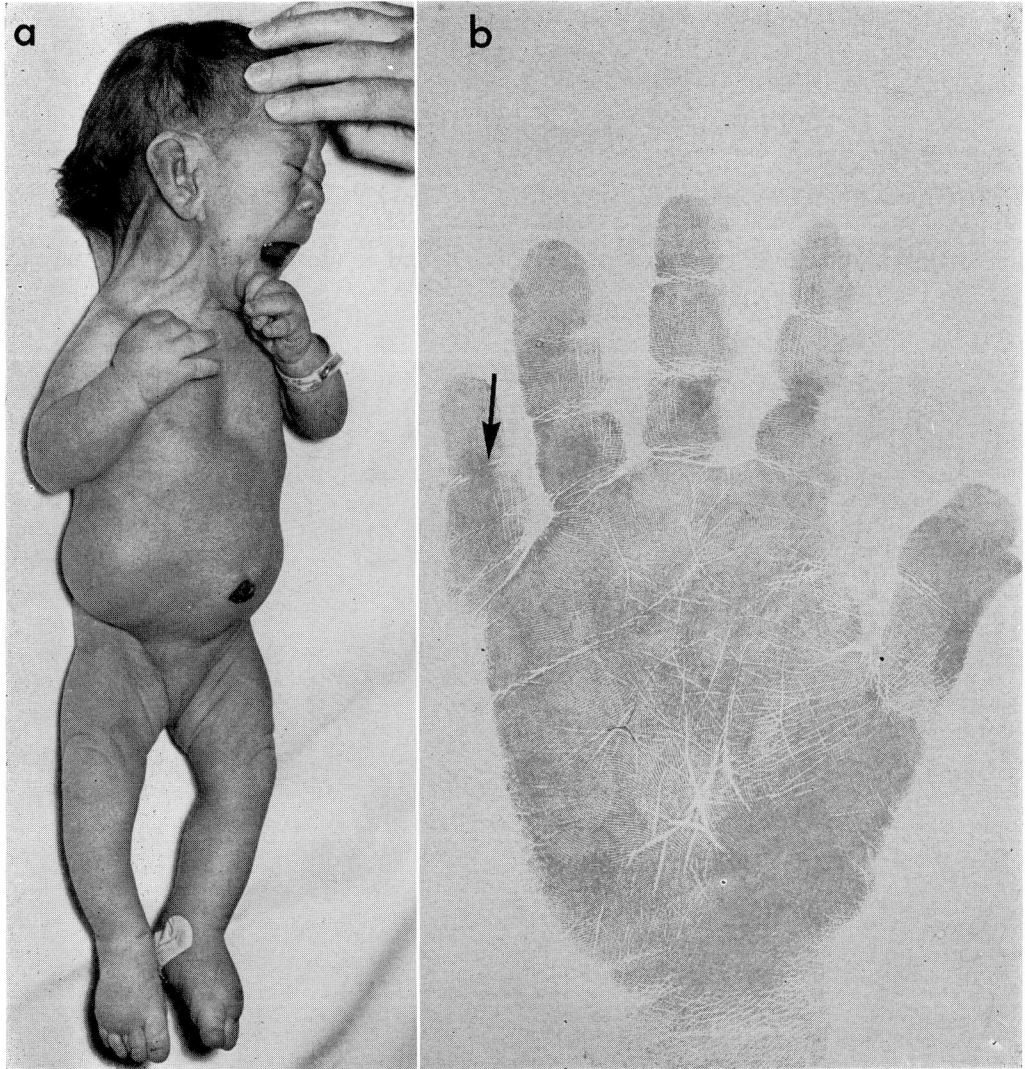

Fig. 22. Newborn with Bonnevie-Ullrich-Turner syndrome. Note low-set ears, small mandible, webbed neck and congenital lymphangiectatic edema of the hands and feet. (From Uchida and Soltan, op. cit. Courtesy of Dr. Uchida and the Saunders Company.)

Fig. 23. Palm print of patient with the Bonnevie-Ullrich-Turner syndrome. The arrow points to single crease on the fifth digit. (From Uchida and Soltan, op. cit. Courtesy of Dr. Uchida and the Saunders Company.)

pattern. The major features in the newborn female suspected of having Bonnevie-Ullrich-Turner syndrome are the following: hypertelorism; epicanthal folds; high arched palate; micrognathia; elongated or deformed ears; webbed neck; lymphedema of the dorsal aspects of the hands and feet; renal malformations; congenital heart disease (usually coarctation of the aorta); short tubular bones of hands and feet; and small nails. Gonodal dysplasia is the characteristic finding on laparotomy. Mild psychomotor retardation is an inconsistent find-

ing. Lymphedema of the feet of a newborn should alert one to this syndrome, for this has been a most reliable sign in our experience. The somatic features of this syndrome are variable. A newborn female has recently been diagnosed at our hospital with the features of arthrogryposis multiplex congenita, and chromosome analysis revealed XO monosomy[25]. Dermatoglyphic findings in Bonnevie-Ullrich-Turner syndrome reveal Simian creases, single creases on the fifth digit (Fig. 23), and bilateral distal triradii may be

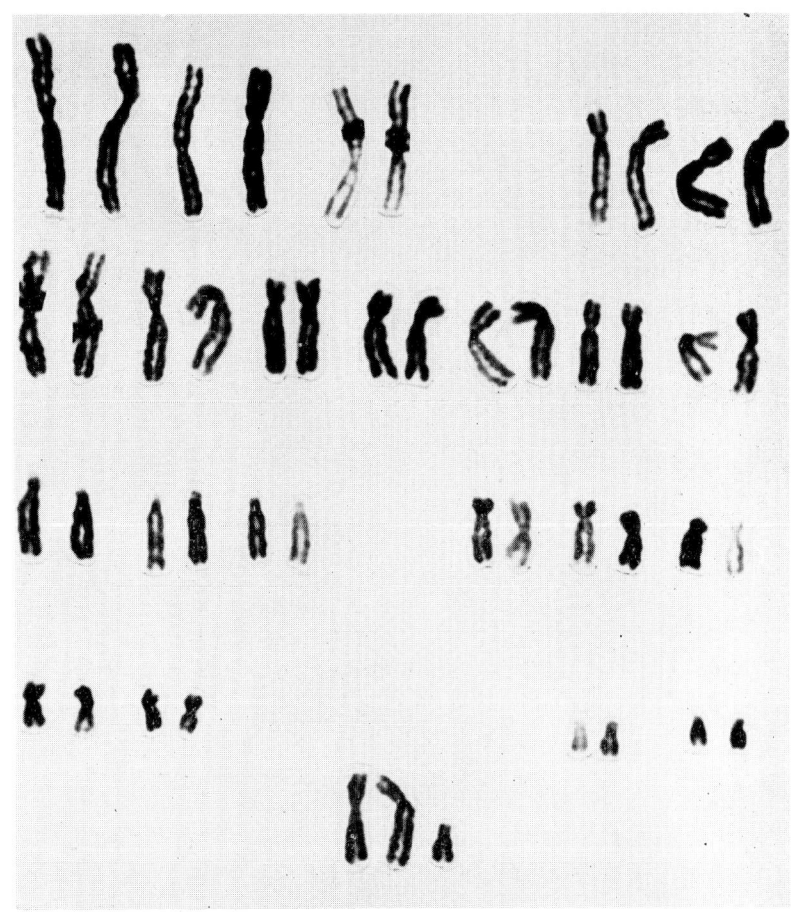

Fig. 24. Karyotype of a patient with Klinefelter syndrome. Note the extra chromosome X in the sex chromosome group. Classification according to Patau[39].

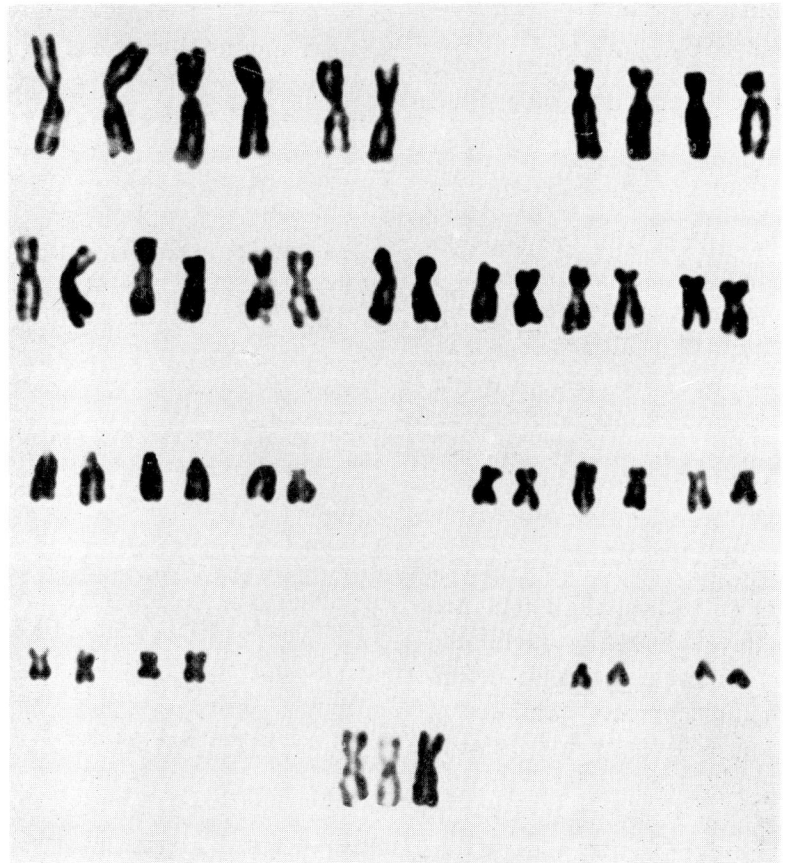

Fig. 25. Karyotype of a patient with trisomy X syndrome. Note three X-chromosomes in the sex chromosome group. Classification according to Patau[39].

present[53]. The XO condition is the only monosomic state found in man.

KLINEFELTER SYNDROME

Little will be said of this syndrome because it is almost impossible to suspect this condition clinically in the newborn. In 1942, Klinefelter described a syndrome in postpuberal males consisting of small testes with tubular hyalinization, azoospermia and gynecomastia. Also noted were high concentrations of urinary gonadotropins and low concentrations of urinary 17-keto-steroids. Soon it was noted that these patients were chromatin positive[43]. Jacobs and Strong[21] in 1959 noted forty-seven chromosomes and an XXY chromosome complement (Fig. 24). Although impossible to diagnose clinically in the newborn, it is possible to note small phallus in prepuberal males as well as mental retardation, although these are both inconsistently present. The frequency of chromatin positive male newborns is 1.96 to 3.10 per 1000 (Caucasian) live births[35]. A variety of genotypes may be present, but it is accepted that the XXY is the common denominator of all cases for the development of testicular dysgenesis.

TRISOMY X

Forty-five cases of XXX have been reported since Jacobs and co-workers first reported a female with trisomy X and chromatin-two positive buccal smear in 1959[7] (Fig. 25). There is no distinct clinical picture in the neonate. Menstrual disorders are common, as is mental retardation. Hypertelorism, hypotonia, micrognathia and low-set ears present in the newborn lead to a suspicion of a possible chromosome aberration. The incidence in newborn females is rare.

SUMMARY

Knowledge of variations in the incidence of maldevelopment has facilitated discovery of its causes. Precise definitions of maldevelopment and exact information on its frequency are necessary in order to understand factors which determine chromosomal aberrations. It is important that more cases be reported.

Each of the chromosomal aberrations represents a specific genetic imbalance which upsets the normal process of embryonic differentiation. For each, the total pattern of resultant anomalies will, with rare exception, allow for a clinical diagnosis. The total pattern of anomalies, minor and major, should be considered. No single anomaly is pathognomonic. There may be a wide variability in patients having the same syndrome. The "cri du chat" seems to be pathognomonic when noted early in infancy. As the patient grows older, the cry becomes more difficult to characterize. Accuracy in diagnosis is essential. It is hoped that the features mentioned in this chapter will help to focus the attention of the

physician upon a more accurate evaluation of the total pattern of anomalies in order to arrive at a specific clinical diagnosis.

REFERENCES

1. Bergman, S., Flodstrom, I., Ansehn, S.: Cri du chat. Lancet, 1:768, 1965.
2. Book, J. A., Atkins, L., and Santesson, B.: Some new data on autosomal aberrations in man. Path. Biol. (Paris), 11:1159-1162, 1963.
3. Breg, W. R., Steele, M. W., Eidelman, A. I., Lion, D. J., and Terzakis, T. A.: A ring chromosome-5 in a newborn infant with the cri du chat syndrome. Proceedings of the Society for Pediatric Research, 67, May 4-6, 1965.
4. Buhler, E. M., Buhler, V. R., and Stalder, G. R.: Deletion of chromosome-18. Lancet, 1:170, 1964.
5. Cavalieri, S.: La sindrome della voce da gatta. Osp. Inf. "Alessondri" Verona. Fracastro, 57:369-371, 1964.
6. Collman, R. D., and Stoller, A.: A survey of mongolism and congenital anomalies of the central nervous system in Victoria. New Zeal. Med. J., 64:24-28, 1962.
7. Day, R. W., Larson, W., and Wright, S. W.: Clinical and cytogenic studies in a group of females with XXX sex chromosome complements. J. Pediat., 64:24-26, 1964.
8. Dumars, R. W., Gaskill, C., and Kitzmiller, N.: Cat cry syndrome. Amer. J. Dis. Child., 108:538-542, 1964.
9. Edwards, J. H., Harnden, D. G., Cameron, A. H., Crosoe, V. M., and Wolff, O. H.: A new trisomic syndrome. Lancet, 1:787-788, 1960.
10. Ford, C. E., Jones, R. W., Polani, P. E., de Almeida, J. C., and Breggs, J. H.: A sex chromosome anomaly in a case of gonadal dysgenesis. Lancet, 1:711-713, 1959.
11. Gerald, Park: Personal communication, 1964.
12. German, J., MacIntyre, M. N., and de Grouchy, J.: Autoradiography of group 4-5 chromosomes in "cri du chat" syndrome. Cytogenetics (Basel), 3:347, 1964.
13. de Grouchy, J., Arthins, M., Salmon, C., Lamy, M., and Thieffry, S.: Le syndrome du cri du chat. Ann. Genet. (Paris), 7:No. 1, 1964.
14. de Grouchy, J., Lamy, M., Theffry, S., Arthins, M., and Salmon, C.: Deletion du chromosome 18. C. R. Acad. Sci. (Paris), 256:1028, 1963.

15. Hall, B.: Mongolism in newborns. Acta Paediat. (Suppl.), **153**:84, 1964.

16. Hansemann, D.: Virchow. Arch. Path. Anat., **123**:356-359, 1891. (Reference given by Ford and Hammerton, 1956.)

17. Hecht, F., Bryant, J. S., Motulsky, A. G., and Giblett, E. R.: The no. 17-18 (E) trisomy syndrome. J. Pediat., **63**:605, 1963.

18. Huehns, E. R., Lutzner, M., and Hecht, F.: Neutrophile projections in trisomy D$_1$. Lancet, **1**:589, 1964.

19. Hustinx, W. J.: An X-ring chromosome in a Turner patient without a specific peripheral localization. Proc. XI Int. Congr. Genet., **1**:313, 1963.

20. Hustinx, T. W. J., and Wijffels, J. C. H. M.: "Cri du chat" syndrome. Lancet, **II**:135, 1965.

21. Jacobs, P. A., and Strong, J. A.: A case of human intersexuality having a possble XXY sex-determining mechanism. Nature (London), **183**:302, 1959.

22. Juberg, R. C., Adams, S., Venema, W. J., and Hart, M. G.: Multiple congenital anomalies associated with a ring-D-chromosome: A new autosomal syndrome. Proceedings of the May 1965 meeting of the Society for Pediatric Research. Univ. of Michigan Medical School, 1965, p. 69.

23. Kundrat, H.: Arrhinencephalie als Typische art von Missbildung. Graz, von Leuscher und Lubensky, 1882.

24. LaPolla, J. J.: Parental age in mongolism. Unpublished data.

25. LaPolla, J. J., and Wander, H.: Arthrogyposis and Turner's Syndrome. Unpublished data.

26. Lejeune, J., Gautier, M., and Turpin, R.: E'tude the chromosomes somatiques de neuf infants mongoliens. C. R. Acad. Sci. (Paris), **248**:1721-1730, 1959.

27. Lejeune, J., LaFourcade, J., Berger, R., and Turpin, R.: Malodie "du cri chat" et sa "Neciproque". C. R. Acad. Sci. (Paris), **258**:5026, 1964.

28. Lejeune, J., LaFourcade, J., Berger, R., and Turpin, R.: Le syndrome du cri du chat. C. R. Acad. Sci. (Paris), **258**:5767, 1964.

29. Lejeune, J., LaFourcade, J., deGrouchy, J., Berger, R., Goutier, M., Salmon, C., and Turpin, R.: Deletion partielle du bras court du chromosome 5; Individualisation d'un novel etat morbide. Sem. Hop. Paris, No. 25: 1079 (April 14), 1964.

30. Lejeune, J., LaFourcade J., Berger, R., Vialatte, J., Boeswillwald, M., Seringe, P., and Turpin, R.: Trois cas de deletion partielle du

bras cort d'un chromosome-5. C. R. Acad. Sci. (Paris), **257**:3098-3110, 1963.

31. Lindsten, J., and Tillinger, F. G.: Self-perpetuating ring chromosome in a patient with gonadal dysgenesis. Lancet, **I**:593, 1962.

32. London Report: The London conference on the normal human karyotype. Cytogenetics (Basel), **2**:264, 1963.

33. MacIntyre, M. N., Staples, W. I., LaPolla, J., Hempel, J. M.: The cat cry syndrome. Amer. J. Dis. Child., **108**:538, 1964.

34. MacLean, Harnden, D. G., Court Brown, W. M., Bond, J., and Mantle, D. J.: Sex-chromosome abnormalities in newborn babies. Lancet, **I**:286, 1964.

35. MacLean, N., Mitchell, J. M., Harnden, D. G., and Williams, J.: A survey of sex-chromosome abnormalities among 4514 mental defectives. Lancet, **I**:293, 1962.

36. Marden, P. M., Smith, D. W., and McDonald, M. J.: Congenital anomalies in the newborn infant, including minor variations. J. Pediat., **64**:357-367, 1964.

37. McCracken, J. S., Gorden, P. R.: Cat cry syndrome. Lancet, **I**:23-, 1965.

38. Painter, T. S., Studies in mammalian spermatogenesis. The spermatogenesis of man. J. Exp. Zool., **37**:291-295, 1923.

39. Patau, K.: Identification of chromosomes. In Yunis, J. J. (ed.): Human Chromosome Methodology. New York, Academic Press, 1965, pp. 155-185.

40. Patau, K., Smith, D. W., Therman, E., Inhorn, S. L., and Wagner, H. P.: Multiple congenital anomaly caused by an extra autosome. Lancet I, 790, 1960.

41. Patau, K., Therman, E., and Inhorn, S. L.: DNA replication pattern in the cat cry syndrome (Abstract). Amer. Soc. Hum. Genet. (Boulder), 20, 1964.

42. Penrose, L. S.: Mongolism. Brit. Med. Bull., **5**:404, 1961.

43. Plunkett, E. R., and Barr, M. L.: Testicular dysgenesis affecting the seminiferous tubules principally, with chromatin-positive nuclei. Lancet, **II**:853, 1956.

44. Polani, P. E.: Turner's syndrome and allied conditions; clinical features and chromosome abnormalities. Brit. Med. Bull., **17**:200, 1961.

45. Punnett, H. H., Carpenter, G. G., and DiGeorge, A. M.: The cat cry syndrome. Lancet, **II**:588, 1964.

46. Ricci, N., Ventimiglia, B., Dallapiccola, Franceschini, F., and Preto, G.: "Cri du chat" syndrome. Lancet, **I**:1279, 1965.

47. Rosenfield, R. L., Breibart, S., Isaacs, H., Klenit, H. D., and Mellman, W. J.: Trisomy

18 syndrome. Amer. J. Med. Sci., **244**:763, 1962.

48. Schmid, W.: The cat cry syndrome. Cytogenetics (Basel), **2**:175, 1963.

49. Shaw, M. W., Cohen, M. M., and Hildebrandt, H. M.: A familial 4/5 reciprocal translocation resulting in partial trisomy 13. Amer. J. Hum. Genet., **17#1**:54, 1965.

50. Smith, D. W.: Autosomal abnormalities. Amer. J. Obstet. Gynec. Symposium on Congenital Defect, 1964, p. 1057.

51. Smith, ibid., p. 1062.

52. Smith, ibid., p. 1064.

53. Uchida, I. A., and Soltan, H. C.: Evaluation of dermatoglyphics in medical genetics. Pediat. Clin. N. Amer., **Vol. 10#2**:409, 1963.

54. Uchida, I. A., Wang, H. C., and Mcrae, R.

N.: Deletion of chromosome 18 (Abstract). Amer. Soc. Hum. Genet. (Boulder), 1964, p. 32.

55. Van Dyke, H. E., Valdmanis, A., and Mann, J. D.: A patient with deletion of chromosome 18. Amer. J. Hum. Genet. (Boulder), **16**:364, 1964.

56. Wolf, V., Porsch, R., Baitsch, H., and Reinwein, H.: Deletion on short arms of a B chromosome without "cri du chat" syndrome. Lancet, **I**:769, 1965.

57. Yunis, J. J.: Human chromosome in disease. In Yunis, op. cit., p. 220.

58. Yunis, J. J., Hook, E. B., and Mayer M.: Identification of the mongolism chromosome by DNA replication analysis. Amer. J. Hum. Genet. (Boulder), **17**:191, 1965.

The Methodology of Cytogenetics: Identification of Chromosomal Karyotypes

JENÖ E. SZAKACS, M.D., IRENE ROECKEL, M.D., AND
ROBERT C. NORTHCUTT, M.D.

INTRODUCTION

The role of chromosomes in the hereditary processes has been studied extensively during the last sixty years in many species. Human chromosomes, although very small and difficult to handle, were eventually correctly counted in 1956 by two groups of investigators[3, 14]. By 1959, constant chromosomal aberrations were described in Down's, Kleinfelter's and Turner's syndromes[6, 5, 4]. These early results stimulated the development of practical methods for cytogenetic studies applicable to clinical medicine. Chromosomes were obtained from dividing cells directly from tumors, or from effusions, from long-term tissue cultures of fibroblasts and bone marrow preparations. In 1960, a method to obtain chromosomes from dividing peripheral blood leukocytes was described by Moorhead[9] and his associates, following Nowell's discovery that a phytohemagglutinin obtained from red kidney beans stimulates mitosis of leukocytes. Improvements and simplifications[8] on the original method are practically as numerous as the laboratories where chromosome cultures are being prepared. In the experience of the authors, the techniques described by Scherz and Louro[13] and the method published by The Radiation Exposure Evaluation Laboratory of the U.S. Naval Hospital, Bethesda[12, 16], have proved satisfactory. Essentially, the methods consist of incubation of peripheral leukocytes in a culture medium containing phytohemagglutinin that stimulates a burst of mitoses in the lymphocytes. Mitosis then is blocked in metaphase with addition of colchicine. The cells are exposed to hypotonic salt solution which allows separation of chromosomes from the metaplate cluster, and are fixed in that state. The chromosomes are obtained in a flat plane on slides from the fixed cell either by an air- or blaze-drying. Counting and identification of the chromosomes are accomplished under the oil immersion lens of a microscope using phase contrast or, more commonly, after staining.

Schematic diagram of chromosomes to depict morphologic characteristics utilized in karyotyping is shown on Figure 1. The fine structure is sometimes visible in human chromosomes, and the schematic diagram by Wilson[15] serves well to indicate the primary constriction (centromere) as well as a secondary constriction between the satellite and centromere.

The normal complement of human chromosomes from a preparation of peripheral leukocytes is shown in Figure 2. Two of each of the chromosomes

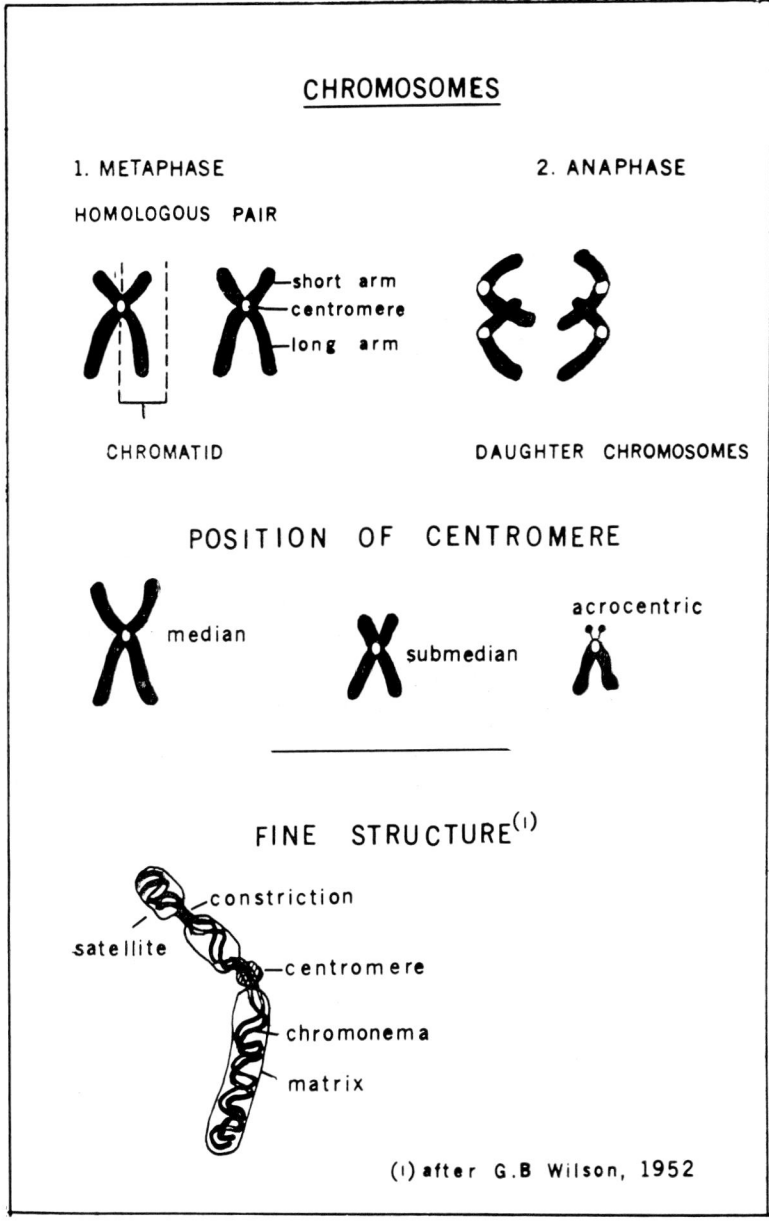

Fig. I

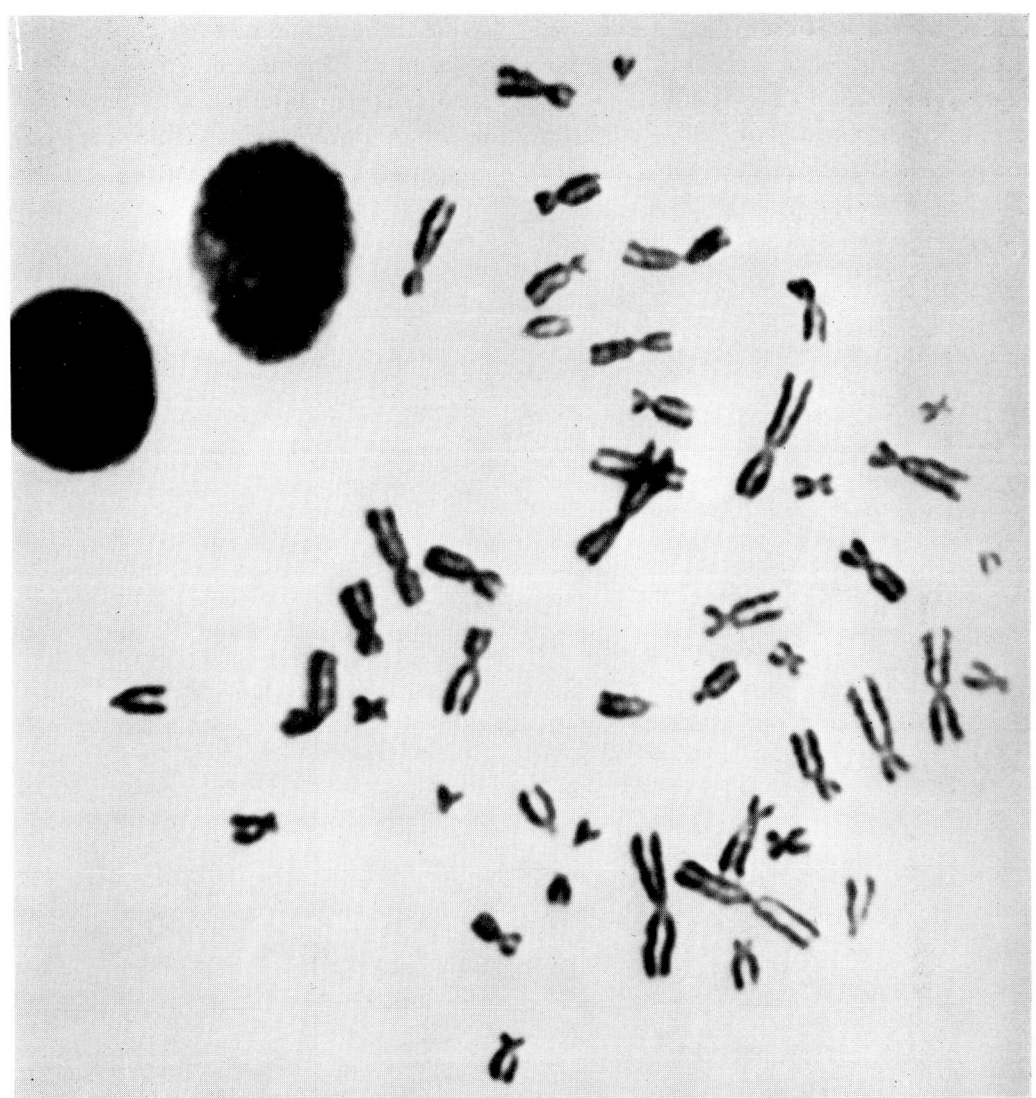

Fig. 2

are alike and can be paired, except for the sex chromosomes in the male. The pairs are referred to as "homologous chromosomes," and one of each pair is transmitted from the father, the other from the mother. The normal complement is twenty-two sets of homologous chromosomes per cell that are called "autosomes" in opposition to the sex chromosomes. The sex chromosomes referred to as X and Y are quite different in size. The normal male cell contains one X and one Y chromosome (XY), while that of the female contains two X chromosomes (XX). The total count of chromosomes is forty-six. It is easiest to obtain the count by dividing the field into smaller areas by drawing lines across as illustrated in Figure 3 and then counting each subdivision separately and totalling the results.

The twenty-two pairs of autosomes show considerable differences in size and in the position of their centromere, the point of attachment of the two chromatids. These differences are not random, but highly reproducible from cell to cell and characteristic of the species.

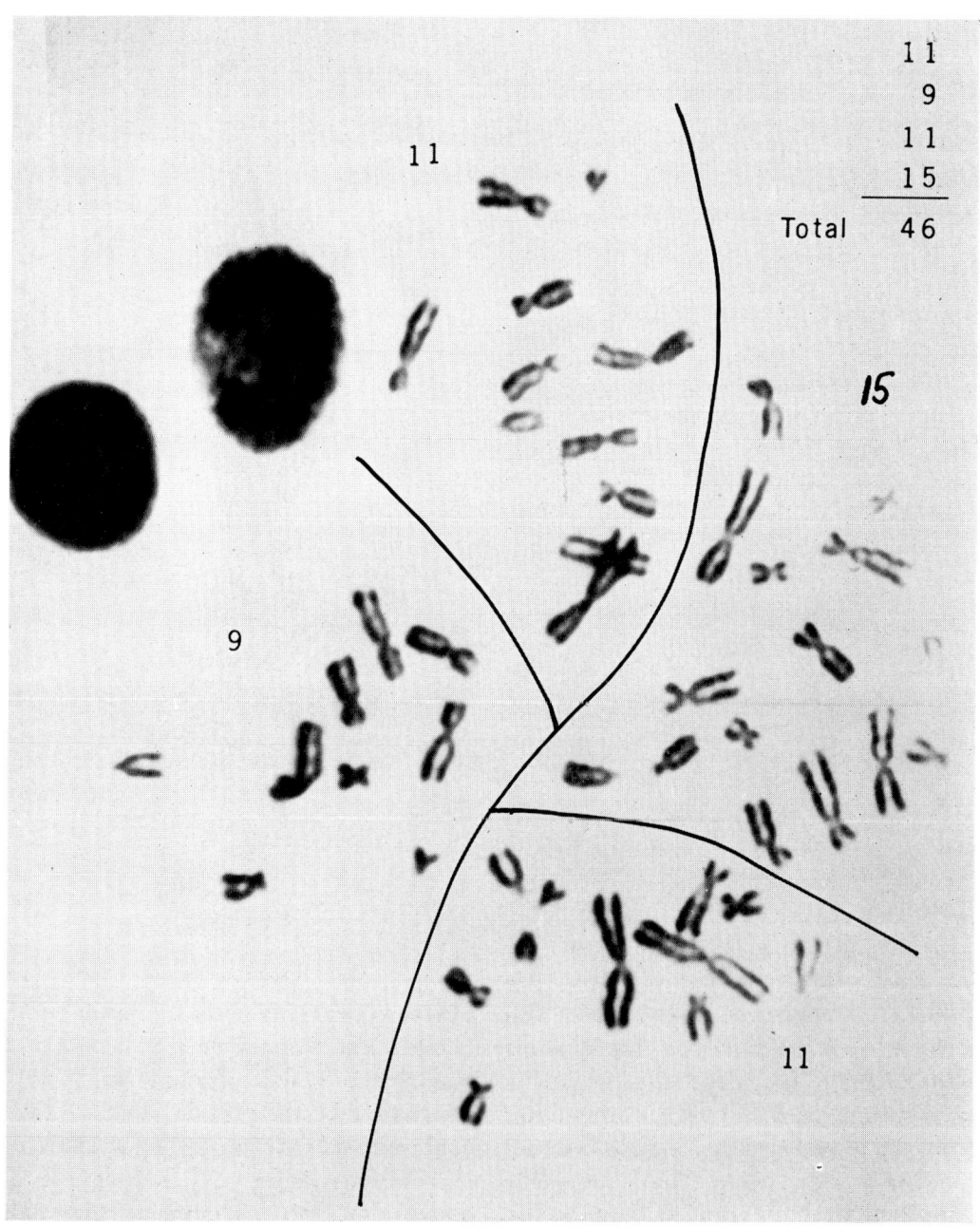

Fig. 3

It is self-evident that a systematic arrangement of the chromosomes would greatly facilitate identification of a group or individual chromosomes. An internationally accepted Standard System of Nomenclature was first proposed in Denver by a study group in 1960[2].

THE DENVER SYSTEM

Based on length of chromosomes and the position of the centromere, the autosomes are numbered from 1 to 22 in descending order of length. In such an arrangement the chromosomes form seven distinguishable groups. In addition, a number of individual chromosomes are shaped so that they can be definitely identified (1, 2, 3, 16, Y). The characterization of the seven groups is described in Table I.

The groups are also referred to by letters from A to G corresponding relatively to Group 1-3 through Group 21-22, in recent publications[10, 11]. A systematized array of the chromosomes of a single cell is referred to as a karyotype. An idealized chromosome set designed on the basis of measurements performed on chromosomes obtained from many cells is referred to as an "idiogram." Such an idiogram, illustrated in Figure 4 prepared after B. Lennox[7] according to the Denver System, is a useful introduction to karyotyping. The two numbers next to each pair represent the chromosome length ratio and the centromeric index. For example, Chromosome 1 represents 85/1000 of the total length of the chromosomes from a cell containing one X chromosome, and 48/100 is the ratio of the length of the shorter arm to the whole length of the chromosome itself.

TABLE I CONSPECTUS OF HUMAN MITOTIC CHROMOSOMES[2]

Group	1- 3	Large chromosomes with approximately median centromeres. The three chromosomes are readily distinguished from each other by size and centromere position.
Group	4- 5	Large chromosomes with submedian centromeres. The two chromosomes are difficult to distinguish, but Chromosome 4 is slightly longer.
Group	6-12	Medium-sized chromosomes with submedian centromeres. The X chromosome resembles the longer chromosomes in this group, especially Chromosome 6, from which it is difficult to distinguish. This large group is the one which presents major difficulty in identification of individual chromosomes.
Group	13-15	Medium-sized chromosomes with nearly terminal centromeres ("acrocentric" chromosomes).
Group	16-18	Rather short chromosomes with approximately median (in Chromosome 16) or submedian centromeres.
Group	19-20	Short chromosomes with approximately median centromeres.
Group	21-22	Very short, acrocentric chromosomes. The Y-chromosome is similar to these chromosomes.

KARYOTYPING

There are some useful landmarks to facilitate karyotyping.

1. Chromosomes of Group 1-3, or A, the largest chromosomes, can be identified at first sight and numbered.

2. Group 21-22, or G, and the Y chromosome if present, being the smallest and acrocentric, are easily counted and

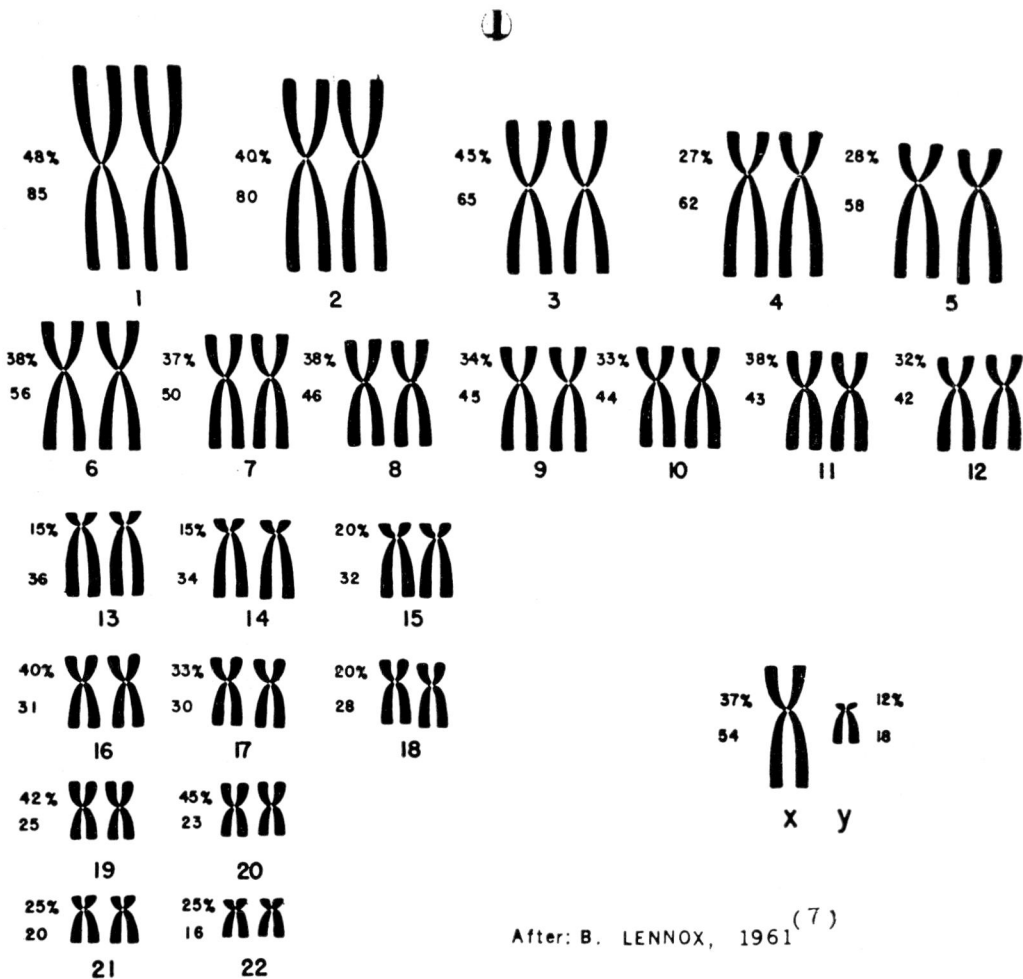

Fig. 4

identified as a group. Four are normally seen in the female, five in the male.

3. Group 13-15, or D, are medium-sized but also acrocentric (often referred to as the large acrocentrics). There are six chromosomes in all in this group with a definite "wishbone" shape.

4. From the remaining complement the two largest chromosomes with a pincer shape are identified as Group 4-5, or B.

5. The small x-shaped chromosomes are grouped as 19-20, or F.

6. Group 16-18, or E, and Group 6-12, or C, are classified by size as best as possible.

In Figure 5, the chromosomes are lettered according to the groups to which they belong. Chromosome pairs 1, 2, 3, 16 and possibly Y can be so marked as they are distinctive enough to be identified with certainty. The rest of the chromosomes are best arranged in order of decreasing length in the karyotype without an effort for numerical identification.

At this point, obtaining a karyotype is only a matter of cutting out the picture and mounting the images according to the idiogram of Lennox. The completed karyotype of a normal male example is illustrated in Figure 6.

DIRECT COUNTING

Karyotyping is the most illustrative way of demonstrating aberrations in the chromosome complement of a cell. A variation in chromosome complement from cell to cell, however, is detectable only by counting at least thirty mitoses. It is advantageous to count first the easily recognized small acrocentrics. A normal number in this count immediately rules out trisomy G (mongol), now believed to be Trisomy 22. Next, the large acrocentrics are counted. A

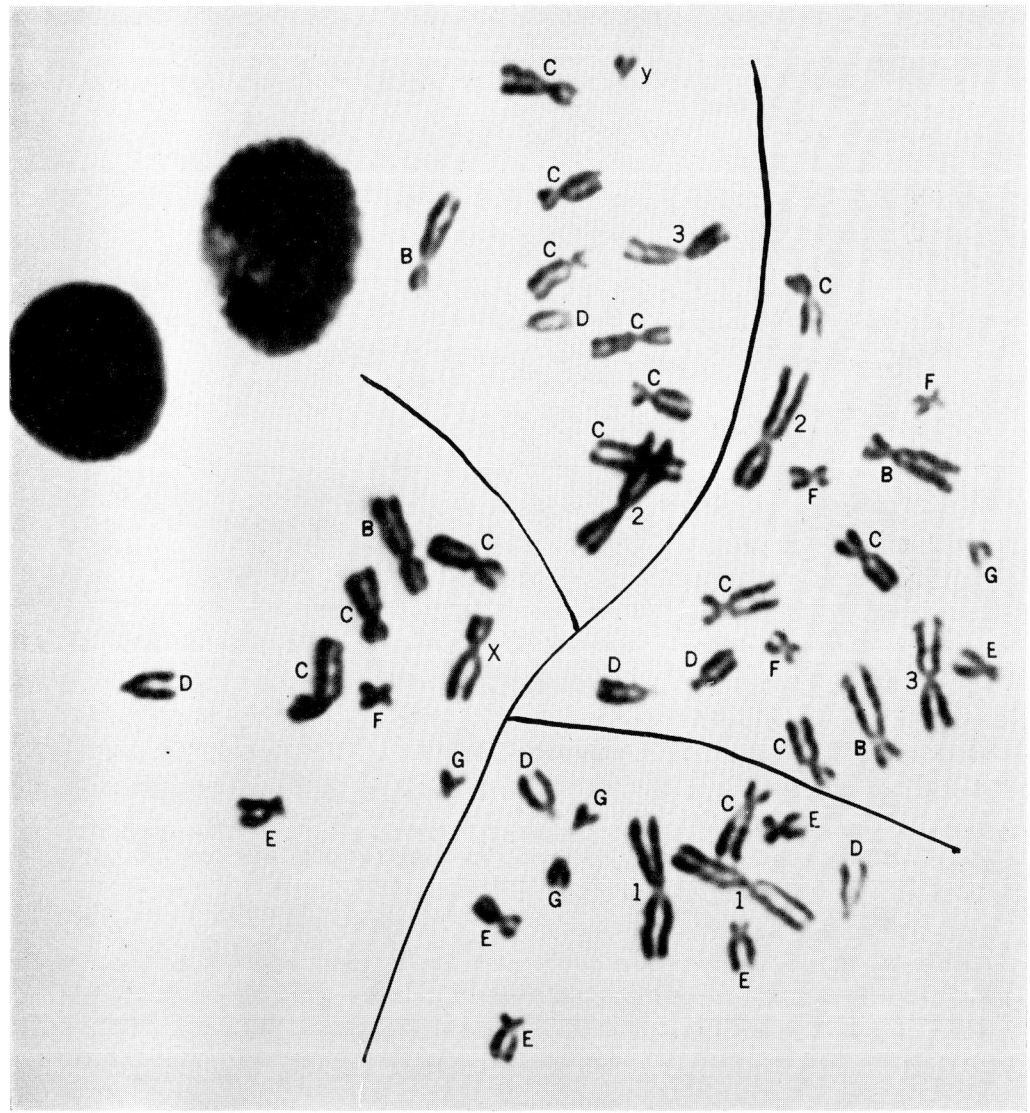

Fig. 5

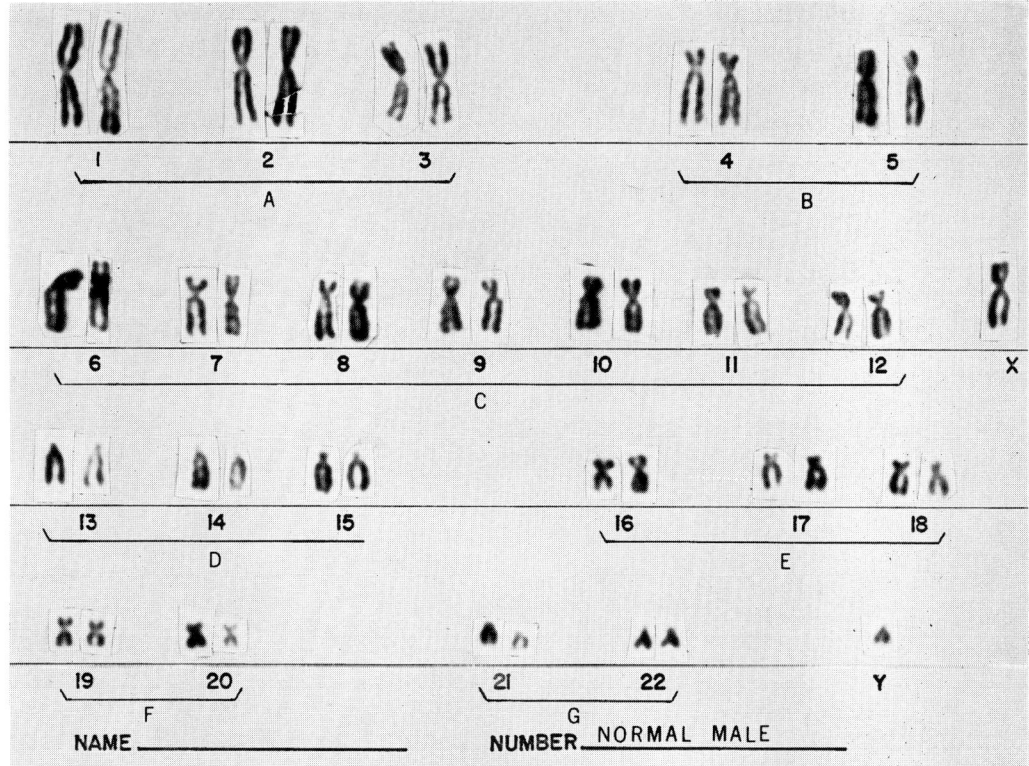

Fig. 6

normal number rules out Trisomy 18. The total number is counted finally to determine a modal number of the chromosomes. A representative mitosis is then photographed and processed for the karyotype. Should the patient have two or more types of chromosomal distribution as observed by different total count or variation in numbers within groups, a karyotype of each cell type should be prepared. For example, a patient with XO/XX chromosome complement is a mosaic female with Turner's syndrome. The total count in a portion of her mitoses will be forty-five, in the rest, forty-six. By patient counting and karyotyping it is possible to characterize even the more complicated mosaics.

Identification of individual chromosomes within the groups is difficult and requires special techniques, such as autoradiographic identification of DNA replication time and its rate, in addition to some more careful morphologic studies[11]. With the stepwise karyotyping procedure, much of the described and all of the more common aberrations of clinical significance can be identified.

INTERPRETATION OF RESULTS

Even with the best technique, only major alterations such as the absence of a chromosome or the excess of one or more can be detected immediately. With careful study, other gross structural abnormalities such as translocation

TABLE II*

Chromosomal Disorder	Karyotype	Possible Mechanism	Sex Ratio	Approximate Incidence
Autosomal disorders				
Down's syndrome (21 trisomy) 3 types	47/21 trisomy		slightly oftener males	1.6:1,000
1. Standard/ regular	47/21 trisomy	nondisjunction, failure chromo-mosome 21 to separate during maternal gametogenesis; non-familial; chromosomal accident		1:600 or 700
2. Translocation	46/21 trisomy (1 no. 21 attached to 15 chromosome)	familial (translocation)		5 to 10% Down's patients
3. Mosaic	2 sets chromosomes: 1 normal, other 47/21 trisomy	non-familial; error in mitotic division of an early embryonic cell		Extremely rare
18 trisomy	47/18 trisomy	altered gestation timing; accidental development of sperm or egg	oftenest female	0.23:1,000
D$_1$ trisomy	47/13-15	accidental development of sperm or egg	oftenest female	0.45:1,000
Sex chromosome anomalies				
Klinefelter's syndrome	usually 47/XXY found: XXYY, XXXY, XXXYY, XXXXY and occasional mosaicism	nondisjunction	males	1:500 general pop. 1:100 in mentally retarded
Turner's syndrome	45/xo; sometimes mosaicism with 1 set of normal chromosomes	nondisjunction	females	1:10,000
Unusual patterns	XXX, XXXX, XXXXX have been found	nondisjunction	females	

*After GUSTAFSON, S. H., and COURSIN, B. D.: *The Pediatric Patient.* Philadelphia, Lippincott, p. 28, 1964.

of genetic material from one chromosome to another have been detected, in 15/21 translocation, for example. Loss of genetic material can be identified if it is massive enough for detection, as in the cat cry syndrome. In this syndrome, part of the short arm of a chromosome 5 is missing. The (Ph[1]) Philadelphia chromosome is a small autosomic chromosome of Group 21-22 which has lost approximately one half of its long arm. Other acquired aberrations can be observed after deep X radiation and possibly in some cases of virus infections. A tabulation of the better understood syndromes is included in Table II.

An independent way of detecting numerical aberrations of chromosomes is based on counting sex chromatin of epithelial cell nuclei from buccal scrapings. Barr[1] has studied extensively the relationship of X chromosomes to sex chromatin and to the drumstick-shaped nuclear appendages in leukocytes. In general, one less nuclear chromatin clump is seen per nucleus than the number of X chromosomes present. If a cell population with different numbers of nuclear chromatin clumps are obtained from a patient, the possibility of a mosaic is to be entertained.

REFERENCES

1. Barr, M. L., and Carr, D. H.: Sex chromatin, sex chromosomes and sex anomalies. Canad. Med. Ass. J., 83:979-986, 1960.

2. Denver Study Group: A proposed standard system of nomenclature of human mitotic chromosomes. Eugen. Quart., 7:96-100, 1960.

3. Ford, C. E., and Hamerton, J. L.: The chromosomes of man. Nature (London), 178:1020, 1956.

4. Ford, C. E., et. al.: A sex chromosome anomaly in a case of gonadal dysgenesis (Turner's syndrome). Lancet, 1:711-713, 1959.

5. Jacobs, P. A., and Strong, J. A.: A case of human intersexuality having a possible XXY sex-determining mechanism. Nature (London), 183:302, 1959.

6. Lejeune, J., Gautier, M., and Turpin, R.: Etude des chromosomes somatiques de neuf enfants mongoliens. C. R. Acad. Sci. (Paris), 248:1721-1722, 1959.

7. Lennox, B.: Chromosomes for beginners. Lancet, 1:7185-1046-1051, 1961.

8. Mellman, W. J.: Human peripheral blood leukocyte cultures. In Yunis, J. J. (ed.): Human Chromosome Methodology. New York, Academic Press, 1965, pp. 21-49.

9. Moorhead, P. S., et al.: Chromosome preparations of leukocytes cultured from human peripheral blood. Exp. Cell Rev., 20:613-616, 1960.

10. Patau, K.: The identification of individual chromosomes, especially in man. Amer. J. Hum. Genet., 12:250-276, 1960.

11. Patau, K.: Identification of chromosomes. In Yunis, op cit., pp. 155-186.

12. Radiation Exposure Evaluation Laboratory, U.S. Naval Hosp.: A method for human chromosome analysis using whole blood. Bethesda, Maryland, 1965.

13. Scherz, R. G., and Louro, J. L.: A simple method for making chromosome slides. Amer. J. Clin. Path., 40:222-225, 1963.

14. Tjio, J. H., and Levan, A.: The chromosome number of man. Hereditas (Lund), 42:1, 1956.

15. Wilson, G. B.: Outline of Genetics. Michigan State University Press, Figure 1, page 4.

16. Northcutt, R. C., Mella, G. W., and Dickson, L.: The analysis of human chromosomes. Post grad. Med., 39:285-294, 1966.

The Methodology of Cytogenetics: Techniques for Chromosome Culture

JENÖ E. SZAKACS, M.D., IRENE ROECKEL, M.D., AND ROBERT C. NORTHCUTT, M.D.

INTRODUCTION

Short-term peripheral leukocyte cultures can be performed with standard laboratory equipment available in most clinical laboratories. The technique, however, is by no means simple. The procedure includes six basic steps.

1. Concentration of leukocytes from venous blood may be obtained by passive settling of the red cells. The settling may be accelerated by agglutinating the RBC with phytohemagglutinins or by centrifugation.

2. The incubation of leukocytes in culture media may be performed with or without additional enrichment (bovine serum). Addition of phytohemagglutinin enhances mitotic activity.

3. The blocking of mitosis is performed by the addition of colchicine. The exposure time and concentration of colchicine influences the degree of contraction of the chromosomes.

4. The clumps of chromosomes in the metaphase plates are dispersed by the addition of hypotonic saline, diluted serum or protein solutions.

5. The quality and amount of dispersion of the chromosomes is influenced by the concentration of acetic acid during fixation.

6. Spreading the chromosomes on microscope slides may be accomplished by gentle squashing, by air-drying or by a flame-drying technique.

In addition to these basic steps, the preparations may be stained by the Giemsa or Orcein stains.

Two methods are presented in this chapter: the method of Moorhead et al.[1] as modified by Scherz and Louro[2]; and the method used at the U.S. Naval Hospital, Bethesda, Maryland.

MOORHEAD METHOD MODIFIED BY SCHERZ AND LOURO[1-3]

PRINCIPLE

Leukocyte-rich plasma is obtained by allowing the red cells to settle. The plasma is then inoculated into an artificial culture medium containing phytohemagglutinin and incubated for three days. Mitosis then is blocked in metaphase by the addition of colchicine. Slides are prepared by blaze-drying. Staining is with Wright's stain.

Reagents

1. *Bacto-phytohemagglutinin M or P* (Difco).

2. *Sterile water,* 5 ml ampules (diluent for reagent 1).

3. *Heparin* (1000 units per ml).

4. *Culture mediums, TC 199 or NCTC 109* (Difco).

5. *Colchicine* (USP) or *Colcimide* (Ciba). The colchicine is diluted with buffered saline solution (reagent 5) to provide a concentration of 40 µg per ml of saline.

6. *Buffered saline solution* (diluent for reagent 5). Stock buffered saline is prepared as follows: (a). Approximately 1.4 gm of calcium chloride is dissolved in 200 ml of distilled water; (b). Eighty gm NaCl, 4 gm KCl, 0.6 gm KH_2PO_4 • $2H_2O$, 0.6 gm Na_2HPO_4 • $2H_2O$ are dissolved in 100 ml of 0.2 per cent phenol red aqueous solution, and the volume is adjusted to 800 ml with distilled water. Solutions (a) and (b) are combined, and water is added to make 1100 ml.

    The working buffered solution is obtained by diluting the stock solution 1:10, and sterilizing it under 10 lbs of steam pressure (115 C) for ten minutes.

7. *Sodium citrate,* 1.12 per cent aqueous solution (w/v).

8. *Fixing solution* (1:3 glacial acetic acid:methanol), freshly mixed.

9. *Wright's stain.*

10. *Absolute alcohol.*

11. *Xylene.*

12. *Permount* (mounting medium).

13. *Penicillin G,* aqueous crystalline, 2000 units per ml.

14. *Streptomycin sulfate,* aqueous, 2 mg per ml.

Procedure

Collection of specimen

Ten ml of venous blood are drawn into a heparinized syringe and transferred without foaming into a sterile screw cap tube. (Caution: Hemolysis interferes with the procedure.) The tubes are placed upright in a refrigerator for two to three hours to allow sedimentation of red cells.

Planting

Five ml of culture medium (TC 199 or NCTC 109) and 0.05 ml bacto-phytohemagglutinin are placed in a 2 oz sterile bottle. The addition at this point of 100 units of aqueous crystalline penicillin (0.05 ml) and 10 mg of streptomycin sulfate (0.05 ml) is optional.

Approximately 2 ml of leukocyte-rich plasma is aspirated from the specimen and added to the culture medium. The bottle is stoppered and gently agitated.

Incubation

Incubation may be started immediately at 37.5 C for sixty-eight to seventy-two hours, or it may be postponed for as long as three days, if the bottle is refrigerated.

At the end of the first incubation period (seventy hours) 0.25 ml of colchicine in saline is added to the culture.

The culture is gently mixed and incubated for four more hours.

Cell Preparation

1. The culture is poured into a graduated 15 ml conical centrifuge tube and centrifuged for ten minutes at 800 rpm. The supernatant is decanted.

2. Ten ml of warm (37 C) 1.12 per cent sodium citrate solution is placed in the original culture bottle and gently agitated to remove any cells that adhere to the glass.

3. Several drops of citrate solution are added from the culture bottle to the cell button in the centrifuge tube. The cells are suspended by gentle agitation, then the rest of the citrate solution is added.

4. The cell suspension is further incubated from fifteen to twenty-five minutes at 37.5 C.

Fixation

1. The cell suspension is centrifuged at the end of the incubation period for ten minutes at 800 rpm and the supernatant is discarded.

2. The cell button is dispersed by adding dropwise the freshly prepared cold fixing solution (reagent 8) until approximately 5 ml of fixative have been added.

3. The suspension is centrifuged and the supernatant fixative is discarded. Fixative is added as in the previous steps two more times. The cells are then ready for preparation of slides.

Spreading by Blaze-Drying

1. Slides are prepared by cleaning with 70 per cent alcohol. (Only *new* glass slides should be used.)

2. With a Pasteur pipette, four to five small drops are placed on the slide and allowed to spread.

3. The slide is immediately ignited with a Bunsen burner or a match.

4. The blaze is allowed to extinguish itself.

5. The few remaining drops of moisture are shaken off by tapping the slide.

6. The slide is allowed to dry completely before staining.

Staining

Wright's stain is used in the customary manner.

Permanent Mounting

The slides are dipped in absolute alcohol and then twice in xylene. The cover slide is attached with permount. The slides prepared by this technique are adequate for karyotyping and direct counting of chromosomes.

THE REEL METHOD[4, 5]

INTRODUCTION

This method for chromosome analysis has proved to be successful in the Radiation Exposure Evaluation Laboratory of the U.S. Naval Hospital, Bethesda, Maryland. The principles are the same as previously described. More emphasis is placed on treatment of the cells with hypotonic salt solution in order to disperse the chromosomes from the metaphase plate. Blaze-drying and staining of chromosomes with Giemsa "blood" stain complete the preparation.

REAGENTS

1. *Tissue culture medium TC-109 or TC-199* (Difco).

2. *Bacto-phytohemagglutinin P* (Difco).

3. *Sterile water*, 5 ml ampule (diluent for reagent 2).

4. *Fetal bovine serum* (sterile).

5. *Penicillin-G*, aqueous crystalline 2000 units per ml.

6. *Streptomycin sulfate* aqueous, 2 mg per ml.

7. *Heparin sodium*, solution 1000 units per ml (free of phenol).

8. *Colcimide* (Ciba). One vial (1 mg) of colcimide is dissolved in 25 ml of TC-109 in a sterile rubber-stoppered bottle to allow aseptic entry. Two drops of this solution are used per culture.

9. *Fibrinolysin*, human.

10. *Hank's Balanced Salt Solution*, adjusted to pH 7.4 with sodium bicarbonate. 9.9 gm of Difco's Dried Hank's BSS are dissolved in 1000 ml of distilled water. The temperature is brought to 37 C and the pH is adjusted to 7.4.

11. *Fixing solution.* One part glacial acetic acid, three parts methanol freshly mixed, chilled to 4 C.

12. *Staining solution*: Giemsa "blood" stain, 10 ml; ammonium hydroxide, 0.15 N, 3 ml; distilled water to make 100 ml.

13. *Acetone*

14. *Xylene*

PROCEDURE FOR CULTURING

Preparation of Nutrient Medium

The following are added in sequence to 10 ml of TC-109 or TC-199 tissue culture medium in a sterile, 1 oz bottle:

The contents of the bottle are gently mixed and the temperature is brought to 37 C.

Preparation of the Culture

Using a 10 ml glass syringe, 1 ml of heparin solution followed by peripheral venous blood are aspirated up to the 10 ml mark. Further aspiration of 1 or 2 ml of air clears the needle of blood. The syringe is placed with needle capped and upright into a rack and incubated at 37 C for thirty to sixty minutes, (time required for 2 ml of plasma to appear by gravity sedimentation). When a sufficient amount of leukocyte-rich plasma is available, the needle is bent, and one ml of plasma is injected into the bottle containing the nutrient medium.

Incubation

The cultures are incubated for seventy-two hours upright at 37 C. (Incubation time is reduced to eighteen to thirty-six hours for leukocyte cultures from patients with leukemia and for bone marrow cultures.) Incubation time is counted from the time of inoculation of the culture.

HARVESTING THE CULTURE

1. At seventy-two hours incubation, two drops of colcimide are added from the stock solution to each culture. The final concentration of colchicine is about 10^{-6} molar. Following the colchicine, 1000 units of human fibrinolysin are

Phytohemagglutinin-P (reconstituted), 0.025-0.035 ml
Fetal bovine serum, 1 ml
Penicillin-G, 500 units
Streptomycin, 0.5 μg

added and, after gentle mixing, incubation is continued.

2. At seventy-four hours to eighty hours incubation, the cultures are poured into graduated centrifuge tubes and centrifuged for ten minutes at 800 rpm. The supernatant is discarded by aspiration.

3. The cells are gently re-suspended in 5 ml of Hank's Balanced Salt Solution; the tubes are centrifuged as before; and the salt solution is discarded. The volume of the cell "button" at this time should be about 0.5 ml. If this is not the case, the volume is adjusted by adding Hank's solution or by removing the excess amount of the sediment.

4. Triply distilled water (2.5 ml) is added, and the tubes are allowed to stand for twenty-five minutes. The suspension is again centrifuged as before and as much of the supernatant is removed as possible.

5. Five ml of chilled (4 C) fixing solution (acetic acid: methanol, 1:3) are added and allowed to stand for ten minutes. The sediment is agitated gently and then centrifuged at 1400 rpm for ten minutes. The supernatant is discarded. Fixing solution is added the same way two more times followed by centrifugation. It is observed that better results are obtained if the last exposure to the fixing solution is extended from twelve to twenty-four hours.

Preparation of Slides

The cells are suspended in 5 ml of fresh fixative and then centrifuged for ten minutes at 1400 rpm. The supernatant is discarded. Fixing solution is added again and, after centrifugation, decanted to a 1.5 ml total volume. The cells are now re-suspended by gentle agitation.

Standard microscopic slides are dipped in distilled water and removed. Two drops of cell suspension are placed on each wet slide. The slides are placed in the flame of a Bunsen burner until dry (1 to 4 seconds). This flattens and spreads the groups of chromosomes. Overheating produces artefacts and reduces the affinity for stain.

Staining of Slides

1. Staining with Giemsa stain is recommended by placing the slides for one hour in the staining solution (Reagent 12).

2. Dehydration is accomplished by dipping five times in acetone. The slide is then immersed in acetone: xylene, 1:1 for three minutes and cleaned in two changes of xylene for five minutes.

Photomicroscopy

Basically, the photomicrographic techniques with the light microscope in cytogenetic work are aimed at producing suitable photographic records of chromosomes, their parts and their appendages. The production of a clear, dense, well-focused negative of a suitable chromosome spread at high magnification fulfills these requirements. The human chromosomes vary in size from about 1.5 to 10 μ in length; and chromomeres and satellites may be as small as 0.2 μ, which approaches the theoretical limit of resolution of a visible light system. The microscopic and photographic system used, from the lighting and optics to the production of the final photograph, must at all times minimize the losses of optical quality and resolution.

A suitable film for this work should produce a dense high-contrast negative with a fine grain to allow adequate enlargement. The black and white films used to obtain the intermediate grays so important with tissue sections find little application but may be used; these usually include Plus-X, Panatomic-X and Adox KB-14. The best films currently available in our experience have been 35 mm Kodak High Contrast Copy Film, and 4 inch x 5 inch Kodak Contrast Process Panchromatic Sheet Film. These are fine grain, high-contrast films which produce excellent dense negatives.

These films provide no problem in regard to processing, inasmuch as any fine-grain developer such as Kodak D-11, DK-50 or Microdol may be used. The sensitivity spectrum is panchromatic and allows the use of any stain or filter system. Currently, the most commonly used chromosome stains are Aceto-Orcein, Feulgen and Giemsa, all of which have significant red color. To improve contrast, a green filter should be used which also provides a secondary gain of being an eyesaver during the long hours spent viewing through the microscope. The Kodak Wratten filter 58 or 58-B, and the Zeiss VG and "Green Interference Filter" are the most suitable for this purpose.

Enlargements to 5 inch x 7 inch made on Kodak F-3 or F-4 papers have proved to be satisfactory. Overlap of individual chromosomes at times is unavoidable. Several identical prints should be made at the same magnification from each negative in order to allow cutting out each one of the overlapping chromosomes for karyotyping.

REFERENCES

1. Moorhead, P. A., et. al.: Chromosome preparations of leukocytes cultured from human peripheral blood. Exp. Cell. Res., **20**:613-616, 1960.
2. Tjio, J. H., and Whang, J.: Chromosome preparations of bone marrow cells without prior in vitro culture or in vivo colochicine administration. Stain Tech., **37**(1):17-20, 1962.
3. Scherz, R. G., and Louro, J. J.: A simple method for making chromosome slides. Amer. J. Clin. Path., **40**:222-225, 1963.
4. Radiation Exposure Evaluation Laboratory, U.S. Naval Hosp.: A Method for human chromosome analysis using whole blood. Bethesda, Maryland, 1965.
5. Northcutt, R. C., Mella, G. W. and Dickson, L.: The analysis of human chromosomes. Post Grad. Med., **39**:285-294, 1966.

Index

H

M

N